URINE

pH	4.5–8 (av. 6)
Sodium	75–200 mg/24 hr
Potassium	25–100 mEq/L
Ammonia	20–70 mEq/L
Creatinine	1–2 g/24 hr
Urea	25–35 g/24 hr
Uric acid	0.6–1 g/24 hr
Glucose	0
Protein	0–150 mg/24 hr (trace)
Acetone	0
Bilirubin	0
Hemoglobin/cells	0
Casts	0
Bacteria	<10,000/mL
Appearance	clear, pale yellow

CEREBROSPINAL FLUID (CSF)

Appearance	clear, colorless
Pressure	70–180 mm H_2O
Albumin	11–48 mg/100 mL
Glucose	50–75 mg/100 mL
Cells	occasional WBC
Bilirubin	0

Pathophysiology
for the
HEALTH-
RELATED
Professions

Barbara E. Gould, M.Ed.

School of Health Sciences
Seneca College of Applied Arts and Technology
Toronto, Ontario, Canada

Pathophysiology
for the
HEALTH-
RELATED
Professions

W.B. SAUNDERS COMPANY
A Harcourt Health Sciences Company
Philadelphia   London   New York   St. Louis   Sydney   Toronto

W.B. SAUNDERS COMPANY
A *Harcourt Health Sciences Company*

The Curtis Center
Independence Square West
Philadelphia, Pennsylvania 19106

Library of Congress Cataloging-in-Publication Data

Gould, Barbara E.
  Pathophysiology for the health-related professions / Barbara
Gould.

        p.   cm.

  Includes bibliographical references and index.

  ISBN 0–7216–5954–3

  1. Physiology, Pathological.   I. Title.
  [DNLM: 1. Pathology.   QZ 140 G696p 1997]

  RB113.G64   1997   616.07—dc20

  DNLM/DLC   96–42341

Pathophysiology for the Health-Related Professions   ISBN 0–7216–5954–3

Printed in the United States of America.

Last digit is the print number: 9   8   7

To my family, for their continued love and support
To my friends and colleagues, who have each had a unique role in the development of this text
To my students, who have taught me so much

Preface

In recent years, many of the health-related professions have developed more formal academic programs that include a core course in general pathophysiology. This textbook provides an introduction to the fundamentals of pathophysiology for students in a variety of health-related programs. Because such students present with a diversity of backgrounds and needs, this book focuses on essential concepts of disease processes such as inflammation and infection and includes a selection of common disorders. The content is presented in a concise fashion and is accompanied by numerous illustrations to add clarity and interest. Understanding this basic information enables the student to apply that knowledge to other disorders that will be encountered in practice. It is hoped that students will enjoy studying these topics and proceed with enthusiasm to more detailed studies in their individual specialities.

The textbook is organized into three major sections:
Section I—fundamental concepts and processes in pathophysiology

- Introductory chapter includes terminology and basic cellular changes.
- Covers topics such as inflammation and healing, tumors, abnormal immune responses.
- Immediate clinical application provided by an example of a specific disease for each topic.

Section II—relationship of developmental stages and other factors to pathophysiology

- Physiologic changes related to adolescence, pregnancy, and aging.
- Specific disorders associated with developmental stages.
- Other factors such as stress, substance abuse, or pain that may be significant in disease processes or affect the care of such individuals.

Section III—specific disorders, traditionally organized by body systems

- Selection based on incidence and occurrence, as well as the need to present a variety of pathophysiologic processes.

- For major disorders, information provided on pathophysiology, etiology, clinical manifestations, significant diagnostic tests, common treatment modalities, and potential complications.

In addition, *Ready References* are located inside the book covers and at the end of the book. These include normal values for blood, cerebrospinal fluid, and urine; a review of anatomic terms with accompanying illustrations; a pH scale; blood clotting factors and times; selected numerical conversions for temperature, weights, and volumes; definitions of common abbreviations and acronyms; and a brief description and illustrations of some diagnostic tests such as ultrasound and magnetic resonance imaging. It is hoped that these resources will facilitate student study time.

This content provides the practitioner in a health-related profession with the prerequisite knowledge to recognize and understand a patient's problems, limitations and the implications of treatment measures; to reduce exacerbating factors; to participate in preventive programs; and to be an effective member of a health care team. Individual instructors may emphasize certain aspects or topics, as is most appropriate for students in a specialty area.

A number of features related to the presentation of information in this textbook should be mentioned. These include the following:

- Brief *reviews* of normal anatomy and physiology at the beginning of each chapter, essentially to remind students of the factors that are frequently affected by pathologic processes. Additional review material such as the pH scale or the location of body cavities may be found in the Ready Reference section.
- Frequent *cross-references* in the text, to enable students to review quickly and to understand interrelationships more readily. This feature is also helpful to instructors who may need to limit course content to particular chapters.
- Numerous *illustrations*, including flow charts, schematic diagrams, and photographs, clarify and rein-

force textual information as well as offer an alternative visual learning mode, particularly when complex processes are involved. Illustrations are fully labeled including anatomic parts and pathologic changes.

- *Tables* summarize information or offer comparisons, which are helpful to the student in discriminating more significant information and for review purposes.
- Basic *diagnostic tests and treatment measures* strengthen the comprehension of pathophysiology.
- *Questions* are presented to the student throughout the text, as "Thinkabout Questions" following each small section of information and as study questions at the end of each chapter. Questions may relate to factual information, potential applications, or the integration of several concepts. These questions are helpful in alerting a student to points initially overlooked or useful for student self-evaluation before proceeding to a new section. They may also serve as a tool for review and test preparation. Brief answers are provided in the Instructor's Manual.
- Brief, adaptable *case studies* with questions are incorporated at the end of each chapter and are intended to provide a basis for discussion in a tutorial, an assignment, or an alternative learning mode. Specific clinical applications may be added for each professional group.
- *Concise, readable* style with sufficient scientific and medical terminology to help the student acquire a professional vocabulary, without overwhelming or impeding the learning process in a student who comes with little scientific background.
- *Key terms* are listed at the beginning of the chapter, and most terms are defined when initially used in the text.
- Lists of *anatomic terms* and combining forms, *abbreviations,* and *acronyms* facilitate student learning. Because of the broad scope of pathophysiology, a medical dictionary is a useful adjunct for any student in the health-related professions.

Certain guidelines were developed to facilitate the use of this textbook by students in different health-related professions. The recipient of care or service is referred to as a patient. Every effort has been made to present current information and concepts simply but accurately. The presence of numeric values within textual information often confuses students and detracts from the basic concepts being presented; therefore, numbers are included only when they promote understanding of a principle. When a topic refers to a group of related disorders, discussion focuses on either a typical representative of the group or the general characteristics of the group. Suggested diagnostic tests and treatments are not individualized or necessarily complete but are presented generally to assist the students' application of the pathophysiology and to provide students with an awareness of the impact of certain diseases on a patient and of possible modifications in the care required. Students need to understand that these areas are subject to constant change as research and technology advances, and, as well, are dependent on the resources available in a particular geographic region. Diagnostic tests increase student cognizance of the extent of data collection and sifting that may be necessary before making a diagnosis as well as the importance of monitoring the course of a disease or the response to treatment. Information regarding adverse effects of treatment is included when there may be potential problems such as high risk for infection or special precautions required for members of the health care team. At some time, patients may be involved in clinical research trials for new drugs, tests, or procedures. It is helpful for students to have an opportunity during their course to assess new developments, recognize change, or project new possibilities. In this text, drugs are referred to by generic name, and examples provided are suggested only as commonly used representatives of a drug classification. In some disciplines, rapid changes in terminology have occurred, creating difficulty for some students. For example, current terms such as chemical dependency or cognitive impairment have many synonyms, and some of these are included to enable students to relate to a more familiar phrase.

A NOTE TO STUDENTS

This textbook has been written to facilitate your learning, and I hope you find it useful, enjoyable, and a stimulus to acquire additional knowledge. General pathophysiology provides a considerable foundation of information for you to apply in your specialty area and a powerful tool in your care of any patient. I trust the illustrations are helpful in developing an understanding of complex disease processes. There are many learning aids included in this textbook, so before you begin your course, take a few moments to examine the list of contents, the insides of the front and back covers, and the Ready Reference section at the back of the book. Read the introduction in Chapter 1, and glance over several chapters to acquaint yourself with the convenient illustrations and questions. Note that review material to refresh your memory and fill in any gaps is available at the beginning of each chapter.

Many scientific and medical terms are defined within the text, and numerous cross-references are included to help you to utilize this book fully. Perhaps in the practical component of this program you may find it necessary to look up a diagnosis in this textbook before you have studied the topic in class. Each chapter is quite readable before lectures occur, and the tables and illustrations provide useful summaries for you to consolidate information following class or for review purposes. The questions and case studies are helpful in preparing for examinations, and you may use these as models to create additional questions for self-evaluation. As you move through this book, I suggest you note any information that you think is significant in your specialty area or is of special interest to you for any reason. Such relationships build more links in your memory banks! Whenever possible, check the current journals in your area for updates, and add to your notes. Because health-related professionals must require a specific knowledge base for safe practice, it is essential to comprehend your course material thoroughly, and I hope that this textbook expedites the process. I wish you success and pleasure in your chosen profession.

I welcome your comments and suggestions, which may be forwarded to me through the publisher.

Acknowledgments

I would like to thank the W.B. Saunders Company, which gave me the opportunity to develop this textbook, and the staff for their guidance and expertise during the process. In particular, I am grateful to Selma Kaszczuk, Senior Editor, who initiated the project and carried it through to reality; to Scott Weaver, Developmental Editor, who coordinated the many activities and patiently provided immense support for all facets of its development; to Ruth Low and Lee Ann Draud, Copy Editors, who refined the final version of the text; to Lori Irvine, Production Manager, who organized the final stages; to Nicholas Rook, who designed the book; and to all those who worked quietly behind the scenes.

Many individuals reviewed chapters and offered advice in specialty areas. Their comments and assistance were most appreciated. In particular, I would like to recognize the time, effort, and expertise contributed by Gwen Buttle, R.N., B.Sc.N, M.Ed., Health Sciences, George Brown College of Applied Arts and Technology; and Margaret Heilig, R.N., B.N.Sc., Health Educator, The Gage Transition to Independent Living, West Park Hospital, Toronto. The significant information and helpful suggestions extended by each of the following individuals have been of inestimable value in the evolution of this textbook: Margaret Carter, Respiratory Therapy, The Michener Institute for Applied Health Sciences, Toronto; William Cornish, B.Sc.Phm., Drug Information Center, Department of Pharmacy, Sunnybrook Health Science Center, University of Toronto; Patricia Cross, B.Sc.(PT), Dip. P & OT, Director, Physiotherapy and Speech Pathology Services, St. Mary's of the Lake Hospital, Kingston, Ontario; Ruthanna Dyer, Ph.D., Professor, Health Sciences, Seneca College of Applied Arts and Technology, Toronto; Cheryl Emmerson, ECEDH (Dip), B.A. (Psych), Health Sciences, Early Childhood Education, Humber College of Applied Arts and Technology, Toronto; Jacqueline Jury, B.Sc., M.A., Speech Language Pathologist, Childrens' Treatment Center, Peterborough, Ontario; Dr. Miriam Kaufman, Teen Clinic, The Hospital for Sick Children and Assistant Professor of Pediatrics, University of Toronto; Elisabeth King, Laboratory Coordinator, North York General Hospital, Toronto; Dr. Susan King, Division of Infectious Diseases, The Hospital for Sick Children and Associate Professor of Pediatrics, University of Toronto; Dr. Ali Kisselbach, Director of Laboratories, North York General Hospital, Toronto; Vinh Le, Librarian, Seneca College of Applied Arts and Technology; the staff of the Drug Information Center, Ontario College of Pharmacy; Cheryl Palmer-Wickham, Nurse-Manager, Regional Cancer Treatment Center, Ontario Cancer Treatment and Research Foundation, Sunnybrook Health Science Center, Toronto; the staff of the Renal Transplant unit at The Toronto Hospital (General Division); Mary Rowell, R.N., Dip.N.Ed., B.A. (Phil), M.A. (Medical Ethics and Law) of the Department of Bioethics, The Hospital for Sick Children, Toronto; Ann Topple, Nuclear Medicine, Michener Institute for Applied Health Sciences, Toronto; Marjorie Wilson, R,P.T.; Elaine Wood, R.N., B.Sc.N., Seneca College of Applied Arts and Technology; Dr. Philip Wyatt, Medical Director, Genetics Program, North York General Hospital, Toronto. I am most grateful to the unknown reviewers commissioned by W.B. Saunders for their evaluations and advice that proved so valuable in the preparation of final drafts.

I am most grateful to the following for providing photographs: Paul Emmerson, Toronto and Patricia Hall, B.Sc.N., M.Ed., Chair, School of Health Sciences, Seneca College of Applied Arts and Technology, Toronto; Dr. Christine MacAdam, Radiologist, Department of Medical Imaging, North York General Hospital, Toronto; Ellen Mak-Tam, Cytogenetics Department, North York General Hospital, Toronto; Dr. Mercer Rang, Division of Orthopedics, The Hospital for Sick Children, Toronto; Dr. Ralph Shaw, M.A., FRCP(C), Pathologist, Department of Laboratories, North York General Hospital, Toronto. Recognition is due all those who accepted the challenge of converting my sketches and charts into figures using computer graphics, including Adrienne, Craig, Eric, Glenn, Jennifer, Jerry, Sandy, and Terry. And many thanks to Cherryl Ramesar who spent many hours in word processing and preparing tables. To many other individuals who have contributed through past and present interactions to this textbook, I extend my appreciation.

Writing this textbook has been a wonderful experience for me—challenging, sometimes overwhelming, exhilarating, and a great learning opportunity. This endeavor would not have been possible without the continued interest and enthusiasm of many friends, colleagues, and family, for which I am most grateful.

Contents

BASIC CONCEPTS OF DISEASE PROCESSES

CHAPTER

1

Introduction to Pathophysiology

KEY TERMS

• •

anaerobic	homeostasis	lysis	microscopic
autopsy	hypoxia	lysosomal	morphologic
biopsy	inflammation	metabolism	probability
endogenous	ischemia	microorganisms	

HEALTH AND DISEASE

Disease may be defined as a deviation from the *normal* state of health or from a state of *wellness.* The World Health Organization includes physical, mental, and social well-being in its definition of health. Disease develops when significant changes occur in the body, leading to a state in which **homeostasis** cannot be maintained. In normal conditions frequent minor changes occur in the body, the compensation mechanisms respond, and homeostasis is quickly restored. A state of health is difficult to define because the genetic differences among individuals as well as the many variations in life experiences and environmental influences create a variable base. The context in which health is measured is also a consideration. A person who is blind can be in good general health. Injury or surgery may create a temporary impairment in a specific area, but the person's overall health status is not altered.

When one is defining "normal" values for health indicators such as blood pressure or pulse, the figures used usually represent an *average* or a small *range* of values. These figures represent the values expected in a typical individual but are not an absolute criterion. Among normal healthy individuals, the actual figures may be adjusted for factors such as age and activity level. For example, blood pressure usually increases slightly with age. Well-trained athletes often have a slower pulse or heart rate than the average person. Also, small daily fluctuations in blood pressure occur as the body responds to minor changes in activity or body position. It is therefore impossible to state a single figure as the only normal value. Likewise, a discussion of a specific disease in a text presents a general description of the typical characteristics of that disease, but some variations in the clinical picture can be expected to occur in any individual.

Terms Used in Pathophysiology

Pathophysiology involves the study of *functional* or physiologic changes in the body that result from disease processes. As such, pathophysiology includes some aspects of *pathology,* the laboratory study of cell and tissue changes associated with disease. These laboratory studies, which are particularly useful in establishing the *cause* of a disease, make use of tissue specimens from **biopsy,** surgical specimens, or examination after death **(autopsy).** Analysis of body fluids is another essential diagnostic tool. The study of pathophysiology utilizes knowledge of the normal structure and function of the human body, or *anatomy and physiology.* This basic knowledge is particularly important when a disease affects

3

several organs or systems in the body. For example, kidney disease often affects cardiovascular function, and the significance of these effects on another system can be more easily understood when knowledge of normal physiology can be applied to the altered function. A disease or condition usually involves changes at the organ or system (*gross*) level as well as at the cellular or **microscopic** level. Pathophysiology focuses on the effects of abnormalities at the organ level, but cellular changes are usually integral to a full understanding of these effects. Pathophysiologic changes at a particular site depend largely on the basic causes of disease, whether it be an infection, a neoplasm, or a genetic defect.

Following are a few terms used in the discussion of disease processes. Not all of these terms can be used appropriately in any one disorder. A *diagnosis* refers to the identification of a specific disease. *Etiology* concerns the causative factors in a particular disease. There may be one or several causative factors. Etiologic agents include congenital defects, inherited disorders, microorganisms such as viruses or bacteria, immunologic dysfunction, metabolic derangements, degenerative changes, malignancy, burns and other trauma, and nutritional deficiencies. When the cause of a disease is unknown, it is termed *idiopathic*. In some cases, a treatment, a procedure, or an error may cause a disease, which is then described as *iatrogenic*. Examples are a bladder infection caused by catheterization or bone marrow damage due to a prescribed drug. In some cases, a difficult decision must be made about a treatment that does involve an additional risk. The term *predisposing factors* encompasses the tendencies that promote development of a disease in an individual. A predisposing factor indicates a *high risk* for the disease but not certain development. For example, predisposing or high-risk factors may include age, gender, an inherited factor, or a certain dietary component. *Prevention* of disease is closely linked to etiology. Preventive measures include vaccines, use of dietary modifications, and cessation of potentially harmful activities such as smoking, as well as the provision of information about these activities that allows individuals to make better choices.

Epidemiology is the science of tracking the pattern or occurrence of disease. Epidemiologic records include data on the transmission and distribution of diseases and are particularly important in the control of infectious diseases and environmentally related disease. For example, this information is used to determine the components of the influenza vaccine to be administered each year based on the currently active strains and geographic movement of the influenza virus. Major data collection centers are the Centers for Disease Control and Prevention (CDC) in Atlanta, Georgia and Ottawa, Canada. The *incidence* of a disease indicates the number of new cases noted within a stated time period. *Communicable* diseases are infections that can be spread from one person to another. *Notifiable* or *reportable* diseases must be reported by the physician to certain designated authorities. This list of diseases changes over time and is intended to protect the public health. Such infections as measles and human immunodeficiency virus (HIV) or acquired immune deficiency syndrome (AIDS) may be included in some jurisdictions. *Epidemics* occur when there are many cases of an infectious disease within a given area, whereas *pandemics* involve high numbers of cases in several regions and perhaps worldwide.

In describing the characteristics of a particular disease, certain terms are standard. *Pathogenesis* refers to the development of the disease or the sequence of events involved in the tissue changes. An *acute* disease indicates a sudden illness with marked signs such as high fever, whereas a *chronic* disease is a milder but long-term illness. Some conditions exist in a *subclinical* state in which the pathologic changes occur, but no obvious manifestations are exhibited by the patient, perhaps because of the great reserve capacity of some organs. For example, kidney damage may progress to an advanced stage of renal failure before signs are manifested. The *onset* of a disease may be *sudden* and obvious or *acute*, or *insidious*, best described as a gradual progression with only vague or very mild signs. There may be several stages in the development of a single disease. Frequently there is an initial *latent* or "silent" stage, in which no clinical signs are evident. In infectious diseases this may be referred to as the *incubation* period; it may last for a day or so or may be prolonged, perhaps for days or weeks. The *prodromal* period comprises the time in the early development of a disease when one is aware of a change in the body, but the signs are nonspecific—for example, fatigue, loss of appetite, or headache. This threatening feeling often develops in the early stage of infections.

The *manifestations* of a disease are the clinical evidence or effects, the signs and symptoms, of disease. These manifestations, such as redness and swelling, may be *local* or found at the site of the problem. Or manifestations may be *systemic* general indicators of illness, such as fever. *Signs* are objective indicators of disease that are obvious to someone other than the subject. An example of a sign is a fever or skin rash. *Symptoms* are subjective feelings, such as pain or nausea. *Lesion* is the term used to describe a specific local change in the tissue. Such a change may be microscopic, as when liver cells are examined for pathologic change, or highly visible, such as a blister observed on the skin. A *syndrome* is a collection of signs and symptoms that usually occur together in response to a certain condition. *Diagnostic* tests are laboratory tests that assist in diagnosis. These tests may also be used for monitoring the response to treatment or the progress of the disease. Such tests may involve chemical analysis of body fluids, examination of tissues and cells from specimens (e.g., biopsies or body secretions), identification of microorganisms in body fluids or tissue specimens, or radiologic examination of the body.

The *course* or progress of a disease may be marked by *remissions* and *exacerbations*. During a remission, the manifestations of thc disease subside, whereas during an exacerbation the signs increase. A *precipitating* factor is a condition that triggers an acute episode such as a seizure in an individual with a seizure disorder. *Complications* are new secondary or additional problems that arise after the original disease begins. For example, following a heart attack, a person may develop congestive heart failure, a complication. *Therapy* or therapeutic interventions are treatment measures used to promote recovery. They may include surgery, drugs, or behavioral change. *Sequelae* describe the potential outcome of the primary disease, such as scar tissue and its effects. *Convalescence* is the period of recovery and return to the normal healthy state; it may last for several days or months. *Prognosis* defines the **probability** for recovery. The probability figures used in prognosis are based on averages, and there may be considerable variation among affected individuals. *Morbidity* indicates the disease rates within a group; this term is sometimes used to indicate the functional impairment that certain diseases inflict on the population. *Mortality* figures indicate the number of deaths resulting from a particular disease.

Thinkabout 1–1

Define the following terms: idiopathic, prodromal, manifestation, systemic sign, prognosis, exacerbation.

Cellular Adaptations

The cells have mechanisms by which they can adapt their growth and differentiation to altered conditions in the body. Some minor alterations, such as increases in breast and uterine tissue during pregnancy, are normal adaptations by the body. Tissues are frequently modified as a response to hormonal stimulation or to environmental stimuli such as irritation. Frequently such changes are reversible after the stimulus is removed. Abnormal changes are not necessarily a precursor to permanent tissue damage or to the development of tumors or cancer, but it is important to determine the cause of any abnormality in the early stages and to monitor such growth to reduce the risk of serious consequences.

Atrophy refers to a decrease in the *size* of cells, resulting in a reduced tissue mass (Fig. 1–1). Causes include reduced use of the tissue, insufficient nutrition, and aging. An example is the shrinkage of skeletal muscle that occurs when a limb is immobilized in a cast for several weeks.

Hypertrophy refers to an increase in the *size* of individual cells, resulting in an enlarged tissue mass. This increase may be due to additional work by the tissue, for example, the effect of consistent exercise on skeletal muscle. Excessive hormonal stimulation may also stimulate growth of cells.

Hyperplasia is an increased *number* of cells resulting in an enlarged tissue mass. In some cases, hypertrophy and hyperplasia occur simultaneously, as in the uterine enlargement that occurs during pregnancy. Hyperplasia may be a compensatory mechanism to meet increased demands, or it may be pathologic when there is a hormonal imbalance. In certain instances, there may be an increased risk of cancer with developing hyperplasia.

Metaplasia occurs when one mature type of cell is replaced by a different mature cell type. This change may result from a deficit of vitamin A. Metaplasia may be an adaptive mechanism that provides a more resistant tissue—for instance, when stratified squamous epithelium replaces ciliated columnar epithelium in the respiratory tract of cigarette smokers. Although the new cells present a stronger barrier, they cause loss of function because cilia are no longer present on the simpler squamous cells.

Dysplasia is the term applied to tissue in which the cells vary in size and shape, large nuclei are frequently present, and the rate of mitosis is increased. This situation may result from chronic irritation or infection, or it may be a precancerous change. Detection of dysplasia is the basis of routine screening tests for atypical cells such as the Pap smear (Papanicolaou test on cervical cells).

Anaplasia refers to cells that are undifferentiated and have variable nuclei and cell structure and numerous mitotic figures. Anaplasia is associated with malignancy or cancer and is the basis for grading a tumor.

Neoplasm means new growth and commonly called a tumor. There are two types of tumors, benign and malignant. Malignant neoplasms are referred to as *cancer*. Benign tumors do not necessarily become malignant. Benign tumors are usually considered less serious because they do not spread and are not life-threatening unless they are found in certain locations. The characteristics of each tumor depend on the specific type of cell from which the tumor arises, resulting in a unique appearance and growth pattern.

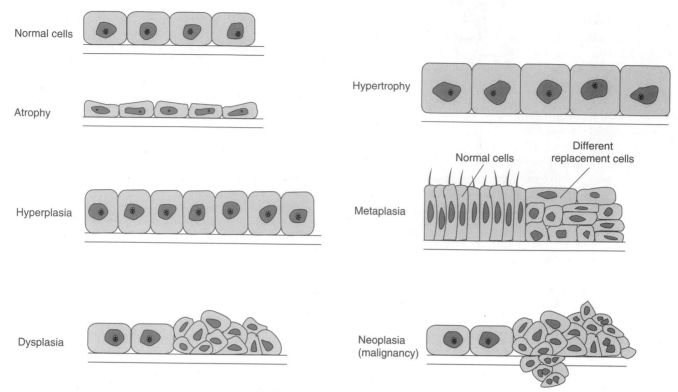

FIGURE 1-1. Abnormal growth patterns.

Thinkabout 1-2

Differentiate between hypertrophy, hyperplasia, and dysplasia.

Cell Damage and Necrosis

There are many ways of injuring cells in the body. The most common cause of injury is a deficit of oxygen **(ischemia),** which interferes with cell **metabolism.** Decreased oxygen in the tissue may occur locally because of a blocked artery or systemically because of respiratory impairment. Cells with a high demand for oxygen, such as those of the brain, heart, and kidney, are quickly affected by **hypoxia** (decreased oxygen in the tissue). A severe oxygen deficit interferes with energy (ATP) production in the cell, leading to loss of the sodium pump at the cell membrane as well as loss of other cell functions. An increase in sodium ions inside the cell leads to swelling of the cell and eventually rupture. At the same time, **anaerobic** metabolism occurs in the cell, leading to a decrease in pH and further metabolic impairment. A deficit of other essential nutrients such as vitamins may also damage cells because normal metabolic processes cannot take place.

Another common cause of cellular damage is physical injury related to thermal (heat) or mechanical pressures. Infectious diseases cause cell injury through the actions of **microorganisms** such as bacteria and viruses. Radiation exposure may damage cells by interfering with their blood supply or directly altering their chemical constituents, creating toxic materials inside the cells. Chemicals from both the environment and from inside the body **(endogenous** chemicals) may damage cells, either by altering cell membrane permeability or by producing other reactive chemicals called free radicals that continue to damage cell components. Some genetic defects or inborn errors of metabolism can lead to abnormal metabolic processes. This altered metabolism leads to toxic accumulations of lipids or proteins that ultimately destroy the cells.

In general, the *initial* cell damage causes an alteration in a metabolic reaction, which leads to a *loss of function* of the cell. As the amount of damage increases, **morphologic** or structural changes occur in the cell as well. These may involve cellular swelling if the cell membrane is affected or accumulations of lipid inside the cell if metabolic derangements are present. If the factor causing the damage is removed quickly, the cell may be able to recover and return to its normal function. If the noxious factor remains, the damage becomes irreversible and the cell dies. Following cell death, the nucleus of the cell disintegrates. The cells undergo **lysis** or dissolution, releasing **lysosomal** enzymes, which cause **inflammation** and damage to nearby cells. If a large number of cells have died, the released enzymes can diffuse into the blood, providing clues that can be detected by diagnostic tests that indicate the type of cells damaged and therefore the site and source of the problem.

Necrosis is the term used when a group of cells die. The process of cell death varies with the cause of the damage and the type of tissue involved. For example, liquefaction necrosis refers to the process by which dead cells liquefy under the influence of cell enzymes. This process occurs in bacterial infections in which a cavity or an ulcer may develop in the infected area (Fig. 1–2). Coagulative necrosis occurs when the cell proteins are altered or denatured and the cells retain some form for a time after death. This process typically occurs in a myocardial infarction (heart attack) when a lack of oxygen causes cell death. *Infarction* is the term applied to an area of dead cells resulting from lack of oxygen. When a large number of cells in an area die, the functional loss can be significant. For example, when part of the heart muscle is infarcted or dies, that area can no longer contract to pump blood. One other concern with cell death is that necrotic tissue can provide a good medium for infection by microorganisms. Such an infection may occur in the intestines or in a limb where bacteria are normally present. *Gangrene* is an area of necrotic tissue that has been invaded by bacteria. Gangrenous tissue may have to be removed surgically to prevent the spread of infection to other parts of the body. After tissue dies, it is eventually replaced either by tissue regenerated from nearby similar cells or by connective tissue or scar tissue that fills the gap.

Specific types of cells die at different rates. Brain cells die quickly (4 to 5 minutes) when deprived of oxygen, whereas heart muscle can survive for approximately 30 minutes. Formerly, death of the body (somatic death) was assumed to occur when heart action and respiration ceased. Now, because cardiac and respiratory function can be maintained artificially, the diagnosis of death is more complex. Currently, *brain death* provides the criteria for somatic death. Brain death is based on the lack of any electrical activity in any neurons in the brain as demonstrated by electroencephalography (EEG) and by the absence of responses (see Chapter 20).

The Study of Pathophysiology

Pathophysiology builds on a knowledge of anatomy and physiology because it is based on a loss of or a change in normal structure and function. There are basic pathophysiologic concepts related to inflammation or infection, for example, that are common to many diseases. The use of these building blocks facilitates the study of specific diseases.

In this text, to provide a comprehensive overview of disease processes the focus is on major diseases, with other disorders added when appropriate. The principles illustrated by these diseases can then be applied to other diseases encountered in practice. In addition, a general approach is used to describe diseases in which there may be several subtypes. For example, only one type of glomerulonephritis is described in the text, acute poststreptococcal glomerulonephritis, which represents the many forms of glomerulonephritis.

There are other considerations in the study of pathophysiology. New developments are occurring constantly. New causes of disease are discovered, better diagnostic tests are perfected, and new drugs are formulated. Reports from health professionals are gathered, leading to new research or signaling a warning about predisposing conditions or treatments. Constant updating of information is required. The etiology and predisposing factors to specific diseases are being used in the development of more effective preventive programs. Prevention includes maintaining vaccinations and encouraging participation in screening programs (e.g., genetic

FIGURE 1–2. Pulmonary tuberculosis. (Drawing by Margot Mackay, University of Toronto Faculty of Medicine, Department of Surgery, Division of Biomedical Communications, Toronto. Reprinted from Walter JB: An Introduction to the Principles of Disease, 3rd ed. Philadelphia, W. B. Saunders, 1992.)

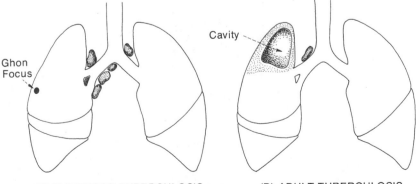

(A) CHILDHOOD TUBERCULOSIS   (B) ADULT TUBERCULOSIS

or blood pressure testing). As more community health programs develop and increased amounts of information are disseminated to the public, health care workers become more involved in responding to questions and promoting preventive measures.

During the study of pathophysiology, many implications can arise from a list of signs and symptoms or a prognosis. Technology has advanced tremendously in the past few years. Sophisticated and expensive diagnostic tests are now available. The availability of these tests, however, also depends on the geographic location of individuals, including their access to large, well-equipped facilities. More limited resources may restrict the number of diagnostic tests available to an individual, or a long waiting period may be necessary before testing and treatment are available. Many tests, including DNA testing and genetic information, are handled by computer, and these results may be available to many individuals. This development is helpful in some ways in that it avoids duplicate testing, but it also gives rise to questions about the confidentiality and potential use or abuse of such information. The ethics of anonymous testing or mandatory testing for certain disorders is another issue of concern to health care professionals.

In many cases, the manifestations of a disease follow from the pathophysiology, as does the treatment. Recognition of potential complications or untoward reactions in an early stage by any member of the health care team can often prevent serious consequences for the patient. Individuals are now better informed and are encouraged to question health professionals about their case. Thus, a solid knowledge base enables health professionals to meet such demands.

New treatments are constantly being developed. Some of these measures raise new hope in terminally ill patients, even when the treatments are still experimental. Current technology provides an opportunity to prolong life through the use of various machines, many advances in surgery, and the use of organ transplants. Legal and ethical issues about fetal tissue transplants and genetic engineering remain to be addressed. In these developing areas, the goal is still to reduce the incidence of disease. The concerns that exist are directed toward the means by which this goal is accomplished and the potential of this new technology for abuse. Questions have also been raised about the allocation of resources for treatment. Treatments such as heart transplants or in vitro fertilization (test-tube babies) are costly. The public health dilemma is the choice between a high-cost treatment for one person or low-cost treatment for many persons, given the limited amount of funding available. Many options other than traditional therapies are now available. Treatment by acupuncture or naturopathy may be preferred. These options may replace traditional therapies or may be used in conjunction with them. A patient may seek an alternative mode of treatment if the initial traditional treatment is not totally successful.

The health care team has become larger as more specialty groups have formed. Each group has a unique interest in the study of pathophysiology. The care given by individual team members can affect the disease process in the patient and the care provided by other team members. Sharing significant information and updating knowledge can benefit both the patient and the health professional.

CHAPTER
2
Inflammation and Healing

KEY TERMS

• •

abscess	exudates	intra-articular	permeability
acute	fibrinogen	ischemia	phagocytosis
adhesions	fibrinous	isoenzymes	purulent
chemical mediators	fibroblast	leukocytosis	pyrogens
chemotaxis	glucocorticoids	lysosomal	regeneration
chronic	granulation tissue	macrophage	resolution
collagen	granuloma	mitosis	scar
contracture	hematocrit	necrosis	serous
diapedesis	hematopoiesis	neutrophil	stenosis
ESR (erythrocyte	hydrostatic pressure	osmotic pressure	ulcer
sedimentation rate)	hyperemia	perforation	vasodilation

BRIEF REVIEW OF NORMAL CAPILLARY EXCHANGE

Usually all capillaries are not open in a particular capillary bed unless the cells' metabolic needs are not being met by the blood supply to the area. Precapillary sphincters composed of smooth muscle restrict blood flow through some channels. Movement of fluid, electrolytes, oxygen, and nutrients out of the capillary at the arteriolar end is based on the net **hydrostatic pressure** (the difference between hydrostatic and **osmotic pressures**) inside the capillary (essentially arterial pressure) (Fig. 2–1). Differences in concentration of dissolved substances in the blood and interstitial fluid promote diffusion of electrolytes, glucose, oxygen, and other nutrients across the capillary membranc. Blood cells and plasma proteins normally remain inside the capillary. At the venous end of the capillary, where capillary hydrostatic pressure is decreased, fluid, carbon dioxide, and other wastes return to the blood. Excess fluid and

9

INFLAMMATION

1. Injury
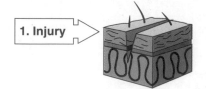

2. Cells release chemical mediators
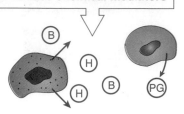

3. Vasodilation – increased blood flow
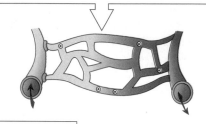

NORMAL

Arteriole
Precapillary sphincter   Venule
Open capillary
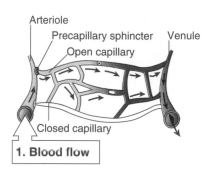
Closed capillary

1. Blood flow

2. Normal fluid shift
Protein remains in blood
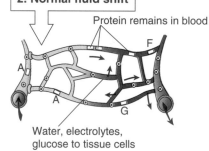
Water, electrolytes, glucose to tissue cells

4. Increased capillary permeability
Protein and water leave capillary – form exudate
Water
Water, electrolytes

5. Leukocytes move to site of injury
Leukocyte
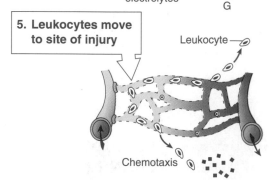
Chemotaxis

3. Cells remain in blood
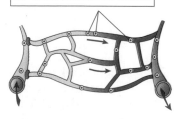

6. Phagocytosis – preparation for healing
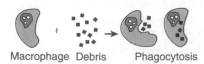
Macrophage   Debris   Phagocytosis

⊙ = Cell
$\overline{\underset{A}{\square}}$ = Albumin
$\overline{\underset{G}{\square}}$ = Globulin
$\overline{\underset{F}{\square}}$ = Fibrinogen

Ⓑ = Bradykinin
Ⓗ = Histamine
Ⓟ Ⓖ = Prostaglandin

FIGURE 2–1. Comparison of normal capillary exchange and inflammatory response.

any protein are recovered from the interstitial area by means of the lymphatics.

INFLAMMATION

The inflammatory response is a basic concept in pathophysiology. You have probably observed the inflammatory process resulting from a cut, an insect bite, an infection, or a small burn on your body. Inflammation is a normal defense mechanism in the body and is intended to localize and remove the injurious agent. The signs and symptoms of inflammation serve as a *warning* of a problem, which may be hidden within the body.

Definition

Inflammation is the body's response to tissue injury. Disorders are named using the ending *-itis* for inflammation. The root word is usually a body part or tissue—for example, tendinitis or colitis.

Thinkabout 2–1

What term would indicate inflammation of the stomach?

Causes

Inflammation is associated with many types of tissue injury. Causes include direct damage (cuts, sprains), chemicals such as acids, **ischemia** and cell necrosis or infarction, allergic reactions, physical agents (thermal injuries or burns, radiation), foreign bodies (splinters or dirt), and infection.

ACUTE INFLAMMATION

Pathophysiology

The inflammatory process is basically the same regardless of the cause. The severity of the inflammation may vary with the specific situation. Tissue injury damages cells. Mast cells and platelets release **chemical mediators** such as histamine, serotonin, prostaglandins, and leukotrienes into the interstitial fluid and blood (see Fig. 2–1). These chemicals affect blood vessels and nerves in the area. Note that many anti-inflammatory drugs and antihistamines reduce the effects of some of these chemical mediators.

Although nerve reflexes at the site of injury cause immediate transient vasoconstriction, the rapid release of chemicals results in local **vasodilation,** which increases blood flow in the area **(hyperemia)** Capillary **permeability** also increases, allowing plasma proteins to shift into the interstitial space along with more fluid. Vasodilation and increased permeability make up the "vascular response" to injury. The increased fluid dilutes any toxic material at the site, while the globulins serve as antibodies, and fibrinogen forms a fibrin mesh around the area to localize the injurious agent.

During the "cellular response," leukocytes are attracted **(chemotaxis)** to the area of inflammation as damaged cells release their contents. The chemicals at the site of injury act like magnets for cells. Leukocytes and their functions are summarized in Table 2–1. First **neutrophils** (polymorphonuclear leukocytes, PMNs) and later monocytes and macrophages collect along the capillary wall (marginate) and then move through the wider separations in the wall **(diapedesis)** into the interstitial area. There they destroy and remove foreign material, microorganisms, and cell debris by **phagocytosis,** thus preparing the site for healing. When phagocytic cells die at the site, **lysosomal** enzymes are released that damage the nearby cells and prolong inflammation. If an immune response or blood clotting occurs, these processes also enhance the inflammatory response.

As excessive fluid and protein collects in the interstitial compartment, blood flow in the area decreases, and fluid shifts out of the capillary are reduced. Severely reduced blood flow can decrease the nutrients available to the undamaged cells in the area and prevent the removal of wastes. This may cause more severe damage to the tissue.

TABLE 2–1 Function of Cellular Elements in the Inflammatory Response	
Leukocytes	**Activity**
Neutrophils	Phagocytosis of microorganisms
Basophils	Release histamine leading to inflammation
Eosinophils	Numbers are increased in allergic responses
Lymphocytes	
T lymphocytes	Active in cell-mediated immune response
B lymphocytes	Produce antibodies
Monocytes	Phagocytes
Macrophages	Active in phagocytosis. These are mature monocytes that have left the blood

Thinkabout 2–2

Using the information just given, predict the signs and symptoms of inflammation.

Local Effects

Increased blood flow into the damaged area causes redness and warmth. Swelling or edema results from the shift of protein and fluid into the interstitial space. Pain results from the increased pressure of fluid on the nerves, especially in enclosed areas, and the local irritation of nerves by chemical mediators. Loss of function may develop if the cells lack nutrients, for example, liver cells, or if swelling interferes mechanically with an action, for example, joint movement.

Inflammatory **exudate** refers to the interstitial fluid formed in the affected area. The characteristics of the exudate vary with the cause of the trauma. **Serous,** or watery, exudates consist primarily of fluid with small amounts of protein and cells. Common causes are allergic reactions or burns. **Fibrinous** exudates are thick and sticky and have a high cell and fibrin content. This type of exudate increases the risk of scar tissue in the area. **Purulent** exudates are thick, yellow-green in color, and contain more leukocytes and cell debris as well as microbes. Typically, this type of exudate indicates *bacterial infection,* and the exudate is often referred to as *pus.* An **abscess** is a localized pocket of pus in a solid tissue (e.g., around a tooth or in the brain). Blood may be present in the exudate if blood vessels have been damaged.

Systemic Effects

Other general manifestations of inflammation include malaise, fatigue, headache, and anorexia. *Fever* or *pyrexia* (low-grade or mild) is common if inflammation is extensive. Fever results from the release of **pyrogens** or fever-producing substances (e.g., interleukin-1) from white blood cells (WBCs) or macrophages. If infection has caused the inflammation, fever can be severe, depending on the particular organism. However, high fever can be beneficial if it impairs the growth and reproduction of a pathogenic organism. Pyrogens circulate in the blood and cause the body temperature control system (the thermostat) in the hypothalamus to be reset at a higher level.

Heat-production mechanisms such as shivering are activated to increase cell metabolism. Involuntary cutaneous vasoconstriction (characterized by pale, cool skin) reduces heat loss from the body, and voluntary curling up of the body conserves heat. These mechanisms continue until the body temperature reaches the new higher setting (Fig. 2–2).

Thinkabout 2–3

Predict the changes that occur when the cause of a fever is removed. That is, think about how you have felt with a fever, and how the processes are reversed to lower body temperature.

Diagnostic Tests

Refer to the *normal values* shown on the inside front cover of this book.

Leukocytosis, an elevated **erythrocyte sedimentation rate (ESR),** and increased plasma proteins and cell enzymes in the serum are nonspecific changes; they do not indicate the particular cause or site of inflammation (Table 2–2). They provide helpful screening and monitoring information when a problem is suspected. In patients with leukocytosis there is often an increase in *immature* neutrophils, commonly referred to as a shift to the left. A *differential* count (the proportion of each type of WBC) may be helpful in distinguishing viral infection from bacterial infection. Allergic reactions commonly produce eosinophilia. Examination of a peripheral blood smear may disclose significant numbers of abnormal cells, another clue when one is seeking the cause of a problem. Increased circulating plasma proteins (**fibrinogen,** prothrombin, and alpha-antitrypsin) result from a response in the liver that increases protein synthesis. *Cell enzymes* and **isoenzymes** may be elevated in the blood in the presence of severe inflammation and **necrosis.** This sign may be helpful in locating the site of the necrotic cells that have released the enzymes. Some of the enzymes are not tissue specific. For example, aspartate aminotransferase (AST, formerly serum glutamic-oxalosetic transaminase [SGOT]) is elevated in liver disease and in the acute stage of a myocardial infarction (heart attack). However, the isoenzyme CK-MB is specific for myocardial infarction. The enzyme alanine aminotransferase (ALT) is specific for the liver.

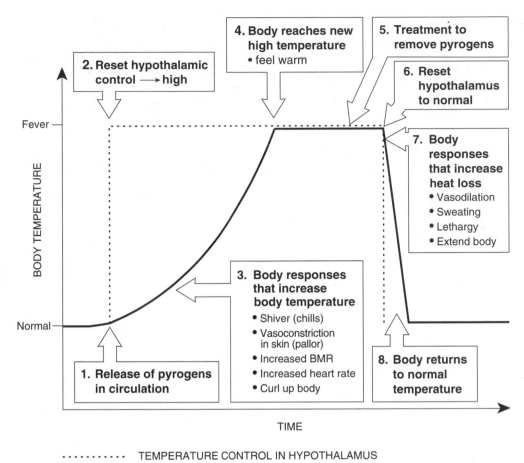

2. Reset hypothalamic control → high

4. Body reaches new high temperature
• feel warm

5. Treatment to remove pyrogens

6. Reset hypothalamus to normal

7. Body responses that increase heat loss
• Vasodilation
• Sweating
• Lethargy
• Extend body

3. Body responses that increase body temperature
• Shiver (chills)
• Vasoconstriction in skin (pallor)
• Increased BMR
• Increased heart rate
• Curl up body

1. Release of pyrogens in circulation

8. Body returns to normal temperature

BODY TEMPERATURE

Fever

Normal

TIME

- - - - - - - - - - TEMPERATURE CONTROL IN HYPOTHALAMUS

—————— BODY TEMPERATURE

FIGURE 2-2. The course of a fever.

Course of the Inflammatory Response

If the cause of the inflammatory response is a brief exposure to a damaging agent, for instance, touching a hot object, the response often subsides in approximately 48 hours. Vascular integrity is recovered, and excess fluid and protein are recovered by the lymphatic capillaries and returned to the general circulation. The manifestations of inflammation gradually decrease. Otherwise, inflammation persists until the causative agent is removed (Fig. 2–3).

TABLE 2-2	Changes in the Blood with Inflammation
Leukocytosis	Increased numbers of white blood cells, especially neutrophils
Differential count	Proportion of each type of white blood cell altered
Plasma proteins	Increased fibrinogen and prothrombin
Increased ESR	Elevated plasma proteins increase the rate at which red blood cells settle in a sample
Cell enzymes	Released from necrotic cells: may indicate the site of inflammation

"Blocking" enzymes are present in the body to prevent an excessive response to injury. However, the amount of tissue destruction (necrosis) that occurs depends on the specific cause of the trauma and the factors contributing to the inflammatory response. Extensive necrosis may lead to **ulcers** or erosion of tissue. For example, gingivitis or stomatitis in the oral cavity often leads to painful ulcerations in the mouth.

Potential Complications

Infection is common because microorganisms can more easily enter a tissue when the barrier (skin or mucosa) is damaged and the blood supply is impaired. Foreign bodies such as dirt often introduce microbes directly, and some microbes resist phagocytosis. Inflammatory exudate provides an excellent medium for organisms to reproduce and colonize an area.

Ulcers may result from severe or prolonged inflammation because cell necrosis and lack of regeneration cause erosion of tissue. This in turn can lead to complications such as **perforation** of viscera or development of extensive scar tissue.

Skeletal muscle spasm or strong muscle contractions may be initiated by inflammation resulting from musculoskeletal injuries such as sprains, tendinitis, or fractures. Spasm is likely to force a joint out of its normal alignment, thus causing additional pressure on the nerves and increasing the pain.

Local complications depend on the site of inflammation. For example, inflammation in the lungs may impair expansion of the lungs and diffusion of oxygen. Inflammation of a joint may decrease its range of movement.

CHRONIC INFLAMMATION

Chronic inflammation may develop following an **acute** episode of inflammation when the cause is not completely eradicated. Or it may develop insidiously owing to **chronic** irritation, specific bacteria, or abnormal immune responses.

Pathophysiology

Characteristics of chronic inflammation include less swelling but more lymphocytes, **macrophages,** and **fibroblasts** than in acute inflammation. More collagen

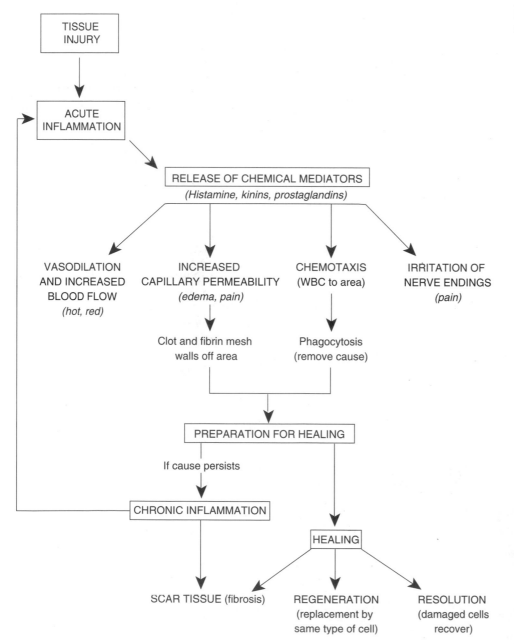

FIGURE 2-3. The course of inflammation and healing.

TABLE 2–3	The Use of Aspirin
Advantages	**Disadvantages**
Anti-inflammatory	Allergies are common, includ-
Antipyretic (reduces fever)	ing skin rash and asthma
Analgesic (reduces pain)	Causes ulcers in mouth and
	stomach; take with food or use
	enteric-coated tablets
	Prolongs blood-clotting time,
	which can be significant with
	high doses and long-term use

is produced in the area, resulting in more fibrous scar tissue forming. **Granulomas** may develop when an area is walled off by fibrous tissue but the cause has not been removed, as in tuberculosis. Frequently, more tissue destruction occurs with chronic inflammation.

TREATMENT OF INFLAMMATION

Aspirin (acetylsalicylic acid, ASA) has long been used as an anti-inflammatory agent, sometimes in very large doses. This drug decreases prostaglandin synthesis at the site of inflammation. The advantages and disadvantages of aspirin are presented in Table 2–3.

Thinkabout 2–4

Based on your knowledge of the normal physiology of the stomach, why would intake of food or milk with a drug reduce the risk of nausea and irritation in the stomach?

Nonsteroidal anti-inflammatory drugs (NSAIDs) such as fenoprofen, ibuprofen, and piroxicam are used extensively to treat inflammation involving the musculoskeletal system, both injuries and long-term problems such as rheumatoid arthritis. Many of these agents block prostaglandin synthesis, thus decreasing the inflammation and pain associated with tissue injury. The side effects are similar to those of aspirin, but they are less severe. These drugs are available as oral medications.

Glucocorticoids, or steroidal anti-inflammatory drugs, can be administered as oral tablets, as creams and ointments for topical application, or as injections, both local and systemic. Examples include prednisone (oral), triamcinolone (topical), methylprednisolone (**intra-articular**—into joint), dexamethasone (intramus-

cular [IM], intravenous [IV]) injections, and beclomethasone dipropionate (Beclovent [inhaler]). These are synthetic chemicals that are related to the naturally occurring glucocorticoids in the body such as hydrocortisone. The structure of the drug has been altered to enhance its anti-inflammatory action and reduce the other effects of the hormone. This category of drugs is extremely valuable in the treatment of many disorders. Glucocorticoids decrease capillary permeability and enhance the effectiveness of the hormones epinephrine and norepinephrine in the system. Thus, the vascular system is stabilized. These drugs also reduce the number of leukocytes and mast cells at the site, decreasing the release of histamine and prostaglandins. In addition, glucocorticoids block the immune response.

However, with long-term use and high dosages of glucocorticoids, marked *side effects* occur similar to Cushing's disease (see Chapter 21). These side effects (or adverse effects) should be considered when one is taking a medical history from a patient because they may complicate the care of the person. Side effects include atrophy of lymphoid tissue and reduced numbers of WBCs, leading to an increased risk of infection and a decreased immune response. Catabolic effects include osteoporosis (bone demineralization), muscle wasting, delayed healing, tendency to breakdown of skin and mucosa (e.g., peptic ulcer), and retarded growth in children, all of which result from decreased protein synthesis and decreased regeneration of tissue. Retention of sodium and water often leads to high blood pressure and edema. Increased intake of glucocorticoids affects the normal feedback mechanism in the body, reducing the normal secretion of glucocorticoids. Therefore, sudden cessation of the medication or the presence of increased stress may cause adrenal crisis (similar to shock) because insufficient glucocorticords are available in the body.

To lessen the risk of serious side effects, it is best to limit prescription of glucocorticoids to the treatment of acute episodes with minimal dosages. Intermittent drug-free time periods ("drug holidays") are recommended during long-term therapy. Whenever the drug is discontinued, the dosage should be gradually decreased over a period of days to allow the body's natural secretions to increase to normal levels. Adrenocorticotropic hormone (ACTH) therapy is used for long-term therapy in many cases because it stimulates the patient's glands to produce more cortisol. The risk of adrenal shock is less because glandular atrophy does not occur.

Hot and cold applications may be helpful. Cold applications are useful in the early stage of acute inflammation. Local vasoconstriction decreases edema and pain. The use of hot or cold applications during long-term therapy and recovery periods depends on the particular situation. In some instances, for example, acute rheumatoid arthritis, heat and moderate activity may improve the circulation in the area, thereby removing excess fluid, pain-causing chemical mediators, and waste metabolites as well as promoting healing.

Other treatment measures, including physiotherapy, may be necessary to maintain joint mobility, although splints may be required during acute episodes to prevent **contractures.** Rest and adequate nutrition and hydration are important. Other drugs such as analgesics for pain and antibiotics to prevent secondary infection may be required.

HEALING

Types of Healing

Healing of a wound area can be accomplished in several ways.

Resolution is the process that occurs when there is minimal tissue damage. The damaged cells recover, and the tissue returns to normal within a short period of time, for example, after a mild sunburn.

Regeneration is the healing process that occurs in damaged tissue in which the cells are capable of **mitosis.** The damaged tissue is replaced by identical tissue from the proliferation of nearby cells. This type of healing may be limited if the organization of a complex tissue is altered. For instance, sometimes fibrous tissue develops in the liver, distorting the orderly arrangement of cells, ducts, and blood vessels. Although nodules of new cells form, they do not contribute to the overall function of the liver.

Thinkabout 2–5

Which types of cells can regenerate? Which cannot regenerate?

Repair by **scar** *or fibrous tissue* formation takes place when there is extensive tissue damage or the cells are incapable of mitosis or in the presence of chronic inflammation. Complications such as infection prolong the inflammatory period and lead to scar tissue. The wound area must be filled in and covered by some form of tissue.

The repair process begins following injury when a *blood clot* forms and seals the area. Inflammation devel-

ops in the surrounding area. After 3 to 4 days, foreign material and cell debris have been removed by phagocytes, monocytes, and macrophages, and then **granulation tissue** grows into the gap from nearby connective tissue (Fig. 2–4).

Granulation tissue is highly vascular and appears moist and pink or red in color. It contains many new capillary buds from the surrounding tissue. This tissue is very fragile and is easily broken down by microorganisms or stress on the tissue.

Thinkabout 2–6

What happens if you pull a scab off a wound too early?

At the same time as the cavity is being filled in, nearby *epithelial* cells undergo mitosis, extending across the wound from the outside edges inward. Within a few days, fibroblasts enter the area, stimulated by macrophage activity, and produce **collagen,** a protein, that is the basic component of scar tissue and provides strength for the new repair. Gradually, cross-linking and shortening of the collagen fibers promote formation of a tight, strong scar. The capillaries in the area decrease, and the color of the scar fades from red to white. Scar tissue is not normal, functional tissue, nor does it contain specialized structures such as hair follicles or glands.

Thinkabout 2–7

Which would heal more rapidly—a surgical incision in which the edges have been stapled together or a large jagged tear in the skin and subcutaneous tissue? Why?

Factors Affecting Healing

A small gap in the tissue results in complete healing within a short period of time and with minimal scar

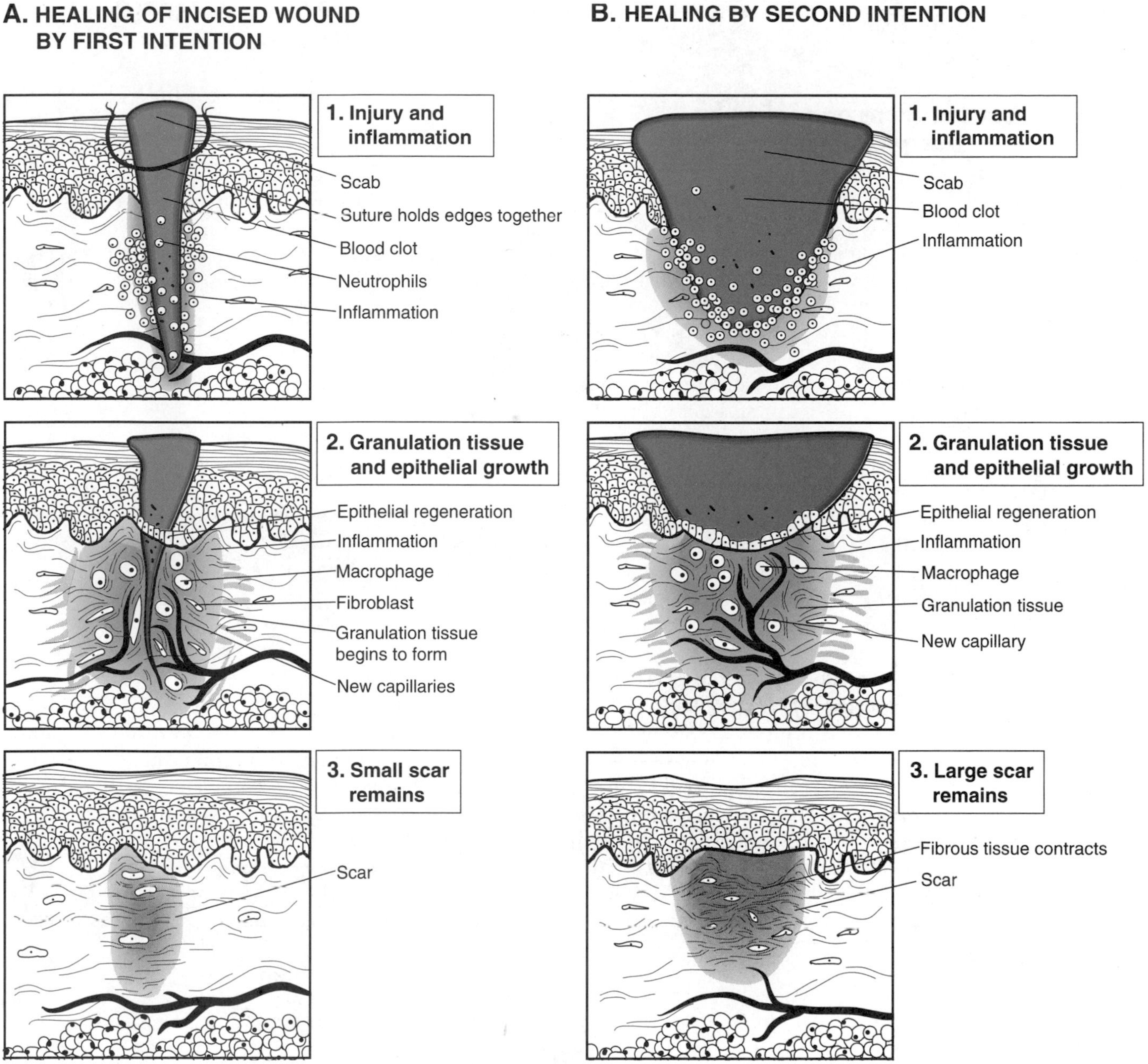

A. HEALING OF INCISED WOUND BY FIRST INTENTION

1. Injury and inflammation

- Scab
- Suture holds edges together
- Blood clot
- Neutrophils
- Inflammation

2. Granulation tissue and epithelial growth

- Epithelial regeneration
- Inflammation
- Macrophage
- Fibroblast
- Granulation tissue begins to form
- New capillaries

3. Small scar remains

- Scar

B. HEALING BY SECOND INTENTION

1. Injury and inflammation

- Scab
- Blood clot
- Inflammation

2. Granulation tissue and epithelial growth

- Epithelial regeneration
- Inflammation
- Macrophage
- Granulation tissue
- New capillary

3. Large scar remains

- Fibrous tissue contracts
- Scar

FIGURE 2–4. The healing process.

tissue formation. A large or deep area of tissue damage requires a prolonged healing time and results in a large scar.

Healing is *promoted* when

- nutrition is good and includes ample protein and vitamins A and C
- the blood supply is good, supplying oxygen and nutrients
- the wound area is clean and undisturbed during healing
- no complications are present during healing

Healing is *delayed*

- in the elderly, in whom circulation is impaired and a lower metabolic rate reduces mitosis
- when foreign material is present or infection develops
- when circulatory problems are present
- if the wound is exposed to radiation, which reduces all mitosis
- in the presence of dehydration or poor nutrition
- if excessive mobility, bleeding, or hematoma formation occurs

- in the presence of insulin deficit or excess glucocorticoids

Complications of Healing by Scar Formation

LOSS OF FUNCTION. Loss of function results from the loss of normal cells and the lack of specialized structures and normal organization in scar tissue. For example, if scar tissue replaces normal skin, that area will lack hair follicles, glands, and sensory nerve endings.

CONTRACTURES AND OBSTRUCTIONS. Scar tissue is nonelastic and tends to shrink over time. This process may decrease the range of movement of a joint and eventually may result in fixation and deformity of the joint or contracture (Fig. 2–5). Physiotherapy or surgery may be necessary to break down the fibrous tissue and improve mobility. Shortening of the scar tissue may also cause shortening or narrowing (**stenosis**) of structures, particularly tubes or ducts. For example, if the esophagus were shortened, malposition of the stomach (hiatal hernia) or a narrowed esophagus, causing obstruction during swallowing (Fig. 2–6), could result.

ADHESIONS. Adhesions are bands of scar tissue that join two surfaces that are normally separated. Common examples are adhesions between loops of intestine or between the pleural membranes. Such adhesions usually result from inflammation or infection in the cavities. Adhesions prevent normal movement of the structures and may cause distortion or twisting of the tissue.

ULCERATION. Blood supply may be impaired around the scar, resulting in further tissue breakdown and ulceration.

EXAMPLE OF INFLAMMATION AND HEALING

Burns

Burns are a common cause of tissue injury and inflammation. They may be mild or cover only a small area, or they may be severe and life-threatening if an extensive area of skin is involved. Burns may be caused by direct contact with a heat source or by chemicals, radiation, or electric shock. Any burn injury causes an acute inflammatory response.

Thinkabout 2–8

From your own experience and the information just given, describe the appearance and sensation of a thermal burn (e.g., a burn resulting from touching a hot object).

Burns are classified by the depth of damage and the percentage of body surface area involved. *Partial-thickness burns* damage part of the epidermis and dermis (Fig. 2–7). *Superficial partial-thickness* burns (first-degree) damage the epidermis. They usually are red and painful but heal readily without scar tissue. Examples include a sunburn or a mild scald.

Deep partial-thickness burns (second-degree) involve the destruction of the epidermis and part of the dermis.

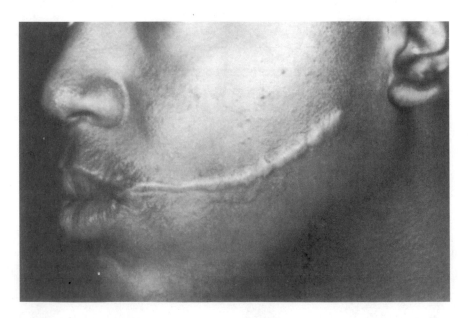

FIGURE 2–5. Complications of scar tissue. Example of scar tissue that may cause contractures with time. (From Peacock EE: Wound Repair, 3rd ed. Philadelphia, W.B. Saunders, 1984.)

A. ESOPHAGEAL SCARRING AND OBSTRUCTION

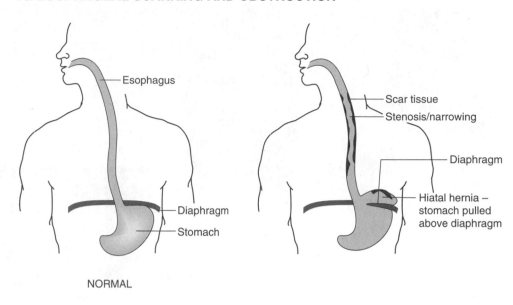

Esophagus

Scar tissue

Stenosis/narrowing

Diaphragm

Diaphragm

Hiatal hernia –
stomach pulled
above diaphragm

Stomach

NORMAL

B. ADHESIONS AND TWISTING OF THE INTESTINES

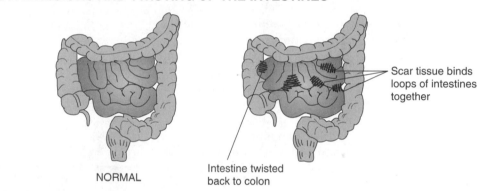

Scar tissue binds
loops of intestines
together

FIGURE 2-6. Effects of scar
tissue.

NORMAL

Intestine twisted
back to colon

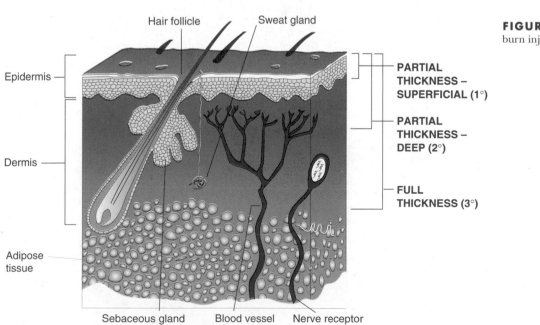

Hair follicle

Sweat gland

FIGURE 2-7. Classification of
burn injury by depth.

Epidermis

**PARTIAL
THICKNESS –
SUPERFICIAL (1°)**

**PARTIAL
THICKNESS –
DEEP (2°)**

Dermis

**FULL
THICKNESS (3°)**

Adipose
tissue

Sebaceous gland   Blood vessel   Nerve receptor

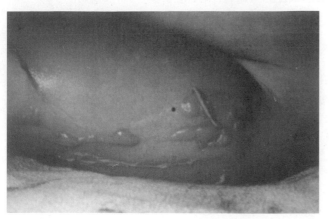

FIGURE 2–8. Partial-thickness burn showing inflammation and blisters. (From Monahan FD, Drake T, Neighbors M: Nursing Care of Adults. Philadelphia, W.B. Saunders, 1994.)

The area is red, edematous, perhaps blistered, and often hypersensitive and painful during the inflammatory stage (Fig. 2–8). The dead skin gradually sloughs off, and healing may occur by regeneration if the area is small and complications do not occur. These burns easily become infected, causing additional tissue destruction and scar tissue formation.

Full-thickness burns (third- and fourth-degree) result in destruction of all skin layers and perhaps deeper tissues as well. The burn wound area is coagulated or charred and therefore is hard and dry on the surface. Initially, it may be painless due to destruction of the nerves. Under the surface an inflammatory response occurs. Burns are very painful until healing is complete. Skin grafts taken from another part of the body are required to reduce the amount of scarring because few cells are available for regeneration at the burn site. Metabolic needs are high during the healing period, and increased dietary intake of protein and carbohydrates is required. The recovery period for severe burns may involve months or years of therapy, and it may be accompanied by many complications.

The percentage of body surface area (BSA) burned provides a guideline for fluid replacement needs as well as other therapeutic interventions. Complicated charts are provided in burn units for the accurate assessment of BSA. The "rule-of-nines" is a rapid calculator. In this estimate, body parts are assigned a value of nine or a multiple of nine. The head and each arm is estimated at 9 percent. Each leg is calculated at 18 percent. The anterior surface of the trunk is given a value of 18 percent, and the posterior surface is also 18 percent. The groin area at 1 percent brings the total BSA to 100 percent. These figures are approximations and can be adjusted. For example, because a young child has a larger head and shorter limbs, an adjustment is required. The parts can be broken down also.

For example, the distal part of the arm (elbow to hand) accounts for 4.5 percent of BSA, and the chest surface can be assessed at 9 percent BSA.

Thinkabout 2–9

a. Draw a line sketch of the body and mark burns on the right arm and right leg. What percentage of BSA has been burned?
b. Calculate the approximate size of the burned area in a person who is burned on the face, chest, and upper arm.

POTENTIAL COMPLICATIONS OF BURNS

- *Fluid imbalance.* If the inflammatory response occurs over a large area of the body, a massive amount of fluid, protein, and electrolytes can shift from the blood into the interstitial space.

Thinkabout 2–10

Predict how this fluid shift would affect blood volume and blood pressure. If you have had a severe sunburn, did you experience a dizzy feeling when you suddenly stood up?

In patients with extensive inflammation over a large area, a fluid imbalance arises, with edema in one area (interstitial tissue) but a fluid deficit in another area (blood). This fluid shift results in low blood pressure (hypovolemic shock) and an increased **hematocrit** due to hemoconcentration.

- *Anemia* is common in burn patients because many erythrocytes are destroyed or damaged in the burned area. Subsequently, protein loss continues, and bone marrow may be depressed, preventing adequate **hematopoiesis.**

- *Infection* is common with burns owing to loss of the protective skin barrier and to the presence of normal flora deep in the hair follicles and glands beneath the burn wound.

- *Local effects* may complicate burns. For example, thermal injury to the respiratory mucosa may impair ventilation and predispose to infection.
- *Scar tissue* occurs even with skin grafting and impairs function as well as appearance. Long-term use of elasticized garments and splints may be necessary to reduce scarring.

- *Growth of children* is often affected both during the acute phase, when metabolic needs are compromised, and at a later time, when additional surgery or grafts may be required to accommodate growth.

STUDY QUESTIONS

Answers to study questions are found in the instructor's manual.

INFLAMMATION

1. Explain why a cast placed around a fractured leg in which extensive tissue damage has occurred might be too tight after 24 hours.

2. Explain why such a cast might become loose in 3 weeks.

3. List specific reasons why the inflammatory response is considered a body defense mechanism.

4. Explain why leukocytosis, a differential count, and elevated ESR are useful data but are of limited value.

5. Explain how acute inflammation predisposes to development of infection.

6. How does the presence of thick, cloudy, yellowish fluid in the peritoneal cavity differ from the normal state?

7. If a large volume of fluid has shifted from the blood into the peritoneal cavity, how would this affect blood volume and hematocrit?

8. Explain how acute inflammation impairs movement of a joint.

9. Why might a client be asked to discontinue ASA prior to extensive oral surgery (e.g., multiple tooth extractions)?

10. Explain why a young child taking prednisone (glucocorticord) for chronic kidney inflammation is at high risk for infection and might need prophylactic antibiotics.

HEALING

11. When part of the heart muscle dies, how does it heal?

12. How would the new tissue affect the strength of the heart contraction?

13. Suggest several reasons why healing is slow in the elderly.

14. Explain how scar tissue could affect the function of the
    a. Small intestine
    b. Brain
    c. Cornea of the eye
    d. Mouth
    e. Lungs (try to find more than one point!)

BURNS

15. Explain why immediate neutralization or removal of a chemical spilled on the hand minimizes burn injury.

16. Describe some of the factors that would promote rapid healing of this burn.

17. If the hand receives a full-thickness burn, describe how its function could be impaired after healing.

CHAPTER

3

Abnormal Immune Responses

KEY TERMS

antibiotics	erythema	monocytes	pruritic
antigens	fetus	mononuclear	secondary
autoantibodies	genes	phagocytic system	specific
bronchoconstriction	hypogammaglobulinemia	mutate	splenectomy
chromosome	hypoproteinemia	phagocytosis	stem cells
colostrum	leukotrienes	placenta	thymus
complement	lysis	prophylactic	titer
cytotoxic	mast cells	prostaglandins	vesicles

REVIEW OF THE IMMUNE SYSTEM

Purpose of the Immune System

The immune system is a major defense mechanism in the body. Defense mechanisms that the body uses to protect itself may be specific or nonspecific. One nonspecific or general defense mechanism in the body is the mechanical barrier such as skin and mucous membrane (often called the first line of defense) that blocks entry of bacteria or harmful substances into the tissues (Fig. 3–1). Associated with these mechanical barriers

are unique body secretions that contain enzymes or chemicals that destroy foreign material. The second line of defense includes the nonspecific processes of phagocytosis and inflammation (see Chapter 2). **Phagocytosis** is the process by which neutrophils and macrophages, the "vulture cells," randomly engulf and destroy bacteria or foreign debris. The third line of defense, the immune system, is the **specific** defense mechanism in the body. It provides protection by stimulating a specific response following exposure to unique foreign matter. In recent years, much effort has been expended on research on the immune system in an

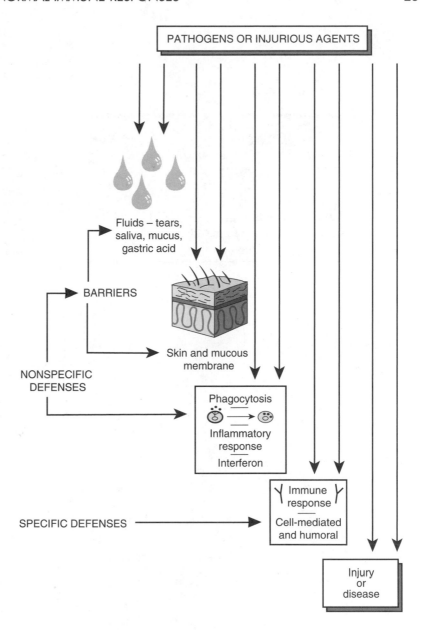

FIGURE 3-1. Defense mechanisms in the body.

effort to increase understanding of the process and create ways to strengthen this defense mechanism. Thus, new information is constantly coming forward.

The Immune Response

Because of unique **antigens** on the surface of an individual's cells, that person's immune system can distinguish *self* from *nonself* (foreign) and can thus detect and destroy unknown material. Normally, the immune system ignores self cells. The immune system *recognizes* a specific invader (antigen), develops a specific *response* to that foreign material (for example, antibody), and remembers that particular invader if it enters the body again. It is similar to a surveillance system warning of attack and the subsequent mobilization of an army for defense. Note that a person must have been exposed to the specific foreign material and must have developed immunity to it (such as antibodies) before this defense is effective. This response is usually repeated each time the person is exposed to a particular substance because the immune system has *memory* cells. In destroying foreign material, the immune system is assisted by general defense mechanisms such as phagocytosis and the inflammatory response. By removing the foreign material, the immune system also plays a role in preparing injured tissue for healing. Because cancer cells are abnormal, the immune system should be able to identify these cells as unwanted and remove them, thus playing an important role in the prevention and treatment of cancer (see Chapter 5).

Components of the Immune System

The immune system consists of the lymphoid structures, the immune cells, and the tissues concerned with immune cell development. Many chemical mediators have essential functional roles as well. The lymphoid structures, including the lymph nodes, the spleen and tonsils, the intestinal lymphoid tissue, and the lymphatic circulation form the basic structure within which the immune response can function (Fig. 3–2). The immune cells, or lymphocytes, as well as macrophages provide the specific mechanism for the identification and removal of alien material. The bone marrow and thymus have roles in the development of the cells. The blood and circulatory system provide a major transpor-

Thinkabout 3–1

a. Using your knowledge of the body, give two examples of a body secretion that acts as a defense and describe the active components of each.

b. List two areas of the body where a mucous membrane is a defensive barrier.

c. From the information given previously, explain how the immune system is limited in its defensive ability, especially in a young child.

FIGURE 3–2. Structures in the immune system.

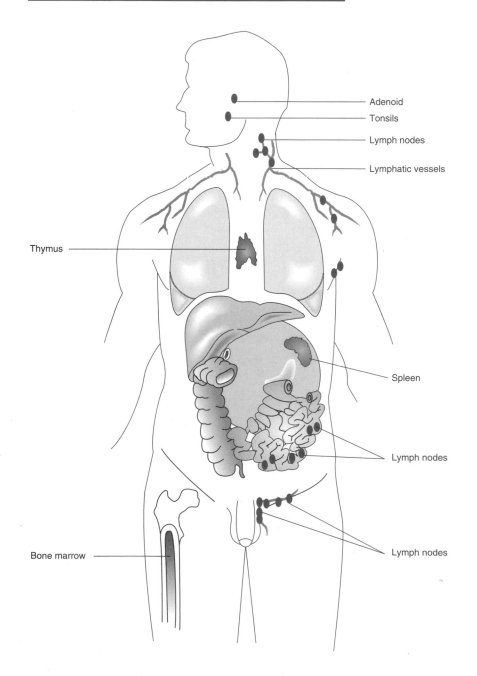

Adenoid
Tonsils
Lymph nodes
Lymphatic vessels
Thymus
Spleen
Lymph nodes
Lymph nodes
Bone marrow

tation and communication network for the immune system. The major components and their functions are summarized in Table 3–1.

Antigens are either foreign substances or cell markers that are unique (except in identical twins) in each individual. They are usually composed of complex proteins or polysaccharides. These substances activate the immune system to produce *antibodies.* The antigens on an individual's cells are inherited from the parents. Antigens are coded by a large group of **genes** called major histocompatibility complex (MHC) genes on **chromosome** 6 (see Chapter 7). Owing to the large number of possible combinations of genes that may be inherited from the parents, it is unlikely that two individuals would ever have identical antigens. Human leukocyte antigens (HLA) were first detected on the cell membranes of leukocytes. These antigens are important in providing a close match in tissues that are to be transplanted. Antigens provide the means by which the immune system distinguishes self from nonself. The immune system can also *tolerate* self-antigens. In other words, the system does not recognize antigens in its own host body as foreign.

CELLS

The *macrophage* is critical in the implementation of the immune response. Macrophages develop from **monocytes** (see Chapter 16), part of the **mononuclear phagocytic system** (formerly called the reticuloendothelial system). Macrophages occur throughout the body in such tissues as the liver, lungs, and lymph nodes. They are large phagocytic cells that intercept and engulf foreign material and then process and present the antigen from the foreign material to the lymphocytes, thus initiating the immune response (Fig. 3–3). Macrophages also secrete chemicals such as monokines and interleukins (see Table 3–1) that play a role in the activation of additional lymphocytes and in the inflammatory response, which often accompanies an immune response.

The primary cell is the *lymphocyte,* one of the *leukocytes* or white blood cells produced by the bone marrow (see Chapter 16). Lymphocytes are termed *immunocompetent* cells—cells that have the special function of recognizing and reacting with antigens in the body. The two groups of lymphocytes, T lymphocytes and B lymphocytes, determine which type of immunity will be initiated, either cell-mediated immunity or humoral immunity. *T lymphocytes (T cells)* arise from **stem cells** in the bone marrow and then travel to the **thymus** for further differentiation. *Cell-mediated immunity* develops when T lymphocytes recognize antigen on the surface of macrophages, become sensitized, and directly destroy the invading antigen (see Fig. 3–3). These sensitized or specially programmed T cells then reproduce, creating

TABLE 3–1 Major Components of the Immune System and Their Functions

Antigen	Foreign substance or component of cell that stimulates immune response
Antibody	Specific protein produced in humoral response to bind with antigen
Autoantibody	Antibodies against self-antigen; attacks body's own tissues
Thymus	Gland located in the mediastinum, large in children, decreasing size in adults. Site of maturation and proliferation of T lymphocytes
Lymphatic tissue	Contains many lymphocytes. Filters body fluids, removes foreign matter
Bone marrow	Source of stem cells, lymphocytes, and maturation of B lymphocytes
Cells	
Neutrophils	White blood cells for phagocytosis; nonspecific defense; active in inflammatory process
Basophils	White blood cells: bind IgE, release histamine in anaphylaxis
Eosinophils	White blood cells: participate in allergic responses
Monocytes	White blood cells: migrate from the blood into tissues to become macrophages
Macrophages	Phagocytosis; process and present antigens to lymphocytes for the immune response
Mast cells	Release chemical mediators such as histamine in connective tissue
B lymphocytes	Humoral immunity-activated cell becomes an antibody-producing plasma cell or a B memory cell
Plasma cells	Develop from B lymphocytes and secrete specific antibodies
T lymphocytes	White blood cell: cell-mediated immunity
Cytotoxic T cells	Destroy antigens, cancer cells, virus-infected cells
Memory T cells	Remember antigen and quickly stimulate immune response on reexposure
Helper T cells	Activate B and T cells
Suppressor T cells	Control or limit specific immune response
Chemical Mediators	
Complement	Group of inactive proteins in the circulation that, when activated, stimulate the release of other chemical mediators, promoting inflammation, chemotaxis, and phagocytosis
Histamine	Released from mast cells and basophils, particularly in allergic reactions. Causes vasodilation and increasd vascular permeability or edema, contraction of bronchiolar smooth muscle, and pruritus
Kinins (bradykinin)	Cause vasodilation and increased permeability (edema), and pain
Prostaglandins	Group of lipids with varying effects. Some cause inflammation-vasodilation and increased permeability, and pain
Leukotrienes	Group of lipids derived from mast cells and basophils, which cause contraction of bronchiolar smooth muscle and have a role in development of inflammation
Cytokines	Includes lymphokines, monokines, and interleukins; produced by macrophages and activated lymphocytes; stimulate activation and proliferation of B and T cells (communication between cells); involved in inflammation and fever and leukocytosis
Chemotactic factors	Attract phagocytes to area of inflammation

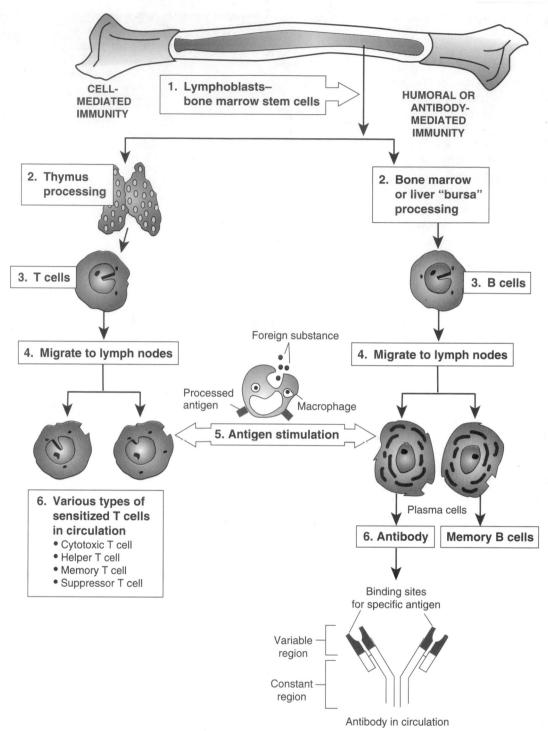

FIGURE 3–3. Development of cellular and humoral immunity.

an "army" to battle the invader, and they also activate other T lymphocytes and B lymphocytes. T cells are primarily effective against virus-infected cells, fungal and protozoal infections, cancer cells, and foreign cells such as transplanted tissue. There are a number of subgroups of T cells, each of which has a specialized function in the immune response (see Table 3–1). The **cytotoxic,** or killer T, cells, destroy the target cell by binding to the antigen and releasing damaging chemicals such as monokines and lymphokines, which may destroy foreign cell membranes or cause an inflammatory response, attract macrophages to the site, stimulate the proliferation of more lymphocytes, and stimulate hematopoiesis. Phagocytic cells then clean up the debris. Memory T cells remain in the lymph nodes for years, ready to activate the response again if the same invader returns.

The *B lymphocytes* or *B cells* are responsible for *humoral immunity* through the production of *antibodies* or *immunoglobulins.* B cells are thought to mature in the bone marrow and then proceed to the spleen and lymphoid tissue. After exposure to antigen, and with the assistance of T lymphocytes, they become antibody-producing plasma cells (see Fig. 3–3). B lymphocytes act primarily against bacteria and viruses that are outside body cells. B memory cells that provide for repeated production of antibodies as needed also form.

ANTIBODIES OR IMMUNOGLOBULINS

Antibodies or immunoglobulins are proteins. Each has a unique sequence of amino acids on a common base and binds to the specific matching antigen, destroying it. This specificity of antigen for antibody, similar to a key fitting into a lock, is a significant factor in the development of immunity to various diseases. Antibodies are found in the general circulation, forming the globulin portion of the plasma proteins, as well as in lymphoid structures. There are five classes of immunoglobulins, each of which has a special structure and function (Table 3–2). Immunoglobulin G (*IgG* or *gamma globulin*) is the major component of the immunoglobulin pool that circulates in body fluids. This group includes antibacterial and antiviral antibodies as well as antibodies to bacterial toxins. These antibodies can cross the **placenta** from mother to **fetus,** offering important protection to the newborn. Sometimes gamma globulin is administered to individuals as a prophylactic measure following exposure to a pathogen or to minimize the effects of an infection—for

example, hepatitis B, measles, or poliomyelitis. Immunoglobulin M (*IgM*) develops early in the course of an infection and then subsides as IgG levels rise. Immunoglobulin A (*IgA*) acts as a defense on mucous membranes, occurring in saliva and secretions in the respiratory and digestive tracts. It is present in **colostrum,** the early breast milk, and passes maternal antibodies to the newborn. Immunoglobulin E (*IgE*) is primarily bound to mast cells and is involved in hypersensitivity reactions. Immunoglobulin D (*IgD*) appears to be related to B-cell activity in some way.

Thinkabout 3–2

> a. Describe two differences between B lymphocytes and T lymphocytes.
> b. Where is IgG found in the body?
> c. Which lymphocyte has a role in both cell-mediated and humoral immunity?
> d. Describe the development of antibodies to a specific antigen.

COMPLEMENT SYSTEM

The **complement** system is frequently activated during an immune reaction with IgG or IgM. Complement involves a group of inactive proteins circulating in the blood. When an antigen-antibody complex binds to the first complement component, C1, a sequence of activating steps occurs (similar to a blood clotting cascade). This results eventually in the destruction of the antigen by phagocytosis or by **lysis** when the cell membrane is destroyed. Complement activation also initiates an inflammatory response.

CHEMICAL MEDIATORS

A number of chemical mediators such as histamine or interleukin may be involved in an immune reaction, depending on the particular circumstances. These chemicals have a variety of functions, perhaps signaling a cellular response or causing cellular damage. A brief summary is provided in Table 3–1.

Diagnostic Tests

Tests may assess the levels and functional quality (qualitative and quantitative) of serum immunoglobu-

TABLE 3–2 Immunoglobulins and Their Functions	
IgG	Most common antibody in the blood, produced in both primary and secondary immune responses; activates complement; includes antibacterial, antiviral, and antitoxin antibodies. Crosses placenta, creates passive immunity in newborn
IgM	Bound to B lymphocytes in circulation and is usually the first to increase in the immune response; activates complement; forms natural antibodies; is involved in blood ABO type incompatibility reaction
IgA	Found in secretions such as tears, saliva, mucous membranes and in colostrum to provide protection to newborn child
IgE	Binds to mast cells in skin and mucous membranes; when linked to allergen, causes release of histamine and other chemicals, resulting in inflammation
IgD	Attached to B cells; activates B cells

lins or the **titer** of specific antibodies. Identification of antibodies may be required for such purposes as detecting Rh blood incompatibility (indirect Coombs' test) or screening for human immunodeficiency virus (HIV) infection (enzyme-linked immunosorbent assay [ELISA]). During hepatitis B infection, changes in the levels of antigens and antibodies take place, and these changes can be used to monitor the course of the infection (see Chapter 18). The number and characteristics of the lymphocytes in the circulation can be examined as well. Extensive HLA typing is required to complete tissue matching prior to transplant procedures. Many new and improved techniques are emerging, and more details on these techniques may be found in references on serology or diagnostic methods.

The Process of Acquiring Immunity

The immune response is a normal defense mechanism by which the body adapts to the presence of foreign material. *Natural* immunity is species specific. For example, humans are not susceptible to infections common to many other animals. *Innate* immunity is gene specific and is controlled by factors such as race, as evident from the increased susceptibility of North American aboriginal people to tuberculosis

When a person is first exposed to an antigen, a *primary* response occurs, during which the antigen is recognized and processed, and subsequent development of antibodies or sensitized T lymphocytes is initiated (Fig. 3–4). This process may take several days or weeks and can be monitored using serum antibody titer. Following the initial rise in titer, the level of antibody falls. If there is a repeat exposure to the same antigen, even years later, the memory cells stimulate a rapid and extensive **secondary response,** producing many matching antibodies or T cells very quickly.

When a single strain of bacteria or virus causes a disease, the affected person usually has only one episode of the disease because the specific antibody is retained in the memory. Young children are subject to many infections until they establish a pool of antibodies. As one ages, the number of infections declines. However, when there are many strains of a bacteria or virus causing a disease, for example, the common cold, which has more than 100 causative organisms, each with slightly different antigens, an individual never develops antibodies to all the organisms and therefore he or she has recurrent colds. The influenza virus, which affects the respiratory tract, has two antigenic forms, type A and type B. These viruses have various strains that **mutate** or change slightly over time. For this reason, a new influenza vaccine is manufactured each year, its

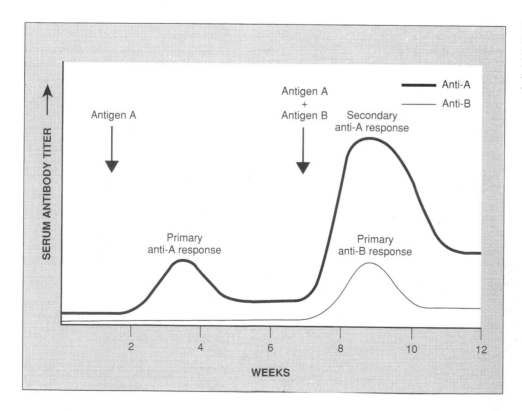

FIGURE 3–4. Graph illustrating primary and secondary immune responses. (From Abbas AK, Lichtman AH, Paber JS: Cellular and Molecular Immunology. Philadelphia, W.B. Saunders, 1991.)

TABLE 3–3	Types of Acquired Immunity			
Type	**Mechanism**	**Memory**	**Example**	
Natural active	Pathogens enter body and cause illness; antibodies form in host	Yes	Person has chickenpox one time	
Artificial active	Vaccine (live or attenuated organisms) is injected into person. No illness results, but antibodies form	Yes	Person has measles vaccine and gains immunity	
Natural passive	Antibodies passed directly from mother to child to provide temporary protection	No	Placental passage during pregnancy or ingestion of breast milk	
Artificial passive	Antibodies injected into person (antiserum) to provide temporary protection or minimize severity of infection	No	Gamma globulin if recent exposure to microbe	

composition based on the current antigenic form of the virus most likely to cause an epidemic of the disease.

Thinkabout 3–3

a. Predict why a person usually has chickenpox only once in a lifetime but may have influenza many times.

b. Why is the secondary response to an antigen faster and greater than the primary response?

There are four ways to acquire immunity (Table 3–3). Active immunity develops when the person's own body develops antibodies or T cells in response to a specific antigen introduced into the body. This process takes a few weeks, but the result usually lasts for years because memory B and T cells are retained in the body. *Active natural immunity* may be acquired by direct exposure to an antigen, for example, when a person has an infection. *Active artificial immunity* develops when a specific antigen is purposefully introduced into the body. For example, a *vaccine* is a solution containing dead or weakened (attenuated) organisms that stimulate the immune system to produce antibodies but do not result in the disease itself. A *toxoid* is an altered or weakened bacterial toxin that acts similarly. A *booster* is an additional immunization, given perhaps 5 or 10 years later, that "reminds" the immune system of the antigen and promotes a better secondary response. A schedule of immunizations for children may be found in a pediatric reference.

Passive immunity occurs when antibodies are transferred from one person to another. These are effective immediately but offer only temporary protection because memory has not been established in the recipient, and the antibodies are gradually removed from the circulation. There are also two forms of passive immunity. *Passive natural immunity* occurs when IgG is transferred from mother to fetus across the placenta. Breast milk also supplies maternal antibodies. These antibodies protect the infant for the first few months of life. *Passive artificial immunity* results from the injection of antibodies from a person or animal into a second person. An example is the administration of rabies antiserum or snake antivenom. Sometimes immunoglobulins are administered to an individual who has been exposed to an organism but has not been immunized in order to reduce the effects of the infection (for example, hepatitis B).

Thinkabout 3–4

a. Explain why a newborn infant is protected from infection by the measles virus immediately after birth but later will be given measles vaccine.

b. Explain the differences between active artificial immunity and passive natural immunity.

IMMUNODEFICIENCY

Causes of Immunodeficiency

Immunodeficiency results from a loss of function, partial or total, of one or more components of the immune system. The problem may be acute and short-

TABLE 3–4 Examples of Immunodeficiency Disorders

Deficit	Primary	Secondary
B cell (humoral)	Hypogammaglobulinemia (congenital)	Kidney disease with loss of globulins
T cell (cell-mediated)	Thymic aplasia	Hodgkin's disease (cancer of the lymph nodes)
	DiGeorge's syndrome	AIDS (HIV infection); temporary with some viruses
B- and T-cell	Inherited combined immunodeficiency syndromes (CIDS)	Radiation, immunosuppressive drugs, cytotoxic drugs (cancer chemotherapy)
Phagocytes	Inherited chronic granulomatous diseases (CGD)	Immunosuppression (glucocorticoid drugs, neutropenia); diabetes (decreased chemotaxis)
Complement system	Inherited deficit of one or more components	Malnutrition (decreased synthesis)
		Liver disease—cirrhosis

term, or it may be chronic. Deficits may be classified by etiology or component. *Primary* deficiencies involve a basic developmental failure somewhere in the system, for example, in the bone marrow or thymus, or in the synthesis of antibodies. Many defects result from a genetic or congenital abnormality and are first noticed in infants and children. There may be associated problems that affect other organs and systems in the body. Examples include an inherited X-linked hypogammaglobulinemia or a developmental defect called DiGeorge's syndrome. *Secondary* or acquired immunodeficiency refers to loss of the immune response due to specific causes and may occur at any time during the lifespan. These causes include infection, particularly viral infection, malnutrition, **splenectomy,** liver disease (**hypoproteinemia**), use of *immunosuppressive* drugs in clients with organ transplants, and radiation and chemotherapy for cancer treatment. Immunodeficiency associated with cancer is a result of malnutrition and blood loss as well as the effects of treatment, all of which depress bone marrow production of leukocytes (see Chapter 5). Glucocorticoid drugs such as prednisone, a common long-term treatment for chronic inflammatory diseases as well as for cancer, cause decreased leukocyte production, atrophy of lymph nodes, and suppression of the immune response (see Chapter 2) Also, it is thought that severe stress, physical or emotional, may cause a temporary immunodeficiency state owing to high levels of glucocorticoid secretion in the body. Another well-known cause of secondary immunodeficiency is acquired immunodeficiency syndrome (AIDS) or HIV infection, in which the human immunodeficiency virus type 1 attacks T lymphocytes (see Chapter 4), decreasing their number and function and leaving the patient vulnerable to infection and cancer.

Types of Immunodeficiency

Immunodeficiencies can be the result of a problem involving any component of the immune system. Be-

cause of a deficit of stem cells, bone marrow dysfunction interferes with both humoral and cell-mediated immunity. A deficit of protein or B-cell impairment may result in **hypogammaglobulinemia** or insufficient antibodies in the circulation. Cells, either lymphocytes or phagocytes, may be reduced in number or function. Dysfunction of T lymphocytes or phagocytes or disorders affecting the complement system may interfere with an effective immune response. Examples of deficiency states are summarized in Table 3–4.

Effects of Immunodeficiency

Immunodeficiency states predispose to the development of *opportunistic* infections, which may involve multiple organisms. These infections are difficult to treat successfully. They often arise from normal flora of the body—for example, fungal or candidal infection in the mouth of someone whose normal defenses are impaired. Sometimes severe, life-threatening infections result from unusual organisms that are normally not pathogenic or disease-causing, such as *Pneumocystis carinii*. Therefore, it is essential that **prophylactic antibiotics** be administered to anyone in an immunodeficient state before undertaking an invasive procedure that carries an increased risk of organisms entering the body. This includes any procedure in which there is direct access to blood or tissues, for example, a tooth extraction, and especially procedures in areas where normal flora are present (see Chapter 4). There also appears to be an increased incidence of cancer in persons who have impaired immune systems, probably related to the decrease in immune surveillance and the failure to destroy malignant cells quickly.

Treatment

Replacement therapy using gamma globulin is helpful. Bone marrow or thymus transplants are possible, but success with these has been limited.

Thinkabout 3–5

Explain why a person whose blood test shows an abnormally low leukocyte count should be given penicillin prior to a tooth extraction.

TISSUE AND ORGAN TRANSPLANT REJECTION

Replacement of damaged organs or tissues by healthy tissues from donors is occurring more frequently as the success of such transplants improves. Skin, corneas, kidneys, lungs, hearts, and bone marrow are among the more common transplants. Transplants differ according to donor characteristics, as indicated in Table 3–5. In most cases, transplants, or grafts, involve the introduction of foreign tissue from one human, the donor, into the body of the human recipient *(allograft)*. Because the genetic makeup of the cells is the same only in identical twins, the obstacle to complete success has been that the immune system of the recipient then responds to the foreign tissue, *rejecting* and destroying it. Rejection is a complex process, primarily involving a type IV cell-mediated hypersensitivity reaction (see next section on hypersensitivity reactions), but also a humoral response, both of which cause inflammation and tissue necrosis. The rejection process eventually destroys the organ, so transplanted organs usually have to be replaced after a few years. To achieve a successful transplant, a good match of blood type and the many HLA antigens on the lymphocytes of both donor and recipient is required.

One type of rejection occurs when the host or recipient's immune system rejects the graft (host-versus-graft disease [HVGD]), a possibility with kidney transplants. Rejection may occur at any time. Hyperacute rejection occurs immediately after transplantation when circulation to the site is reestablished, usually in patients who have preexisting antibodies for some reason, perhaps from blood transfusions. The blood vessels are affected, resulting in lack of blood flow to the transplanted tissue. Acute rejection develops after several weeks when unmatched antigens cause a reaction. Chronic or late rejection occurs after months or years, with gradual degeneration of the blood vessels. Sometimes the graft tissue containing T cells attacks the host cells (graft-versus-host disease [GVHD]), as may occur in bone marrow transplants. Survival time of a transplant is increased when the HLA match is excellent, when the donor is living, and when immunosuppressive drugs are taken on a regular basis. Corneas and cartilage are avascular tissues, and therefore rejection is not a problem with these transplants.

Immunosuppression techniques are used to reduce the immune response and prevent rejection. The common treatment involves drugs such as cyclosporine, azathioprine (Imuran), and prednisone, a glucocorticoid. The use of cyclosporine has been very successful in reducing the risk of rejection, but dosage must be carefully monitored to prevent kidney damage. A new form of cyclosporine, Sandimmune-Neoral, provides better absorption and more consistent blood levels, thereby reducing the adverse effects. Also, many new drugs are under investigation in clinical trials. The major concern with any immunosuppressive drug is the high risk of *infection,* because the normal body defenses are now limited. Infections often involve opportunistic organisms, which usually are not pathogenic. Individuals with diabetes frequently require transplants of kidneys and other tissues, and this group is already at risk of infection because of vascular problems (see Chapter 21). Also of note is the increased incidence of certain cancers, including lymphomas, skin and lip cancer, and Kaposi's sarcoma in people taking immunosuppressive drugs. Also dental professionals should be aware of the high incidence of gingival hyperplasia in patients using cyclosporine.

TABLE 3–5	Types of Tissue or Organ Transplants
Allograft (homograft)	Tissue transferred between members of the same species but may differ genetically—e.g., one human to another human
Isograft	Tissue transferred between two genetically identical bodies—e.g., identical twins
Autograft	Tissue transferred from one part of body to another part on the same individual—e.g., skin or bone
Xenograft (heterograft)	Tissue transferred from a member of one species to a different species—e.g., pig to man

Thinkabout 3–6

Explain why immunosuppressive drugs should be taken on a regular and permanent basis following a transplant.

TABLE 3–6 Types of Hypersensitivities

Type	Example	Mechanism	Effects
I	Hay fever; anaphylaxis	IgE bound to mast cells; release of histamine and chemical mediators	Immediate inflammation and pruritus
II	ABO blood incompatibility	IgG or IgM reacts with antigen on cell—complement activated	Cell lysis and phagocytosis
III	Autoimmune disorders: SLE, glomerulonephritis	Antigen-antibody complex deposits in tissue—complement activated	Inflammation, vasculitis
IV	Contact dermatitis	Antigen binds to T-lymphocyte; sensitized lymphocyte releases lymphokines	Delayed inflammation
	Transplant rejection		

HYPERSENSITIVITY REACTIONS

Hypersensitivity or allergic reactions are unusual immune responses to normally innocuous substances that cause tissue damage. There are four basic types of hypersensitivity (Table 3–6), which differ in the mechanism causing tissue injury.

Type I Hypersensitivity—Allergy

Allergies are very common and appear to be increasing in incidence and severity. They take many forms, including skin rashes, hay fever, vomiting, and anaphylaxis. The tendency toward allergic conditions is inherited, and the manifestations of such allergies in families are referred to as *atopic* hypersensitivity reactions. The antigen is often called an *allergen*. The specific allergen may be a food, a chemical, pollen from a plant, or a drug. One person may be allergic to a number of substances, and these may change over time. Common allergenic foods include shellfish, nuts, and strawberries. Hypersensitivities occur frequently with drugs such as ASA (aspirin), penicillin, sulfa, and local anesthetics. Cross-allergies are common, and therefore an allergy to one form of penicillin means that an individual is allergic to all drugs in the penicillin family.

CAUSATIVE MECHANISM

Type I hypersensitivity begins when an individual is exposed to a specific allergen and for some reason develops IgE antibodies from B lymphocytes. These antibodies attach to **mast cells** in specific locations (Fig. 3–5), creating *sensitized* mast cells. Mast cells are connective tissue cells that are present in large numbers in the mucosa of the respiratory and digestive tracts. On reexposure to the same allergen, the allergen attaches to the IgE antibody on the mast cell, stimulating the release of chemical mediators such as histamine from granules within the mast cells (see Table 3–1). These chemical mediators cause an inflammatory reaction involving vasodilation and increased capillary permeability at the site (e.g., the nasal mucosa), resulting in swelling and redness of the tissues. This initial release of histamine also irritates the nerve endings, causing itching or mild pain. Other chemical mediators, including **prostaglandins** and **leukotrienes,** are released at the site in a second phase of the reaction, and these cause similar effects. If the sensitized (IgE) mast cells are located in the nasal mucosa, the antibody reaction causes the typical signs of hay fever. If sensitization occurs in the respiratory mucosa in the lungs, the chemical mediators also cause **bronchoconstriction** (contraction of the bronchiolar smooth muscle) and release of mucus in the airways, resulting in obstruction of the airways, or asthma.

CLINICAL SIGNS AND SYMPTOMS

The signs and symptoms of an allergic reaction occur on the second or any subsequent exposure to the specific allergen, since the first exposure to allergen causes only the formation of antibodies and sensitized mast cells. The target area becomes red and swollen, there may be **vesicles** or blisters, and usually the area is highly **pruritic** or itchy.

HAY FEVER OR ALLERGIC RHINITIS. As mentioned earlier, an allergic reaction in the nasal mucosa causes frequent sneezing, copious watery secretions from the nose, and itching. Because the nasal mucosa is continuous with the sinuses and conjunctiva of the eyelid, the eyes are frequently red, watery, and pruritic as well. Hay fever is usually seasonal because it is related

Thinkabout 3–7

a. Why is an inflammatory response not present on the first exposure to an allergen?

b. Explain how a hay fever medication containing a vasoconstrictor and a drug that blocks the action of histamine could decrease the allergic response.

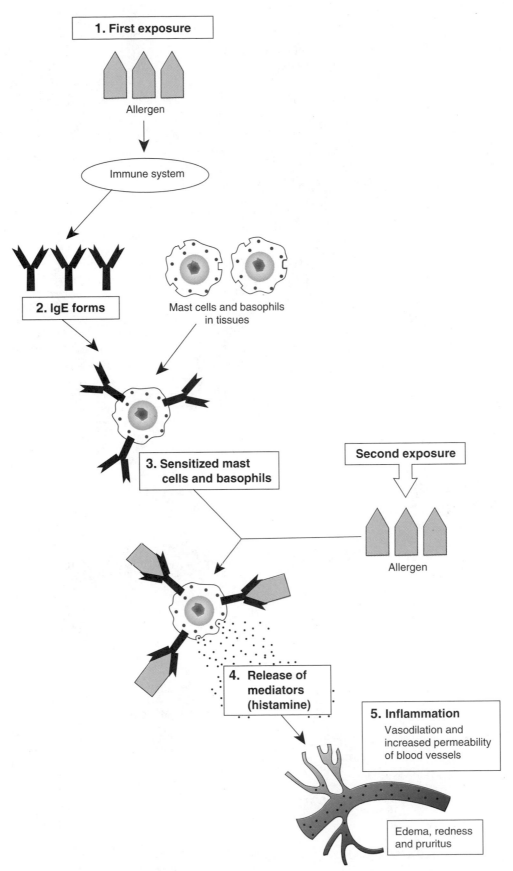

FIGURE 3-5. Type I hypersensitivity reaction—allergy.

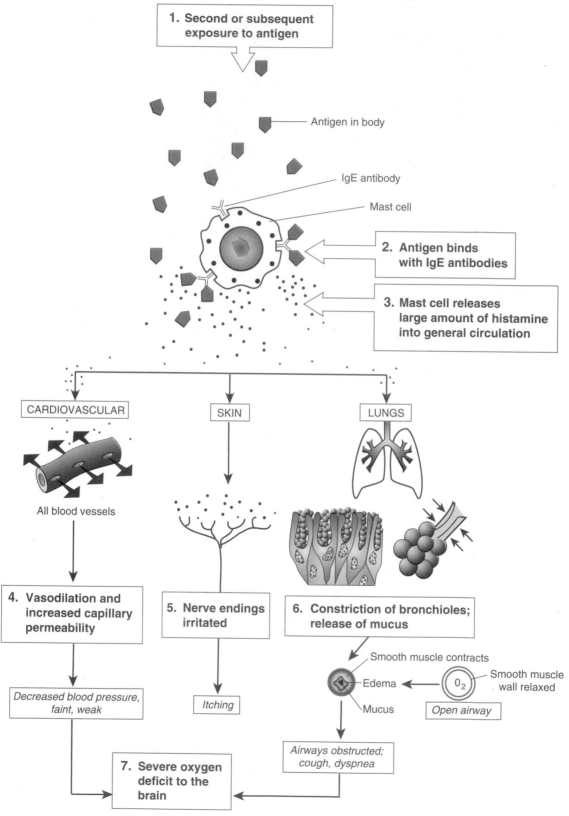

FIGURE 3-6. The effects of anaphylaxis (type I hypersensitivity reaction).

to plant pollens in the air, but some people are susceptible to multiple allergens and can exhibit signs at any time of year.

FOOD ALLERGIES. Food allergies may be manifested in several ways. When an inflammatory reaction occurs in the digestive tract mucosa, the inflammatory response results in nausea, vomiting, or diarrhea. In some cases, food allergies cause a rash on the skin called hives, which are large, hard, raised red masses that are highly pruritic. In severe cases, these hives also occur on the pharyngeal mucosa and may obstruct airflow; therefore, it is important to watch for respiratory difficulty associated with skin rash.

ATOPIC DERMATITIS OR ECZEMA. Eczema is a skin rash common in infants and young children and may occur on the face, trunk, or extremities. It is associated with ingested foods, irritating fabrics, and a dry atmosphere. There may be remissions as the child develops, and the condition may recur in adulthood.

ASTHMA. A lung disorder, asthma may result from an allergic response in the bronchial mucosa that interferes with airflow. Asthma is covered in more detail in Chapter 17. Frequently, a triad of atopic conditions including hay fever, eczema, and asthma occurs in family histories.

ANAPHYLAXIS OR ANAPHYLACTIC SHOCK

Anaphylaxis is a severe, life-threatening, systemic hypersensitivity reaction. Commonly caused by insect stings, ingestion of nuts or shellfish, or administration of penicillin or local anesthetic injections, the reaction usually occurs within minutes of the exposure.

PATHOPHYSIOLOGY. Large amounts of chemical mediators are released from mast cells into the general circulation very quickly, resulting in two serious problems. General vasodilation occurs with a sudden, severe decrease in blood pressure. In the lungs, edema of the mucosa and constriction of the bronchioles occur, obstructing airflow (Fig. 3–6). The extensive lack of oxygen that results from both respiratory and circulatory impairment causes loss of consciousness within minutes.

CLINICAL SIGNS AND SYMPTOMS. The initial manifestations of anaphylaxis include a generalized itching sensation over the body, coughing, and difficulty in breathing. This is quickly followed by feelings of weakness, dizziness, or fainting and a sense of fear and panic (Table 3–7). Edema may be observed around the eyes, lips, tongue, hands, and feet. Hives or urticaria may appear on the skin. General collapse soon follows with loss of consciousness.

EMERGENCY TREATMENT. Emergency treatment consists of an injection of epinephrine, which acts to increase blood pressure by stimulating the sympathetic nervous system; it causes vasoconstriction and increases the rate and strength of the heartbeat. This drug also relaxes the bronchiolar smooth muscle, opening the airway. If available, oxygen should be administered immediately. Persons who have experienced anaphylactic reactions often carry an injectable epinephrine with them because there are only seconds or minutes between the exposure to the allergen and the body's collapse. First-aid treatment for shock and immediate transport to a hospital are essential.

Thinkabout 3–8

Give three reasons why anaphylaxis is a serious problem.

TREATMENT

Skin tests can be performed to determine the specific cause of an allergy. This procedure involves injecting a minute amount of antigen intradermally and observing any **erythema** or redness, which indicates a positive skin reaction. In many cases, the person with an allergy can determine the contributing factors by observation and keeping a log of daily events. Avoidance of the sus-

TABLE 3–7 Signs and Symptoms of Anaphylaxis	
Manifestation	Rationale
Skin: pruritus, warmth, hives	Histamine and chemical mediators irritate sensory nerves
Respiration: difficulty in breathing, cough, wheezing, tight feeling	Chemical mediators cause contraction of smooth muscle in bronchioles, edema, and increased secretions, leading to narrow airways and lack of oxygen
Cardiovascular: decreased blood pressure with rapid, weak pulse, perhaps irregular	Chemical mediators cause general vasodilation, leading to low blood pressure; sympathetic nervous system responds by increasing rate
Central nervous system: anxiety and fear (early); weakness, dizziness, and loss of consciousness	Sympathetic response; lack of oxygen to the brain due to low blood pressure and respiratory obstruction

pected antigen or prevention will keep the person symptom free. Desensitization treatments involving repeated injections of very small amounts of antigen to create a blocking antibody may reduce the allergic response.

Antihistamine drugs are useful in the early stages of an allergic reaction because they block the response of the tissues to the released histamine (blocking histamine-1 receptors on cells). Glucocorticoids or cortisone derivatives may be used for severe or prolonged reactions because they reduce the immune response and stabilize the vascular system (see Chapter 2). By reducing inflammation, these drugs minimize scar tissue. Glucocorticoids can be administered by injection or orally, or they can be applied topically to the skin.

Type II—Cytotoxic Hypersensitivity

In type II hypersensitivity, often called cytotoxic hypersensitivity, the antigen is present on the cell membrane (Fig. 3–7). The antigen may be a normal component or foreign. Circulating IgG antibodies react with the antigen, causing destruction of the cell, either by releasing cytolytic enzymes related to complement activation or by phagocytosis. An example of this reaction is the response to an incompatible blood transfusion (see Chapter 16). A person with type A blood has A antigens on his red blood cells and anti-B antibodies in his blood. A person with type B blood has anti-A antibodies. If type B blood from a donor is added to the recipient's type A blood, the antigen-antibody reaction will destroy the red blood cells (hemolysis) in the type A blood (see Fig. 3–7). Another type of blood incompatibility involves the Rh factor, which is discussed in Chapter 9.

Type III—Immune Complex Hypersensitivity

In this type of reaction, the antigen combines with the antibody, forming a complex, which is then deposited in tissue, often in blood vessel walls, and also activates complement (Fig. 3–8). This process causes inflammation and tissue destruction. A number of diseases are now thought to be caused by immune complexes, including glomerulonephritis (see Chapter 19) and rheumatoid arthritis (see Chapter 22). *Serum sickness* refers to the systemic reaction that occurs when immune complex deposits occur in many tissues. With improved technology, it is less common today. An *Arthus* reaction is a localized inflammatory and tissue necrosis that results when an immune complex lodges in the blood vessel wall, causing vasculitis. One example is "farmer's lung," a reaction to molds inhaled when an individual handles hay.

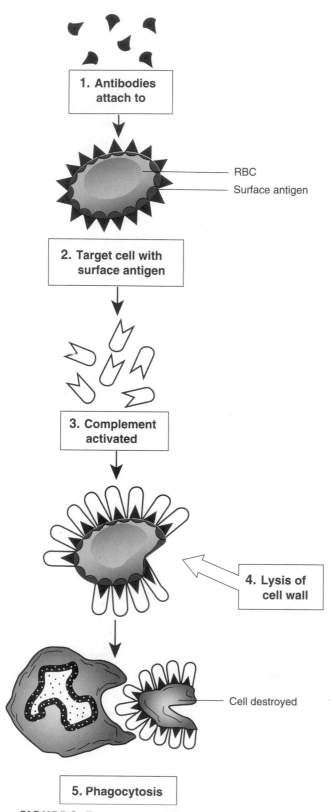

1. Antibodies attach to

RBC
Surface antigen

2. Target cell with surface antigen

3. Complement activated

4. Lysis of cell wall

Cell destroyed

5. Phagocytosis

FIGURE 3–7. Type II hypersensitivity—cytotoxic reaction.

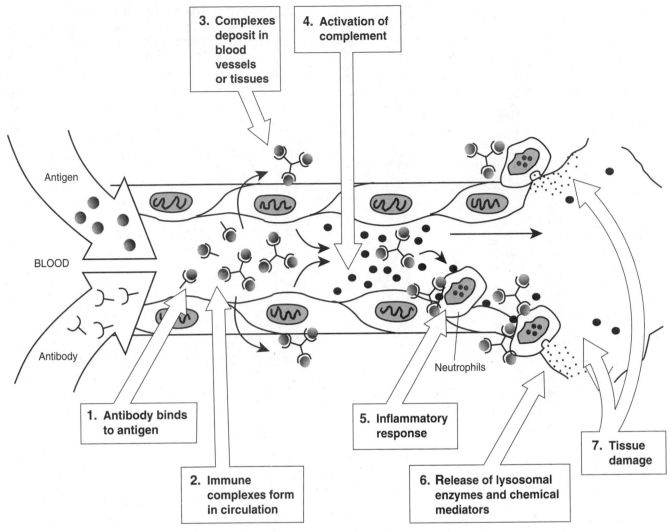

3. Complexes deposit in blood vessels or tissues

4. Activation of complement

Antigen

BLOOD

Antibody

Neutrophils

1. Antibody binds to antigen

2. Immune complexes form in circulation

5. Inflammatory response

6. Release of lysosomal enzymes and chemical mediators

7. Tissue damage

FIGURE 3-8. Type III hypersensitivity—immune complex reaction.

Type IV—Cell-Mediated or Delayed Hypersensitivity

Type IV hypersensitivity is a delayed response by sensitized T lymphocytes to antigens, resulting in release of lymphokines or other chemical mediators that cause an inflammatory response and destruction of the antigen (Fig. 3–9). The tuberculin test (e.g., the Mantoux skin test) uses this mechanism to check for prior exposure to the organism causing tuberculosis. Once in the body, this mycobacterium has the unusual characteristic of causing a hypersensitivity reaction in the lungs. When a small amount of antigen is injected into the skin of a previously sensitized person, an area of inflammation develops, indicating a positive test. This positive reaction does not necessarily indicate active infection, but it does indicate exposure of the body to the tuberculosis organism at some prior time.

Contact dermatitis, or an allergic skin rash, is caused by a type IV reaction to direct contact with a chemical. Such chemicals include cosmetics, dyes, soaps, and metals. Of importance to health workers is the high frequency of sensitivity to latex products and to metals such as nickel, which are frequently found in instruments used by health professionals. Such sensitivities are usually indicated by the location of the rash. The skin is red and pruritic, and vesicles and a serous exudate may be present at the site. Other examples include skin reactions to plant toxins such as those in poison ivy. These skin reactions usually do not occur immediately after contact. As mentioned earlier in this chapter, organ transplant rejection belongs in this cat-

Thinkabout 3–9

a. Compare type II and type IV hypersensitivity reactions, giving examples of the cause and the mechanism of each.

b. Briefly explain how a cream containing a form of cortisol (glucocorticoid) relieves the signs and symptoms of a contact dermatitis.

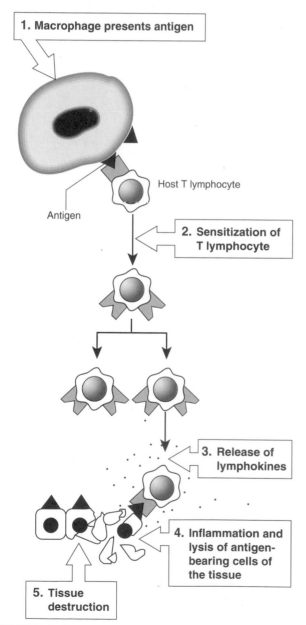

1. Macrophage presents antigen

Host T lymphocyte

Antigen

2. Sensitization of T lymphocyte

3. Release of lymphokines

4. Inflammation and lysis of antigen-bearing cells of the tissue

5. Tissue destruction

FIGURE 3–9. Type IV hypersensitivity—cell-mediated delayed hypersensitivity.

AUTOIMMUNE DISORDERS

Mechanism

Autoimmune disorders occur when certain individuals develop antibodies to their own tissues, and these antibodies attack the individual's tissues. The term **autoantibodies** refers to antibodies against self-antigens. Self-antigens are usually tolerated by the immune system, and there is no response to one's own antigens. This is fortunate because one cannot avoid exposure to one's own antigens. When self-tolerance is lost, the immune system is unable to differentiate self from foreign material. The antigen-antibody reaction leads to inflammation and necrosis of tissue (Fig. 3–10). There is greater recognition of autoimmune disorders now than formerly. Some of these disorders affect single organs or tissues, for example, Hashimoto's thyroiditis and myasthenia gravis, and some, such as systemic lupus erythematosus, are generalized.

Example: Systemic Lupus Erythematosus

Systemic lupus erythematosus (SLE) affects primarily women and becomes manifest between the ages of 20 and 40. It has a familial occurrence. The name of this systemic or generalized disorder is derived from the characteristic facial rash, which is erythematous and occurs across the nose and cheeks, resembling the markings of a wolf (lupus) (Fig. 3–11). It is a chronic inflammatory disease that affects a number of systems, and therefore it can be difficult to diagnose and treat. The specific cause has not been established, but it appears to be multifactorial and includes genetic, hormonal (estrogen levels), and environmental (ultraviolet light exposure) factors. The condition is becoming better known as more cases are identified in the early stages. The course is progressive and is marked by remissions and exacerbations. Certain drugs may cause a lupus-like syndrome.

PATHOPHYSIOLOGY

SLE is characterized by the presence of large numbers of circulating autoantibodies against DNA, platelets, erythrocytes, nucleic acids, and other nuclear materials (antinuclear antibodies [ANAs]). Immune complexes, especially those with anti-DNA antibody, are deposited in connective tissues anywhere in the body, activating complement and causing inflammation and necrosis. Vasculitis, or inflammation of the blood vessels, develops in many organs, impairing blood supply to the tissue. The resultant ischemia (inadequate oxygen for the cells) leads to further inflam-

NORMAL IMMUNE RESPONSE

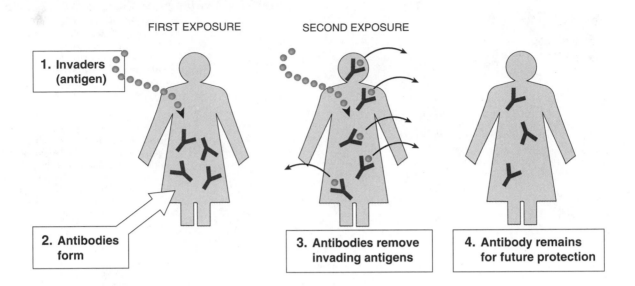

AUTOIMMUNE DISEASE

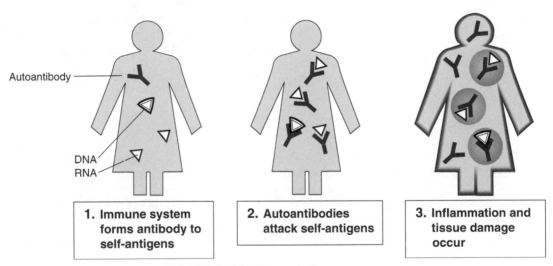

FIGURE 3-10. The autoimmune process.

mation and destruction of the tissue. The process commonly involves several areas at once, including the kidneys, lungs, heart, brain, skin, joints, and digestive tract. Diagnosis is based on the presence of multiple system involvement (a minimum of four areas) and laboratory data.

CLINICAL SIGNS AND SYMPTOMS

The clinical presentation varies greatly because different combinations of effects develop in each indi-

vidual. Common signs and symptoms are listed in Table 3–8.

DIAGNOSTIC TESTS

The presence of numerous ANAs, especially anti-DNA, and lupus erythematosus (LE) cells in the serum points to the presence of SLE. LE cells are mature neutrophils containing nuclear material. Complement levels are low, and the erythrocyte sedimentation rate (ESR) is high, indicating the inflammatory response.

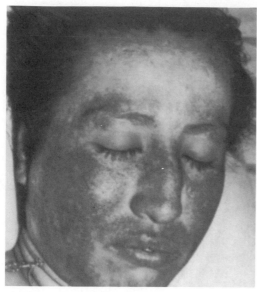

FIGURE 3–11. Butterfly rash in systemic lupus erythematosus. (From Moschella SL, Hurley JH [eds]: Dermatology, 3rd ed. Vol. I. Philadelphia, W.B. Saunders, 1992.)

TABLE 3–8	Common Manifestations of Systemic Lupus Erythematosus
Joints	**Polyarthritis,** with swollen painful joints, without damage; arthralgia
Skin	Butterfly rash with erythema on cheeks and over nose or rash on body; **photosensitivity**—exacerbation with sun exposure
	Ulcerations in oral mucosa
	Hair loss
Kidneys	Glomerulonephritis with antigen-antibody deposit in glomerulus, causing inflammation with marked proteinuria and progressive renal damage
Lungs	Pleurisy—inflammation of the pleural membranes, causing chest pain
Heart	Carditis—inflammation of any layer of the heart, commonly pericarditis
Blood vessels	Raynaud's phenomenon—periodic vasospasm in fingers and toes, accompanied by pain
Central nervous system	Psychoses, depression, mood changes, seizures
Bone marrow	Anemia, leukopenia, thrombocytopenia

Frequently, counts of erythrocytes, leukocytes, lymphocytes, and platelets are low. Additional immunologic tests may be required to confirm the diagnosis.

TREATMENT

Treatment usually consists of prednisone (glucocorticoid) to reduce the immune response and subsequent inflammation. High doses may be used during an exacerbation, but the dose should be reduced when the person is in remission. Additional therapy may be required for specific system involvement. Avoidance of sun exposure and excessive fatigue assists in preventing exacerbations.

STUDY QUESTIONS

1. Describe the role of the macrophage in the immune response.

2. State the origin and purpose of lymphocytes.

3. Compare active natural immunity and passive artificial immunity, describing the causative mechanism and giving an example.

4. What is the purpose of a booster vaccination?

5. Describe the purpose of gamma globulins.

6. Where is IgA found in the body?

7. Describe two types of immune deficits.

8. Explain the process by which an attack of hay fever follows exposure to pollen.

9. Explain why anaphylaxis is considered life-threatening.

10. Describe the pathophysiology of a type III hypersensitivity reaction.

11. Define an autoimmune disease, and explain how the causative mechanism differs from a normal defense.

12. Describe two factors that promote a successful organ transplant.

CHAPTER

4

Infection

KEY TERMS

• •

anaerobic	fimbriae	neutropenia	purulent
antiseptics	leukocytosis	obligate	seizures
autoclaving	leukopenia	pandemics	septicemia
culture	lymphadenopathy	parasite	sterilization
disinfectants	lymphopenia	pathogens	toxins
endemic	monocytosis	pili	unicellular
epidemics	mutation	prosthetic	virulent

REVIEW OF MICROBIOLOGY

Microorganisms

Infectious diseases result from invasion of the body by microorganisms such as bacteria, viruses, fungi, helminths, or protozoa. There are many variations among these organisms and their ability to cause disease. Not all microorganisms are **pathogens** or disease causing. Detailed classifications of organisms with their names are available in microbiology references.

Microorganisms vary widely in their growth needs, and their specific requirements may form the basis for identification tests. The need for oxygen, carbohydrate, a specific pH or temperature, or a living host varies with the particular organism. These factors play a role in determining the site of infection in the human body because each organism seeks a hospitable environment. For example, the organism causing tetanus is an **anaerobic** bacterium that thrives in the absence of oxygen and therefore can cause infection deep in dead tissue. Successful **culture** of organisms in

41

a laboratory depends on finding the optimal environment.

Types of Microorganisms

BACTERIA

Bacteria are **unicellular** organisms that do not require living tissue to survive. Bacteria vary in size and shape and are classified and named accordingly. The major groups are the *bacilli,* or rod-shaped organisms, the *spirals,* which include spirochetes and vibrios, and the *cocci,* or spherical forms (Fig. 4–1*A*). Cocci are further categorized by their characteristic groupings; for example, *diplococci* are pairs, *streptococci* are chains, and *staphylococci* are clusters. These structural variations allow for rapid identification.

Most bacteria have an outer *cell wall,* which protects them and provides a specific shape (see Fig. 4–6). A bacterium has one of two types of cell wall, *gram-positive* or *gram-negative,* which differ in their chemical composition. This difference can be quickly determined in the laboratory using *Gram's stain* and provides a means of identification and classification for bacteria. This classification is useful in selecting appropriate antibiotic therapy. For instance, penicillin acts on the cell wall of gram-positive bacteria. Because human cells do *not* have cell walls, a drug such as penicillin does not damage human cells but is effective against bacteria.

Inside the bacterial cell wall is a *cell membrane,* which

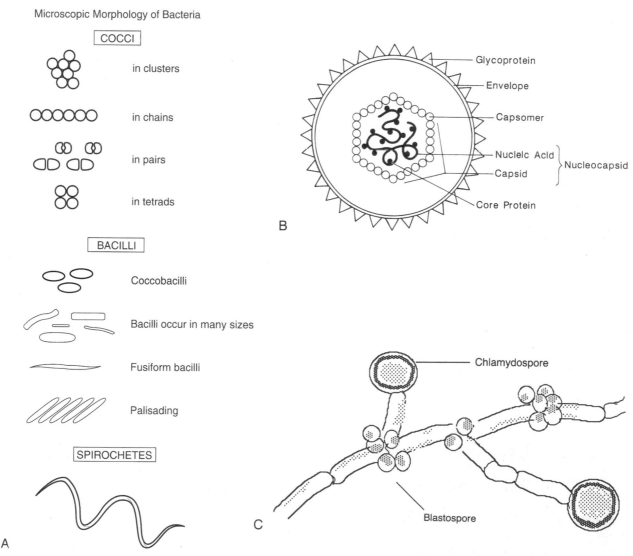

FIGURE 4–1. Types of microorganisms. *A,* Bacteria. *B,* Virus. *C,* Fungus. (*A* from Mahon CR, Manuselis G: Textbook of Diagnostic Microbiology. Philadelphia, W.B. Saunders, 1995. *B* and *C* from Nisengard RJ, Newman MG: Oral Microbiology and Immunology, 2nd ed. Philadelphia, W.B. Saunders, 1994.)

controls movement of nutrients and other materials in and out of the organism. Some bacteria also have an external *capsule* or *slime layer*, which offers additional protection to the organism and also interferes with phagocytosis. Some species are motile because of one or more rotating *flagellae* attached to the body. Several species can form *spores* (endospores), a form of the bacterium with a coat that is highly resistant to heat and other adverse conditions. These bacteria can survive long periods in this state but cannot reproduce when in spore form. Later, when conditions improve, the bacteria resume a vegetative state and then can reproduce. Tetanus and botulism are two examples of dangerous infections caused by spore-forming bacteria.

The bacterium contains *cytoplasm* within which are contained the chromosome (DNA), ribosomes (RNA), and plasmids (DNA fragments that are important in drug resistance). These constituents provide for the metabolism, growth, reproduction, and unique characteristics of the bacterium. Because a bacterium is a simple organism and lacks a nuclear membrane around the chromosome, it is classified as prokaryotic.

VIRUSES

A virus is a very small **obligate** intracellular **parasite** that requires a *living* host cell for replication. The need of viruses for living tissue complicates any laboratory procedure involving viruses. When it is extracellular, a virus particle is called a *virion*. It consists of a *protein* coat, or capsid, and a core of *either* DNA or RNA (Fig. 4–1*B*). This nucleic acid content provides one method of classification of viruses. When a virus infects a person, it attaches to a host cell, and the core material with its chromosomes enters the cell. Viral DNA or RNA takes over control of the host cell, using its capacity for cell metabolism to synthesize protein and begin the replication of the virus (Fig. 4–2). The new viruses are then released, usually with destruction of the host cell, and they in turn infect nearby cells. However, some viruses are *latent;* they enter host cells and do not begin to replicate until later. There are frequently many strains of one type of virus, and viruses tend to *mutate,* or change slightly with replication. Both of these factors make it difficult for a host to develop adequate immunity to a virus. Certain intracellular viruses may also change host cell chromosomes, thus leading to the development of malignant cells or cancer. Because of their unique characteristics, viruses are difficult to control. They can hide inside human cells, and they lack metabolic processes or structures that can be attacked by drugs. Because they mutate easily, it is difficult to maintain effective antibodies against viruses.

Thinkabout 4–1

Compare three aspects of a bacterium and a virus.

CHLAMYDIA, RICKETTSIAE, AND MYCOPLASMA

These three groups of microorganisms have some similarities to both bacteria and viruses. All require living cells for reproduction. *Chlamydial* infection is a common sexually transmitted disease that causes sterility in women. *Rickettsiae* are transmitted by insects and cause diseases such as typhus and Rocky Mountain spotted fever. *Mycoplasmal* infection is a common cause of pneumonia.

FUNGI

Fungal or mycotic infection results from single-celled yeasts or multicellular molds. These consist of chains of cells, which form a variety of structures (Fig. 4–1*C*). Their growth is promoted by warmth and moisture, and they commonly cause infection on the skin or mucosa. Only a few fungi are pathogenic, causing such infections as tinea pedis (athlete's foot) or candida (thrush). Fungi are also a source of antibiotic drugs.

PROTOZOA

Protozoa are eukaryotic or more complex organisms; they are unicellular, mobile, lacking a cell wall, but have interesting shapes. Some diseases caused by protozoan infection include trichomoniasis, malaria, and amebic dysentery.

Normal Flora

Many areas of the body, such as the skin and the mouth, have a resident population of microorganisms. Different sites host different varieties. These microbes are not pathogenic under normal circumstances but may cause disease if they are transferred to another location in the body or if the balance among the varieties is not maintained (e.g., one variety becomes dominant), or if the body's defenses are impaired (e.g., in immunodeficiency states). Such infections are termed *opportunistic*. Normal flora are usually helpful in preventing other invading organisms from establishing a

A. DIFFERENT SHAPES OF VIRUSES

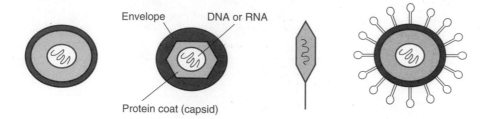

Envelope   DNA or RNA

Protein coat (capsid)

B. VIRAL REPLICATION

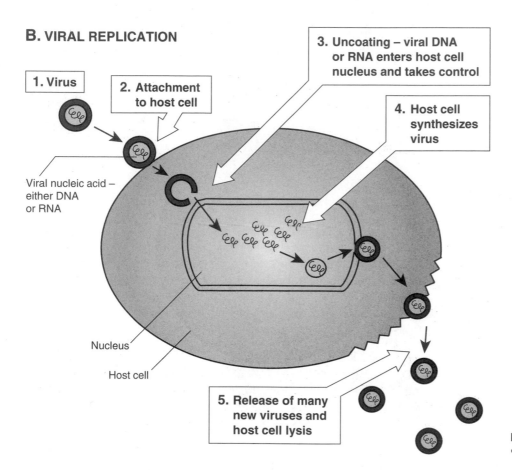

1. Virus

2. Attachment to host cell

3. Uncoating – viral DNA or RNA enters host cell nucleus and takes control

4. Host cell synthesizes virus

Viral nucleic acid – either DNA or RNA

Nucleus

Host cell

5. Release of many new viruses and host cell lysis

FIGURE 4-2. *A,* Different shapes of viruses. *B,* Viral replication.

colony. Certain organisms in the intestinal tract are of great benefit to the host in the synthesis of vitamin K and in some digestive processes. Some areas of the body such as the lungs, bladder, and stomach lack normal flora or are sterile under normal circumstances, and properly obtained specimens from these areas should not contain microorganisms (Table 4–1).

Thinkabout   4–2

Normal flora reside in the glands and hair follicles of the skin as well as on the surface. Predict the possibility of totally removing all organisms from the skin by scrubbing the hands with a brush.

PRINCIPLES OF INFECTION

Infectious diseases may occur in single individuals, in localized groups, and in **epidemics** or **pandemics.**

TABLE 4–1	Location of Normal Flora
Normal Flora Present	**Sterile Area**
Skin	Blood, cerebrospinal fluid
Nose, throat	Lungs
Mouth, colon, rectum	Stomach
Vagina	Uterus, fallopian tubes, ovary
Distal urethra and perineum	Bladder and kidney

Certain infections are **endemic** to an area, consistently occurring in that population. Knowledge of the methods of transmission of microorganisms and of methods of control is essential for the prevention of infection.

Transmission

A chain of events occurs during the transmission of infecting organisms from one person to another (Fig. 4–3). The *reservoir,* or source of infection, may be a person with an obvious active infection in an acute stage or a person who is asymptomatic and shows no clinical signs or symptoms. The latter may be in the early incubation stage of infection, or the person may be a *carrier* of the organism and never develop infection. Hepatitis B is an example of an infection that is often transmitted by unknown carriers or persons who have a subclinical form of infection that is very mild, with few or no manifestations. The reservoir may also be an animal or contaminated water, soil, food, or equipment.

The mode of transmission from the reservoir to the new host may be direct contact with no intermediary, such as sexual intercourse. Indirect contact involves an intermediary such as a contaminated hand or food, or a *fomite,* an inanimate object that carries organisms such as facial tissue or bed linen. In some cases, there are several stages in transmission. For example, shellfish can be contaminated by human feces. The microorganisms in the shellfish are then ingested and cause infection in another human. *Droplet* transmission occurs

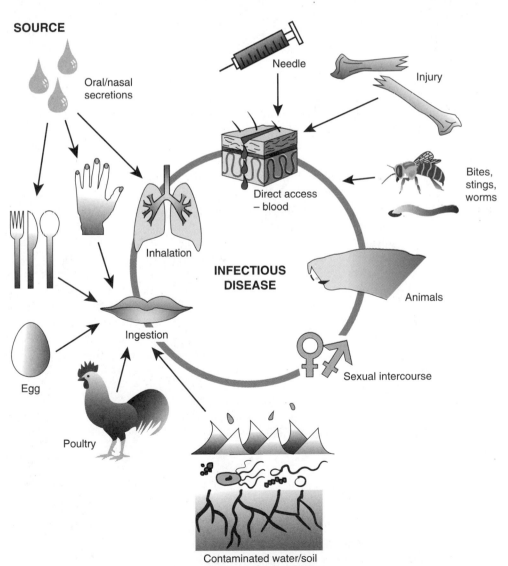

FIGURE 4–3. Transmission of infection.

SOURCE

Oral/nasal secretions

Needle

Injury

Direct access – blood

Bites, stings, worms

Inhalation

INFECTIOUS DISEASE

Animals

Ingestion

Sexual intercourse

Egg

Poultry

Contaminated water/soil

TABLE 4-2 Host Resistance and Microbial Pathogenicity

Increased Host Resistance	Increased Microbial Pathogenicity
Intact skin and mucous membrane	Production of exotoxins and endotoxins
Body secretions—stomach acid, tears	Production of destructive enzymes
Nonspecific phagocytosis	Spore formation
Effective inflammatory response	Entry of large number of organisms into body
Absence of disease	Presence of bacterial capsule
Effective immune system	
Interferon production (virus)	

when respiratory or salivary secretions containing pathogens such as influenza or tuberculosis are expelled from the body. These organisms from these secretions may fall on nearby objects, or they may remain airborne. Insects or animals may serve as an intermediary in *vector*-borne diseases such as malaria. *Nosocomial* refers to infection acquired in a hospital or health-care facility by any of these means.

Host Resistance

The healthy individual is quite resistant to infection. With some infections such as tuberculosis, host resistance is a primary factor in determining the risk of exposure (Table 4–2). Factors that decrease host resistance include age (infants and the elderly), immunodeficiency of any type, malnutrition, chronic disease including cardiovascular disease, cancer, and diabetes, severe physical or emotional stress, and inflammation or trauma affecting the skin or mucosa, including burns, lack of protective secretions, bladder catheters, or other invasive procedures. Sometimes infection occurs easily because of a very small break in the skin or mucosa or in an area of inflammation. Establishment of infection in an individual also depends on the effectiveness of the inflammatory response.

Interferons are proteins produced by human host cells in response to viral invasion of the cell. These interferons then influence the activity of nearby host cells, increasing their resistance to viral invasion and interfering with viral replication. Interferons also stimulate the immune system and are used in cancer treatment for this reason.

Pathogenicity of Microorganisms

Host resistance and the ability of a microbe to cause disease often coexist in a delicate balance. In some cases, organisms such as Ebola virus are highly **virulent**

and have the power to cause serious infection, even in a healthy host. Virulence may also be related to the *case fatality rate,* the percentage of deaths occurring in the number of persons who develop the disease. Organisms may directly damage host cells or may release substances that damage host cells or interfere with a host function such as nerve conduction.

Organisms are predisposed to **mutation.** Slight changes in the organism may occur spontaneously or in response to environmental conditions including the presence of drugs. When bacteria or viruses mutate, antibodies that matched the earlier form are no longer effective, so the individual is no longer protected. Vaccines or drugs are unlikely to be effective against the new form. This is why a new influenza vaccine must be administered each year.

Pathogenicity may depend on the structural characteristics of the organism, such as a slime capsule that resists phagocytosis. Many bacteria secrete toxins. There are two types of **toxins,** exotoxins and endotoxins. *Exotoxins* are usually produced by gram-positive bacteria and diffuse through body fluids. They have a variety of effects, often interfering with nerve conduction, such as the *neurotoxin* from the tetanus bacillus, and other toxins may affect capillary permeability. Exotoxins do stimulate antibody or antitoxin production and when treated can be used as toxoids (see Chapter 3). *Endotoxins* are present in the cell wall of gram-negative organisms and are released after the organism dies. Endotoxins may cause fever and general weakness, or they may have serious effects on the circulatory system, causing increased capillary permeability, loss of vascular fluid, and *endotoxic shock,* a serious complication of infection (see Chapter 16).

The ability of organisms to attach to tissue by means of projecting **pili** or **fimbriae** can be important to the establishment of an infection. Certain organisms tend to establish infection in particular areas of the body; for example, streptococci are common in respiratory and ear infections. Certain organisms produce substances that increase the organism's invasiveness such as collagenase or hyaluronidase, which break down connective tissue. Other organisms produce substances that de-

Thinkabout 4–3

a. Differentiate exotoxins from endotoxins.

b. Describe three factors that enhance host resistance, and three factors that promote pathogenicity of an organism.

stroy certain cells, such as *leukocidin,* which acts against phagocytic white blood cells.

Control of Transmission

Isolation of an infected person is rarely carried out now, and there are fewer diseases that must be reported to government bodies. It is advisable for anyone with an infection to use general precautions to prevent transmission by body fluids. This includes minimizing the effects of coughing and sneezing when in close contact with other people. However, it is now evident that contaminated oral and nasal secretions are more dangerous when they are on the hands or facial tissues. The use of appropriate condoms is essential to prevent the spread of sexually transmitted disease. It is important to know the mode of transmission to recognize the dangers, but frequently there is more than one mode. Also, the number of organisms transmitted at any one time can be an important factor in the establishment of infection. *Universal precautions* are encouraged in which all blood, body fluids, and wastes are considered "infected" in any client regardless of condition. Gloves and other protective apparel are then used to reduce the transmission of organisms in either direction, that is, from patient to caregiver and from caregiver to patient. Guidelines have been established for the disposal of such potentially dangerous items as needles, tissue, and waste materials. The *Centers for Disease Control and Prevention (CDC)* can be consulted for advice. *Contaminated food or water or carrier food handlers* should be identified to prevent continued transmission or epidemics of infectious disease. As a precaution, some institutions test stool specimens from food handlers. Some intestinal pathogens can survive in feces outside the body for long periods of time and can contaminate food or water.

Sources and contacts must be identified in some situations, especially when asymptomatic carriers may be present or when travelers may be infected. In some cases, infection can be transmitted before clinical signs are evident in the infected person, and this permits widespread contamination if the lag time is prolonged. For example, there is a prolonged "window" of 3 to 6 months before human immunodeficiency virus (HIV) infection can be identified in persons.

Disinfectants are chemical solutions that are known to destroy microorganisms or their toxins on inanimate objects. The literature on these solutions must be carefully checked to determine the limitations of the specific chemicals as well as the instructions for use. For example, few chemicals destroy spores. Adequate exposure time and concentration of the chemical is required to kill some viruses such as hepatitis B. Other potential problems include inactivation of some chemicals by soap or protein (mucus, blood) or damage to metals or latex materials on instruments by the disinfectant. One of the more effective disinfectants at present is *glutaraldehyde.*

Antiseptics are chemicals applied to the skin that do not usually cause tissue damage, such as isopropyl alcohol-70%. The chemical affects only surface organisms and does not penetrate crevices. Antiseptics reduce the number of organisms in an area but do not destroy all of them. Also, they may be diluted or removed quickly by body secretions. Some antiseptics, such as iodine compounds, cause allergic reactions.

Sterilization destroys microorganisms by exposing them to heat using several methods, such as **autoclaving.** Again, time and temperature are critical to success. Incineration (burning) and autoclaving are effective methods of destroying microbes.

Thinkabout 4–4

Briefly describe four methods of reducing transmission of infection.

DEVELOPMENT OF INFECTION

Onset and Course

Infectious agents can be present in the body for some time before any clinical signs are apparent. The microorganism must gain entry to the body, choose a hospitable site, establish a colony, and begin reproducing (Fig. 4–4). Only if the host defenses are insufficient during this process will infection be established. The *incubation period* refers to the time between entry of the organism into the body and appearance of clinical signs of the disease. Incubation periods vary considerably, depending on the characteristics of the organism, and may be days or months. During this time, the organisms reproduce until there are sufficient numbers to cause adverse effects in the body. The *prodromal period,* which is more evident in some infections than others, follows. This is the time when the infected person may feel fatigued, lose appetite, or have a headache, and usually senses that "something is wrong." Next is the *acute period* when the disease develops fully and the clinical manifestations reach a peak. The *onset* of a specific infection may be insidious if there is a prolonged prodromal period or sudden or acute if the clinical signs appear quickly with severe manifestations. The length of the acute period depends on the virulence of the

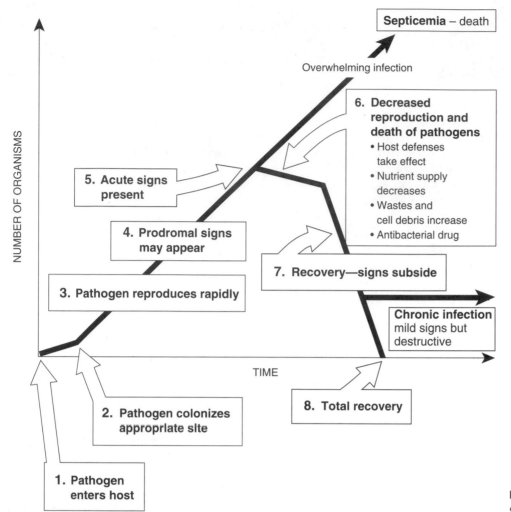

FIGURE 4-4. Onset and course of infection.

particular pathogen and the host resistance. In many cases, the acute period ends when host resistance, perhaps the immune system, becomes effective. Or it may end when sufficient nutrients for the numbers of microbes decline or when they are affected by wastes from dead organisms and necrotic tissue, thus decreasing their reproductive rate. The acute phase is followed by the recovery or convalescent period when signs subside.

There are other alternatives to recovery. In some cases, the infection is not totally eradicated, and some organisms remain in the body, causing *chronic infection.* In these conditions, the clinical signs are mild, although there may be periodic acute episodes. It is important to follow up with tests to ensure that all microorganisms have been destroyed because chronic infection can cause serious tissue damage.

Another alternative is overwhelming systemic infection, or **septicemia,** a situation in which the pathogens are circulating in the blood and reproducing, affecting all systems and threatening life. This may occur with highly virulent organisms, when the body defenses are

compromised, or when the organism is resistant to drugs. *Bacteremia,* in which organisms enter and circulate in the blood in small numbers for a short time, may occur as a transient problem. Usually the circulating phagocytes remove these organisms quickly before they can lodge in a tissue. An exception occurs in the presence of damaged tissue such as a heart valve damaged by rheumatic fever or foreign material such as a **prosthetic** heart valve, on which these organisms quickly tend to lodge and initiate infection.

Thinkabout 4–5

Compare the prodromal period with the acute period of infection, using your own experience as an example (perhaps the last time you had a cold).

TABLE 4–3 Local and Systemic Signs of Bacterial Infection

Local Signs	Systemic Signs
Swelling	Fever
Erythema (redness)	Leukocytosis
Pain	Elevated ESR
Tenderness	Fatigue, weakness
Exudate, **purulent**	Headache, arthralgia

Thinkabout 4–6

List three local signs of infection and three systemic signs and give a rationale for each one.

Clinical Signs and Symptoms of Infection

LOCAL SIGNS

The local signs of infection are usually those of inflammation, pain or tenderness, swelling, redness, and warmth (see Chapter 2). If the infection is due to bacteria, a **purulent** exudate or pus is usually present, whereas a viral infection results in a serous exudate (Table 4–3). There is likely to be tissue necrosis at the site as well. Local lymph nodes may be swollen and tender (lymphadenopathy).

Particular local signs depend on the site of infection. For instance, in the respiratory tract, local signs probably include coughing or sneezing and difficulty in breathing. In the digestive tract, local signs would include vomiting or diarrhea.

SYSTEMIC SIGNS

Systemic signs include signs and symptoms common to significant infections in any area of the body. Fever, fatigue and weakness, headache, and nausea, are all commonly associated with infection. The characteristics of *fever (pyrexia)* may vary with the causative organism. The body temperature may be very high or spiking and may be accompanied by chills (see Chapter 2), or it may be elevated only slightly. In some viral infections, the temperature is subnormal. With severe infection, the nervous system may be affected, resulting in confusion or disorientation, **seizures,** or loss of consciousness.

Variations in the numbers of leukocytes are another general indicator of infection. With bacterial infections, **leukocytosis,** or an increase in white blood cells, is common, whereas viral infections often cause **leukopenia.** Changes in the distribution of types of leukocytes occur as well (differential), depending on the organism, for example, **monocytosis** or **neutropenia.** Neutrophils tend to increase with acute infections, but lymphocytes and monocytes increase with chronic infection. ESR is usually elevated and is a general indicator of inflammation. None of these factors by themselves provides a diagnosis, but they contribute to a final diagnosis.

Diagnostic Tests

Blood tests also are useful in detecting antibodies and confirming a diagnosis, particularly in the case of viral infection. In hepatitis B infections, such tests can also be used to monitor the course of the infection because different antibodies form at various points in the course of this infection.

Organisms can be identified by culture and staining techniques, using specific specimens such as sputum, in patients in whom tuberculosis is suspected. It is important that specimens be procured carefully and examined quickly to achieve an accurate result. Many organisms can be grown easily on specific culture media in the laboratory, whereas other organisms such as viruses require a living host. Blood cultures may be examined to check the distribution of the infecting agent. Frequently, drug sensitivity tests, in which the growth of organisms on a culture plate is measured in the presence of a variety of drugs (Fig. 4–5), are also instituted. Drug therapy is often ordered based on preliminary data and knowledge of the common infections occurring at the particular site, but it is helpful to establish the most effective therapy as soon as possible. Any test that calls for a culture requires several days.

In addition, radiologic examination may be used to identify the site of the infection and may assist in the

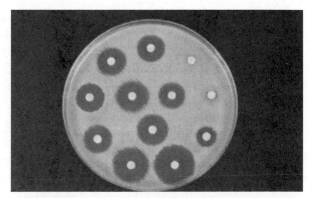

FIGURE 4–5. Culture and sensitivity tests. This species of bacteria is sensitive to all but two of the drugs tested. (From Mahon CR, Manuselis G: Textbook of Diagnostic Microbiology. Philadelphia, W.B. Saunders, 1995.)

identification of the agent. For example, lung congestion localized in one lobe (consolidation) usually indicates a pneumococcal pneumonia.

Antimicrobial Drugs

GUIDELINES FOR USE

It is not always necessary to use drugs to treat an infection because the body's normal defenses are often adequate. Increased use of antimicrobials has resulted in resistance of many organisms to certain drugs and has reduced the opportunity to develop antibodies in individuals. *Drug resistance* has developed in several ways as some bacteria have adapted their metabolism to block the drug action. Some bacteria, such as penicillinase-producing staphylococci, produce enzymes that inactivate certain drugs.

Antimicrobial drugs may be administered prophylactically, prior to any invasive procedure, in high-risk clients (e.g., immunosuppressed patients). Frequently, a *loading* or larger dose is administered initially to achieve effective blood levels quickly. The drug should be taken at regular, evenly spaced intervals over 24 hours to maintain blood levels that are adequate to control and destroy the organisms. Antimicrobial drugs should be taken until the medication is completely gone even if the symptoms have subsided to ensure that the infection is completely eradicated and to prevent the development of resistant organisms. It is important to follow directions for administration with respect to food or fluid intake because many drugs may be inactivated by food. It is best to identify the specific organism and choose the most effective antibiotic. Because many individuals have drug allergies, obtaining a complete drug history is essential, keeping in mind that an allergy usually includes all members of a chemically related group. In viral infections, antiviral agents do not destroy the virus but merely inhibit its reproduction. Antibacterial agents (antibiotics) are *not* effective against viruses. Antibacterials block synthesis of a bacterial cell wall or interfere with bacterial metabolism, but because viruses lack these components, antibacterials have no effect on them. Antibacterial drugs may be given in certain cases of viral infection to reduce the risk of secondary bacterial infection.

CLASSIFICATION

Antimicrobials may be grouped in many ways. This section provides an overview of their classification, but a pharmacology reference should be consulted for details. Antibiotic is an older term and can be misleading. *Antibiotics* are drugs derived from organisms, such as

penicillin from mold. Now many drugs are synthetic. Therefore, one classification refers to the type of microbe against which the drug is active, such as antibacterials, antivirals and antifungals. These drugs are unique to the type of organism and are not interchangeable. Many terms are used to refer to antibacterials. *Bactericidal* refers to drugs that destroy organisms, whereas *bacteriostatic* applies to drugs that decrease the microbe's rate of reproduction and rely on the host defenses to destroy the organisms. *Broad spectrum* refers to antibacterials that are effective against both gram-negative and gram-positive organisms; *narrow-spectrum* agents act against either gram-negative or gram-positive organisms but not both. Narrow-spectrum drugs are often preferred because they are less likely to upset the balance of normal flora in the body, which may result in an overgrowth of one organism and secondary or *superinfection*. For example, following a prolonged course of tetracycline, clients may develop a fungal or candidal infection in the mouth, and women may develop vaginal candidiasis.

MODE OF ACTION

Antibacterial drugs may act in one of four ways. Interference with bacterial cell wall synthesis is a bactericidal mechanism and is seen in drugs such as penicillin (Fig. 4–6). Large doses of such drugs are safe in humans because human cells lack cell walls and are not directly affected by the drug. A second mechanism is an increase in the permeability of the bacterial cell membrane, allowing leakage of bacterial cell contents; this mechanism is exemplified by polymyxin. Some drugs, such as tetracycline, interfere with protein synthesis and reproduction, whereas another group, including the sulfonamides, interferes with the synthesis of essential metabolites.

Antiviral agents decrease the reproduction of viruses inside the host cell but cannot destroy the virus. They control but do not cure infection. These drugs may interfere with attachment of the virus to the host cell, the shedding of the protein coat, or protein synthesis

Thinkabout 4–7

a. Describe two mechanisms by which antibacterial drugs act on microorganisms.
b. Explain the difference between broad-spectrum and narrow-spectrum drugs.

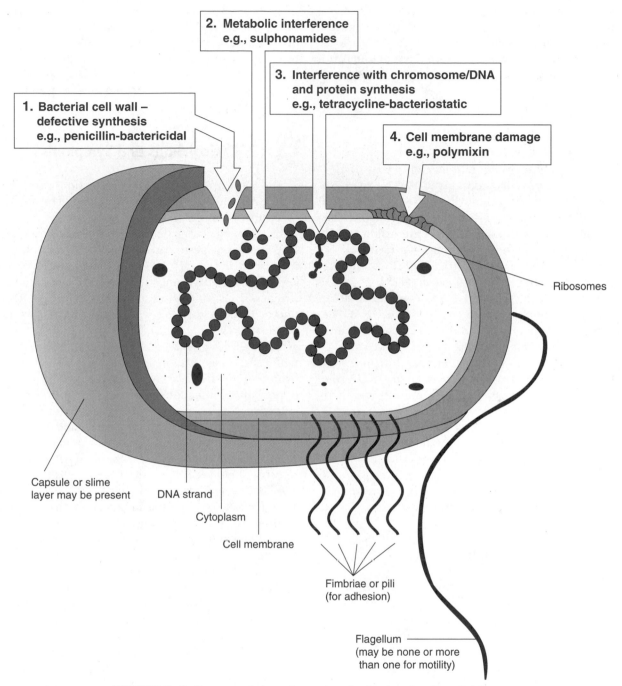

1. Bacterial cell wall –
defective synthesis
e.g., penicillin-bactericidal

2. Metabolic interference
e.g., sulphonamides

3. Interference with chromosome/DNA
and protein synthesis
e.g., tetracycline-bacteriostatic

4. Cell membrane damage
e.g., polymixin

Ribosomes

Capsule or slime
layer may be present

DNA strand

Cytoplasm

Cell membrane

Fimbriae or pili
(for adhesion)

Flagellum
(may be none or more
than one for motility)

FIGURE 4-6. Structure of a bacterium and mode of action of antibacterial drugs.

and viral replication in the host cell. The drugs may be virus specific—for example, acyclovir is effective against herpes simplex virus. Antiviral drugs tend to have significant adverse effects on the host because they alter viral interaction within the host cell.

Antifungal agents may interfere with mitosis in fungi (e.g., griseofulvin), or they may increase fungal membrane permeability (e.g., amphotericin, nystatin). Most antifungal agents are administered topically to skin or mucous membranes.

EXAMPLE OF INFECTION: HUMAN IMMUNODEFICIENCY VIRUS AND ACQUIRED IMMUNODEFICIENCY SYNDROME

HIV is the causative agent of acquired immunodeficiency syndrome (AIDS). AIDS is the stage of active disease. An individual may be HIV positive for some time, even years, before he or she develops AIDS. The infection may not be diagnosed in the early stages because of this latent asymptomatic period. If a patient presents with an unusual infection or cancer such as Kaposi's sarcoma or *Pneumocystis carinii* pneumonia and no other pathology, this often indicates the presence of active HIV infection.

The Agent

HIV refers to human immunodeficiency virus (type I or II), a retrovirus, which contains RNA. The virus is a member of a subfamily, lentivirus, so called because infection develops slowly. Type I HIV is the major cause of AIDS in America and appears to have originated in central Africa, although it now occurs worldwide.

The virus core contains two strands of RNA, and the coat is covered with glycoproteins (see Fig. 4–2). Once inside the host cell, the viral RNA forms viral DNA, which is then integrated with the host cell DNA. The infected cells then produce more virus particles and subsequently die. This virus infects the T-helper (CD4) lymphocytes, leading to a decrease in function and numbers of these cells, which play an essential role in the immune response, both humoral and cell-mediated.

There is a lag time or window before antibodies to the virus develop in the blood; it may be anywhere from 2 weeks to 1 year but averages 3 weeks to 6 months. This creates difficulty in detecting the infection and requires repeated testing in some cases. Research is proceeding on better detection methods.

Transmission

The virus is transmitted in body fluids, such as blood, semen, and vaginal secretions. HIV may be present in other secretions, such as saliva, but transmission in such cases has not been proved. Because of the risk of HIV transmission, blood products are now tested and treated when possible, but there is a slight risk that blood donated by newly infected persons will not test positive for antibodies during the "window" period. Self-protection is essential when one is in contact with body fluids from any source. People who are specific high-risk sources include intravenous drug users (who often share needles) and those with multiple sexual partners. Unprotected sexual intercourse with infected persons (heterosexual as well as homosexual) provides another mode of transmission, particularly in the presence of associated tissue trauma and direct access to the blood. Women are the fastest-growing infected group at this time.

Women may also transmit the virus to a fetus in the uterus. Some infants of infected mothers are infected at birth. Administration of azidothymidine (AZT) to pregnant women is reducing the risk of infant infection. Some infants carry the mother's antibodies for the first few months, but eventually they test negative.

HIV is not transmitted by fomites, such as toilet seats or eating utensils, nor by touching or kissing an infected person, nor by insect bites.

Clinical Signs and Symptoms

The clinical effects of HIV infection vary among individuals and also differ in women and children. This section summarizes the major categories of manifestations. The categories include general manifestations of HIV infection, gastrointestinal effects, neurologic effects, secondary infections, and malignancies. Secondary infections and cancer are caused by the immunodeficiency. Each patient may demonstrate more effects in one or two categories as well as minor changes in the other systems.

Generalized effects include lymphadenopathy, fatigue and weakness, headache, and arthralgia. Gastrointestinal effects seem to be related primarily to opportunistic infections. The signs include chronic severe diarrhea, vomiting, and ulcers on the mucous membranes. Severe weight loss or *wasting* is common, as is excessive fluid loss.

HIV *encephalopathy*, sometimes called AIDS dementia, refers to the direct infection of brain cells by the virus. This may be aggravated by malignant tumors or secondary infection in the brain. Encephalopathy is reflected by progressive cognitive impairment, including confusion, memory loss, loss of coordination and balance, and depression. Eventually, the person cannot talk or move, and seizures or coma may develop.

Secondary infections are common with AIDS. They are frequently multiple, extensive, and opportunistic and may be caused by unusual organisms that are not normally pathogenic. Herpes simplex, a virus, is common, and *Candida*, a fungus, may involve the mouth and extend into the esophagus. In the lungs, *Pneumocystis carinii* is a common cause of severe pneumonia and is frequently the cause of death.

Unusual cancers are another common complication. Kaposi's sarcoma affects the skin, mucous membranes, and internal organs. Skin lesions are purple or brown nonpruritic and painless patches, which eventually become nodular. Lymphomas are another form of malignancy.

Young children with AIDS show developmental delays and neurologic impairment such as spastic paralysis early in life. The life and health care of an infected child are frequently complicated by the illness and perhaps death of the parents. *P. carinii* pneumonia is often the cause of death in children.

Diagnostic Tests

There is a difference between a positive result on an HIV test and a diagnosis of AIDS. HIV infection is determined by using a test for HIV antibodies, such as the enzyme-linked immunosorbent assay (ELISA) for the primary test or the Western blot test, which is usually used to confirm a positive ELISA test. Presently, research is proceeding on a test for the virus itself.

A diagnosis of AIDS depends on a decrease in T-helper (CD4) lymphocytes in the blood as well as **lymphopenia** in the presence of opportunistic infection or certain cancers. B-lymphocytes remain normal, and IgG is increased. Additional tests depend on the particular effects of AIDS in the individual. The CDC has established case definition criteria.

Treatment

Antiviral drugs are given, the best known of which is AZT (azidothymidine or zidovudine). Several new drugs such as saquinavir or ritonavir appear promising in extending lives in clinical studies. Vaccines are a major area of research. The primary focus of treatment is on minimizing the effects of complications, such as infections or malignancy. At the present time, the prognosis is not favorable because active infection develops in time, and the complications are difficult to control.

STUDY QUESTIONS

1. Explain how each of the following contribute to the pathogenicity of bacteria: (a) production of endotoxin, (b) spore formation, (c) presence of a capsule.

2. Predict how each of the following could reduce host resistance to infection: (a) bone marrow damage, (b) circulatory impairment, (c) a puncture wound.

3. Explain two benefits of normal flora.

4. Differentiate infection from inflammation.

5. Describe three ways of reducing transmission of a respiratory infection.

6. Explain (a) why the clinical signs of infection are not present immediately after the microorganism enters the body; (b) why infection can often be cured without drug treatment; (c) why antibacterial agents might be prescribed for an infection.

7. Explain why it is important to take the complete course of antimicrobial medication prescribed.

8. Explain why viral infections are difficult to treat.

9. Differentiate between a diagnosis of HIV-positive and a diagnosis of AIDS.

10. Why are opportunistic infections common with AIDS?

11. State three methods of transmitting HIV and three methods by which the virus is not transmitted.

12. Describe two common complications associated with AIDS.

CHAPTER

5

Neoplasms

KEY TERMS

anemia	DNA	mitosis	prophylactic
antineoplastic	etiologic	mutation	radioisotope
atypical	immunodeficiency	oncology	recurrence
biopsy	infiltrate	nadir	remission
carcinogenesis	leukopenia	palliative	seeding
chromosomes	metastasis	pneumonia	thrombocytopenia
cytologic	micrometastases	prognosis	TPN
differentiation			

REVIEW OF NORMAL CELLS

During its life span, each cell follows the basic cell cycle of growth and reproduction (see Fig. 5–8). The timing of each event varies with the specific cell type. Cells that reproduce rapidly may complete the cycle in 16 to 18 hours. Other cells spend months in one cycle. Cells also vary in degree of **differentiation** and specialization related to the cell's function. Genetic control is exerted through **DNA,** and the daughter cells are identical to the parent cell. If DNA is altered in the parent cell, this **mutation** is passed on to the daughter cells.

Cells vary in lifespan; for example, erythrocytes live for approximately 120 days, and some leukocytes survive only a few days. Epithelial cells usually undergo **mitosis** very rapidly because of the constant "wear and tear" on surface tissues. There are usually several layers of tightly packed cells, the upper layers being sloughed off or shed and replaced by regenerating cells from the lower layers. Some types of cells can increase their reproductive rate on demand, for example, bone injury increases osteoblast activity. Highly specialized cells such as neurons cannot regenerate. Cell reproduction requires an adequate blood supply to the area and sufficient quantities of essential nutrients such as amino acids, glucose, and oxygen. Normally, cell growth and reproduction are controlled by stimuli such as hormones or inhibition by contact with nearby cells.

Thinkabout 5-1

a. Which types of cells have rapid rates of mitosis?
b. Which cells never undergo mitosis?

Cellular aging occurs naturally over time and results in an altered structure of the cell, decreased function, and cell death. The processes of cellular aging and changes in cell control systems are not fully understood. Current theories of aging focus on a limited number of reproductive cycles for a specific tissue.

Changes in DNA can alter cell structure and function or cause cell death. DNA can mutate as a result of exposure to chemicals, viruses, radiation, and other environmental hazards. Rapid rates of mitosis may increase the risk of errors occurring in the **chromosomes,** cell enzymes, or cell components. Mutant cells may lose or change function. Seriously defective cells usually die or are destroyed by the immune system.

BENIGN AND MALIGNANT TUMORS

A neoplasm or tumor is a cellular growth that is no longer responding to normal body controls. The cells continue to reproduce when there is no need. This excessive growth deprives other cells of nutrients. Many neoplasms lack any useful function because they consist of **atypical** or immature cells (see Chapter 1). This expanding mass also creates pressure on surrounding structures. The characteristics of each tumor depend on the specific type of cell from which the tumor arises, resulting in a unique appearance and growth pattern.

Nomenclature

There is a system for naming tumors (Table 5–1). The root word, such as chondro, is the cell of origin, in this case cartilage. The suffix indicates whether the tumor is benign (oma) or malignant (carcinoma, sarcoma). However, a number of neoplastic disorders have acquired unique names that are recognized in medical practice. Examples include Hodgkin's disease, Wilms' tumor, and leukemia.

TABLE 5-1 Tumor Nomenclature		
Root	**Suffix**	**Example**
Fatty tissue: lip-	Benign: -oma	Lipoma: benign tumor of fatty tissue
Gland tissue: adeno-	Malignant epithelial tissue: -carcinoma	Adenocarcinoma: malignant tumor of epithelial lining of a gland
Fibrous tissue: fibro-	Malignant connective tissue: sarcoma	Fibrosarcoma: malignant tumor of fibrous tissue

Thinkabout 5-2

a. What does the term chondroma mean?
b. What term is applied to a malignant bone tumor? (Hint: Bone is osteo.)

Characteristics of Benign and Malignant Tumors

Characteristics of specific tumors vary considerably depending on the cell of origin. The general characteristics of each type are summarized in Table 5–2. *Benign* tumors usually consist of differentiated cells that reproduce at a higher rate than normal. The benign tumor is often encapsulated and does not spread. Tissue damage results from compression of adjacent structures such as blood vessels. A benign tumor is not considered life-threatening unless it is in an area such as the brain where the pressure effect can become critical.

By comparison, *malignant* tumors usually are made up of undifferentiated, nonfunctional cells. The cells tend to reproduce more rapidly than normal. Tumor cells **infiltrate** surrounding tissue and easily break away to spread to other organs and tissues. **Oncology** is the study of malignant tumors, otherwise known as cancer.

MALIGNANT TUMORS—CANCER

Pathophysiology

Most tumors manifest as an enlarging space-occupying mass. The expanding mass compresses nearby blood vessels, leading to necrosis and an area of inflammation around the tumor. Some neoplasms develop very rapidly, whereas others remain in situ for a long time. *In situ* refers to neoplastic cells in a preinva-

	Benign Tumors	Malignant Tumors
TABLE 5–2 Characteristics of Benign and Malignant Tumors		
Cells	Similar to normal cells	Varied in size and shape with large nuclei
	Differentiated	Many undifferentiated
	Mitosis fairly normal	Mitosis marked and atypical
Growth	Relatively slow	Rapid growth
	Expanding mass	Cells not adhesive, infiltrate tissue
	Frequently encapsulated	No capsule
Spread	Remains localized	Invades nearby tissues or metastasizes to distant sites through blood and lymph vessels
Systemic effects	Rare	Often present
Life-threatening	Only in certain locations (e.g., brain)	Yes, by tissue destruction and spread of tumors

Thinkabout 5–3

a. **Cytologic** smears of sloughed cells or a biopsy of the mass may be used in the diagnosis of a lung tumor. State three characteristics that would indicate development of a malignant neoplasm.

b. Irritation in the tissues may stimulate cell mitosis. Explain why recurrent vaginal or cervical infection could interfere with a diagnosis based on an abnormal Pap test (a sample of cervical cells taken to check for malignant changes).

c. Explain why malignant cells are usually not functional.

sive stage of cancer that may persist for months or years and offer an excellent opportunity for early diagnosis of cervical cancer and certain oral cancers.

As a tumor mass enlarges, the inner cells are frequently deprived of blood and nutrients and die. This necrosis can lead to more inflammation and infection at the site. Many tumor cells "trap" nutrients, depriving normal cells and preventing tissue regeneration. Also, tumor cells often secrete enzymes such as collagenase, which break down protein or cells, adding to the destruction. Inflammation and the loss of normal cells lead to a progressive reduction in organ function. Tissue breakdown around a tumor allows tumor cells to

move more easily into surrounding tissues. Malignant cells do not adhere to each other but often break loose from the mass, infiltrating into adjacent tissue. This erosion may be accomplished by mechanical means (pressure) or by secretion of proteolytic enzymes (collagenase).

Grading of tumors is based on the degree of differentiation of the malignant cells—a grade I tumor has well-differentiated cells similar to the original cells, whereas a grade IV tumor is undifferentiated with cells varying in size and shape (anaplasia); this type of tumor is considered highly malignant and likely to progress quickly.

Thinkabout 5–4

a. Why is infection likely to occur at the tumor site?

b. Explain the meaning of undifferentiated cells.

LOCAL EFFECTS OF TUMORS

Obstruction can result when a tumor compresses a duct or passageway from an external position or grows inside a passageway or around a structure (Fig. 5–1). Obstruction may occur in ducts or tubes in the body such as those in the digestive tract. Blood supply or lymphatic flow may be blocked, leading to ulceration and edema. Air flow in the bronchi or nerve conduction may be blocked. Obstructions can cause serious complications for the patient, and therefore prevention of obstruction may form the rationale for continuing palliative treatment.

Pain is not usually an early symptom of cancer but rather occurs when the tumor is well advanced. Pain is a warning of a problem and therefore is helpful if it occurs early. The severity of the pain depends on the type of tumor and its location. Pain may be caused by direct pressure of the mass on sensory nerves, particularly where space is restricted (e.g., bone cancer). Dull, aching pain results from the stretching of a visceral capsule such as occurs in the kidney or liver. Inflammation also contributes to pain because of increased pressure on the nerves and the irritation of nerve endings by chemical mediators (see Chapter 2). Secondary causes of pain include infection, ischemia, and bleeding. Blood can be "irritating" to tissues and can cause pressure on nerves (see Chapter 13).

Ulceration may lead to *necrosis* and infection around the tumor, particularly in areas where normal flora can become opportunistic. For example, infection is likely to be associated with cancer in the oral cavity. Host resistance to microbial invasion is often reduced with cancer.

SYSTEMIC EFFECTS OF CANCER

Weight loss and *cachexia* (severe tissue wasting) occur in many malignancies. Contributing factors include anorexia, fatigue, stress, and the increased demands placed on the body by reproducing tumor cells (nutrient-trapping), altered carbohydrate and protein metabolism, and cachectic factors produced by macrophages in response to the tumor. This debilitation in turn leads to added fatigue and weakness and tissue breakdown.

Anemia or decreased hemoglobin is a common problem resulting from anorexia and decreased food intake, chronic bleeding with iron loss, and bone marrow depression. Anemia decreases the oxygen available to cells, leading to fatigue and poor tissue regeneration.

Systemic infections such as **pneumonia** occur frequently as host resistance declines. Tissue breakdown develops,

FIGURE 5–1. Obstruction by tumors.

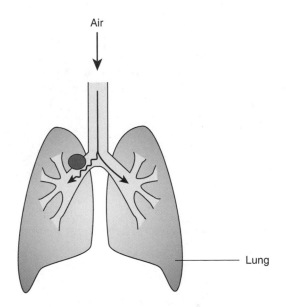

A. TUMOR BLOCKING AIR FLOW IN BRONCHUS

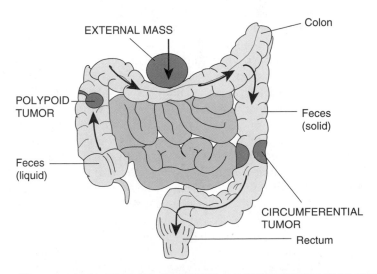

B. TYPES OF TUMOR GROWTH OBSTRUCTING THE COLON

and the immune system is less effective. The host's immobility contributes to infection in the lungs because of stasis of secretions in the lungs and a weaker cough effort.

Paraneoplastic syndromes are additional problems associated with certain tumors, such as lung cancer. Substances are released from the tumor cells that affect neurologic function or blood clotting or have hormonal effects. The cells of a bronchogenic cancer may produce ACTH, leading to the manifestations of Cushing's syndrome in the patient. This syndrome may confuse the diagnosis, complicate the monitoring of the client, and create additional problems for the client.

Bleeding may occur because the tumor cells may erode the blood vessels or cause tissue ulceration. Bone marrow depression may contribute to poor clotting. Chronic bleeding is common in the digestive tract, where the mucosa fails to regenerate quickly. Chronic blood loss leads to iron-deficiency anemia (see Chapter 16).

Thinkabout 5–5

a. Differentiate local from systemic signs of malignant neoplasms and include an example of each.

b. Explain two reasons for each of the following: (1) pain, (2) bleeding, (3) weight loss, and (4) fatigue.

DIAGNOSTIC TESTS

Tests are important in the early detection of cancer and in long-term monitoring subsequent to the diagnosis. All health-care workers should be aware of the early indicators of possible malignancies. Classic warning signs of cancer are publicized by the American Cancer Society. They include weight loss, skin lesions that do not heal, unexplained bleeding, or a change in bowel or bladder pattern. Any health-related professional can play a role in the prevention and early detection of neoplasms. A critical observation can save a life. Sometimes a client may need encouragement to check out a suspicious lesion or change. Routine screening tests and self-examination programs need to be promoted, especially in high-risk clients. Frequent monitoring during and following treatment as well as follow-up is important in assessing the effectiveness of treatment and warning of **recurrence.**

Histologic and *cytologic examinations* are used to evaluate **biopsies** of suspicious masses and to check sloughed cells in specific tissues. An accurate evaluation depends on good technique and preservation of the specimen. *X-ray, ultrasound, magnetic resonance imaging (MRI),* and *computed tomography (CT scans)* are methods of examining changes in tissues or organs (see Ready Reference 3). In some cases **radioisotopes** may be incorporated to trace metabolic pathways and function. Cytologic tests can be used to screen high-risk individuals, to confirm a diagnosis, or to follow a clinical course and monitor change. Tumor markers are substances, enzymes, antigens, or hormones produced by the malignant cell and circulating in the blood or other body fluid. These tumor cell markers can be used to screen high-risk individuals, to confirm a diagnosis, or to monitor the clinical course of a malignancy. Examples include carcinoembryonic antigen (CEA) for colon cancer, human chorionic gonadotropin (HCG) for testicular cancer, alpha-fetoprotein for hepatocellular cancer, and prostate specific antigen (PSA) for prostate cancer. Many of these substances are present with other diseases, and therefore their presence is not diagnostic by itself. Chromosome markers such as Philadelphia chromosome for chronic myelocytic leukemia are also used occasionally.

Blood tests are important both as an indicator of a problem and in monitoring the effects of chemotherapy and radiation. Hemoglobin and erythrocyte counts may be low, a general sign of cancer. In some types of cancer, such as leukemia, the cell characteristics are diagnostic when confirmed by a bone marrow examination. Therapy frequently results in **thrombocytopenia,** erythrocytopenia, and **leukopenia,** and these may limit treatment at some point.

SPREAD OF MALIGNANT TUMORS

Tumors spread by one or more methods depending on the characteristics of the specific tumor cells. They produce *secondary* tumors that are identical to the *primary* (parent) tumor. Many cancers have already spread prior to diagnosis, and it is important to identify this before treatment begins.

Invasion refers to local spread where the tumor cells grow into adjacent tissue, destroying normal cells (Fig. 5–2). The origin of the word cancer is the Latin word meaning "crablike," a good image of an invasive tumor. Tumor cells are loosely attached to other cells and also secrete lytic enzymes that break down tissue.

Metastasis means spread to distant sites by blood or lymphatics. In this case, the tumor cells erode into a vein or lymphatic, travel through the body, and eventually lodge in a hospitable environment to reproduce and create one or more secondary tumors (Fig. 5–3). Only a few tumor cells survive this transfer, but it only takes a few to start a new tumor. Frequently, the first metastasis appears in the regional lymph nodes, which

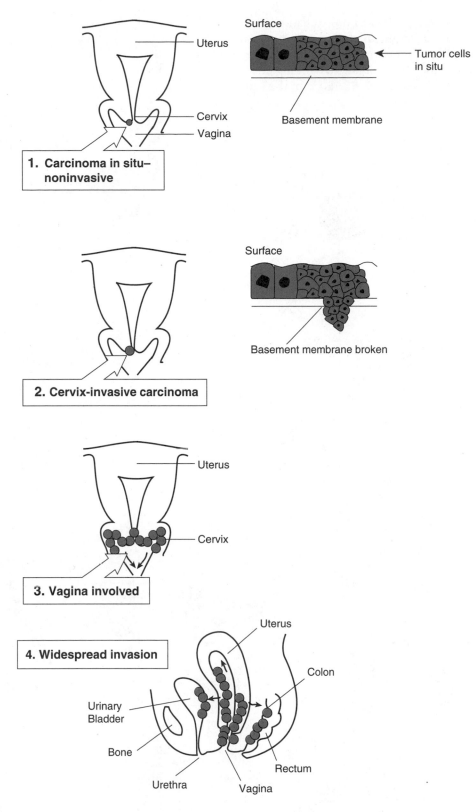

FIGURE 5–2. Invasive carcinoma of the cervix.

localize the tumor cells for a time. These lymph nodes are checked at the time of surgery, and often several are removed. Often, the lymph nodes are removed or treated to eradicate any **micrometastases** that may be missed, particularly in cancers that are known to spread at an early stage (e.g., breast cancer). Many cancers spread by normal venous and lymphatic flow, and therefore the lungs and liver are common secondary sites for many tumors (Fig. 5–4). However, some cancers are more selective and spread to unusual sites.

Seeding refers to the spread of cancer cells in body fluids or along membranes, usually in body cavities. Again, the tumor cells break away and travel easily with movement of fluid and tissue (Fig. 5–5). Malignant cells may also be dislodged from the tumor if excessive handling occurs during diagnostic procedures or surgery, leading to further spread.

Thinkabout 5–6

a. Predict the site of secondary tumors metastasizing from a tumor in the small intestine.

b. Differentiate the process of invasion from that of metastasis.

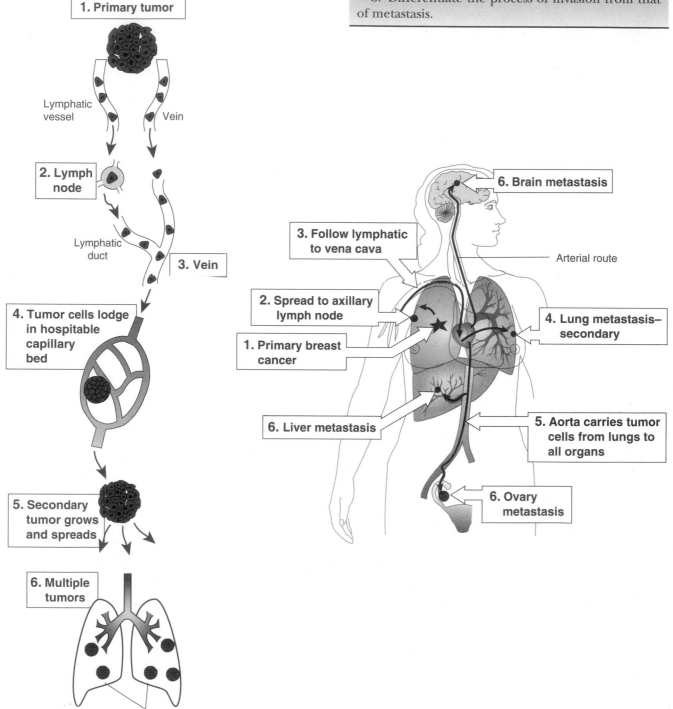

FIGURE 5–3. Metastatic breast cancer.

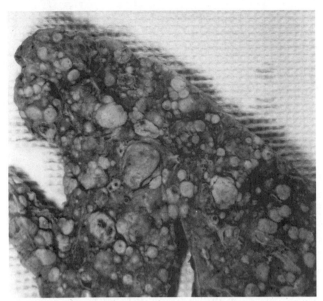

FIGURE 5-4. Metastatic cancer in the liver. (Courtesy of Paul Emmerson, Toronto, Ontario.)

STAGING OF CANCER

Staging of cancer is a classification process applied to a malignant tumor at the time of diagnosis. It may be repeated at critical points. The staging system describes the extent of the disease at the time and therefore provides a basis for treatment and **prognosis.** Staging systems are based on the size of the primary tumor (T), the extent of involvement of regional lymph nodes (N), and the spread (invasion or metastasis) of the tumor (M).

Generally, stage I tumors are small and well localized, easy to treat, and have a good prognosis, whereas stage IV tumors are well advanced, difficult to treat at multiple sites, and have a poorer prognosis (Table 5–3). Subgroups for each grade have also been established.

Etiology

CARCINOGENESIS

Carcinogenesis is the process by which normal cells are transformed into cancer cells. Malignant tumors develop from a sequence of changes over a relatively long period of time. A combination of factors or repeated exposure to a single risk factor predisposes the person to neoplastic changes in the cells. Some specific cancers have well-established risk factors (e.g., bronchogenic carcinoma or lung cancer and cigarette smoking). The multiplicity of developmental steps in carcinogenesis is supported by the fact that not all cigarette smokers develop cancer. It is difficult to establish precise predisposing or causative (**etiologic**) factors because it takes many years to gather sufficient documentation. Also, the incidence of some cancers has changed without adequate explanation. Diagnostic

FIGURE 5-5. Ovarian cancer spread by seeding in the peritoneal cavity.

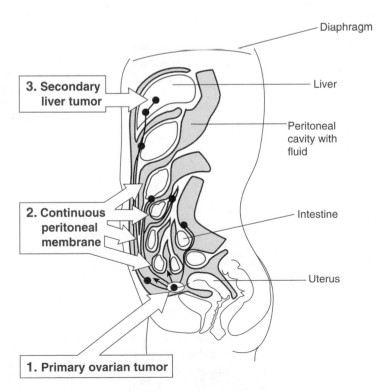

TABLE 5-3 Example of Staging—Breast Cancer		
T = Size of tumor		
N = Involvement of lymph nodes		
M = Pressure of metastasis		
Breast cancer		
Stage 1	T_1—tumor 2 cm or less in diameter	
	N_0—no lymph nodes involved	
	M_0—no metastasis	
Stage 2	T_0 to T_2—tumor less than 5 cm in diameter	
	N_1—nodes involved	
	M_0—no metastasis	
Stage 3	T_3—tumor larger than 5 cm in diameter	
	N_1 or N_2—nodes involved; tumor may be fixed	
	M_0—no metastasis	
Stage 4	T_4—tumor any size but fixed to chest wall or skin	
	N_3—clavicular nodes involved (spread)	
	M_1—metastasis present	

techniques have improved also, which may twist statistics somewhat.

"Initiating" factors cause the first irreversible changes in the cell DNA. Genetic damage or exposure to an environmental risk may cause this first mutation (Fig. 5–6). This initial change does not create an active neoplasm. Exposure to *"promoters"* later causes further changes in DNA, resulting in less differentiation and an increased rate of mitosis. Dysplasia or anaplasia may be evident at this time. This process leads to development of the tumor. Promoters include hormones and chemicals. The prolonged time interval and multiple factors involved complicate efforts by researchers to establish risk factors for cancer.

RISK FACTORS

Risk factors are summarized in Table 5–4. Risk factors associated with geographic areas or ethnic groups may relate to environmental influences or diet as well as genetic variations.

Thinkabout 5–7

Suggest possible reasons for the increased incidence of many cancers in the elderly.

HOST DEFENSES

Cancer suppressor genes present in the body can inhibit neoplastic growth. The immune system appears to offer protection by reacting to non-self antigen on tumor cells. The immune response includes both cell-mediated and humoral immunity (see Chapter 3). T lymphocytes (natural killer cells) and macrophages are involved in immune surveillance and the destruction of "foreign" or abnormal cells. Temporary or long-term **immunodeficiency** has been shown to increase the risk of cancer. For example, human immunodeficiency virus (HIV) infection or acquired immunodeficiency syndrome (AIDS) decreases the number of T lymphocytes. Cancers such as Kaposi's sarcoma and lymphomas occur frequently in AIDS patients.

Treatment

Basic treatment measures are surgery, chemotherapy, or radiation, or a combination thereof, depending on the specific cancer. Hematopoietic cancers such as leukemia are treated by chemotherapy because the cancer cells are dispersed in the blood. Solid tumors are frequently removed by surgery, which is then followed by chemotherapy or radiation (or both) if the tumor cells are sensitive to these.

Treatment may be *curative* if the tumor is small and localized or **palliative** if the cancer is advanced. Palliative treatment is intended to reduce the manifestations and complications related to the cancer and to prolong life. *Adjuvant* therapy is additional **prophylactic** treatment used in cancers that are known to metastasize early in their development, producing secondary tumors that are too small to be detected (micrometastases). For example, following apparent complete removal of a localized breast tumor with no evidence of spread, chemotherapy and radiation are administered as a precaution in case a few cancer cells have broken away to a lymph node or adjacent tissue.

Associated with direct treatment measures is the need to support the client psychologically. The thought of cancer brings great fear and anxiety to clients, fear of death, fear of the treatment and disfigurement, and anxiety related to long-term disability. Many factors are involved. Some clients have a substantial support system, whereas others do not. Treatment can last for months or years, and monitoring continues for a lifetime.

Thinkabout 5–8

Suggest some benefits to the patient for having palliative treatment.

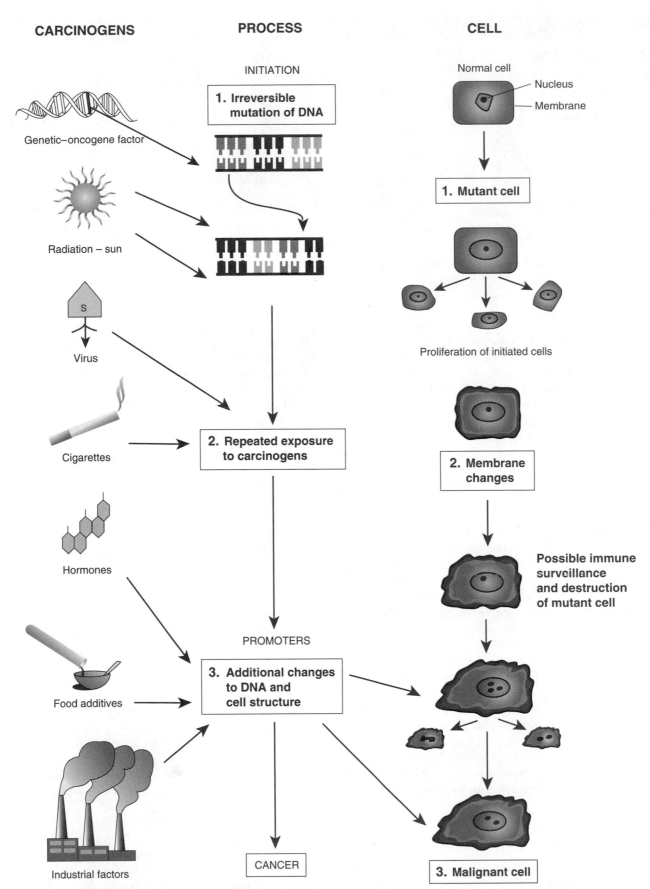

FIGURE 5-6. Multistage carcinogenesis.

TABLE 5–4 Risk Factors

Risk Factors (Carcinogen)	Example
Genetic factors: Oncogenes that regulate all growth	Breast cancer—high family incidence Retinoblastoma—inherited Leukemia—chromosomal abnormalities
Viruses: Oncogenic viruses alter host cell DNA	Hepatic cancer—hepatitis Cervical cancer—papilloma virus (HPV) or herpes simplex II Kaposi's sarcoma—HIV
Radiation: Ultraviolet rays (sun), x-rays, gamma rays, and radioactive chemicals cause cumulative chromosomal damage in cells	Skin cancer—sun exposure Leukemia—radiation exposure
Chemicals: Exposure to both natural and synthetic products in excess may be hazardous; The effects of carcinogenic agents depends on the amount and duration of exposure	Lung cancer—asbestos, nickel Leukemia—solvents (e.g., benzene) Bladder cancer—aniline dyes and rubber

Biologic factors:
  Chronic irritation and inflammation with increased mitosis
  Age—increasing
  Diet—natural substances, additives, or processing methods
	Colon cancer—ulcerative colitis
	Oral cancer—leukoplakia
	Many cancers more common in older persons
	Colon cancer—high fat diet
	Gastric cancer—smoked foods

Hormones	Endometrial cancer—estrogen

Surgery involves the removal of the tumor and surrounding tissue. The tumor cells and the boundaries are checked to confirm the diagnosis and to ensure their complete removal. Removal of a lesion by other methods may not permit histologic diagnosis and grading. In some cases, removal of adequate surrounding tissue may result in a considerable loss and may impair function, for example, skeletal muscle damage or an amputation. Sometimes complete removal of the tumor may be impossible, but reducing the size of the mass may prevent complications and alleviate some symptoms.

Chemotherapy and *radiation therapy* are administered in repeated doses at intervals that maximize tumor cell kill but minimize the effects on normal tissues. Not all cancer cells are destroyed in one treatment. In solid tumors only the surface layers are affected. Between treatments, the tumor may grow slightly (Fig. 5–7). Therefore, treatment continues for a long time, whether curative or palliative.

It is important that any infections, dental problems, or other potential complications be treated prior to commencing therapy. For example, any loose or extensively damaged teeth might be removed, caries and periodontal disease treated, and a good oral hygiene program instituted. During therapy it is risky to implement major procedures because of the tendency toward hemorrhage and the possibility of infection as a result of immunosuppression and poor healing capabilities of the patient.

RADIATION THERAPY

Radiation may be used alone (e.g., for some lymphomas) or combined with other therapies to treat radiosensitive tumors. Radiotherapy causes mutations or alterations in the targeted DNA, thus preventing mitosis or causing immediate cell death. Radiation is most effective on cells undergoing DNA synthesis or mitosis; therefore, it destroys the more rapidly dividing cells in the body, both tumor cells and normal cells. Some types of cancer are radioresistant, or unresponsive to radiation. Radiation may be used prior to surgery or may commence following healing of the surgical site (approximately 6 weeks). There are several methods of administration.

Ionizing radiation consists of either electromagnetic waves such as x-rays or gamma rays (from radioactive substances such as radium or cobalt) or high-energy, penetrating particles (electrons, protons). External sources, such as a cobalt machine, deliver radiation for a short period of time to a specific site in the body. This method frequently requires the client to have daily treatments for a 6-week period on an outpatient basis. Internal insertion of radioactive materials at the tumor site may be used to treat cervical or oral cancers. This is accomplished by sealing the **radioisotope** in a seed or needle and implanting the device at the site. Another method is to instill a radioisotope (e.g., gold-198) in a solution in a body cavity to control excessive inflammatory exudate or blood from the tumor. For certain cancers, radioisotopes may be given orally (e.g., iodine-131 for thyroid cancer) because iodine goes directly to the thyroid gland). These clients must be monitored to ensure that there is no leakage or loss of radioactive materials.

Precautions are required when clients have internal sources of radiation to minimize exposure of other persons. Minimal risk is incurred when the half-life (period when significant radiation is emitted) of a specific radioisotope is short, the cumulative time of exposure is as short as possible, the distance between the

Thinkabout 5–9

a. Is a client "radioactive" after receiving radiation treatment from an external source or machine?

b. Which normal cells are likely to be damaged by radiation?

c. Differentiate internal from external radiation.

source and the individual is great, and shielding materials (e.g., lead aprons), which block penetration by radiation, are utilized.

Adverse effects of radiation depend on the dose and extent of penetration of radiation into the body. Normal cells, which are rapidly reproducing, in the skin and mucosa (epithelial cells), bone marrow, and gonads are also damaged by radiation. Damage to blood vessels (vasculitis) is common. Skin becomes inflamed (as in a

sunburn), and hair loss (alopecia) occurs. The mucosa of the digestive tract is damaged, resulting in some nausea, vomiting, and diarrhea, and the attendant risk of malnutrition and dehydration. Also, inflammation and ulceration in the digestive tract may lead to bleeding, as indicated by melena or hematemesis (blood in the stool or vomitus). With head or neck radiation, the oral mucosa may become ulcerated, and xerostomia (dry mouth) may develop, thereby increasing the risk of damage to teeth.

Bone marrow depression is the most serious effect, and blood cell counts are constantly monitored. Decreased leukocytes increase the risk of infection, decreased platelets may cause excessive bleeding, and decreased erythrocytes contribute to fatigue and tissue breakdown. If blood cell counts are reduced to a critical level, treatment may need to be postponed. Abdominal radiation is likely to damage the ovaries or testes, leading to sterility. In addition, radiation often produces a nonspecific fatigue and lethargy accompanied by mental depression.

Long-term effects of radiation are related to necrosis, inflammation, and scar tissue along the pathway of the

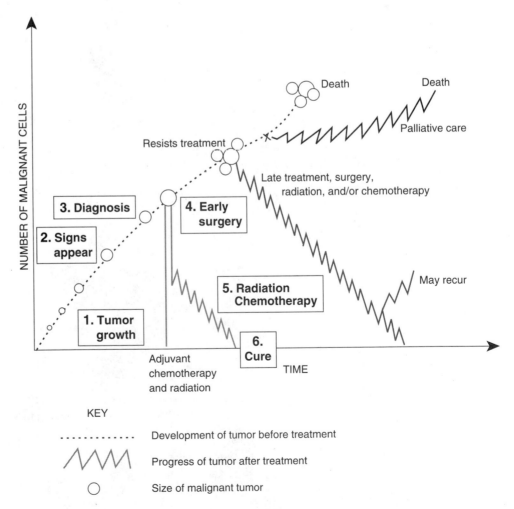

FIGURE 5–7. The effects of treatment on a solid tumor.

radiation and at the tumor site. At some time later, scar tissue may cause adhesions or obstruction and other secondary problems (see Chapter 2).

Thinkabout 5–10

a. List several reasons why the client with cancer may lack adequate nutrition to maintain normal tissues.

b. Why is breakdown of mucous membranes likely to occur in cancer patients?

CHEMOTHERAPY

Some types of cancer cells respond well to **antineoplastic** drugs, while other types of cells are resistant to this therapy. Chemotherapy may be used alone (as in leukemias), or it may be combined with surgery or radiation. Usually therapy commences approximately 6 weeks following surgery, allowing time for some recovery. In most treatment protocols, a combination of two to four drugs each from a different classification are given to a patient at periodic intervals. The classifications include antimitotics, antimetabolites, alkylating agents, and antibiotics. They interfere with protein synthesis and DNA replication at different points in the cell cycle. The choice of drugs and the timing sequence depend on the cell cycle of the tumor cell. When each drug acts at a different point in the cell cycle, the maximum number of tumor cells can be destroyed. Figure 5–8 illustrates the combination of Adriamycin, an antibiotic that acts on cells in the S phase, and the antimitotic vinblastine, which acts on cells in the M stage, along with two nonspecific drugs, bleomycin and dacarbazine. This combination is the ABVD regimen for treating Hodgkin's lymphoma. An example of timing is represented in the older MOPP protocol for treating Hodgkin's lymphoma. Mechlorethamine and

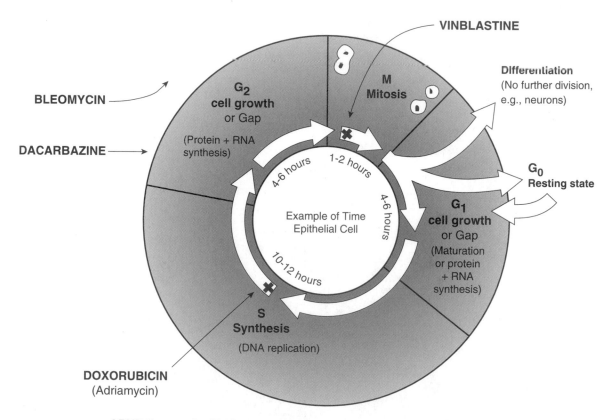

FIGURE 5–8. The cell cycle and chemotherapy.

Oncovin (vincristine) are given intravenously on days 1 and 8 of a cycle. Procarbazine and prednisone are given daily on days 1 to 14. The cycle is repeated every 28 days. Drugs are most effective against the most rapidly reproducing cells and on small tumor masses.

The need to minimize side effects is another factor in choosing the combination. There are a large number of specific protocols, and new ones are being researched constantly in an effort to improve effectiveness and minimize adverse effects. High doses of the drugs are administered to maximize damage to the tumor; then a rest period is provided to allow recovery of normal tissues. A cycle may be repeated at specific weekly or monthly intervals. Many drugs are administered intravenously on an outpatient basis. Sometimes drugs are instilled in body cavities such as the pleural or peritoneal cavity, particularly if bleeding or inflammation is developing. Lower dosages may be used as palliative therapy.

Adverse effects may be quite marked with drug therapy. As with radiation, the normal cells are also damaged, most commonly the skin and mucosa, bone marrow, and gonads. Bone marrow depression is the limiting factor with chemotherapy, and dangerously low blood counts may require transfusions or cessation of therapy until the bone marrow recovers. Blood tests to check cell count must be taken before each treatment. The **nadir,** or point of lowest cell count (neutropenia), may occur at different points in the cycle depending on the particular drug. If the count is too low, treatment may need to be postponed, and antibiotics or hospitalization may be required.

Vomiting may occur during or shortly after treatment owing to direct stimulation by the drug of the emetic or vomiting center in the brain. Vomiting may continue after treatment in response to the mucosal damage in the digestive tract. Antiemetic drugs such as ondansetron may be helpful in decreasing vomiting. Hair loss and breakdown of skin and mucosa occur frequently. Stomatitis and candidal infections are common in the mouth. In addition, some antineoplastic drugs have unique damaging effects in specific areas, for example, fibrosis in the lungs.

Thinkabout 5–11

Suggest several ways by which the treatment of cancer by radiation and chemotherapy may aggravate the problems.

OTHER DRUGS

Information and support for the patient and family is offered by the American Cancer Society as well as by clinics and other support groups. *Hormones* are frequently prescribed in addition to the basic treatment. A glucocorticoid such as prednisone is used to decrease mitosis and to increase erythrocyte counts. For the patient, these drugs improve appetite and a sense of well-being. They also decrease inflammation and swelling around the tumor. Sex hormones are beneficial when tumor growth is dependent on hormone levels. For example, estrogens may slow the growth of prostate cancer. Hormone-blocking agents are often effective in reducing tumors and preventing recurrences. Tamoxifen is an estrogen-blocking agent used in clients with estrogen-dependent breast cancer; it has been particularly useful in postmenopausal women.

Biologic response modifiers (BRMs) are agents that augment the natural immune response in the body to improve surveillance and removal of abnormal cells. Included in this group are a natural product of human cells, interferon, and bacillus Calmette-Guérin (BCG) vaccine (for tuberculosis). BCG vaccine may be injected near the tumor or instilled in a cavity such as the bladder when cancer is present. BCG stimulates the movement of macrophages and T lymphocytes to the site, where they may destroy the tumor cell. These are not first-line treatment at this time.

Analgesics for pain control are an important part of therapy, particularly when cancer is advanced (see Chapter 13). Determining the cause of the pain is important because this determines the therapeutic approach. In some cases, a specific factor such as infection or muscle spasm can be treated, leading to pain reduction. Radiation treatment can relieve nerve compression.

For analgesics, a stepwise approach is frequently adopted. This involves the use of mild drugs in low doses initially, then increasing the dose, then changing to a stronger analgesic, and ultimately using morphine. Very high doses of narcotics may be administered as tolerance builds. Self-administration or implanted units providing continuous infusion are helpful in long-term pain control. Dependency is currently less of a concern, but narcotic analgesics do have a number of significant side effects. These include nausea, constipation, drowsiness, and respiratory depression. Other methods for pain relief may be beneficial, as well as measures that reduce fatigue and anxiety, which can aggravate pain.

NUTRITION

Patients with advanced cancer are often malnourished. Contributing factors include anorexia and vomiting, pain and fatigue, malabsorption due to inflammation in the digestive tract, altered metabolism, and nutrient-trapping by the tumor. These factors may result from the tumor itself or from the effects of chemotherapy and radiation.

It is suggested that measures such as ice and mouth rinses be used to reduce the discomfort of ulcers and inflammation in the mouth. Small amounts of nonirritating and "favorite" foods are better tolerated. These small meals can be planned to be attractive to the patient and to optimize protein and vitamin intake. Pain control and antiemetic drugs may increase appetite. If necessary, total parenteral nutrition (**TPN**) may be used. TPN involves the administration of a nutrient mixture directly into a peripheral vein.

Alternative therapies are sought by many clients in whom the traditional treatments have not been successful. Research continues to study many of these, although trials have not shown much benefit. Examples include Laetrile and Essiac (both of which are folk medicine remedies), megavitamins, and high-dose oxygen therapy.

Prognosis

The death rates for specific cancers vary. For some types of cancer, such as lung cancer, there has been no improvement in the outcome even with aggressive treatment. For other cancers, such as certain leukemias, treatment has become very effective, and survival rates are good. Prognosis in a specific individual is influenced by many factors and so is subject to change.

A "cure" for cancer is generally defined as a 5-year survival without recurrence after diagnosis and treatment. In some cases, several periods of **remission** (no clinical signs) may occur before the disease becomes terminal.

Thinkabout 5–12

a. From your knowledge of normal physiology, explain how good nutrition could reduce the complications or additional problems associated with cancer and its treatment.

b. Suggest some factors other than the obvious clinical test results that could affect the prognosis or outcome for an individual.

EXAMPLES OF TUMORS

These examples are used to illustrate some aspects of cancer. Additional details are provided in the appropriate chapter dealing with the system.

Skin Cancer

Skin cancer is visible, easily diagnosed and treated (by surgery), develops slowly, and has an excellent prognosis. Basal cell carcinoma is the most common form of skin cancer (see Chapter 23). Skin cancers have the highest rate of recurrence and usually arise on the head and neck or back, areas exposed to the sun and irritation. They occur more frequently in individuals with fair skin who are over 40 years of age and live in southern climates. The number of cases is increasing.

The tumor appears as a pearly papule and develops a central ulceration, a "rodent ulcer" (Fig. 5–9). Significant characteristics of the lesion include lack of pain or pruritus (itching) and persistence—the lesion remains and grows slowly. The tumor is slowly invasive.

Thinkabout 5–13

Explain several reasons for the good prognosis with skin cancer.

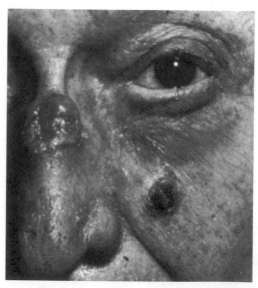

FIGURE 5–9. Example of basal cell carcinoma. (From Arnold HL, Odom RB, James WD: Andrews Diseases of the Skin: Clinical Dermatology. 8th ed. Philadelphia, W.B. Saunders, p. 765.)

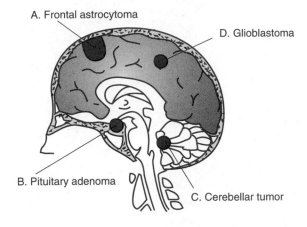

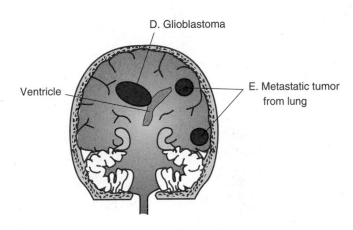

A. Tumor on surface of brain

B. Pituitary tumor causes neurological dysfunction and hormonal abnormalities

C. Cerebellar tumors, even when small, can interfere with brain stem function

D. Tumors in the interior of the brain shift structures and interfere with flow of cerebrospinal fluid

E. Multiple metastases

FIGURE 5-10. Examples of brain tumors.

Ovarian Cancer

Although there are many histologic types of ovarian cancer, this section deals only with the basic concepts. This malignancy occurs often in women 25 to 40 years old with a family history of reproductive cancers.

Ovarian cancer has a poor prognosis because the tumor is hidden in the peritoneal cavity; it is a "silent" tumor (see Fig. 5–5). Presenting (or first) signs appear only when the tumor is well advanced and is large enough to cause pressure on the adjacent structures, such as the bladder or the intestine, or when an inflammatory exudate forms in the abdominal cavity. There are no definite tumor markers to assist in diagnosis. The tumor spreads easily by seeding as cancer cells pass along the peritoneal membranes to the liver and other organs. The cancer also invades the uterus and pelvis. Treatment includes surgery and chemotherapy.

Brain Tumors

Brain tumors may be benign or malignant. Both are space-occupying masses that create pressure inside the skull, and both are serious. Brain tumors, even when small, can cause death if they are located in the brain stem or cerebellum where they can interfere with vital functions such as respiration. Removal of the mass may be fairly easy if it is located on the brain surface but difficult and dangerous if it is located elsewhere (Fig. 5–10). Brain tumors vary histologically and can occur in children as well as adults. Early indications of brain tumors are signs of pressure such as headache, drowsiness, vomiting, visual problems, or impaired motor function (see Chapter 20). Malignant brain tumors do not metastasize outside the central nervous system. However, tumors from the breast or lung or bone can metastasize into the brain, forming secondaries.

STUDY QUESTIONS

1. Explain why severe thrombocytopenia can be life-threatening.

2. Compare benign and malignant neoplasms, describing three differences.

3. How does the zone of inflammation around the tumor contribute to pain?

4. Explain why metastasis can lead to multiple secondary tumors.

5. Why may chemotherapy be recommended for a client when a cure is not likely?

6. Compare basal cell skin cancer and ovarian cancer by (a) presenting signs, (b) spread, and (c) prognosis.

7. Explain why bleeding may occur with cancer.

8. Describe two potential problems resulting from bleeding.

9. Describe the local effects of radiation.

CHAPTER
6

Fluid, Electrolyte, and Acid-Base Imbalances

KEY TERMS

acid
aldosterone
anaerobic
anion
anorexia
antidiuretic hormone (ADH)
arrhythmia
ascites
base
capillary permeability (membrane)

carpopedal spasm
cation
diffusion
diuretic
dysrhythmia
electrocardiogram
extracellular
filtration
homeostasis
hydrogen ions
hydrostatic pressure

hypertonic
hypervolemia
hypothalamus
hypotonic
hypovolemia
interstitial fluid
intracellular
intravascular
isotonic
laryngospasm
milliequivalent (mEq)

nonvolatile metabolic acids
osmoreceptor
osmosis
osmotic pressure
paresthesias
tetany
transcellular
turgor (skin)

FLUID IMBALANCE

Review of Fluid Balance

Water is a major component of the body and is found both within and outside the cells. It is critical to **homeostasis**, the maintenance of a relatively constant and favorable environment for the cells. Water is the medium within which metabolic reactions and other processes take place. It also comprises the transportation system for the body. For example, it carries nutrients into cells and removes wastes, transports enzymes in digestive secretions, and moves blood cells around the body. Without adequate fluid, cells cannot continue to function, and death results. Fluid also facilitates movement of body parts, for example, the joints and the lungs.

Thinkabout 6–1

Suggest several other functions performed by water in the body.

FLUID COMPARTMENTS

Although the body appears to be a solid object, approximately 60 percent of an adult's body weight consists of water, and an infant's body is about 70 percent water (Table 6–1). Female bodies have a lower percentage of body weight as water than males. The elderly and the obese also have a lower proportion of water in their bodies. Individuals with less fluid reserve are more likely to be adversely affected by any fluid imbalance.

Fluid is distributed between the **intracellular** compartment and the **extracellular** compartment, which

TABLE 6–2	Sources and Losses of Water		
Sources (mL)		Losses (mL)	
Liquids	1200	Urine	1400
Solid foods	1000	Feces	200
Cell metabolism	300	Insensible losses	
		Lungs	400
		Skin	500
Total	2500		2500

includes the **intravascular fluid** or blood, the **interstitial fluid** or intercellular fluid cerebrospinal fluid (CSF), and the **transcellular** fluids present in various secretions, such as those in the pericardial (heart) cavity or the synovial (joint) cavities. In an adult male, blood constitutes about 4 percent of body weight and interstitial fluid about 15 percent; the remaining transcellular fluids amount to about 1 percent of total body weight. Water constantly circulates around the body and moves between various compartments. For example, CSF forms continuously from the blood and is reabsorbed back into the general circulation.

Thinkabout 6–2

a. Which body compartment contains the most water?

b. Suggest several other locations where water is found in the body.

MOVEMENT OF WATER

To maintain a constant level of body fluid, the amount of water entering the body should equal the amount of water leaving the body. Fluid is added to the body through the ingestion of solid food and fluids and as a product of cell metabolism (Table 6–2). Fluid is lost in the urine and feces as well as through *insensible* (invisible) losses through the skin (perspiration) and exhaled air. One control of fluid balance is the *thirst* mechanism in the **hypothalamus**, the **osmoreceptor** cells of which sense the internal environment, both fluid volume and concentration, and then promote the intake of fluid when needed. Also, hormones such as **antidiuretic hormone (ADH)** and **aldosterone** control the amount of fluid leaving the body in the urine (see Chapters 19 and 21). ADH promotes reabsorption of water into the blood from the kidney tubules, and aldosterone controls the reabsorption of both sodium ions and water from the kidney tubules.

TABLE 6–1	Fluid Compartments in the Body			
	Volume	Approximate Percentage of Body Weight		
	Adult Male (L)	Male (%)	Female (%)	Infant (%)
Intracellular fluid	28	40	33	40
Extracellular fluid	15	20	14	30
Plasma	(4.5)	(4)	(4)	(4)
Interstitial fluid	(10.5)	(15)	(9)	(25)
Other		(1)	(1)	(1)
Total water	43	60	50	70

Note: In elderly females, water content is reduced to approximately 45% of body weight.

Thinkabout 6–3

Describe how excessive fluid is lost from the body during strenuous exercise on a very hot day and how the body can respond to the loss.

Fluid constantly circulates throughout the body and moves relatively freely between compartments by the processes of **filtration** or **osmosis** (Fig. 6–1). Water is also recycled and conserved under normal conditions. For example, the large volume of water in the digestive secretions (up to 8 liters per 24 hours) that enters the stomach and intestines following a meal is largely reabsorbed from the colon into the blood.

Water moves between the vascular compartment or blood and the interstitial compartment through capillary membranes depending on the relative **hydrostatic** and **osmotic pressures** (see Fig. 6–1). You may view hydrostatic pressure as the "push" and osmotic pressure as the "pull." At the arteriolar end of the capillary, the blood hydrostatic pressure (or blood pressure) exceeds the opposing interstitial hydrostatic pressure and the plasma colloid osmotic pressure (which depends on the concentration of electrolytes and proteins) of the blood, and therefore fluid moves out from (or is "pushed" out of) the capillary into the interstitial compartment. At the venous end of the capillary, the blood hydrostatic pressure is greatly decreased, and

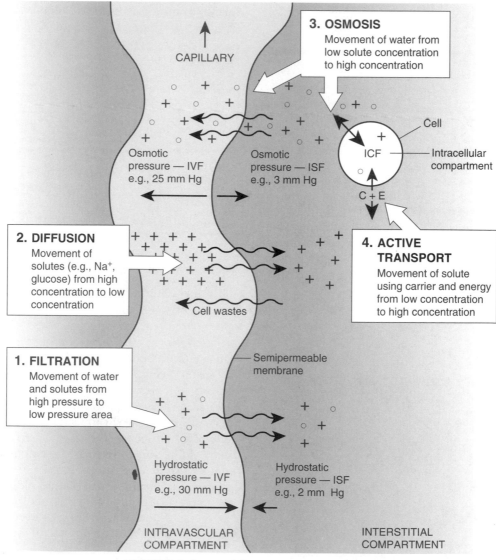

FIGURE 6–1. Movement of water and electrolytes.

therefore fluid tends to shift (or is "pulled") back into the capillary. It is easier to remember the direction of movement if one thinks of the movement of nutrients and oxygen out of the arterial blood toward the cells and the flow of wastes and carbon dioxide from the cell back into the venous blood. Any change in the relative values of hydrostatic pressure or osmotic pressure in the compartments alters the fluid shift. Excess interstitial fluid and any protein can return to the circulation through the lymphatic capillaries.

Movement of water through cell membranes depends on differences in osmotic pressure between the two compartments. As the relative concentrations of electrolytes in the interstitial fluid and intracellular fluid change, the osmotic pressure also changes, causing water to move across the cell membrane by osmosis. For example, if an erythrocyte is placed in a dilute solution (low osmotic pressure), water will enter the cell, causing it to swell and eventually rupture.

Thinkabout 6-4

a. Explain how a very high hydrostatic pressure in the venule end of a capillary affects fluid shift.

b. Explain how a loss of plasma protein affects fluid shift at the capillaries.

c. Explain how a high concentration of sodium ions in the interstitial fluid affect intracellular fluid levels.

Fluid Excess—Edema

Fluid excess occurs in the extracellular compartment and may be **isotonic, hypotonic,** or **hypertonic,** depending on the cause. The tonicity or concentration of solute in the fluid affects fluid shifts between compartments, including the cells. Edema refers to an excessive amount of fluid in the interstitial compartment, which causes a swelling or enlargement of the tissues. Edema may be localized in one area or generalized throughout the body. Depending on the type of tissue and the area of the body, edema may be highly visible or relatively invisible; for example, facial edema is usually visible, but edema of the liver may not be. Edema is usually more severe in *dependent* areas of the body, where the force of gravity is greatest such as the buttocks, ankles, or feet of a person in a wheelchair. Prolonged edema can interfere with venous return, arterial circulation, and cell function in the affected area.

CAUSES OF EDEMA

There are four general causes of edema (Fig. 6–2). The first is *increased capillary hydrostatic pressure,* which prevents return of fluid from the interstitial compartment to the venous end of the capillary, or forces excessive amounts of fluid out of the capillaries into the tissues. The latter is a cause of pulmonary edema, in which excessive pressure, often due to increased blood volume, can force fluid into the alveoli, interfering with respiratory function. Specific causes of edema related to increased hydrostatic pressure include increased blood volume (**hypervolemia**) associated with kidney failure, pregnancy, and congestive heart failure. In pregnancy the enlarged uterus compresses the veins, and when a pregnant woman must stand still for long periods of time, the pressure in the leg veins can become quite elevated, causing edema in the feet and legs. In some people with congestive heart failure the blood cannot return easily through the veins to the heart, raising the hydrostatic pressure in the legs and abdominal organs and causing **ascites,** or fluid in the abdominal cavity.

The second general cause is related to the *loss of plasma proteins,* which results in a decrease in plasma osmotic pressure. Plasma proteins usually remain inside the capillary and very seldom move through the capillary membrane. The presence of fewer plasma proteins allows more fluid to leave the capillary and less fluid to return to the venous end of the capillary. Protein may be lost in the urine through kidney disease, or synthesis of protein may be impaired in patients with malnutrition and malabsorption diseases or with liver disease. Protein levels may drop acutely in burn patients who have large areas of burned skin; the subsequent inflammation and loss of the skin barrier allow protein to leak out of the body.

Frequently *excessive sodium levels* in the extracellular fluid accompany the two causes just mentioned. When sodium ions are retained, they promote accumulation of fluid in the interstitial compartment by increasing the osmotic pressure and decreasing the return of fluid to the blood. Blood volume and blood pressure are usually elevated as well. High sodium levels are common in patients with heart failure, high blood pressure, kidney disease, and increased aldosterone secretion.

The third cause of edema is *obstruction of the lymphatic circulation.* Such an obstruction usually causes a localized edema because excessive fluid and protein are not returned to the general circulation. This situation may develop if a tumor or infection damages a lymph node or if lymph nodes are removed, as they may be in cancer surgery.

The fourth cause of edema is *increased* **capillary permeability**. This usually causes a localized edema also and may result from an inflammatory response or infec-

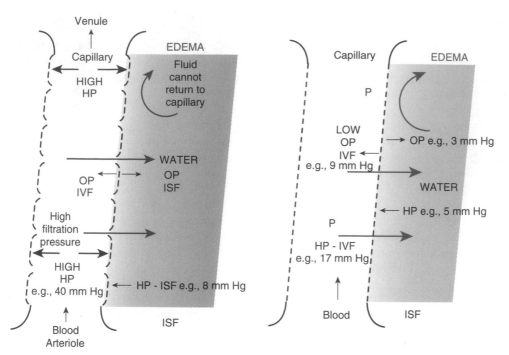

A. HIGH CAPILLARY HYDROSTATIC PRESSURE

B. LOSS OF PLASMA PROTEINS LOW CAPILLARY OSMOTIC PRESSURE

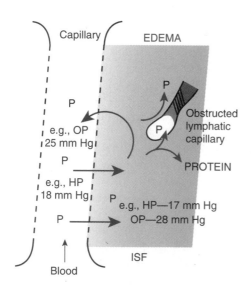

C. LYMPHATIC OBSTRUCTION

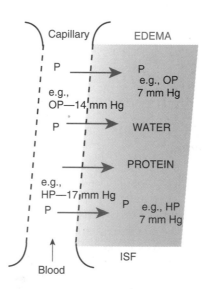

D. INCREASED CAPILLARY PERMEABILITY

P = Protein
HP = Hydrostatic pressure
OP = Osmotic pressure
ISF = Interstitial fluid
IVF = Intravascular fluid

FIGURE 6-2. Causes of edema.

tion (see Chapter 2). In this case, histamine and other chemical mediators released from cells following tissue injury cause increased capillary permeability and increased fluid movement into the interstitial area. Protein also leaks into the interstitial compartment, increasing the osmotic pressure and thus holding more fluid in the interstitial area.

Thinkabout 6–5

a. In some cases of breast cancer, many of the axillary lymph nodes are removed. Why may the arm be edematous?

b. Explain why severe kidney disease may cause generalized edema.

c. Explain why the feet may become swollen when one sits for long periods of time with the legs dangling, but the swelling then decreases when one lies recumbent in bed.

EFFECTS OF EDEMA

A local area of swelling may be visible and may be very pale or red in color, depending on the cause (Table 6–3). *Pitting* edema occurs in the presence of excess interstitial fluid, which moves aside when firm pressure is applied by the fingers. A depression or "pit" remains after the finger is removed. In people with generalized edema there is a significant increase in body weight, which may indicate a problem before there are other visible signs of it. Edema may interfere with function, for example, when it restricts the movement of joints. Edema of the intestinal wall may interfere with digestion and absorption. Edema or accumulated fluid around the heart or lungs impairs the movement and filling of the organ.

Pain may occur if edema exerts pressure on the nerves locally, as with the headache that develops in patients with cerebral edema. If cerebral edema becomes severe, the pressure can impair brain function because of ischemia and can cause death. When viscera such as the kidney or liver are edematous, the capsule is stretched, causing pain.

In people with sustained edema the arterial circulation may be impaired. The increased interstitial pressure may obstruct arterial blood flow into the area, preventing the fluid shift that carries nutrients into the cells. This can prevent normal cell function and reproduction and eventually results in tissue necrosis or the development of ulcers. This situation is evident in individuals with severe varicose veins in the legs—large, dilated veins that have a high hydrostatic pressure. Varicose veins can lead to fatigue, skin breakdown, and varicose ulcers (see Chapter 16). The ulcers do not heal easily because of the continued insufficient blood supply.

Edema can cause complications in many ways. For example, in dental practice, it is difficult to take accurate impressions when the tissues are swollen; dentures do not fit well, and sores may develop that often are slow to heal and become infected because the blood flow is impaired.

Thinkabout 6–6

a. List three signs of edema involving the knee.

b. Explain why persistent edema in a leg could cause weakness and skin breakdown.

c. Explain why rinsing or soaking tissue with a salt and water solution may decrease edema temporarily.

TABLE 6–3 Comparison of Signs and Symptoms of Fluid Excess (Edema) and Fluid Deficit (Dehydration)	
Fluid Excess (Edema)	**Fluid Deficit (Dehydration)**
Localized swelling (feet, hands, periorbital area, ascites)	Sunken, soft eyes
Pale, gray, or red skin color	Decreased skin turgor, dry mucous membranes
Weight gain	Weight loss
Slow, bounding pulse; high blood pressure	Rapid, weak, thready pulse; low blood pressure, orthostatic hypotension
Lethargy, possible seizures	Fatigue, weakness, dizziness, possible stupor
Pulmonary congestion, cough, rales	Increased body temperature, thirst
Laboratory values	Laboratory values
decreased hematocrit	increased hematocrit
decreased serum sodium	increased electrolytes (or variable)
urine: low specific gravity, high volume	urine: high specific gravity, low volume

Note: Signs may vary depending on the cause of the imbalance.

Fluid Deficit—Dehydration

Dehydration refers to insufficient body fluid resulting either from inadequate intake or excessive loss or a combination of the two. Losses are more common and affect the extracellular compartment first. Water can shift within the extracellular compartments. For example, if fluid is lost from the digestive tract because of vomiting, water shifts from the vascular compartment into the digestive tract. If the deficit continues, eventually fluid is lost from the cells.

As a general guide to extracellular fluid loss, a *mild* deficit is defined as a decrease of 2 percent in body weight, a *moderate* deficit as a 5 percent weight loss, and *severe* dehydration as a decrease of 8 percent. This figure should be adjusted for the individual's age, body size, and condition. Dehydration is a more serious problem for infants and elderly people, who lack fluid reserves and the ability to conserve fluid quickly. Also, infants experience not only greater insensible water losses through their proportionately larger body surface area but also an increased need for water owing to their higher metabolic rate. The vascular compartment is rapidly depleted (**hypovolemia**), affecting the heart, brain, and kidneys.

Water loss is often accompanied by a loss of electrolytes and sometimes of proteins, depending on the specific cause. For example, sweating results in a loss of water and sodium chloride. Electrolyte losses can influence water balance significantly because osmotic pressures change between compartments. To restore balance, electrolytes as well as fluid must be replaced. Isotonic dehydration refers to a proportionate loss of fluid and electrolytes, hypotonic dehydration to a loss of more electrolytes than water, and hypertonic dehydration to a loss of more fluid than electrolytes. The latter two types of dehydration cause signs of electrolyte imbalance and influence the movement of water between the intracellular and extracellular compartments (see the next section of this chapter, Electrolyte Imbalances).

CAUSES OF DEHYDRATION

Common causes of dehydration include vomiting and diarrhea, both of which result in loss of numerous electrolytes and nutrients such as glucose as well as water. Drainage or suction of any portion of the digestive system can also result in deficits. Excessive sweating with loss of sodium, and diabetic ketoacidosis with loss of fluid, electrolytes, and glucose in the urine also cause dehydration. Occasionally, insufficient water intake may be a cause in an elderly or unconscious person.

EFFECTS OF DEHYDRATION

Initially, dehydration involves a decrease in interstitial and intravascular fluids. These losses may produce direct effects such as dry mucous membranes in the mouth or decreased skin **turgor** or elasticity (see Table 6–3). Also, blood pressure is reduced, the pulse is weak, and the person feels fatigued. The body attempts to compensate for the fluid loss by increasing thirst, increasing the heart rate, and constricting the cutaneous blood vessels, leading to pale and cool skin. Urine output is decreased, and specific gravity is high (more concentrated) as a result of renal vasoconstriction and increased secretion of ADH and aldosterone. The hematocrit increases, indicating a higher proportion of red blood cells to water in the blood. As the brain cells lose water, decreasing mental function, confusion, and loss of consciousness develop.

Thinkabout 6–8

Describe three signs or symptoms of dehydration that are direct effects, and three signs that indicate the occurrence of compensation.

Thinkabout 6–7

a. Explain briefly why an infant is more vulnerable than an adult to fluid loss.

b. If more sodium is lost from the extracellular compartment than water, how will fluid move between the cell and the interstitial compartment?

Third-Spacing: Fluid Deficit and Fluid Excess

Third-spacing refers to a situation in which fluid shifts out of the blood into a body cavity or tissue where it is no longer available as circulating fluid. Examples include peritonitis, the inflammation and infection of the peritoneal membranes, and burns, in which extensive inflammation of the skin and underlying tissues causes fluid to shift out of the blood, causing edema. The result of this shift is a fluid deficit in the vascular compartment (hypovolemia) and a fluid excess in the interstitial space. Until the cause is removed, fluid remains in the "third space"—in the body but not a functional part of the circulating fluids.

Thinkabout 6-9

Based on the information given previously on fluid excess and fluid deficit, describe three signs and symptoms of third-spacing related to a large burn area.

ELECTROLYTE IMBALANCES

Sodium Imbalance

REVIEW OF SODIUM

Sodium (Na^+) is the primary **cation** (positively charged ion) in the extracellular fluid (Table 6–4). It **diffuses** between the vascular and interstitial fluids. Sodium transport across the cell membrane is controlled by the sodium-potassium pump or active transport, and therefore sodium levels are high in the extracellular fluids and low inside the cell. Sodium is actively secreted into mucus and other body secretions. It exists in the body primarily in the form of the salts sodium chloride and sodium bicarbonate. It is ingested in food and beverages, usually in more than adequate amounts, and is lost from the body in perspiration, urine, and feces. Sodium levels in the body are controlled by the kidneys through the action of aldosterone.

Sodium is important for the maintenance of extracellular fluid volume through its effect on osmotic pressure because it makes up approximately 90 percent of the solute in extracellular fluid. Sodium also is essential in the conduction of nerve impulses (Fig. 6–3) and in muscle contraction.

It is important to note the relative changes of electrolytes and fluids associated with the individual's specific problem to put the actual serum value in perspective. For example, excessive sweating may result in a low serum sodium level if proportionately more sodium is lost than water or if only water is used to replace the loss. If an individual loses more water than sodium in perspiration, the serum sodium level may be high.

HYPONATREMIA

Normal blood levels are presented inside the front cover. Hyponatremia refers to a serum sodium concentration of below 135 **mEq** per liter or 135 mmol per liter.

Causes of Hyponatremia

A sodium deficit can result from direct loss of sodium from the body or from an excess of water in the extracellular compartment, resulting in dilution of sodium. Common causes of low serum sodium levels include excessive sweating, vomiting and diarrhea, use of certain **diuretic** drugs combined with low-salt diets, insufficient aldosterone, adrenal insufficiency, renal failure, excess ADH secretion, or excessive water intake.

Thinkabout 6-10

a. A high fever is likely to cause deep, rapid respirations, excessive perspiration, and higher metabolic rate. How would this affect the fluid and electrolyte balance in the body?

b. List several reasons why drinking a fluid containing water, glucose, and electrolytes might be better than drinking plain water after vomiting.

Effects of Hyponatremia

Low sodium levels impair nerve conduction and result in fluid imbalances in the compartments. Manifestations include fatigue, muscle cramps, and abdominal

TABLE 6-4	Distribution of Major Electrolytes	
Ions	**Intracellular (mEq/L)**	**Blood (mEq/L)**
Cations		
Sodium (Na^+)	10	142
Potassium (K^+)	160	4
Calcium (Ca^{++})	Variable	5
Magnesium (Mg^{++})	35	3
Anions		
Bicarbonate (HCO_3^-)	8	27
Chloride (Cl^-)	2	103
Phosphate (HPO_4^-)	140	2

Note: There are variations in "normal" values among individuals.

The concentration of electrolytes in plasma varies slightly from that in the interstitial fluid or other types of extracellular fluids.

The number of anions, including those present in small quantities, is equivalent to the concentration of cations in the intracellular compartment (or in the plasma) in order to maintain electrical neutrality (equal negative and positive charges) in any compartment.

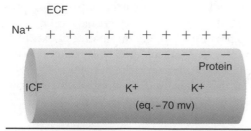

1. Polarization
Resting state of semipermeable membrane

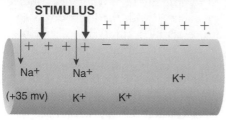

2. Depolarization
Stimulus opens Na⁺ channels
Na⁺ moves into cell

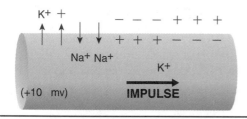

3. Repolarization
As impulse moves along membrane, Na⁺ channels close and K⁺ channels open allowing K⁺ to move outward

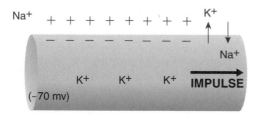

4. Repolarization
Channels close. Sodium-potassium pump returns Na⁺ outside cell and K⁺ inside cell

FIGURE 6–3. Conduction in a neuron.

discomfort or cramps with nausea and vomiting (Table 6–5). Decreased osmotic pressure in the extracellular compartment may cause a fluid shift into cells, resulting in hypovolemia and decreased blood pressure. The swelling of brain cells may cause confusion, headache, weakness, or seizures (Fig. 6–4).

TABLE 6–5 Signs of Sodium Imbalance

Hyponatremia	Hypernatremia
Anorexia, nausea, cramps	Thirst, tongue and mucosa are dry and sticky
Fatigue, lethargy, muscle weakness	Weakness, lethargy, agitation
Headache, confusion, seizures	Edema
Decreased blood pressure	Elevated blood pressure

HYPERNATREMIA

Hypernatremia is an excessive sodium level in the blood and extracellular fluids (above 145 mEq per liter).

Causes of Hypernatremia

Excess sodium results from ingestion of large amounts of sodium without proportionate water intake or a loss of water from the body that is faster than the loss of sodium. Specific causes include insufficient ADH, which results in a large volume of dilute urine (diabetes insipidus), loss of the thirst mechanism, watery diarrhea, or prolonged periods of rapid respiration.

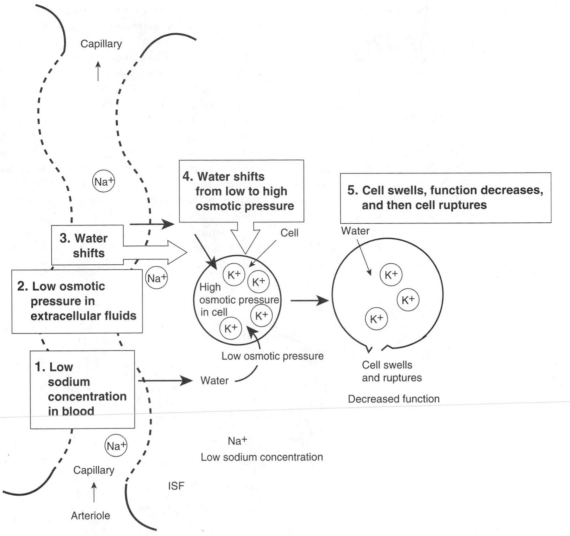

FIGURE 6-4. Hyponatremia and fluid shift into cells. ISF, Interstitial fluid.

Thinkabout 6–11

Hypernatremia accompanied by an elevated hematocrit value indicates what fact about body fluids?

Effects of Hypernatremia

The major effect of hypernatremia is a fluid shift out of the cells owing to the increased osmotic pressure of interstitial or extracellular fluid; this effect is manifest by weakness, agitation, and firm subcutaneous tissues (see Table 6–5). Thirst increases, and the mucous membranes become dry and rough. ADH is secreted, result-ing in decreased urine output. Note that the manifestations can change depending on the cause of the problem: If the cause of hypernatremia is fluid loss due to lack of ADH, urine output would be high.

Thinkabout 6–12

a. Compare the effects of excessive aldosterone with those of excessive ADH on serum sodium levels.

b. List the signs and symptoms common to both hyponatremia and hypernatremia and also any signs that differentiate the two states.

Potassium Imbalance

REVIEW OF POTASSIUM

Potassium (K^+) is a major intracellular cation, and therefore serum levels are very low (3.5 to 5 mEq per liter or 3.5 to 5 mmol per liter), whereas the intracellular concentration is about 160 mEq per liter (see Table 6–4). It is difficult to assess total body potassium by measuring the serum level. Potassium is ingested in foods and is excreted primarily in the urine under the influence of the hormone aldosterone. Foods high in potassium include bananas, citrus fruits, tomatoes, and lentils; potassium chloride tablets may be taken as a supplement.

Potassium levels are also influenced by the acid-base balance in the body, acidosis tending to shift potassium ions out of the cells into the extracellular fluids, and alkalosis tending to move more potassium into the cells (Fig. 6–5). With acidosis, many hydrogen ions diffuse from the blood into the interstitial fluid because of the high hydrogen ion concentration in the blood. When these hydrogen ions move into the cell, they displace potassium out of the cells to maintain electrical neutrality. Then the excess potassium ions in the interstitial fluid diffuse into the blood, leading to hyperkalemia. The reverse process occurs with alkalosis. Acidosis also promotes hydrogen ion excretion by the kidneys and retention of potassium in the body. The hormone insulin also promotes movement of potassium into cells (see Chapter 21).

Potassium assists in the regulation of intracellular fluid volume and has a role in many metabolic processes in the cell. It is also important in nerve conduction and

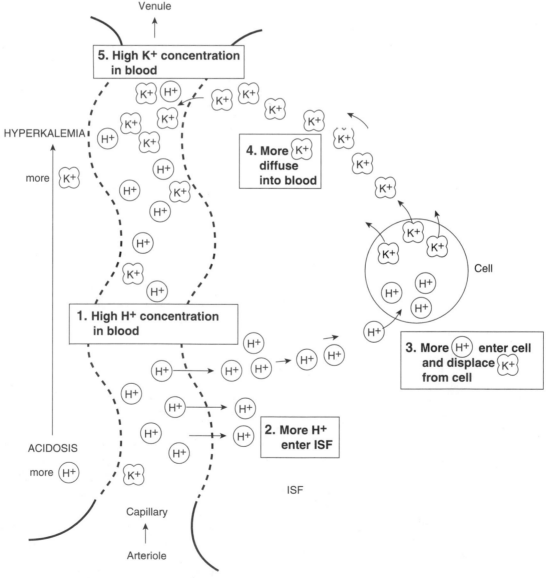

FIGURE 6–5. Relationship of hydrogen and potassium ions. ISF, Interstitial fluid.

muscle contractions, determining the membrane potential (see Fig. 6–3). Most important, abnormal potassium levels, both high and low, have a significant and serious effect on the contractions of cardiac muscle, which can be seen on the **electrocardiogram** (ECG) and ultimately can cause cardiac arrest.

HYPOKALEMIA

In hypokalemia the serum level of potassium is below 3.5 mEq per liter or 3.5 mmol per liter.

Causes of Hypokalemia

Low serum potassium levels may result from excessive losses from the body due to diarrhea, diuresis associated with certain **diuretic** drugs, or the presence of excessive aldosterone or glucocorticoids in the body (in Cushing's syndrome, in which glucocorticoids have some mineralocorticoid activity, retaining sodium and excreting potassium). Patients with heart disease who are being treated with certain diuretic drugs such as furosemide may have to increase their intake of potassium in food or take a potassium supplement because hypokalemia may increase the toxicity of heart medications such as digitalis. Other causes of hypokalcmia include decreased dietary intake, which may occur with alcoholism or starvation diets, and the treatment of diabetic ketoacidosis with insulin.

Effects of Hypokalemia

Hypokalemia interferes with neuromuscular function, and the muscles become less responsive to stimuli, as shown by fatigue and muscle weakness commencing in the legs. **Paresthesias** such as "pins and needles" develop. Decreased digestive tract motility causes decreased appetite (**anorexia**) and nausea. In people with severe potassium deficits, the respiratory muscles become weak, leading to shallow respirations. Cardiac **dysrhythmias** are serious, typically showing ECG pattern changes (Fig. 6–6) that indicate prolonged repolarization, and eventually may lead to cardiac arrest (see Chapter 16). In severe cases, renal function is impaired, owing to failure to concentrate the urine, and increased urine output (polyuria) results.

HYPERKALEMIA

In hyperkalemia the serum level of potassium is above 5 mEq per liter or 5 mmol per liter.

Causes of Hyperkalemia

Causes of high serum potassium levels include renal failure, deficit of aldosterone, and use of "potassium-sparing" diuretic drugs, which prevent potassium from being excreted in adequate amounts. Intracellular potassium may leak into the extracellular fluids in patients with tissue damage such as crush injuries or burns. Prolonged or severe acidosis may displace potassium from cells (see Fig. 6–5).

Effects of Hyperkalemia

Muscle weakness is common, progressing to paralysis as hyperkalemia advances and impairs neuromuscular activity (Table 6–6). Fatigue, nausea, and paresthesias are common also. The ECG shows cardiac dysrhythmias (see Fig. 6–6), which may progress to cardiac arrest.

Thinkabout 6–13

a. Compare the manifestations of hyponatremia and hypokalemia.
b. Why is any small potassium imbalance considered a serious problem?

Calcium Imbalance

REVIEW OF CALCIUM

Calcium (Ca^{++}) is a very important extracellular cation. Calcium is ingested in food, especially milk products, and stored in bone, and it is excreted from the body in the urine and feces. Calcium balance is controlled by parathyroid hormone (PTH) and calcitonin (see Chapter 21) but is also influenced by vitamin D (Table 6–7) and phosphate ion levels. For example, low blood calcium levels stimulate the secretion of PTH, which increases calcium absorption from the digestive tract and kidneys and promotes resorption from bone. Vitamin D may be ingested or synthesized in the skin in the presence of ultraviolet rays, but then it must be activated in the kidneys. It promotes calcium movement from bone and intestines into blood. Calcium and phosphate ions in the extracellular fluid have a reciprocal relationship. For example, if calcium levels are high, phosphate is low. The product of calcium and phosphate concentrations is a constant value. If levels of both calcium and phosphate rise, crystals of calcium phosphate precipitate in soft tissue. The measured or biologically active form of calcium is the ionized form, which is not attached to plasma protein or complexed with other ions such as citrate. Alkalosis can decrease the number of free calcium ions, causing hypocalcemia.

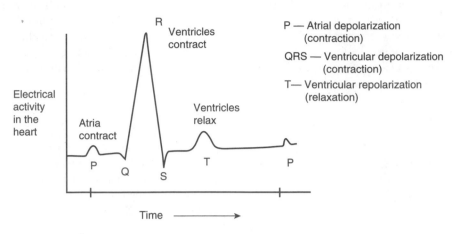

R
Ventricles
contract

Electrical
activity
in the
heart

Atria
contract

Ventricles
relax

P   Q   S   T   P

Time ———→

P — Atrial depolarization
    (contraction)
QRS — Ventricular depolarization
    (contraction)
T — Ventricular repolarization
    (relaxation)

A. NORMAL ELECTROCARDIOGRAM

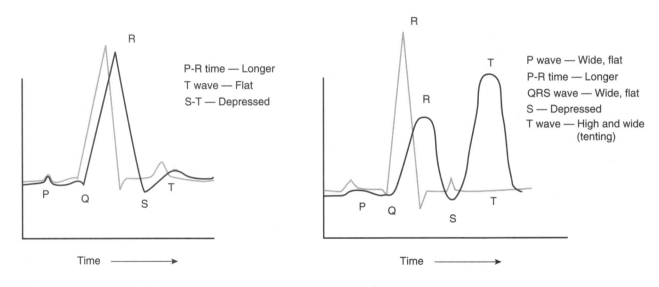

R

P   Q   S   T

Time ———→

P-R time — Longer
T wave — Flat
S-T — Depressed

R

T

R

P   Q   S   T

Time ———→

P wave — Wide, flat
P-R time — Longer
QRS wave — Wide, flat
S — Depressed
T wave — High and wide
    (tenting)

B. HYPOKALEMIA   **C. HYPERKALEMIA**

FIGURE 6-6. Schematic representation of the effects of potassium imbalance on the heart.

TABLE 6-6	Signs of Potassium Imbalance
Hypokalemia	**Hyperkalemia**
Anorexia, nausea, constipation	Nausea, diarrhea
Fatigue, muscle weakness, leg cramps	Muscle weakness, paralysis beginning in legs
Shallow respirations	
Paresthesias	Paresthesias—fingers, toes, face, tongue
Postural hypotension	
Cardiac arrhythmias, cardiac arrest	Arrhythmias, cardiac arrest
Polyuria and nocturia	Oliguria
Serum pH elevated—7.45 (alkalosis)	Serum pH decreased—7.35 (acidosis)

TABLE 6-7	Causes of Hypocalcemia
Cause	**Rationale**
Decreased parathyroid hormone	Decreased intestinal absorption of calcium
Decreased dietary intake of calcium	Decreased supply
Malabsorption syndrome	Decreased intestinal absorption of Vitamin D or calcium
Vitamin D deficit— decreased dietary intake, malabsorption syndrome, decreased activation of vitamin	Decreased absorption and utilization of calcium
Elevated serum phosphate levels	Increased urinary excretion of calcium
Alkalosis	Increased binding of calcium to protein

Calcium has many important functions. It provides the structural strength essential for bones and teeth. Calcium ions maintain the stability of nerve membranes, controlling the permeability and excitability needed for nerve conduction, and are required for muscle contractions. Calcium ions are necessary for many metabolic processes and enzyme reactions such as those involved in blood clotting.

Thinkabout 6–14

When nerve membranes become more permeable, is the nerve more or less easily stimulated?

HYPOCALCEMIA

In hypocalcemia, the serum calcium level is below 2.2 mmol per liter.

Causes of Hypocalcemia

Causes of hypocalcemia include hypoparathyroidism, malabsorption, deficient serum albumin, or increased serum pH. In patients with renal failure, hypocalcemia results from retention of phosphate ion, which causes loss of calcium; also, vitamin D is not activated, thereby decreasing the intestinal absorption of calcium.

Effects of Hypocalcemia

Low serum calcium levels increase the permeability and excitability of nerve membranes, leading to spontaneous stimulation of skeletal muscle. This leads to muscle twitching, **carpopedal spasm** (a typical contraction of the fingers), and hyperactive reflexes (Table 6–8). Chvostek's sign, spasm of the lip or face when the face is tapped in front of the ear, and Trousseau's sign, carpopedal spasm when a blood pressure cuff blocks

circulation to the hand, both indicate low serum calcium and **tetany,** or skeletal muscle spasm. Severe calcium deficits may cause **laryngospasm,** which obstructs the airway. Paresthesias are common as well as abdominal cramps. Heart contractions become weak owing to insufficient calcium for muscle action, conduction is delayed, **arrhythmias** develop, and blood pressure drops. Note that the effects of hypocalcemia on *skeletal muscle* and *cardiac muscle* differ. Skeletal muscle spasms result from the increased irritability of the nerves associated with the muscle fibers, whereas the contraction of cardiac muscle (which lacks nerves) is directly affected by the calcium deficit. Also, adequate calcium is stored in the skeletal muscle cells to provide for contractions, whereas contraction of cardiac muscle relies on available extracellular calcium ions passing through the calcium channels.

Thinkabout 6–15

Explain the different effects of low serum calcium on skeletal muscle and cardiac muscle.

HYPERCALCEMIA

In hypercalcemia the serum calcium is above 2.5 mmol per liter.

Causes of Hypercalcemia

Excessive serum levels of calcium frequently result from uncontrolled release of calcium ions from the bones due to neoplasms, hyperparathyroidism, or prolonged immobility. Malignant bone tumors may directly destroy the bone, and some tumors, such as bronchogenic carcinoma, may secrete PTH. Immobility may decrease stress on the bone, leading to demineralization. Hypercalcemia may also result from increased intake of calcium due either to excessive vitamin D or excess dietary calcium. Milk-alkali syndrome, associated with increased milk and antacid intake, may also elevate serum calcium levels.

Effects of Hypercalcemia

High serum calcium levels depress neuromuscular activity, leading to muscle weakness, loss of muscle tone, lethargy, and stupor, often with personality changes, anorexia, and nausea (see Table 6–8). High calcium levels interfere with the function of ADH in the kidneys,

TABLE 6–8 Signs of Calcium Imbalance	
Hypocalcemia	**Hypercalcemia**
Tetany—involuntary skeletal muscle spasm, carpopedal spasm, laryngospasm	Apathy, lethargy
	Anorexia, nausea, constipation
Tingling fingers	Polyuria, thirst
Mental confusion, irritability	Arrhythmias, prolonged strong cardiac contractions, increased blood pressure
Arrhythmias, weak heart contractions	

Note: Effects on bone depend on the cause of the calcium imbalance.

resulting in less absorption of water and polyuria. Cardiac contractions increase in strength, and arrhythmias may develop. If hypercalcemia is severe, blood volume drops, renal function decreases, nitrogen wastes accumulate, and cardiac arrest may ensue.

Effects on bone vary with the cause of hypercalcemia. If excess PTH is the cause, bone density will be decreased, and spontaneous (pathologic) fractures may occur, particularly in the weight-bearing areas, causing bone pain. If intake of calcium is high, PTH levels will be low, and more calcium will be stored in the bone, maintaining bone strength.

Thinkabout 6–16

Describe the effect of each of the following conditions on serum calcium levels and on bone density: (1) hyperparathyroidism, (2) renal failure, and (3) very large intake of vitamin D.

Other Electrolytes

MAGNESIUM

Magnesium (Mg^{++}) is an intracellular ion that has a normal serum level of 0.7 to 1.1 mmol per liter. About 50 percent of total body magnesium is stored in bone. Serum levels are linked to both potassium and calcium levels. Magnesium is found in green vegetables and is important in many enzyme reactions as well as in protein and DNA synthesis. Hypermagnesemia is a rare occurrence.

Hypomagnesemia

Magnesium deficits frequently result from malabsorption or malnutrition. Low serum levels may also occur with the use of diuretics, diabetic ketoacidosis, hyperparathyroidism, and hyperaldosteronism.

Low serum magnesium leads to neuromuscular hyperirritability, with tremors or chorea (involuntary repetitive movements), insomnia, personality changes, and an increased heart rate with arrhythmias.

PHOSPHATE

Phosphate ion (HPO_4^{--} and $H_2PO_4^-$), is located in the bone primarily but circulates in both the intracellular and extracellular fluids. The serum level is normally 0.85 to 1.45 mmol per liter. It is important in bone and tooth mineralization and in many metabolic processes, particularly those involving the cellular energy source, adenosine triphosphate (ATP). Phosphate serves as a buffer system for acid-base balance and has a role in the removal of hydrogen ions from the body through the kidneys. Phosphate is also an integral part of the cell membrane. As indicated earlier, phosphate levels are linked reciprocally with serum calcium levels.

Hypophosphatemia

Low serum phosphate levels may result from malabsorption syndromes, diarrhea, or excessive use of antacids. Alkalosis and hyperparathyroidism are other causes.

Neurologic function is impaired with low serum phosphate, causing tremors, weak reflexes (hyporeflexia), paresthesias, confusion and stupor, anorexia, and difficulty in swallowing (dysphagia). The blood cells function less effectively—oxygen transport decreases and clotting and phagocytosis decrease.

Thinkabout 6–17

Explain how serum calcium levels are affected by low phosphate levels.

Hyperphosphatemia

High serum phosphate often results from renal failure. Tissue damage or cancer chemotherapy may cause release of intracellular phosphate. The manifestations of hyperphosphatemia are the same as those of hypocalcemia.

CHLORIDE

Chloride ion (Cl^-) is the major extracellular **anion** with a normal serum level of 98 to 106 mmol per liter. Chloride ion tends to follow sodium because of the electrical charge on the ions. Therefore, high sodium levels often lead to high chloride levels. Chloride and bicarbonate ions, both negatively charged, can exchange places as the blood circulates through the body to maintain acid-base balance (see the next section of this chapter, Acid-Base Balance). As bicarbonate ions are used up in binding with metabolic **acids**, chloride ions diffuse out of the red blood cells into the serum to maintain the same number of negative ions in the blood (Fig. 6–7). The reverse situation can also occur when serum chloride levels decrease, and bicarbonate ions leave the erythrocytes to maintain electrical neutrality. Thus, low serum chloride leads to high serum bicarbonate, or alkalosis. This situation may be referred to as a chloride shift.

Hypochloremia

Low serum chloride is usually associated with alkalosis in the early stages of vomiting when hydrochloric acid is lost from the stomach.

Thinkabout 6–18

a. Give one cause of hypomagnesemia.
b. Give one cause of hyperphosphatemia.
c. List and describe two signs of hypophosphatemia.

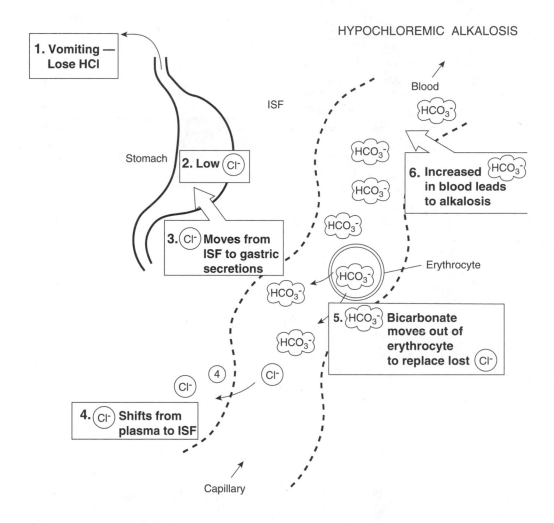

FIGURE 6–7. Schematic representation of chloride-bicarbonate shift with vomiting.

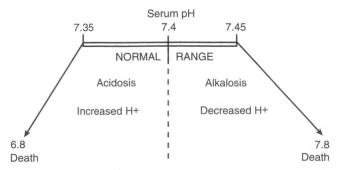

FIGURE 6-8. The hydrogen ion and pH scale.

ACID-BASE IMBALANCE

Review of Acid-Base Balance

Acid-base balance is very important in the body because cell enzymes can function only within a very narrow pH range. *The normal serum pH range is 7.35 to 7.45.* Death usually results if serum pH is below 6.8 or above 7.8 (Fig. 6–8). For example, a pH of below 7.35 depresses central nervous system function and decreases all cell enzyme activity.

When serum pH is below 7.4, more hydrogen ions (H^+) are present, and acidosis results. A serum pH of above 7.4 is more basic, indicating alkalosis or the presence of fewer **hydrogen ions.** The body normally has a tendency toward acidosis, or a lower pH, because cell metabolism is constantly producing carbon dioxide (CO_2 or carbonic acid, H_2CO_3) or **nonvolatile metabolic acids** such as lactic acid, ketoacids, sulfuric acid, or phosphoric acid. Lactic acid results from the **anaerobic** (without oxygen) metabolism of glucose, ketoacids result from incomplete oxidation of fatty acids, and protein metabolism may produce sulfuric or phosphoric acid.

Thinkabout 6–19

a. When hydrogen ions are decreased, is the pH higher or lower?
b. State the optimal range of serum pH for normal cell function.

Control of Serum pH

There are three control or compensation mechanisms for pH. As the blood circulates through the body, the cells use nutrients, and metabolic wastes, including acids, diffuse into the blood (Fig. 6–9). First, the buffer pairs circulating in the blood respond to pH changes immediately; second, the respiratory system can alter carbon dioxide levels in the body by changing the respiratory rate (see Chapter 17); and third, the kidneys can modify the excretion rate of acids and the production and absorption of bicarbonate ion (see Chapter 19). Note that the lungs can change only the amount of carbon dioxide (equivalent to the amount of carbonic acid) in the body. The kidneys are slow to compensate for a change in pH but are most effective because they can excrete all types of acids and can also adjust serum bicarbonate levels.

Thinkabout 6–20

How does the respiratory rate change when more hydrogen ions enter the blood, and how does this change affect acid levels in the body?

BUFFER SYSTEMS

To control serum pH, several buffer systems are present in the blood. A buffer is a combination of a weak acid and its alkaline salt. The components react with any acids or alkali added to the blood, neutralizing them and maintaining a relatively constant pH. There are four major buffer pairs in the body: the sodium bicarbonate-carbonic acid system, the phosphate system, the hemoglobin system, and the protein system. The bicarbonate system is the major extracellular fluid buffer and is used clinically to assess a client's acid-base status. The principles of acid-base balance are discussed here using the bicarbonate pair. Specific figures are not used because the emphasis is on the basic concepts.

THE BICARBONATE-CARBONIC ACID BUFFER SYSTEM AND MAINTENANCE OF SERUM pH

The bicarbonate system is composed of carbonic acid, which arises from the combination of carbon dioxide with water, and bicarbonate ion, which is present as sodium bicarbonate. The balance of bicarbonate ion (HCO_3^-), a **base**, and carbonic acid (H_2CO_3) levels is controlled by the respiratory system and the kidneys (see Fig. 6–9). Cell metabolism produces carbon dioxide, which diffuses into the blood, where it

$$\text{lungs: } CO_2 + H_2O \Longleftrightarrow H_2CO_3 \Longleftrightarrow H^+ + HCO_3^- \text{ : kidneys}$$

$$\text{lungs: carbon dioxide + water} \Longleftrightarrow \text{carbonic acid} \Longleftrightarrow \text{hydrogen ions + bicarbonate ions : kidneys}$$

reacts with water to form carbonic acid, which can then dissociate to form hydrogen ions and bicarbonate ions. In the lungs, this reaction can be reversed to form carbon dioxide, which is then expired along with water, thus reducing the total amount of carbonic acid or acid in the body. In the kidneys, the reaction needed to form more hydrogen ions is promoted by enzymes; the resultant hydrogen ions are excreted in the urine, and the bicarbonate ions are returned to the blood to restore the buffer levels.

To maintain serum pH within the normal range, 7.35 to 7.45, the *ratio* of bicarbonate ion to carbonic acid (or carbon dioxide) must be *20:1*.

$$\frac{HCO_3^-}{H_2CO_3} \rightarrow \frac{20}{1} \rightarrow pH = 7.4$$

As one component of the ratio changes, the other component must change proportionately to maintain this ratio and thus serum pH. For instance, if respiration is impaired, causing an increase in carbon dioxide in the blood, the kidneys must increase serum bicarbonate levels to compensate for the change. The actual concentrations are not critical as long as the proportions are sustained. It may help to remember that the bicarbonate part or alkali part of the buffer ratio is 20,

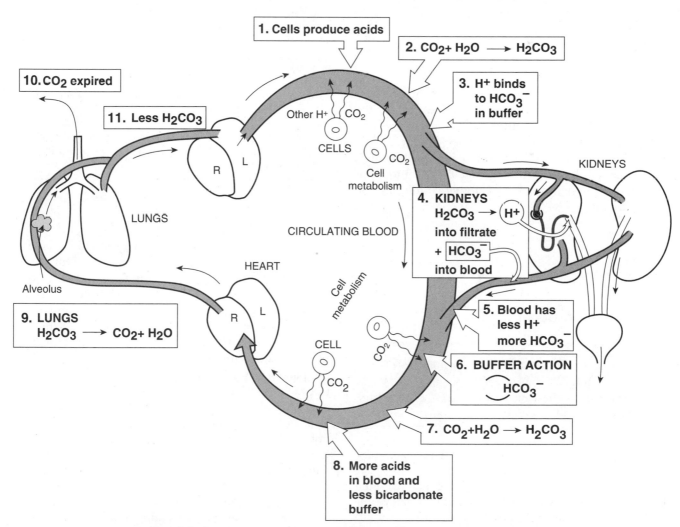

FIGURE 6-9. Changes in acids, bicarbonate ion, and serum pH in circulating blood.

the higher figure, because more bicarbonate base is required to neutralize the acids constantly being produced by the body cells.

Thinkabout 6–21

If bicarbonate ion is lost from the body, how will carbonic acid levels change?

RESPIRATORY SYSTEM

When serum carbon dioxide or hydrogen ion levels increase, chemoreceptors stimulate the respiratory control center to increase the respiratory rate, thus removing more carbon dioxide or acid from the body. When alkalosis develops, the respiratory rate decreases, thus retaining more carbon dioxide and increasing acid levels in the body.

RENAL SYSTEM

The kidneys can also reduce the acid content of the body by exchanging hydrogen for sodium under the influence of aldosterone and can remove acids by combining them with ammonia and other chemicals. The kidneys also provide the bicarbonate ion for the buffer pair as needed. Urine pH may range from 4.5 to 8.0 as the kidneys compensate for metabolic conditions and dietary intake.

Thinkabout 6–22

a. Reduced blood flow through the kidneys for a long time will have what effect on serum pH? Why?
b. How would the lungs and kidneys respond to the ingestion of large quantities of antacids?

A number of laboratory tests can determine acid-base balance. These tests include arterial blood gases (ABGs), base excess or deficit, or anion gap, and details about them may be found in laboratory manuals. Some normal values are listed inside the front cover.

Acid-Base Imbalance

There are four basic types of acid-base imbalance (Table 6–9). An increase in hydrogen ions or a decrease in serum pH results in acidosis, which can result either from an increase in carbon dioxide levels (acid) due to respiratory problems or from a decrease in bicarbonate ions (base) because of metabolic or renal problems. The first category is termed respiratory acidosis (increased carbon dioxide), and the second is called metabolic acidosis (decreased bicarbonate ions).

Alkalosis refers to an increase in serum pH or decreased hydrogen ions and may be respiratory alkalosis if increased respirations cause a decrease in carbon dioxide (less acid), or metabolic alkalosis if serum bicarbonate increases.

Imbalances may be acute or chronic. In some situations, combinations of imbalances may occur; for example, metabolic acidosis and respiratory alkalosis can occur simultaneously.

Thinkabout 6–23

State the name or category of the imbalance resulting from each of the following: (1) increased respiratory rate, (2) renal failure, (3) excessive intake of bicarbonate.

COMPENSATION

The *cause* of the imbalance is determined by the first change in the ratio (Fig. 6–10). Respiratory disorders are always represented by an initial change in carbon dioxide. All other problems are metabolic and result from an initial change in bicarbonate ions. The *compensation* is assessed by the subsequent change in the second part of the ratio (Table 6–10) and requires function by body systems not involved in the cause. For example, if a patient has a respiratory disorder causing acidosis, the lungs cannot compensate effectively, but the kidneys can. As long as the ratio of bicarbonate to carbonic acid is maintained at 20:1 and serum pH is normal, the imbalance is said to be compensated. If the kidneys and lungs cannot compensate adequately, the ratio changes, and serum pH moves out of the normal range, thus affecting cell metabolism and function. At this point, the imbalance is called decompensated. Examples of acid-base imbalance are given in Table 6–10.

TABLE 6–9 Acid-Base Imbalances

	Acidosis	Alkalosis
Respiratory		
Causes	Slow shallow respirations	Hyperventilation
	Respiratory congestion	
Effect	Increased P_{CO_2}	Decreased P_{CO_2}
Compensation	Kidneys excrete more hydrogen ion and reabsorb more bicarbonate	Kidneys excrete less hydrogen ion and reabsorb less bicarbonate
Laboratory	Elevated P_{CO_2}	Low P_{CO_2}
	Elevated serum bicarbonate	Low serum bicarbonate
	Compensated—serum pH = 7.35 to 7.4	Compensated—serum pH = 7.4 to 7.45
	Decompensated—serum pH <7.33	Decompensated—serum pH >7.47
Metabolic		
Causes	Shock	Vomiting (early stage)
	Diabetic ketoacidosis	Excessive antacid intake
	Renal failure	
	Diarrhea	
Effect	Decreased serum bicarbonate ion	Increased serum bicarbonate ion
Compensation	Rapid, deep respirations	Slow, shallow respirations
	Kidneys excrete more acids and increase bicarbonate absorption	Kidneys excrete less acid and decrease bicarbonate absorption
Laboratory	Low serum bicarbonate	Elevated serum bicarbonate
	Low P_{CO_2}	Elevated P_{CO_2}
	Compensated—serum pH = 7.35 to 7.4	Compensated—serum pH = 7.4 to 7.45
	Decompensated—serum pH <7.33	Decompensated—serum pH >7.47

Thinkabout 6–24

a. In an individual with very low blood pressure or circulatory shock, blood flow to the cells is very poor, resulting in increased lactic acid. Briefly describe the compensations that will take place.

b. As long as compensation maintains the 20:1 bicarbonate to carbonic acid ratio, what is the serum pH?

c. What changes in the bicarbonate ratio and serum pH indicate that decompensation has occurred?

ACIDOSIS

Causes

Respiratory acidosis, in which there is an increase in carbon dioxide levels, may occur in patients with acute problems such as pneumonia, airway obstruction (aspiration or asthma), or chest injuries, and in those taking drugs such as opiates, which depress the respiratory control center. Chronic respiratory acidosis is common in people with chronic obstructive pulmonary diseases (COPD) such as emphysema. Decompensated respiratory acidosis may develop if the impairment becomes severe or if, for example, a patient with a chronic problem develops an additional infection.

Metabolic acidosis is associated with a decrease in serum bicarbonate levels resulting from excessive loss of bicarbonate ions or increased use of bicarbonate. Diarrhea is a common cause of metabolic acidosis due to loss of bicarbonate in the intestinal secretions. Bicarbonate is used up quickly when large amounts of acids are produced in the body because the buffer bicarbonate binds with such acids until they can be removed by the kidneys (see Fig. 6–10). For example, lactic acid may accumulate if blood pressure decreases and insufficient oxygen is available to the cells, or diabetics may produce large amounts of ketoacids that use up bicarbonate ions (see Chapter 21). The other common cause of metabolic acidosis is renal disease or failure, in which decreased excretion of acids and decreased production of bicarbonate ion occur (see Chapter 19). In people with renal failure, compensation by the lungs is inadequate because the lungs can remove only carbon dioxide, not other acids, nor can they produce bicarbonate. Therefore, a treatment such as dialysis is required to maintain serum pH.

Decompensated metabolic acidosis may develop when an additional factor interferes with compensation. For example, a person with severe diarrhea may become so dehydrated that the kidneys receive little blood and cannot function adequately, causing decompensation.

Effects of Acidosis

The direct effects of acidosis are manifested by the nervous system, which is depressed. Headache, lethargy,

A. NORMAL

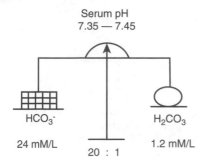

Serum pH
7.35 — 7.45

HCO$_3^-$
24 mM/L   20 : 1   H$_2$CO$_3$
1.2 mM/L

$$\frac{\text{Serum bicarbonate}}{\text{Carbonic acid}} = \frac{24}{1.2} = \frac{20}{1} \rightarrow \text{Serum pH — 7.4}$$

B. RESPIRATORY ACIDOSIS

1. CAUSE — Respiratory problem causes increased CO$_2$ retention → ↑ H$_2$CO$_3$ in blood

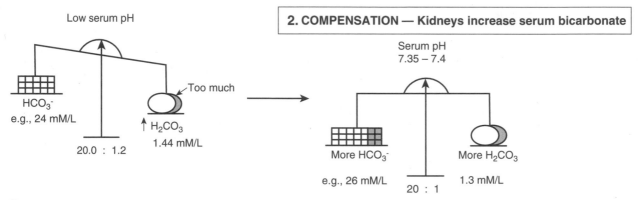

Low serum pH

HCO$_3^-$
e.g., 24 mM/L

Too much
↑ H$_2$CO$_3$
1.44 mM/L

20.0 : 1.2

2. COMPENSATION — Kidneys increase serum bicarbonate

Serum pH
7.35 – 7.4

More HCO$_3^-$
e.g., 26 mM/L   20 : 1   More H$_2$CO$_3$
1.3 mM/L

C. METABOLIC ACIDOSIS

1. CAUSE — Loss of bicarbonate ions
Excessive production of acids > **Decreased serum bicarbonate**

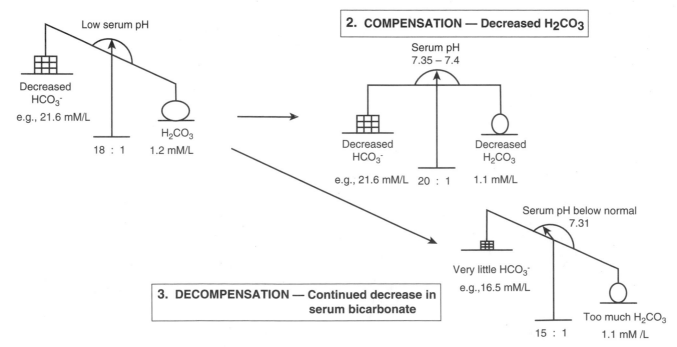

Low serum pH

Decreased
HCO$_3^-$
e.g., 21.6 mM/L

H$_2$CO$_3$
1.2 mM/L

18 : 1

2. COMPENSATION — Decreased H$_2$CO$_3$

Serum pH
7.35 – 7.4

Decreased
HCO$_3^-$
e.g., 21.6 mM/L   20 : 1   Decreased
H$_2$CO$_3$
1.1 mM/L

Serum pH below normal
7.31

Very little HCO$_3^-$
e.g.,16.5 mM/L

Too much H$_2$CO$_3$
15 : 1   1.1 mM /L

3. DECOMPENSATION — Continued decrease in serum bicarbonate

FIGURE 6-10. Changes in blood gases with acidosis.

TABLE 6–10 Examples of Acidosis	
Respiratory Acidosis—Individual with Emphysema Retaining CO_2	
Stage 1: Kidneys compensate for slight increase in P_{CO_2} by increasing excretion of acids and production of bicarbonate	No change in serum levels
Stage 2: Increased retention of CO_2 Respiratory acidosis	Elevated P_{CO_2}
Stage 3: Compensation. Kidneys reabsorb more bicarbonate ions	Elevated serum bicarbonate
Stage 4: Abnormal serum values indicate problem and compensation adequate to maintain ratio and normal serum pH: Compensated respiratory acidosis	$$\frac{H_2CO_3}{HCO_3^-} = \frac{2}{40} \rightarrow \frac{1}{20}$$ serum pH = 7.35
Stage 5: Patient acquires pneumonia, and much more CO_2 is retained. Also, kidneys cannot maintain compensation. Ratio is no longer normal, and serum pH drops below the normal range: Decompensated respiratory acidosis	$$\frac{H_2CO_3}{HCO_3^-} = \frac{3}{30} \rightarrow \frac{1}{10}$$ serum pH = 7.31 CNS depression, coma
Metabolic Acidosis—Individual with Diabetic Ketoacidosis Due to Insulin Deficit	
Stage 1: Slight increase in production of ketoacids. Kidneys increase excretion of acids	No change in serum values
Stage 2: More ketoacids produced than kidneys can excrete quickly, and acids bind with or "use up" buffer bicarbonate: Metabolic acidosis	Low serum bicarbonate
Stage 3: Respirations become rapid and deep to remove CO_2. Kidneys compensate by excreting more acids and reabsorbing more bicarbonate but cannot keep up with the increasing ketoacids added to the blood.	Low P_{CO_2}
Stage 4: Abnormal serum values indicate the problem and compensation adequate to maintain ratio and normal serum pH: Compensated metabolic acidosis	$$\frac{HCO_3^-}{H_2CO_3} = \frac{10}{\frac{1}{2}} \rightarrow \frac{20}{1}$$ serum pH = 7.35
Stage 5: Ketoacids continue to increase in the blood at a faster rate, and the kidneys have decreased function owing to dehydration. Therefore, the problem becomes more severe and compensation is inadequate. The ratio is not maintained, and serum pH drops below the normal range: Decompensated metabolic acidosis	$$\frac{HCO_3^-}{H_2CO_3} = \frac{5}{\frac{1}{2}} \rightarrow \frac{10}{1}$$ serum pH = 7.31

weakness, and confusion develop, leading eventually to coma and death. Compensations are manifested by deep rapid breathing (Kussmaul's respirations) and secretion of urine with a low pH (e.g., 5).

ALKALOSIS

Respiratory alkalosis results from hyperventilation, usually caused by anxiety, high fever, or an overdose of ASA (aspirin). Head injuries or brainstem tumors may lead to hyperventilation. Stress-related alkalosis may develop quickly and is best treated by rebreathing exhaled air from a paper bag placed over the face because renal compensation is slow to take place.

Metabolic alkalosis, in which there is an increase in serum bicarbonate ion, commonly follows loss of hydrochloric acid from the stomach either in the early stages of vomiting or with drainage from the stomach. Other potential causes are hypokalemia (see the earlier section of this chapter on electrolyte imbalances) and excessive ingestion of antacids.

Effects of Alkalosis

Alkalosis increases the irritability of the nervous system, causing restlessness, muscle twitching, tingling and

numbness of the fingers, and eventually tetany, seizures, and coma.

Thinkabout 6–25

a. For each of the following situations, list the kind of acid-base imbalance likely to occur: (1) chest injury with fractured ribs, (2) infection with high fever, (3) diarrhea.

b. Describe the effect of metabolic acidosis on the respirations and on the central nervous system.

c. If respiratory acidosis develops because of congestion in the lungs, why might the respiratory rate increase but not be effective in maintaining normal serum pH?

d. In the situation described in c, what compensations would help to maintain normal serum pH?

e. If serum pH decreases to 7.1 because of severe renal disease, explain the change that has occurred in the buffer pair and the effect of this change on the central nervous system.

EXAMPLES OF IMBALANCES

CASE STUDIES

CASE STUDY A
Vomiting

Mr. KB is 81 years old and has had gastritis with severe vomiting for 3 days. He has a history of heart problems and is presently feeling dizzy and lethargic. His eyes appear sunken, his mouth is dry, he walks unsteadily, and he complains of muscle aching, particularly in the abdomen. He is thirsty but is unable to retain food or fluid. A neighbor has brought Mr. KB to the hospital, where examination shows that his blood pressure is low, and his pulse and respirations are rapid. Laboratory tests demonstrate elevated hematocrit, hypernatremia, decreased serum bicarbonate, serum pH 7.35, and urine of high specific gravity (highly concentrated).

This case study illustrates a combination of fluid, electrolyte, and acid-base imbalances. Specific laboratory values are not given to focus on the basic concepts. For clarity, this case study will be discussed in two parts, the early stage and the advanced stage of the imbalances. Further information about the specific problems involved is given in each part and is followed by a series of questions.

PART A—DAY 1. Initially, Mr. KB lost water, sodium in the mucus content, and hydrogen and chloride ion in the hydrochloric acid portion of the gastric secretions.

Thinkabout 6–26

Which compartments are likely to be affected in this case by early fluid loss?

Alkalosis develops for two reasons, the first being the direct loss of hydrogen ions and the second being the effects of chloride ion loss. When chloride ion is lost in the gastric secretions, it is replaced by chloride from the serum (see Fig. 6–7). To maintain equal numbers of cations and anions in the serum, chloride ion and bicarbonate ion can exchange places when needed. Therefore, more bicarbonate ions shift into the serum from storage sites in the erythrocytes to replace the lost chloride ions. More bicarbonate ions in the serum

raise serum pH, and the result is "hypochloremic alkalosis."

Thinkabout 6–27

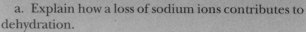

a. Explain how a loss of sodium ions contributes to dehydration.

b. Describe the early signs of dehydration in Mr. KB.

c. What serum pH could be expected in Mr. KB following this early vomiting?

d. Describe the compensations for the losses of fluid and electrolytes that should be occurring in Mr. KB.

e. Explain why Mr. KB may not be able to compensate for losses as well as a younger adult.

PART B—DAY 2–3. As Mr. KB continues to vomit and is still unable to eat or drink any significant amounts, loss of the duodenal contents occurs, which includes intestinal, pancreatic, and biliary secretions. No digestion and absorption of any nutrients occurs.

Losses at this stage include water, sodium ions, potassium ions, and bicarbonate ions. Also, intake of glucose and other nutrients is minimal. Mr. KB shows elevated serum sodium levels.

Thinkabout 6–28

a. Explain why serum sodium levels appear to be high in this case.

b. Explain how high serum sodium levels might affect the intracellular fluid.

c. Using your knowledge of normal physiology, explain how continued fluid loss is likely to affect: (1) blood volume, (2) cell function, (3) kidney function.

d. Given Mr. KB's history, why might potassium imbalance have more serious effects on him?

After a prolonged period of vomiting, metabolic acidosis develops. This change results from a number of factors:

- loss of bicarbonate ions in duodenal secretions
- lack of nutrients leading to catabolism of stored fats and protein with production of excessive amounts of ketoacids
- dehydration and decreased blood volume leading to decreased excretion of acids by the kidney
- decreased blood volume leading to decreased tissue perfusion, less oxygen to cells, and increased anaerobic metabolism with increased lactic acid
- increased muscle activity and stress leading to increased metabolic acid production

These factors lead to an increased amount of acids in the blood, which bind with bicarbonate buffer and result in decreased serum bicarbonate and decreased serum pH or metabolic acidosis.

Thinkabout 6–29

a. List several reasons why Mr. KB is lethargic and weak.

b. Predict the serum level of carbon dioxide or carbonic acid in this case.

c. If Mr. KB continues to lose body fluid, why might serum pH decrease below 7.35?

d. If serum pH drops below 7.35, what signs would be observed in Mr. KB?

e. Describe the effect of acidosis on serum potassium levels.

f. Mr. KB will be given replacement fluid therapy. Why is it important that sodium and potassium be given as well as water?

CASE STUDY B
Diarrhea

Baby C, 3 months old, has had severe watery diarrhea accompanied by fever for 24 hours. She is apathetic and responds weakly to stimulation. The condition has been diagnosed as viral gastroenteritis.

Thinkabout 6–30

a. List the major losses resulting from diarrhea and fever.

b. List other signs or data that would provide helpful information.

c. Explain several reasons why infants become dehydrated very quickly.

CASE STUDY C
Nephrotic Syndrome

S, age 5, has idiopathic nephrotic syndrome (nephrosis). He has generalized edema with a puffy face, distended abdomen, and edematous legs. He has gained weight but has eaten very little during the past week and has been quite irritable and lethargic. His blood pressure is normal. Laboratory tests indicate high levels of albumin, lipids, and hyaline (protein) casts in the urine, which has a high specific gravity. Blood tests show hypoalbuminemia and elevated cholesterol levels.

Thinkabout 6–31

a. State the cause of idiopathic nephrotic syndrome

b. Describe the change in the nephron that leads to albuminuria.

c. Describe the characteristics of the blood and urine that distinguish nephrotic syndrome.

d. Explain how hypoalbuminemia causes generalized edema.

e. Explain why S is retaining sodium and water.

f. Explain why skin breakdown is common in patients with prolonged edema.

STUDY QUESTIONS

1. Describe the locations of intracellular and extracellular fluids.

2. Which makes up the higher proportion of body fluid, intracellular fluid or extracellular fluid?

3. How does the proportion of fluid in the body change with age?

4. Why does dehydration affect cell function?

5. What is the function of sodium ion in the body?

6. Describe the effect of hypernatremia on extracellular fluid volume? Intracellular fluid volume?

7. State the primary location (compartment) of potassium.

8. How are sodium and potassium levels controlled in the body?

9. Describe the signs and symptoms of hypocalcemia.

10. Describe how a deficit of vitamin D would affect:

    (a) bones, (b) serum calcium level

11. Explain how hypochloremia affects acid-base balance.

12. State the normal range of pH for:

    (a) blood, (b) urine

13. Describe how very slow, shallow respirations are likely to affect

    (a) P_{CO_2}, (b) serum pH

14. State three possible causes of metabolic acidosis.

15. A diabetic is producing excess amounts of ketoacids.

    a. Describe the effects of this on serum bicarbonate levels and serum pH.

    b. Explain the possible compensations for this imbalance.

    c. Describe the signs of this compensation.

    d. The respirations that accompany metabolic acidosis are frequently called Kussmaul's respirations or "air hunger." What is the purpose of such respirations?

APPLICATION QUESTIONS

16. Emergency personnel, paramedics: A person is found unconscious. He is wearing a Medicalert bracelet for diabetes, and his breath has the typical odor of acetone (ketoacids).

    a. Predict his serum pH and the rationale for this prediction. Why would bicarbonate be administered as soon as possible?

    b. Predict his serum potassium level.

    c. How does insulin administration affect serum potassium?

    d. This person probably became very dehydrated as the ketoacidosis developed. What heart rate and pulse characteristics would you expect to be present?

17. Fitness personnel: Prolonged strenuous exercise usually leads to an increase in lactic acid. Given your knowledge of normal circulation, explain why it is helpful to have a cool-down period with mild exercise rather than total rest immediately after strenuous exercise, as well as fluid intake.

18. Respiratory function following surgery: General anesthetics, narcotic analgesics for pain, and pain often lead to slow, shallow respirations after surgery. Predict the effects on the partial pressure of carbon dioxide. Also, circulation is frequently slow, and oxygen levels are somewhat reduced. How would all these factors affect serum pH?

SECTION II

ALTERED STATUS/ GROWTH AND DEVELOPMENT

CHAPTER 7

Congenital and Genetic Disorders

KEY TERMS

allele	expression	meiosis	polygenic
amniocentesis	gene	mitosis	RNA
anomaly	genotype	mutation	teratogenic
autosome	heterozygous	neonate	trisomy
chromosome	homozygous	organogenesis	
co-dominant	incomplete dominant	penetration	
DNA	karyotype	phenotype	

REVIEW OF GENETIC CONTROL

Genetic information for each cell is stored on **chromosomes**, of which there are twenty-three pairs in each human cell. Twenty-two pairs are **autosomes**, and they are numbered when arranged by size and shape in a **karyotype** (see Fig. 7–3). The twenty-third pair consists of the pair of sex chromosomes; males have XY, and females have XX chromosomes. A male child receives the X chromosome from his mother and a Y chromosome from his father. A female child receives an X chromosome from each parent. During **meiosis** in humans, each sperm and each ovum receive only 23 chromosomes. When the ovum is fertilized by the sperm, the resulting zygote has 46 chromosomes, or 23 pairs containing an assortment of the parents' genetic information. Because so many combinations of **genes** are possible, it is most unlikely that any two persons will have the same genes and **DNA** (deoxyribonucleic acid). Therefore, DNA is considered a unique identifying characteristic for an individual.

The chromosomes are made up of many genes, which are matched for a function (**allele**) at a specific location on the paired chromosomes. A gene is a DNA "file" that contains information about protein synthesis in the cell. All cells in an individual's body contain the same chromosomes and genetic content (**genotype**), although not all genes are active in each cell. Research is being directed toward "mapping" all the genes on particular chromosomes and identifying the role of each gene (Fig. 7–1). Around 6000 genetic conditions have been determined so far, and it is estimated that there are a total of 50,000–100,000 genes on the human chromosomes. The *International Human Genome Project* is a worldwide project conducted by geneticists that aims to identify and map all the genes on every chromosome. When a specific gene for a pathologic condition is identified, a DNA analysis follows, leading to the development of a simple blood test to screen individuals for the presence of that specific gene. Recent discoveries have included the gene for early-onset Alzheimer's disease. In the past 5 years, genes have been located for

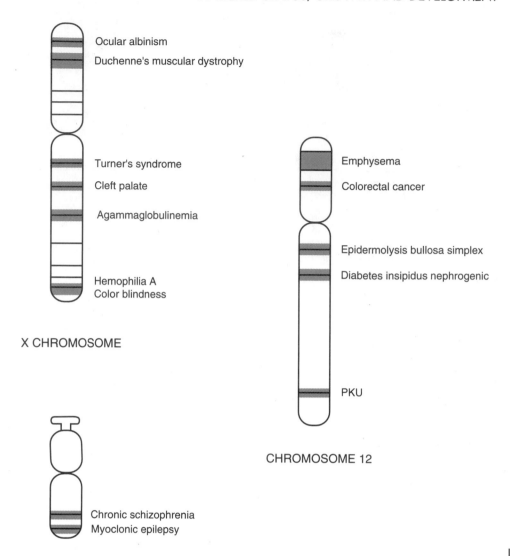

X CHROMOSOME

CHROMOSOME 12

CHROMOSOME 21

FIGURE 7-1. Examples of general gene locations on chromosomes.

diseases such as familial colon cancer, Huntington's disease, and early-onset breast cancer.

Genes control all physical characteristics such as eye color, color blindness, and metabolic processes. An alteration in a gene frequently causes a disease. Inheritance of different types of genes for both normal characteristics and disease characteristics follows specific patterns or Mendelian laws. These patterns include recessive and dominant traits and can be predicted using Punnett squares (Fig. 7–2). Traditionally, recessive genes are represented by small letters and dominant genes by capital letters.

Genes are composed of DNA strands, which determine the function of all cells in the body. **RNA** (ribonucleic acid) provides the communication link with DNA during the actual synthesis of proteins and helps to maintain control of cell activity. During embryonic and fetal development, when cells are undergoing **mitosis,** the chromosomes replicate, and each daughter cell receives DNA identical to that in the parent cell. There-

fore, the same genetic information is carried forward unless there is an error in the process of meiosis or mitosis. Such a **mutation** may be spontaneous or may result from exposure to harmful substances such as radiation or drugs.

Thinkabout 7–1

a. How many chromosomes does a human cell contain?

b. Which pair number represents the sex chromosomes?

c. Which parent passes on the Y chromosome to the child?

d. Describe a gene.

CONGENITAL DEFECTS

Congenital defects are disorders present at birth. Such defects include genetic or inherited disorders and developmental disorders, which usually result from exposure to a damaging agent during fetal development. The defect may be limited to one organ, or it may affect many functions.

Genetic disorders may result from a single-gene trait or from a chromosomal defect, or they may be multifactorial. A few examples are listed in Table 7–1. Single-gene disorders are caused by a defect in one gene; this mutant gene is passed on the chromosome to subsequent generations following the specific inheritance pattern for that gene. In some cases, the **expression,** or effect (**phenotype**), of an altered gene produces clinical signs that vary in severity depending on the **penetration** or activity of the gene. Clinical signs of genetic disorders are not always present at birth but may occur months or years later. However, children with genetic disorders do constitute a significant percentage of those who require hospital and community care.

Chromosomal defects usually result from an error during meiosis, when the DNA fragments are displaced or lost, thus altering genetic information. Such errors are a common cause of spontaneous abortions during the first trimester. Chromosomal defects are found in approximately 7 in 1000 births.

A. AUTOSOMAL RECESSIVE DISORDERS – Example: Cystic fibrosis

B. AUTOSOMAL DOMINANT DISORDERS – Example: Huntington's chorea

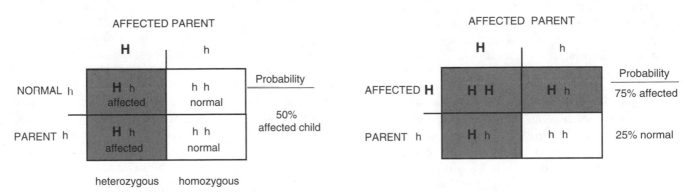

C. X-LINKED RECESSIVE DISORDERS – Example: Duchenne's muscular dystrophy

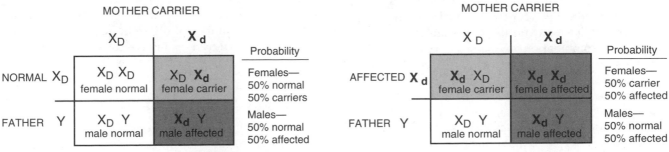

FIGURE 7-2. Inheritance patterns with Punnett squares.

TABLE 7–1 Examples of Genetic Disorders and Their Inheritance

Single-Gene Disorders
Autosomal dominant disorders
  Adult polycystic kidney disease
  Huntington's chorea
  Familial hypercholesterolemia
  Marfan's syndrome
Autosomal recessive disorders
  Color blindness
  Cystic fibrosis
  Phenylketonuria
  Tay-Sachs disease
X-linked recessive disorders
  Hemophilia A
Multifactorial Disorders
Anencephaly
Cleft lip and palate
Clubfoot
Congenital heart disease
Myelomeningocele
Schizophrenia
Chromosomal Disorders
Cri-du-chat syndrome
Monosomy X (Turner's syndrome)
Polysomy X (Klinefelter's syndrome)
Trisomy 18 (Edward's syndrome)

Developmental defects may be spontaneous errors or may result from exposure to environmental factors in utero. The DNA of the embryonic cells may be altered easily because rapid mitosis and differentiation take place in the first few months. Maternal nutrition may affect development. Low folic acid levels in the mother are a factor in the occurrence of spina bifida. **Teratogenic** agents, agents that cause damage during embryonic or fetal development, are often difficult to define. Many reports must be collated before a cause is suspected. Often the reports do not point to a single factor, and scientific experiments on humans to verify the data are not ethically feasible. The effects of the drug thalidomide were not realized for a long time, and during this time many children were born with missing limbs. Since then, women have been advised to refrain from using drugs or chemicals during the child-bearing years unless a physician recommends them

Many disorders, affecting approximately 10 percent of the population, are multifactorial. They may be **polygenic** (caused by multiple genes), or they may be the result of an inherited tendency toward a disorder that is expressed following exposure to certain environmental factors. A combination of factors is required for the problem to be present, whether at birth or later in life. Frequently the predisposing factors of a disorder such as atherosclerosis (heart and vascular disease), certain cancers (e.g., breast cancer), or schizophrenia (a psychiatric disorder) includes a *familial tendency*, which means that family members have an increased risk of developing the disorder, but not every family member will have the disease.

Genetic disorders have social and psychological implications. Decisions about whether or not to bear children with the risk of such disorders frequently create ethical dilemmas for society as well as for families. Parents have difficulty in adjusting to the birth of a child with an unanticipated defect and may need continued assistance with the care of the child and any associated feelings of guilt.

Thinkabout 7–2

a. Are genetic disorders always recognized at birth?
b. Differentiate congenital from genetic defects.
c. Differentiate a multifactorial disorder from a chromosomal disorder.

GENETIC DISORDERS

Single-Gene Disorders

Single-gene disorders are commonly classified by inheritance pattern, the major groups being recessive, dominant, and X-linked recessive. Examples are given in Figure 7–2. When considering the probability that a certain child will be affected, it should be remembered that the risk is present in each pregnancy. For example, if the first child has Duchenne's muscular dystrophy, all subsequent children will not necessarily be normal because the abnormality has already been expressed. The situation is similar to the probability of having a boy or a girl, which is approximately 50 percent with each pregnancy, even if the parents have already produced four boys!

A single gene may control a limited function such as color-blindness, or it may have widespread effects, as in cystic fibrosis or Marfan's syndrome. It is also important to realize that certain functions such as hearing may be affected by a number of different genes; for example, deafness in children is linked to approximately 16 genes.

AUTOSOMAL RECESSIVE DISORDERS

Autosomal recessive disorders include a variety of conditions such as cystic fibrosis, which affects primarily the lungs and pancreas, sickle cell disease, which involves defective hemoglobin, and phenylketonuria (PKU), in which a metabolic enzyme is missing. In recessive disorders, both parents must pass on the defective gene (see Fig. 7–2) to produce an affected (**homozygous**) child. Males and females are affected equally. If the child is **heterozygous** (that is, if one normal gene and one defective gene are present in the allele), then that child is a carrier and shows no clinical signs of disease. In each pregnancy, the probability of inheritance of a recessive gene from two carrier parents is 25 percent; the risk of passing on one recessive gene (from two carrier parents), resulting in a carrier child, is 50 percent, and there is a 25 percent chance that the child will inherit no recessive genes and will be normal.

Many of these recessive gene disorders result from enzyme deficits that cause toxic metabolites to accumulate inside cells, interfering with cell function and possibly causing death. These disorders may also be called *inborn errors of metabolism*. Interestingly, some of these defective genes appear to provide additional resistance to certain diseases. For example, carriers of the sickle cell gene in Africa have demonstrated increased resistance to malaria.

Some genes do not wholly fit either the recessive or the dominant pattern. For example, the gene for sickle cell disease may also be referred to as **incomplete dominant** because heterozygotes may display some clinical signs (sickle cell trait), whereas homozygotes show the full range of expression (sickle-cell anemia).

clinically until mid-life, and because diagnostic tests are not always available, the defective gene may already have been passed on to the next generation before the disease is diagnosed. Examples are Huntington's chorea, a degenerative condition of the brain, and polycystic kidney disease, which results in kidney failure.

Occasionally two dominant genes are both expressed in an individual. An example of such **codominant** genes is expressed by type AB blood.

X-LINKED RECESSIVE DISORDERS

Sex-linked disorders are usually carried by the X or female sex chromosome. They are recessive but are manifested in heterozygous males who lack the matching normal gene on the Y chromosome. Females are carriers (without clinical signs) when they have a heterozygous pair. Examples of X-linked recessive disorders include hemophilia A and Duchenne's muscular dystrophy.

Carrier females have a 50 percent chance of producing an affected male child and an equal chance of producing a carrier female child with each pregnancy. An affected male will transmit the defect to all his daughters, who become carriers, whereas his sons will neither be affected nor be carriers (the male passes only the normal Y chromosome to his sons).

Thinkabout 7–3

a. State the probability of a child of two carrier parents being affected by Tay-Sachs disease.
b. State the probability that a child will be the carrier of a recessive gene when the mother is a carrier and the father is normal.

AUTOSOMAL DOMINANT DISORDERS

In autosomal dominant disorders, the presence of the defect in only one of the alleles produces clinical expression of the disease. An affected parent has a 50 percent probability of passing the disorder on to each child regardless of sex (see Fig. 7–2). There are no carriers, and unaffected persons do not transmit the disorder.

Some of these conditions do not become evident

Thinkabout 7–4

a. Marfan's syndrome is transmitted by a dominant gene. State the probability that a child with an affected parent will have the disorder.
b. With an X-linked recessive disorder carried by the mother, state the probability of a male child being affected and of a female child being affected.
c. Hemophilia A is transmitted by an X-linked recessive gene. With an affected father, what are the probabilities that a child will have the disease? With an affected father and a carrier mother, what are the probabilities?

Chromosomal Disorders

Chromosomal abnormalities frequently result in early spontaneous abortions as well as in congenital abnormalities. During meiosis, genes are often redistributed during the process of "crossover" or spindle for-

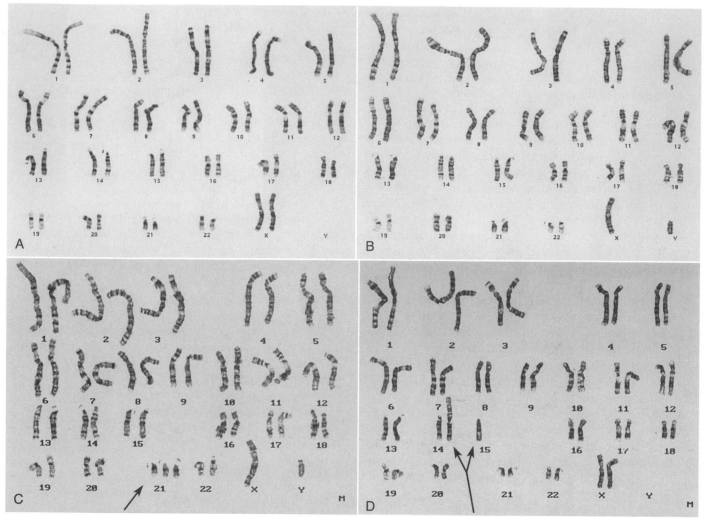

FIGURE 7–3. Examples of karyotypes. *A,* Normal female (46, XX). *B,* Normal male (46, XY). *C,* Male with Down's syndrome or trisomy 21 (47, XY, + 21). *D,* Female with translocation involving chromosomes 14 and 15 (45, XX, t (14q15q). (Courtesy of Cytogenetics Laboratory, North York General Hospital, Toronto, Ontario.)

mation. There may be an error in chromosomal duplication or reassembly, resulting in abnormal placement of part of the chromosome, altered structure, or an abnormal number of chromosomes. These birth defects are more common when the mother is over age 35.

Down's syndrome is an example of a **trisomy**, in which there are three chromosomes rather than two at the 21 position; it is therefore called trisomy 21 (Fig. 7–3). An individual with Down's syndrome therefore has 47 chromosomes. A less common form of Down's syndrome exists when part of a chromosome is shifted to another location (translocation). Monosomy X, or Turner's syndrome, occurs when only one sex chromosome, the X chromosome, is present. This person has only 45 chromosomes. Other common chromosomal abnormalities occur when parts of chromosomes are rearranged or lost during replication.

Thinkabout 7–5

Differentiate a chromosomal disorder from a single-gene disorder.

Multifactorial Disorders

Multifactorial disorders are disorders involving a number of genes or genetic influences combined with environmental factors. Common examples include cleft

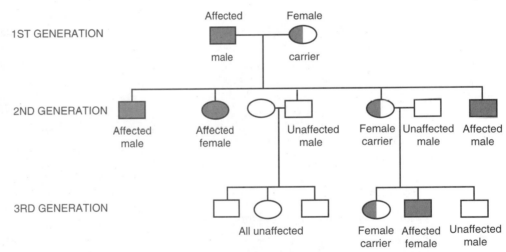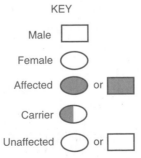

palate, congenital hip dislocation, congenital heart disease, and hydrocephalus. These disorders tend to be limited to a single localized area. The same defect is likely to recur in siblings, but there is no increased risk of occurrence of other defects.

If the genetic tendency can be documented, avoidance of certain environmental factors or close monitoring of the individual may minimize the risk of development of the disease. For example, a familial tendency has been noted in breast cancer, especially in close relatives, and periodic breast examinations are recommended in women in such families. In colon cancer, which also has a familial pattern, dietary changes may reduce the risk of development of this cancer. Familial incidence can be determined by using a family pedigree and tracing the incidence of the disorder through several generations (Fig. 7–4). Pedigrees may be developed for any genetic disorder.

DEVELOPMENTAL DISORDERS

Much concern has been expressed recently about exposure to negative environmental influences during pregnancy and even before pregnancy, when exposure to factors such as radiation may cause changes in the sperm or ova. Evidence has been gathered about the damaging effects on the fetus of alcohol (fetal alcohol syndrome), cigarette smoking (low birthweight), radiation, drugs, cocaine abuse, and maternal infections. TORCH is an acronym applied to screening checks for high-risk maternal infections—*t*oxoplasmosis, *o*ther (hepatitis B, mumps, rubeola, varicella, gonorrhea, syphilis), *r*ubella, *c*ytomegalovirus, and *h*erpes. Chemicals such as mercury in food and water, as well as many drugs, can cross the placental barrier and damage the rapidly dividing cells of the embryo and fetus.

Because many chemicals and drugs are thought to be possibly teratogenic or harmful, and because it is difficult to establish proof of such harm, it is recommended that women avoid exposure to any drugs, chemicals, or radiation during the child-bearing years. In most cases, the damage to the embryo occurs before pregnancy is suspected.

Exposure to harmful influences in the first two weeks of embryonic life usually results in the death of the embryo. The most critical time is the first two months of development when the cells are dividing rapidly and differentiating, **organogenesis** is taking place, and the basic body parts are forming (Fig. 7–5). Changes in the basic cells at this time have far-reaching effects. The

FIGURE 7–4. Illustration of a family pedigree for an X-linked recessive trait.

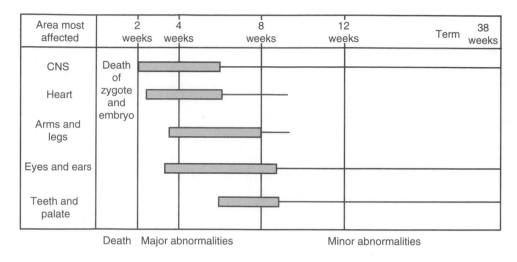

Area most affected	2 weeks	4 weeks	8 weeks	12 weeks	Term	38 weeks
CNS	Death of zygote and embryo					
Heart						
Arms and legs						
Eyes and ears						
Teeth and palate						

Death   Major abnormalities   Minor abnormalities

☐ Major effect
── Minor effect

FIGURE 7–5. Effects of teratogens during pregnancy.

effects of exposure depend on the stage of development at the precise time of the exposure. In addition to **anomalies,** or developmental abnormalities, exposure to damaging substances such as cocaine may cause premature birth, a high risk of further illness in the infant (low birthweight or increased respiratory problems), and increased risk of sudden infant death syndrome.

Cerebral palsy is an example of the kind of brain damage that can occur before, during, or immediately after birth. The cause may be insufficient oxygen, the toxic effects of excessive bilirubin, or trauma. The effects may be localized or may involve several areas of the brain.

Thinkabout 7–6

a. At which stage of pregnancy does the highest risk of central nervous system damage occur?

b. State five substances that are thought to be teratogenic.

c. Why is it safer to avoid contact with any possible teratogenic substance during the child-bearing years?

DIAGNOSTIC TOOLS

Diagnostic tests are available that can detect some abnormalities in carriers, during the prenatal period,

immediately after birth, or later in life when a disorder is suspected. Tests are not available for many disorders because the cause may not yet have been identified. Also, it would be an enormous task and very expensive to screen all pregnancies for all disorders. Testing is recommended for those who have a family history of a specific disease and for women over 35 years of age.

Screening programs for carriers are available for many disorders, particularly when the disorder has an ethnic basis and therefore manageable numbers. For example, Tay-Sachs disease is common among Ashkenazi Jews, and specific screening programs for this group have been successful in determining the carrier population and have offered reassurance and guidance to many individuals. A simple blood test can detect carriers of sickle cell disease. At the present time, priority in testing is given to families in which high risk is demonstrated in a pedigree (see Fig. 7–4) or when the parents have already had an affected child.

Prenatal diagnosis may offer reassurance to high-risk families or allow them to make an informed decision about an abortion or prepare for the birth of an affected child. Prenatal diagnosis does not ensure the birth of a "perfect child" because testing may not eliminate all possibilities; rather, the tests detect certain defects. For example, ultrasonography can visualize structural anomalies. Chromosomal abnormalities can be detected by growing fetal cells, harvesting them, and then examining the chromosomes or karyotype (see Fig. 7–3). DNA tests, enzyme deficits, and the presence of abnormal constituents such as alpha-fetoprotein (AFP) can also be included in this examination. Methods of prenatal diagnosis include **amniocentesis**, or extraction of amniotic fluid from the uterus, and extraction of a sample of the chorionic villus of the fetus.

Extraction of a sample of blood from the uterine artery can be used to diagnose blood disorders and metabolic disorders. These are invasive procedures and carry a slight risk to the fetus and the mother. The other drawback of prenatal diagnosis is that some tests may not show conclusive results until approximately 16 to 18 weeks into the pregnancy, leaving a long period of uncertainty.

Neonates can be tested immediately after birth for some defects. Mandatory testing is necessary in some jurisdictions for congenital disorders such as PKU and hypothyroidism to prevent mental retardation.

DNA testing can be used to identify individuals because DNA is considered a unique characteristic. This has opened the door to the use of genetic markers in blood and other body fluids by forensic scientists.

Genetic engineering refers to the recent developments in methods of manipulating genes in the laboratory. The goal is to replace a defective gene with a normal one to reduce the risk of genetic defects. Concern has been expressed about the possible abuse of such procedures and the risk of unanticipated changes in the expression of genes.

Thinkabout 7–7

a. Explain why it would be helpful to know if one is carrying a defective gene.

b. Briefly describe two methods of prenatal diagnosis and the purpose of each.

EXAMPLE: DOWN'S SYNDROME

Down's syndrome, or trisomy 21, is a common chromosomal disorder. The risk of bearing a child with Down's syndrome increases with maternal age. For example, a woman at age 30 has a risk of approximately 1 in 1000 of bearing a child with Down's syndrome,

whereas at age 35 the risk increases to approximately 1 in 500 and at age 40 to 1 in 100. Whether this risk is due to damage to the oocytes resulting from degeneration with aging or from environmental agents or other factors is unknown. Recently, it has been suggested that some cases may be of paternal origin.

Down's syndrome affects many areas of the body, although specific effects vary among individuals. The condition is apparent at birth because certain physical characteristics are distinctive (Fig. 7–6). The head is small and has a flat facial profile, the eyes are slanted and there are Brushfield's spots on the iris, and the mouth tends to hang open showing a large protruding tongue and a high-arched palate. The hands are small and have a single palmar (simian) crease. As the child develops, the muscles tend to be hypotonic, the joints are loose, cervical abnormalities and instability are often evident, and stature is short. Developmental stages are delayed. All children are cognitively impaired, but the severity of impairment varies with the individual, and early stimulation programs are helpful. Many children have an assortment of other problems, including visual problems (cataracts, strabismus), hearing problems, obstructions in the digestive tract, congenital heart defects, decreased resistance to infection (immune deficit), and a high risk of developing leukemia. Sexual development is often delayed or incomplete. As the life span has been extended for these children with improved medical care, there has been a marked increase in the development of Alzheimer's disease after 40 years of age.

Thinkabout 7–8

a. How is prenatal diagnosis of Down's syndrome achieved?

b. Can diagnostic tests provide full information on the effects of Down's syndrome in an individual child?

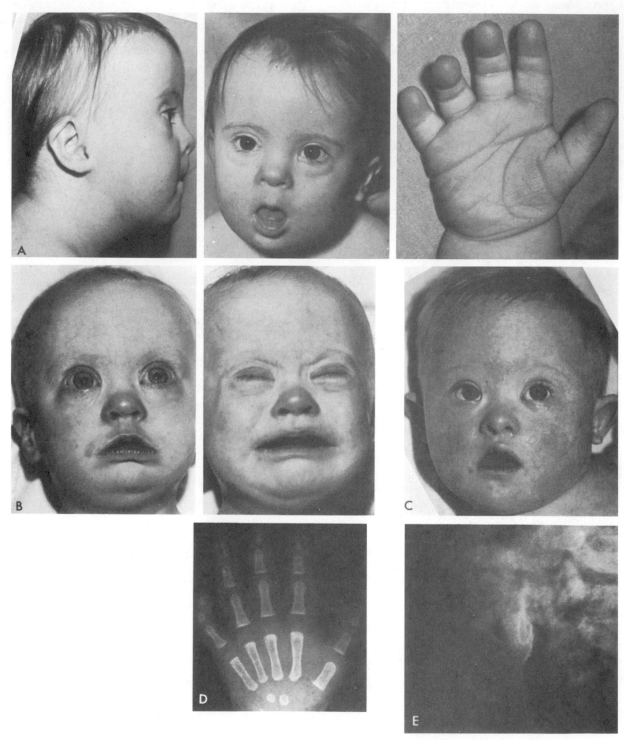

FIGURE 7–6. Down's syndrome. *A*, Young infant. Flat facies, straight hair; protrusion of tongue; single crease on inturned fifth finger. *B*, and *C*, Inner canthal folds. Speckling of iris with lack of peripheral patterning. Small auricles, prominent at right. "Pouting" expression when crying. (*B, C,* from Smith DW: J Pediatr 70:474, 1967.) *D*, Hypoplasia, midphalanx of fifth finger. *E*, Shallow acetabular angle with small iliac wings having the shape of elephant ears. (From Jones KL: Smith's Recognizable Patterns of Human Malformation, 4th ed. Philadelphia, WB Saunders, 1988.)

STUDY QUESTIONS

1. Define homozygous and heterozygous.

2. What is the purpose of a pedigree?

3. Explain why teratogens are difficult to identify.

4. Explain why a woman carrying the gene for hemophilia can produce two hemophiliac sons when she is mated to a normal male.

5. Under what conditions does a female acquire an X-linked recessive disorder?

6. Why are X-linked disorders never passed from a father to a son?

7. What is the probability that a parent carrying a dominant trait will pass that trait on to each child?

8. How can prenatal diagnosis demonstrate the sex of an unborn child?

9. Describe briefly the process of amniocentesis and its purpose.

10. Which of the following can be identified by an abnormal karyotype? sickle cell disease, cystic fibrosis, monosomy X, Tay-Sachs disease, Huntington's chorea?

CHAPTER
8
Health Problems Associated with Adolescence

KEY TERMS

●●●

adhesion	epiphyseal plate or disc	menarche	purulent
amenorrhea	esophagitis	metaphysis	pustule
androgen	estrogen	monosomy	sebaceous
anemia	fixed	osteoporosis	sebum
anomalies	gonadotropin	pathogen	sinus
arrhythmia	gonads	periosteum	testosterone
autoimmune	hypothalamus	pituitary gland	tetany
caries	idiopathic	progesterone	transillumination
effusion	lesion	psychological	
emaciated	leukocytosis	puberty	

REVIEW OF CHANGES IN ADOLESCENCE

Adolescence is a time of major physiologic, psychological, and sociologic changes, a time of transition into adulthood. The period of adolescence is generally considered to begin with the development of secondary sex characteristics around the age of 10 to 12 years and to continue until physical growth is completed at about

age 18. The term **puberty** indicates the onset of reproductive changes, beginning with the appearance of secondary sexual characteristics and the first menstrual cycle in females. There is great variation among individuals in both the timing and the extent of change. In recent years, perhaps because of improved nutrition, maturation has tended to occur at an earlier age.

The biologic changes typical of adolescence result primarily from hormonal activity stimulated by the **hy-**

pothalamus and the **pituitary gland**. The increasing release of **gonadotropins** from the pituitary stimulates the ovaries and testes. The ovaries release ova and the sex hormones **estrogen** and **progesterone**, and the testes begin to produce sperm and release **testosterone**. Although these sex hormones are produced in small quantities by the adrenal cortex during all stages of life, the larger quantities now available from the **gonads** are responsible for the unique types of growth and development that are characteristic of the teen years.

Linear growth is accelerated during the typical adolescent growth spurt. In most males the growth spurt occurs later than in females and usually lasts longer because epiphyseal closure is delayed in males. In recent years both males and females have achieved a greater average height. Any growth retardation usually is apparent prior to adolescence, but if it is evident at this time it can be confirmed by x-rays illustrating an abnormally thin **epiphyseal plate**. Other skeletal changes include the development of a broader pelvis in females and an increase in the width of the shoulders and chest in males. Because of the influence of **androgens** or testosterone (the "muscle-building" steroids), males develop more skeletal muscle than females. In a new form of substance abuse, synthetic androgens are taken by some adolescents to improve body image and performance, without regard for dangerous side effects. The growth changes of adolescence do not occur simultaneously. Limb growth occurs first, then hip and shoulder development, and, lastly, increased skeletal muscle mass. This is why the adolescent may appear awkward and gangly for a time until proportionate and complete maturation is accomplished. Additional factors influencing growth during this period include nutrition, genetic factors, and activity levels. Dietary intake often becomes erratic during this period just when demand is higher for protein and other nutrients. Therefore, it is important for the adolescent to maintain basic nutritional requirements.

Features indicating sexual maturation in females include breast development, onset of menstruation (**menarche**), and the appearance of pubic and axillary hair; fatty (adipose) deposits on the hips, buttocks, thighs, and breasts contribute to the typical female shape. Changes in males include enlargement of the testicles and penis and the development of pubic and axillary hair. Facial hair is also apparent in the male pattern, and additional body hair is common. Voice changes occur in both sexes, but the male voice becomes deeper as the larynx enlarges. The sex hormones also stimulate activity of the **sebaceous** (oil) glands and the sweat glands in the skin in both males and females.

With increasing body dimensions, there is an associated increase in blood volume and in the strength of cardiac contractions, although the pulse rate dimin-

ishes. Both cardiovascular and pulmonary functions reach adult values during adolescence, but usually they do not keep pace with musculoskeletal growth, leading to decreased exercise tolerance and marked fatigue at times in active teens. The basal metabolic rate gradually declines to adult levels during this period.

Thinkabout 8–1

a. List the hormones produced by the ovaries.
b. Describe two major effects of testosterone on the body.

MUSCULOSKELETAL ABNORMALITIES

During the growth spurt, muscular development lags behind skeletal growth; thus, less support is available for the weight-bearing areas. Adequate warm-up before exercise or competitive sports is essential to reduce the risk of injury. Postural abnormalities can easily develop during this growth period. Other factors, such as developmental abnormalities, may predispose an individual to musculoskeletal abnormalities.

Kyphosis and Lordosis

Kyphosis, often called hunchback, is an increase in the convexity of the thoracic spine (Fig. 8–1). Although it may develop in mature adults secondary to disorders such as **osteoporosis** (bone demineralization) and tuberculosis, a milder and reversible form, commonly of postural origin, may occur during the adolescent growth spurt. Teens frequently hunch over, particularly if they are taller than their peers or are self-conscious about breast development. Also, skeletal muscle support may be inadequate temporarily. Exercise and postural change can usually reverse mild deformities, although severe deformity may require surgery or a brace for correction.

Lordosis is an exaggerated concave lumbar curvature, or "swayback." Again, it may accompany musculoskeletal disease, but frequently it develops during the teen growth spurt. Obesity aggravates the tendency toward lordosis because the center of gravity for the body is altered, and postural compensation causes lordosis.

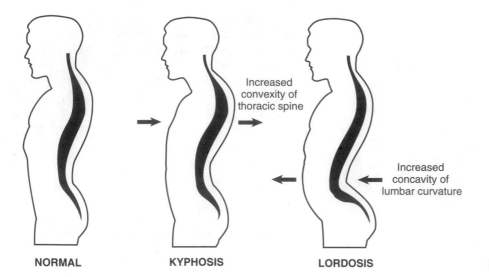

FIGURE 8-1. Kyphosis and lordosis.

Scoliosis

Scoliosis is a lateral curvature of the spine affecting either the thoracic or lumbar area, or both, and it may be accompanied by rotation of the vertebrae (Fig. 8–2). Screening programs offered in many schools aid early diagnosis. Otherwise, it may be noticed when clothes do not fit properly, or the uneven shoulder elevation may become apparent when the child bends forward.

Scoliosis may be classified as structural or functional. *Functional,* nonstructural, or postural scoliosis is secondary to another problem such as unequal leg length or spinal nerve compression. *Structural* scoliosis is a primary spinal deformity, of which a large proportion of cases are **idiopathic** (without known cause), although a genetic factor appears to play a key role. Females are more frequently affected than males. Unequal spinal muscle supports related to partial paralysis, trauma, muscular dystrophy, cerebral palsy, and spinal tumors may lead to loss of the normal curvature. Conditions such as congenital hemivertebra deformity may also alter spinal alignment.

Early effects of abnormal spinal curvature include loss of alignment of the hip and shoulder. Rotation of the vertebrae affects the pelvis and thorax. The ribs can become **fixed** in an abnormal position; if severe, this can restrict ventilation.

In teenagers with milder postural scoliosis, exercise and bracing may be helpful in restoring the normal curvature of the back. However, surgical correction with instrumentation and fusion of the vertebrae is sometimes required, causing restriction of the individual's activity for long periods of time. Unfortunately, even when corrected, complications may occur later in life.

Thinkabout 8–2

a. Compare the abnormal curvatures associated with kyphosis, lordosis, and scoliosis by preparing a chart with a simple line drawing and a brief description of each.

b. Describe the potential complications of scoliosis if it is not treated in the early stage.

Osteomyelitis

Osteomyelitis, an infection of the bone, is more common in younger males than in females. Often a history of sickle cell anemia or of trauma, either an open wound or a soft tissue injury, precedes this condition. The latter can be minor, such as a bruise or a sprain, but the damage leaves the area vulnerable to blood-borne organisms from another site such as a skin boil, an abscess, or sinusitis. In adolescents the common causative organism is *Staphylococcus aureus*, but any **pathogen** may be involved. The most common site of infection in adolescents is the **metaphysis** of the femur or tibia in the leg.

Osteomyelitis causes a local accumulation of purulent exudate or pus, which destroys the bone in the area (see Chapter 4). This exudate creates pressure within the rigid bony structure and causes severe pain owing to pressure on the nerves. The **periosteum** may be lifted or torn off if the pressure becomes excessive (Fig. 8–3). If the infection is not treated quickly, the irritation may stimulate the surrounding bone to develop new bone growth around the infected site, walling off an area of infection and necrotic bone, which then becomes more difficult to treat effectively. Also, if the pressure of the exudate tears the periosteum on the surface of the bone, a **sinus** or passage through the soft tissue may develop, spreading the infection to adjacent tissue. Usually the epiphyseal plate acts as a barrier to joint involvement, although the infection can spread through the joint capsule. However, if the epiphyseal plate or periosteum is damaged, growth may be affected.

Manifestations of osteomyelitis include the local signs of inflammation—swelling, redness, and warmth at the

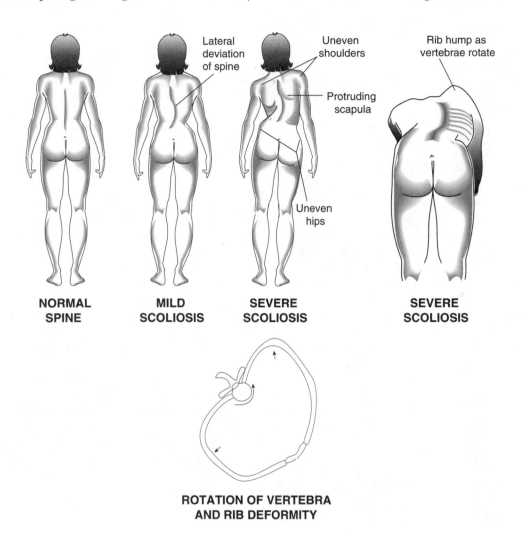

NORMAL SPINE **MILD SCOLIOSIS** **SEVERE SCOLIOSIS** **SEVERE SCOLIOSIS**

Lateral deviation of spine

Uneven shoulders

Protruding scapula

Uneven hips

Rib hump as vertebrae rotate

ROTATION OF VERTEBRA AND RIB DEFORMITY

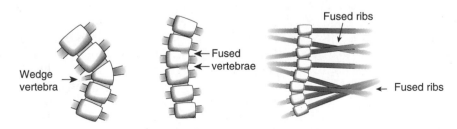

Wedge vertebra

Fused vertebrae

Fused ribs

Fused ribs

SOME CONGENITAL DEFORMITIES CAUSING SCOLIOSIS

FIGURE 8–2. Scoliosis.

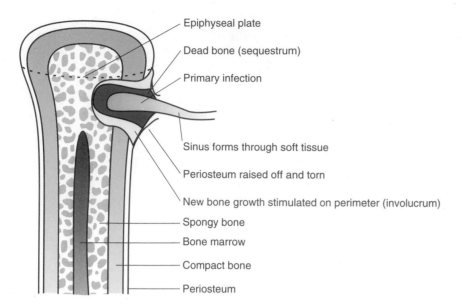

- Epiphyseal plate
- Dead bone (sequestrum)
- Primary infection
- Sinus forms through soft tissue
- Periosteum raised off and torn
- New bone growth stimulated on perimeter (involucrum)
- Spongy bone
- Bone marrow
- Compact bone
- Periosteum

FIGURE 8–3. Osteomyelitis.

site, and pain that increases with movement. There are usually systemic signs of infection as well, including fever, leukocytosis, malaise, and irritability.

Treatment requires aggressive drug therapy with bone-penetrating antimicrobials appropriate for the causative organism. If chronic infection develops, surgery may be necessary to remove necrotic and infected tissue prior to healing.

Thinkabout 8–3

a. List all the manifestations of osteomyelitis.
b. Explain several reasons why early treatment is important.

Juvenile Rheumatoid Arthritis

Juvenile rheumatoid arthritis (JRA) is a group of systemic inflammatory diseases that affect the connective tissue in areas such as the joints. It is somewhat similar to the adult form (see Chapter 22), but has certain distinctive qualities. For example, large joints are frequently involved, and more systemic effects are apparent. The specific cause is not known, although an infectious or **autoimmune** basis has been suggested. It occurs in two age groups, children aged 2 to 5 and those aged 9 to 12 years. Many cases are mild and remain undiagnosed for some time. One or more joints may be involved depending on the specific type of JRA that is present. Usually complete recovery occurs after a few months or years, in most cases with no residual damage.

In JRA the synovial membrane of the joint is inflamed, resulting in swelling and **effusion** in the joint with gradual erosion of the cartilage. Mobility is impaired by the swelling, pain, and occasional muscle spasms. Affected joints are red and swollen in the initial or acute stage; they are often tender to touch and stiff after rest. If the inflammation persists, **adhesions** form, causing fixation and deformity of the joint.

Specific diagnostic tests are not applicable in JRA because rheumatoid factor is usually not present in the child's blood. General signs of inflammation such as **leukocytosis** are present. The course may be marked by remissions and exacerbations, or the signs may persist continuously. Severe cases are marked by more systemic signs such as fever, organomegaly, and rash, and complications such as hip involvement or iridocyclitis (inflammation of the eye) may occur.

Treatment includes nonsteroidal anti-inflammatory drugs (see Chapter 2) and glucocorticoids if needed. Several new chemotherapeutic agents appear promising. Physiotherapy is important to maintain the flexibility, alignment, function, and proper development of the joints. Growth may be impaired during the time of active disease, perhaps related to immobility or to glucocorticoid treatment, but often a catch-up growth spurt follows recovery. In some cases unequal limb growth related to joint involvement may occur, and the individual may never reach his or her original growth potential.

Thinkabout 8-4

a. Explain several ways in which arthritis affects mobility.

b. Explain how long-term arthritis of the legs might affect a child's growth.

EATING DISORDERS

In Western cultures, eating disorders are a common problem in adolescents. Because more children now tend to be obese in early childhood and adolescence, there is an increased focus by many teens on body image combined with a desire to change their bodies. With eating disorders the major medical concern is the effect of poor nutrition on growth and development and on the child's general health status. The incidence of eating disorders is increasing, but often the affected person makes a great effort to conceal the problem, making it more difficult to detect and treat in the early stages. In addition to the physical problems, the psychological and behavioral factors in these disorders need to be addressed. The two major problems are anorexia nervosa and bulimia; they may occur separately or, more frequently, overlap.

Anorexia Nervosa

Anorexia nervosa is an extreme loss of weight in the absence of other disease. Anorexia has two peak periods of onset, first in the early teen years (ages 12 to 14) and again later in the 16- to 17-year age range, with females being most often affected. The **psychological** component is strongly evident in these patients, who typically are young women who are perfectionists and high achievers. This psychological component, combined with a history of family conflict, a confused perception of body image and sexuality, and a morbid fear of "fatness," leads to anorexia. Research is also currently focusing on possible hypothalamic abnormalities related to hunger as well as to other physiologic dysfunctions.

The basic abnormality in anorexia nervosa is a refusal to eat, resulting in extreme loss of weight and malnutrition resulting from self-inflicted starvation. The person may also induce vomiting, take excessive amounts of laxatives, and exercise strenuously to achieve even further weight loss.

The anorexic appears markedly **emaciated**. Other manifestations include **amenorrhea** (lack of menstrual cycles), low body temperature and cold intolerance, low blood pressure and slow heart rate, dry skin and brittle nails, and development of fine body hair (lanugo).

In some cases, anorexia nervosa can be life-threatening. Dehydration can be severe, affecting kidney and cardiovascular function (see Chapter 6). Electrolyte imbalances such as hypokalemia and hyponatremia may cause complications such as cardiac **arrhythmias** (irregular heart rhythms) and cardiac arrest. Hospitalization and long-term psychotherapy with behavioral modification may be necessary to arrest the weight loss and initiate recovery. Many specialized clinics and support groups have been formed to deal with eating disorders.

Bulimia Nervosa

As indicated earlier, bulimia and anorexia may overlap. Bulimia is also common in females but occurs more frequently in older adolescents. Bulimia is characterized by binge-eating followed by purging. Binge-eating consists of ingesting huge amounts of food, usually high in calories, within a very short period of time. This is followed by purging by means of self-induced vomiting and an excessive use of laxatives and diuretics. The cycle may be repeated several times a day or less frequently.

The bulimic often maintains a relatively normal weight, although appropriate levels of individual nutrients may not be sustained, resulting in problems such as **anemia** (low hemoglobin levels). Frequent vomiting causes fluid and electrolyte imbalances, which may cause cardiac arrhythmias or **tetany** or severe abdominal pain. Dental personnel should be aware that recurrent vomiting leads to erosion of tooth enamel (usually on the lingual surface of the maxillary teeth) and increased dental **caries**, tears and ulcers in the oral mucosa, enlarged parotid and submandibular glands, and chronic **esophagitis** with sore throat and difficulty in swallowing. Self-induced vomiting may leave visible scars on the fingers or back of the hand used to stimulate the gag reflex.

Thinkabout 8-5

Prepare a chart comparing anorexia and bulimia according to eating pattern, body weight, and potential complications.

SKIN DISORDERS

Acne Vulgaris

Acne is a very common skin infection in adolescents, particularly in males, although there is a wide variation between mild and severe forms. A number of factors are involved in the development and exacerbation of acne, including hereditary predisposition, increased androgen levels, premenstrual hormonal fluctuations, the application of oily creams, and exposure to increased heat and humidity.

The lesions of acne affect the hair follicles and associated sebaceous glands on the face, neck, and upper trunk. At puberty these glands increase in activity. There are two types of lesions. Comedones, often called whiteheads or blackheads, are noninflammatory collections of **sebum**, sloughed epithelial cells, and bacteria, which clog the gland and prevent normal drainage. These lesions usually resolve without scarring. The second type of lesion involves inflammation and infection and may result in skin damage and scarring. The hair follicles swell and rupture, and *Propionibacterium acnes*, a component of normal flora, breaks down the sebum into irritating fatty acids. Staphylococcal organisms invade, creating a **pustule** (raised red mass containing **purulent** exudate). The lesion is often aggravated by irritation due to the individual picking at or squeezing the mass. Eventually the lesion ruptures, causing local tissue destruction and possibly spreading to nearby areas.

New lesions can be discouraged by decreasing some of the predisposing factors, shampooing and cleaning the area more frequently (but avoiding harsh soaps and scrubbing), improving general nutrition, and avoiding oil-based cosmetics. Peeling agents (benzoyl peroxide, tretinoin) and antibacterial agents (tetracycline) assist in controlling some severe lesions and reducing the cosmetic problem. Dermabrasion may be successful in removing some scars.

Thinkabout 8–6

a. Describe the development of an acneiform lesion.

b. Suggest measures that can reduce the severity of acne.

INFECTION

Infectious Mononucleosis

Infectious mononucleosis is an acute infection caused by the Epstein-Barr virus (in the herpes group), which is common in adolescents and young adults. It is usually mild and self-limiting but occasionally is marked by complications. It is transmitted by direct contact with infected saliva (hence the term "kissing disease"), by airborne droplet, and by blood. The incubation period is approximately 4 to 6 weeks.

The manifestations include sore throat, headache, fever, fatigue and malaise, enlarged lymph nodes and spleen, and a rash on the trunk. There is an increase in lymphocytes and monocytes in the blood, and the heterophil antibody test (Monospot test) is positive.

Possible complications include hepatitis, ruptured spleen, and meningitis. Because no effective treatment for virus infections is available, supportive measures, particularly bed rest, are indicated. As with many viral infections, recovery may be prolonged, and fatigue and malaise may be persistent. Fitness students or trainers should be aware of an important safeguard against rupture of the spleen, that is, ensuring that the spleen has returned to normal size before an individual participates in sports or strenuous exercise programs.

DISORDERS AFFECTING SEXUAL DEVELOPMENT

Chromosomal Disorders

Depending on the manifestations, some genetic disorders are diagnosed early in life, and some are not diagnosed until puberty, when the effects on sexual development become apparent. An example is *Klinefelter's syndrome*, which affects males owing to the presence of an additional X chromosome (XXY instead of XY—see Chapter 7). Although mental retardation is a common finding, most boys are diagnosed at puberty because the testes remain small, sperm are not produced, and secondary male sex characteristics do not develop. *Turner's syndrome*, a **monosomy X** in which one X chromosome is missing, affects sexual development in females and causes other abnormalities as well. **Anomalies** commonly occur in the heart and genitourinary system, growth is retarded, and at puberty the growth spurt, development of secondary sex characteristics, and initiation of the menstrual cycle are lacking. Hormone replacement treatment is beneficial in these girls.

Tumors

When a *testicular tumor* develops in the testes of the adolescent, it is usually malignant (see Chapter 5). It presents as a unilateral hard, heavy mass and often is not painful. It is opaque on **transillumination**. Routine testicular self-examination is helpful in achieving early diagnosis and treatment.

Adenocarcinoma of the vagina, which occurs in adolescent females whose mothers have taken the hormone diethylstilbestrol (DES) during pregnancy to prevent spontaneous abortion is much less common in North America since awareness of the implications of DES therapy has increased, but it provides an example of unanticipated long-term effects of hormone therapy. Early signs include vaginal spotting (blood) and discharge, followed by pain, interference with urination, and a palpable mass. Treatment involves surgery and radiation therapy, in which every effort is made to maintain the structural integrity of the vagina.

Menstrual Abnormalities

Delayed menarche or primary **amenorrhea**, the absence of menstruation after age 17, is usually due to an abnormality in the reproductive organs (structural or hormonal) or an abnormality in the pituitary or hypothalamus. Consistent strenuous physical activity, such as training for competitive sports and certain systemic disorders, such as hypothyroid or diabetes, may also delay menarche.

Dysmenorrhea refers to the discomfort that occurs in varying degrees during the first or second day of menstruation (see Chapter 24). In some girls the pain is incapacitating, and vomiting or fainting may occur. The cramping pain is related to the increased secretion of uterine prostaglandins, which increase muscle contractility and directly irritate the nerve endings, and to the vascular changes and ischemia in the uterine wall that occur as the endometrium is shed. Dysmenorrhea may be treated with hormones or nonsteroidal anti-inflammatory drugs such as ibuprofen (Advil). Popular nonprescription products for dysmenorrhea such as Midol contain ASA, caffeine, and cinnamedrine, a uterine relaxant. Secondary dysmenorrhea usually is related to infection or other pathologies.

STUDY QUESTIONS

1. Briefly describe five changes that indicate sexual maturation in the female.

2. Differentiate structural from functional scoliosis and give an example of a cause of each type.

3. Explain how the signs of osteomyelitis differ from the signs of JRA.

4. How do anorexia and bulimia differ from each other?

5. Explain how anorexia and bulimia can have serious consequences.

6. Explain how scars may develop from acne.

CHAPTER

9

Effects of Pregnancy

KEY TERMS

● ●

abortion	fallopian tube	hypertrophy	progesterone
amniocentesis	fertilization	hypotension	sperm
amniotic fluid	fetus	immunoglobulin	supine
auscultation	gestation	jaundice	teratogens
bilirubin	gingivitis	lactation	thrombus
caries	gravidity	mitotic	trimester
cervix	hematocrit	organogenesis	uterus
chorionic villi	hemolysis	os	vagina
differentiation	human chorionic	ovum	viable
embolus	gonadotropin	parity	zygote
embryo	hyperplasia	peritonitis	
estrogen	hypertension	placenta	

FETAL DEVELOPMENT

Conception or fertilization of the ovum by a sperm takes place in the **fallopian tube**. During the next few hours, the genetic information from the **ovum** and **sperm** are merged in the **zygote** (fertilized ovum), and many rapid **mitotic** divisions occur as the zygote moves along the fallopian tube toward the **uterus**. Implantation of the zygote in the uterine wall is completed approximately 1 week after fertilization, and **differen-**

tiation of cells is apparent as the **placenta** begins to form. The period from 3 to 8 weeks is termed the embryonic stage, and this is a critical time in the development of the new individual. Cells continue to divide rapidly and to differentiate to form the basic functional elements of the various organs (**organogenesis**), systems, and external structures such as the limbs and eyes. By the end of 8 weeks, all organs are formed. For example, the primitive fetal heart is beating at 4 weeks. Exposure of the embryo to any **teratogen** during this time usually causes major widespread damage to the developing structures and leads to congenital abnormalities (see Fig. 7–5). Common teratogens include drugs, viruses, alcohol, and radiation. In some cases, extensive cell necrosis leads to the death of the **embryo**.

After 8 weeks, the term **fetus** is applied to the developing child. Continued growth and differentiation result in completion of many specialized structures. Elementary functions can be observed as the limbs move and amniotic fluid is swallowed. Teratogens have less effect on development during this stage because cell damage occurs primarily in certain tissues that are actively developing at the time of exposure. However, *functional* impairment, particularly in the central nervous system, is a common consequence. During the last trimester in utero, the fetus gains weight, and organs such as the lungs mature. With improved technology and neonatal care, the fetus may be able to survive (remain **viable**) outside the uterus as early as 22 to 23 weeks.

SIGNIFICANT PHYSIOLOGIC CHANGES DURING PREGNANCY

Pregnancy is a normal process in the life cycle. The normal period of pregnancy is divided into three **trimesters**, each approximately 3 months long and each involving significant changes in the mother and the developing fetus. In some individuals, these changes may aggravate preexisting pathologies or precipitate new problems. Good prenatal care is essential to minimize any potential complications. Additional information on various aspects of pregnancy may be found in references on obstetrics.

Diagnosis of Pregnancy

Laboratory diagnosis of pregnancy is based on the presence of **human chorionic gonadotropin** (hCG) in the mother's plasma or urine, using enzyme-linked immunosorbent assay (ELISA)-based tests. The hormone hCG, which is secreted by the **chorionic villi** after implantation of the fertilized ovum in the uterus, can be detected by a simple office or home test. Many typical signs of pregnancy, such as nausea or morning sickness, do not provide absolute confirmation of pregnancy because each could result from other causes.

The *positive* (absolute) signs occur later in the pregnancy and include the fetal heart beat as detected by **auscultation** or ultrasound, fetal movement detected by someone other than the mother, and visualization of the fetus with ultrasound.

The *estimated date of delivery (EDD)* or *estimated date of birth (EDB)* can be calculated easily using Nägele's rule if the first day of the last menstrual period (LMP) is

known. Three months are subtracted from that date, and then 7 days are added to the resulting figure. For example, if the LMP began on October 20, one would subtract 3 months (July 20) and add 7 days, giving an EDB of July 27. Various charts and wheels are available to provide the dates quickly. For women with longer cycles or irregular menstrual cycles, the formula must be adjusted. First pregnancies are often longer.

Gestation refers to the length of time since the first day of the LMP, and equals 280 days (40 weeks) or 10 lunar months. Gestational age is 2 weeks longer than the actual age of the child from the time of **fertilization**—266 days or 38 weeks.

Gravidity and **parity** are terms used to describe a woman's history of pregnancy and childbirth. Gravidity refers to the number of pregnancies, for example, a *primigravida* is a woman who is pregnant for the first time. Parity refers to the number of pregnancies in which the fetus has reached viability (approximately 22 weeks of gestation). A *multipara* has completed two or more pregnancies to the point of fetal viability. Coding systems are available to document histories. For example, a five-digit system records, in sequence, the number of pregnancies, the number of deliveries, the number of premature deliveries, the number of **abortions** of any type, and the number of children living. The history of a woman in her second pregnancy who has one child living and no other experiences would be recorded as 2-1-0-0-1.

Amniocentesis is the withdrawal of a small amount of **amniotic fluid,** including some sloughed fetal cells, from the uterus after 14 weeks. The fluid can be checked for its chemical content and the cells cultured for chromosome analysis. Amniocentesis is recommended when there are signs of abnormality or a history of genetic disorders, or it may be used later in pregnancy to check fetal lung maturity. An alternative process is chorionic villus testing which can take place earlier in pregnancy and is useful for chromosomal examination in high-risk clients.

Physiologic Changes and Their Implications

HORMONAL CHANGES

Levels of **estrogen** and **progesterone** in the maternal blood are increased during pregnancy as the placenta increases its production of these hormones, which are essential to the development of the uterus, maintenance of pregnancy, and preparation of the breasts for **lactation** (milk production). **Hyperplasia** of the thyroid gland and increased production of thyroxine also occur (see Chapter 21), which increases the mother's metabolism.

REPRODUCTIVE SYSTEM CHANGES

Estrogen causes a tremendous increase in the size of the uterus owing to **hypertrophy** of the muscle cells, some hyperplasia, and an increase in fibrous tissue. The number of blood vessels in the uterus is also greatly increased to ensure the adequacy of the blood supply to the fetus. As the fetus and uterus grow, they exert pressure on the surrounding structures (Fig. 9–1). For example, pressure on the bladder and bowel may alter the elimination pattern, and upward pressure on the diaphragm may restrict lung expansion.

Varicose veins frequently develop during pregnancy (see Chapter 16). Either the superficial or the deep veins of the legs may be involved. The superficial veins appear as large, distended purplish veins. They can cause fatigue and aching in the legs. Varicose veins result from restriction of blood flow in the veins to the heart due to the pressure of the uterus, particularly in women who must stand for long periods of time or who are predisposed to this condition by defects in the vein walls or valves. Legs should be elevated whenever possible, and restrictive clothing should be avoided to enhance the flow of venous blood. There is an increased risk of blood clots in these areas, particularly after delivery.

When a pregnant woman lies in a **supine** position, the inferior vena cava may be compressed by the heavy uterus, resulting in decreased venous return to the heart and less cardiac output, leading to potential **hypotension** or low blood pressure. Lying on the left side usually facilitates maternal blood flow back to the heart and increases output to the placenta and the fetus.

Thinkabout 9–1

Explain how the pressure of a large uterus would affect the filling of the bladder and the frequency of urination.

Other changes in the reproductive system include increased vascularity of the **cervix** and **vagina**, resulting in a softening of the tissues (Goodell's sign) and a typical deeper purplish color (Chadwick's sign). Cervical mucus is more abundant and thick and forms a cervical plug to protect the uterine contents from foreign material and microbes. Vaginal secretions increase and become more acidic (pH 3.5–6.0), which is a deterrent to some infecting organisms but when combined with increased glycogen content promotes yeast or monilial infections during pregnancy.

The breasts become larger as the ducts and glands develop preparatory to milk production, and fatty deposits in the breast tissue increase. Bluish veins on the surface become more prominent.

WEIGHT GAIN AND NUTRITION

The average weight gain during pregnancy is 11 to 14 kg or 25 to 30 pounds, much of which occurs in the last trimester. The increased size of the uterus and its contents (the placenta, amniotic fluid, and fetus), the enlarged breasts, the additional blood volume, and stored nutrients or fat all contribute to the weight gain. There is an increased demand for protein, carbohydrate, fat, and minerals to promote tissue development during pregnancy. The metabolic rate of the mother increases in the latter half of pregnancy. However, excess food intake is stored as adipose tissue (fat).

The fetus stores iron in the last trimester to provide for its needs during the first few months after delivery. Adequate calcium is required for fetal bones and teeth. It is a myth that calcium is drawn from the mother's teeth to supply the fetus. Food cravings and fatigue may create nutritional problems and increase dental **caries** of (tooth decay) because the focus is often snack foods

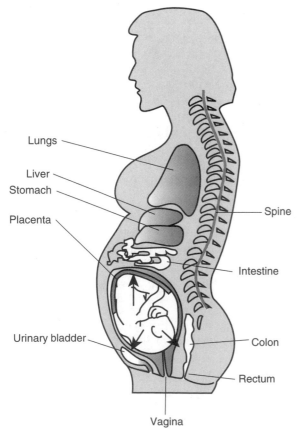

Lungs

Liver

Stomach

Placenta

Spine

Intestine

Urinary bladder

Colon

Rectum

Vagina

FIGURE 9–1. Sagittal section of pregnant woman.

that have a high carbohydrate or fat content but lack other nutrients. Prenatal care should include a dental consultation to ensure good oral hygiene.

The other common complication of pregnancy that may affect dietary control is the development of *diabetes mellitus* during pregnancy (see Chapter 21). Glucose levels in the urine and blood should be monitored in women in whom there is a family history of diabetes.

DIGESTIVE SYSTEM CHANGES

Nausea and vomiting are common in the first trimester because of the hormonal changes that occur in pregnancy. Changes in eating pattern often reduce discomfort. Frequent small meals, avoidance of fatty or spicy foods, and a reduced fluid intake with meals are suggested. Medication is recommended only in severe cases. The combination drug doxylamine-pyridoxine has been studied extensively and appears to be safe. Severe vomiting, or *hyperemesis gravidarum* may lead to dehydration and electrolyte imbalances and may affect nutrition at a critical point in fetal development. Hospital care is advised for these individuals.

Relaxation of smooth muscle in the stomach and intestines by progesterone results in decreased motility in the digestive tract, slow emptying of the stomach, reflux of stomach contents into the esophagus (*heartburn*), and feelings of bloating and abdominal discomfort. The pressure of the expanding uterus interferes with digestive function also. Constipation is common owing to decreased gastric motility and iron supplements. If chronic, constipation may lead to hemorrhoids, which are dilated veins in the rectum. These can become very painful and may bleed or become infected.

Thinkabout 9–2

a. Suggest a reason for maternal weight loss during the first trimester.
b. List three potential effects of excessive intake of foods associated with food cravings.

MUSCULOSKELETAL CHANGES

Marked postural changes occur in the mother as pregnancy progresses. The pelvic joints relax or loosen as hormones prepare the pelvis for delivery, resulting in a loss of stability and a *waddling gait*. The increased abdominal weight leads to a shift in the center of gravity and a tendency toward lordosis or increased lumbar curvature. These changes may lead to backache, particularly if the back and abdominal muscles are weak. Continued regular moderate exercise during pregnancy is helpful in maintaining good posture as well as cardiovascular fitness.

Thinkabout 9–3

Suggest several ways of reducing or preventing backache.

CARDIOVASCULAR CHANGES

Blood volume, including the relative volumes of both fluid and erythrocytes, is greatly increased to meet the metabolic needs of the fetus. For example, blood flow to the uterus and kidneys is increased to supply more oxygen to the fetus and uterine tissue and to remove wastes. Vascular resistance tends to decrease because smooth muscle is relaxed somewhat owing to the effects of progesterone. The heart rate may increase slightly, and blood pressure frequently drops slightly in the first two trimesters but then increases again to normal during the last trimester.

The increased blood volume leads to congestion and edema in many tissues. For instance, there may be nasal congestion, which affects breathing. **Gingivitis** or inflammation of the tissues around the teeth (gums) is common, causing bleeding. Fatigue or stress may impede daily oral hygiene, resulting in more severe *pregnancy gingivitis* and caries.

The increased production of red blood cells for the fetus requires increased iron intake by the mother. Iron supplements are frequently required. Because of a relatively greater increase in fluid, the **hematocrit** decreases slightly, and the woman appears to have a low hemoglobin (physiologic anemia).

Thinkabout 9–4

Using your knowledge of normal blood pressure controls, explain why blood pressure does not rise when blood volume increases during pregnancy.

POTENTIAL COMPLICATIONS OF PREGNANCY

Ectopic Pregnancy

Commonly called tubal pregnancy, an ectopic pregnancy occurs when the fertilized ovum is implanted outside the uterus. The incidence has been increasing recently, perhaps because of an increase in pelvic inflammatory disease or improved diagnosis. In most cases, implantation occurs in the fallopian tube. Spontaneous abortion may follow in the early stages of pregnancy, or the embryo may continue to develop, eventually causing the tube to rupture. This may lead to severe hemorrhage or **peritonitis.** Surgery is the usual treatment, although drug therapy is now being investigated.

Pregnancy-Induced Hypertension: Preeclampsia and Eclampsia

Pregnancy-induced **hypertension** (PIH) is persistently elevated blood pressure (over 140/90) that develops after 20 weeks of gestation and returns to normal following delivery. A specific cause has not been determined. PIH, if not controlled, may lead to damaged blood vessels in tissues such as the kidneys and retina of the eye or to stroke or heart failure. The decreased blood flow to the uterus may cause premature degeneration of the placenta and presents a risk to the fetus. The efficacy of low doses of ASA (aspirin) in controlling PIH continues to be investigated.

Preeclampsia and eclampsia are more serious conditions in which the blood pressure is higher, and kidney involvement is indicated by proteinuria, weight gain, and generalized edema (face, hands, feet, and legs). In some patients, a complication of preeclampsia develops. Known by the acronym HELLP, this condition includes hemolysis, increased serum bilirubin, increased serum liver enzymes, and decreased platelet count. In a few cases, HELLP progresses to coagulation disorders such as disseminated intravascular coagulation, as indicated by excessive bleeding. Preeclampsia may progress to eclampsia in which the blood pressure becomes extremely high, and generalized seizures (grand mal) or coma develop. Immediate hospitalization is required for adequate treatment of eclampsia.

Thinkabout 9–5

Compare the signs of PIH with those of eclampsia.

Placental Problems

Placenta previa occurs when the placenta is implanted in the lower uterus or over the **os**. As the uterus expands and contracts near the end of pregnancy, the placenta is torn, and bleeding occurs. The sign is painless bright red bleeding. Diagnosis is confirmed by ultrasound. Any hemorrhage during pregnancy places both mother and fetus at risk and requires immediate assessment and intervention.

Abruptio placentae refers to premature separation of the placenta from the uterine wall, resulting in bleeding that may or may not be evident vaginally, depending on where the tear occurs. The blood is often dark red, and abdominal pain is common. Abruptio placentae usually occurs during the last trimester.

Thinkabout 9–6

Using your knowledge of normal cardiovascular function, explain why any hemorrhage is serious for both mother and fetus.

Blood Clotting Problems

THROMBOPHLEBITIS AND THROMBOEMBOLISM

Thromboembolism, or blood clots, are more common following childbirth and usually develop in the veins of the legs or pelvis (see Chapter 16). **Thrombus** may form spontaneously (phlebothrombosis), usually because of stasis of blood or increased coagulability of the blood, or the clot may form over an inflamed vein wall (thrombophlebitis). If a piece of the thrombus breaks away (an **embolus**), it will flow with the venous blood to the right side of the heart and then into the lungs, where it will lodge in a pulmonary artery or smaller branch, obstructing blood flow in the lungs. This is a *pulmonary embolus* (see Chapter 17), which, if large, can be very serious and can affect respiratory and cardiovascular function. It is important not to massage a leg that is painful or red until the risk of thrombus has been eliminated.

DISSEMINATED INTRAVASCULAR COAGULATION

Disseminated intravascular coagulation (DIC) is not a primary problem but is a further complication of events such as abruptio placentae and preeclampsia. In DIC an excessive activation of the clotting mechanism occurs, resulting in diffuse blood clots and consumption of all clotting factors. Diagnosis is confirmed by the low serum levels of clotting factors. This situation then leads to hemorrhage. The formation of multiple thrombi causes organ damage, but the signs of DIC are usually related to hemorrhage. Bleeding may occur from the uterus, at injection sites, from the nose or mouth, under the skin (purpura), or internally.

Thinkabout 9–7

Differentiate a thrombus from an embolus.

Rh Incompatibility

Blood incompatibility can develop when the ABO or Rh factor antigens on fetal red blood cells differ from those on maternal blood cells. Rh incompatibility can be more serious when it leads to hemolytic disease of the newborn (erythroblastosis fetalis). Rh incompatibility results when the mother is Rh negative and the fetus is Rh positive. During the first pregnancy there are usually no problems unless the mother has been exposed to Rh-positive blood at some prior time through a blood product or abortion. At the end of the first pregnancy, when the placenta tears during delivery, some Rh-positive fetal blood enters the maternal circulation, causing the formation of antibodies to Rh-positive cells in the mother. During subsequent pregnancies, the maternal Rh antibodies cross to the fetus. The resulting antigen-antibody reaction in the fetus destroys the fetal red blood cells. **Hemolysis** of red blood cells leads to severe anemia or low hemoglobin and possible heart failure and death in the child. Hemolysis also causes high serum **bilirubin** levels in the child, resulting in **jaundice** (yellow color in the eyes and skin) and potential neurologic damage (kernicterus).

If the fetus is experiencing severe hemolysis in utero, an early birth or intrauterine transfusion may be recommended. After birth, an exchange transfusion may be required. When the neonate is jaundiced, phototherapy (exposure of the newborn's body to fluorescent or blue light) can reduce serum bilirubin levels by promoting conjugation of bilirubin and excretion in the bile.

Routine screening of maternal blood for Rh antibodies (indirect Coombs' test) is carried out early in pregnancy and at regular intervals during the pregnancy. If the mother has *not* become sensitized and developed antibodies, for example, during the first pregnancy, she can be given passive immunity at the time of delivery to suppress the immune response temporarily (see Chapter 3). This is done by administering Rh **immunoglobulin** (RhoGAM) to the mother within 72 hours of delivery. This process prevents sensitization of the mother when fetal red blood cells enter her body at this time.

Infection

Localized wound infections are usually contained if they are treated quickly. *Puerperal infection* (childbed fever) is infection of the reproductive tract at any time during the 6 weeks following birth. It may be endogenous (due to vaginal flora) or exogenous (due to causes in the environment). Cervical lacerations or episiotomy repair are vulnerable to infection. Common organisms include group B hemolytic *Streptococcus*, *Escherichia coli*, *Staphylococcus aureus*, mycoplasma, and *Chlamydia trachomatis*.

A predisposition to *endometritis* (inflammation of the uterine lining) may be caused by the separation of the placenta, which leaves raw tissue and allows easy access of organisms from the vagina. Any retained placental fragments also promote infection. Signs of infection include fever, vomiting, lower abdominal pain, and foul discharge from the vagina. The infection may spread to cause *pelvic cellulitis* (infection in the connective tissues or broad ligament of the pelvis) or *peritonitis* (infection of the peritoneal membranes) (see Chapter 18). Peritonitis results from infection that spreads directly along the fallopian tubes into the peritoneal cavity and is a serious complication of childbirth. Peritonitis is manifested by severe pain, high fever, tachycardia, and abdominal distention. Scar tissue resulting from infection that involves the fallopian tubes or ovaries may cause infertility. Pelvic abscess, a localized infection, may persist following peritonitis.

Adolescent Pregnancy

The period of adolescence is a time of growth, change, and maturation in many areas (see Chapter 8). The adolescent has increased nutritional needs to meet the demands of her own growth, and, in addition, dietary intake, physical activity, and hormonal changes are more erratic during this period. Pregnancy at this time is frequently risky because the adolescent may not seek prenatal care early in the pregnancy, and therefore proper nutrition is ignored, the presence of iron-deficiency anemia or any infection is unknown, and assessment of adequate pelvic development does not take place. There may be psychosocial implications, and other factors such as maternal smoking may have to be resolved. Thus, these babies frequently weigh less than normal or are preterm, and the mother has a difficult delivery owing to the immature pelvic structure. For the mother, pregnancy-induced hypertension (high blood pressure) is a common complication. If the adolescent accepts prenatal guidance and support, the pregnancy may proceed with minimal complications.

STUDY QUESTIONS

1. Suggest some possible signs of pregnancy resulting from physiologic changes.

2. Suggest some guidelines for fluid and food intake that would optimize fetal development and minimize complications or discomfort for the mother. Include a rationale for each.

3. Explain how a good fitness program is helpful in several ways during pregnancy.

4. Suggest several signs or symptoms of the development of postpartum infection.

CHAPTER
10
Aging and Disease Processes

KEY TERMS

• •

arteriosclerosis	collagen	kyphosis	periodontal disease
articular cartilage	compliance	mitosis	plaques
atherosclerosis	dyspareunia	neurofibrils	presbyopia
atrophy	fracture	neurotransmitter	retina
autoimmune	frequency	nocturia	sedentary
carcinogen	glaucoma	osteoarthritis	senescence
cataract	incontinence	osteoblastic	xerostomia
cholesterol	intervertebral disc	osteoporosis	

THE AGING PROCESS

Aging begins after birth but becomes more evident at about 30 years of age. **Senescence** refers to the period of life from old age to death. The effects of the aging process vary greatly among individuals and do not necessarily match *chronologic* age. At present more people are living longer largely because of improved social and living standards, improved nutrition, and better health care. Aging is a natural process, but it may be related to pathologic processes. Degenerative changes associated with aging may predispose an individual to certain pathologies, and pathologic changes can hasten aging. This chapter covers only some of the more significant effects of aging that are linked to pathologic problems. For additional information a gerontology reference should be consulted.

With aging a general reduction in function occurs throughout the body at the cellular and organ level, and the body is characterized by a decreased capacity to adapt to change. There are different theories about the causes of aging. One theory suggests that aging is programmed genetically through the cells and that this control directly limits the cell's reproductive capacity. Other possible causes include cellular damage resulting from accumulated wastes and altered protein (amyloid) or lipid (lipofuscin) components or increased **collagen** cross-linkages. Some theories suggest that aging is related to resident latent viruses or to increased **autoimmune** reactions in which the body rejects its own tissues or to other environmental agents that affect cells. It is likely that many factors contribute to the aging process and that these factors vary in individuals.

Cells assume less regular arrangements in tissues later in life. There is a loss of elastic fibers and an increased number of collagen cross-linkages or other abnormal structures in tissues and organs. **Mitosis** or cellular reproduction gradually slows down, resulting in decreased tissue repair. Some cells such as neurons and muscle cells cannot replicate, and when they die function is reduced in these tissues. Certain cells appear to have limits on the number of times they can replicate, and therefore they are not replaced in older individuals. Other cells accumulate wastes or are altered by environmental factors and become less functional. This exposure to numerous environmental factors such as radiation, viral infections, and chemicals over the years leads to an increased risk of cancer in older people.

Thinkabout 10–1

a. List changes in the tissues of the body that occur with aging.

b. List the signs of aging you have noted in individuals of 30 years, 50 years, and 80 years old.

SIGNIFICANT PHYSIOLOGIC CHANGES WITH AGING

Hormonal Changes

Generally, hormone secretions remain relatively constant with advancing age, but the number of tissue receptors may decrease, thus diminishing the body's response to hormones. This effect is apparent in disorders such as type II diabetes mellitus, which is common in older persons. In this condition, sufficient insulin is produced, but because the number of cell receptors is reduced, glucose does not enter the cells (see Chapter 21). In the absence of any pathology, the pituitary, thyroid, parathyroids, adrenals, and pancreas appear to maintain relatively normal function, producing hormones in adequate quantities.

The major natural hormonal change occurs in women at the time of menopause at about age 50, when the ovaries cease to produce estrogen and progesterone; subsequently, serum levels of follicle-stimulating hormone (FSH) and luteinizing hormone (LH) rise in response to natural feedback mechanisms (see Chapter 21). The effects of the decreased estrogen and progesterone will be described in the following sections. Although there is a gradual decrease in testosterone levels in the male, the testes do not totally cease to function.

Reproductive System Changes

Menopause is the term given to the change that occurs in women at around age 50, when the ovaries cease to respond to FSH and LH, resulting in lack of ovulation, cessation of the menstrual cycle, and declining estrogen and progesterone levels. The decreased levels of sex hormones lead to changes such as thinning of the mucosa, loss of elasticity, and decreased secretions in the vagina and cervix. These changes may cause inflammation and **dyspareunia,** or painful sexual intercourse. The pH of the vaginal secretions becomes more alkaline, thus predisposing the woman to recurrent vaginal infections. Breast tissue also decreases in volume. These changes in hormone levels frequently lead to systemic signs such as "hot flashes," which involve periodic sweating or vascular disturbances, and also to headaches, irritability, and insomnia. The effects of menopause may be felt for short or long periods of time (several years) and are more marked in some women than in others. Approximately 25 percent of women experience significant effects. If surgical removal of the ovaries is necessary prior to natural menopause, similar effects will be evident.

In males, testosterone levels decline gradually, the testes decrease in size, sperm production is somewhat reduced, and the glandular secretions of the prostate are decreased, but the older male is capable of fathering a child. The common problem in older males is *benign prostatic hypertrophy* (BPH; see Chapter 19), in which the central part of the gland around the urethra hypertrophies, resulting in some degree of obstruction of the urethra. If urinary flow is significantly impaired, surgery may be necessary.

Cancer of the reproductive organs is more common in both males (prostatic cancer) and females (uterine and breast cancer) in later years and is frequently related to altered hormonal levels. Frequent examinations by a physician in addition to breast self-examination are essential to lessen the risk of advanced malignancy.

Thinkabout 10–2

a. Compare the changes in reproductive hormones and structures that occur in older males and females.

b. Using your knowledge of the normal actions of the sex hormones, suggest some effects of decreased secretion of sex hormones on various body tissues and structures. (You may refer to Chapter 8 on Adolescence for help with hormonal actions.)

Cardiovascular Changes

Age-related changes occur in the cardiac muscle fibers and the connective tissue in the heart. Fatty tissue and collagen fibers accumulate in the heart muscle with aging and may eventually interfere with impulse conduction and cardiac muscle contraction. The size and number of cardiac muscle cells declines, reducing the strength of cardiac contractions. Cardiac muscle fibers do not undergo mitosis and cannot be replaced. Heart valves often thicken and therefore become less flexible and efficient. In some individuals, vascular degeneration causes a decrease in the oxygen supply to the heart muscle and reduces the ability of the heart muscle to utilize oxygen. Thus, cardiac output and cardiac reserve are diminished. Again, a regular fitness program is most helpful in maximizing cardiac function.

The common pathologies of the cardiovascular system are associated with degenerative changes in the arteries, both in the heart and throughout the body (see Chapter 16). Loss of elasticity and accumulation of collagen in the arterial walls result in thickening of the arterial walls, thus limiting expansion of the large arteries and obstructing the lumens of smaller arteries. This leads to **arteriosclerosis** and elevated blood pressure. Also, degenerative changes promote the accumulation of **cholesterol** and lipid in the walls of large arteries, the condition known as **atherosclerosis,** particularly when the individual has elevated blood lipid levels. These lipid plaques obstruct blood flow and predispose to thrombus formation. Atherosclerosis is a common cause of angina, myocardial infarctions (heart attacks), peripheral vascular disease in the legs, and strokes. Dietary changes, including reduced cholesterol intake, and regular exercise programs often reduce blood lipid and cholesterol levels and lessen the risk of vascular degeneration and high blood pressure.

Thinkabout 10–3

a. Based on your general knowledge can you suggest ways of restricting the diet to reduce the risk of cardiovascular problems?

b. Suggest different types of exercise appropriate for older individuals and explain how regular exercise can delay the onset of degenerative changes.

c. Describe the outcome of a blocked artery.

Musculoskeletal Changes

The important change in bone with aging is loss of calcium, which leads to **osteoporosis** (Fig. 10–1). Osteoporosis occurs more frequently in postmenopausal

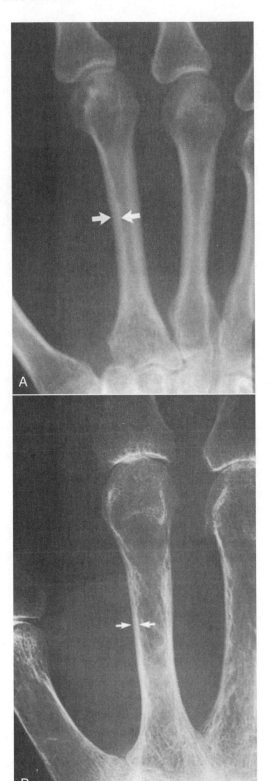

FIGURE 10–1. *A,* Normal metacarpal bone. *B,* Osteoporotic metacarpal bone. (From Helms CA: Fundamentals of Skeletal Radiology, 2nd ed. Philadelphia, WB Saunders, 1995.)

women but can occur in other people as well. Several factors are associated with osteoporosis, including decreased estrogen levels, decreased weight-bearing activity or stress on bone, decreased calcium intake and absorption, and decreased **osteoblastic** activity. Deposition of new bone is reduced, leading to decreased bone mass and density. The bones are often porous and brittle, thus precipitating frequent **fractures**, in areas such as the vertebrae and pelvis. Spontaneous vertebral fractures result in decreased height and **kyphosis** with increased age. As the thoracic curvature increases, the individual compensates by increasing the cervical curvature and tilting the head, leading to a typical hunchback posture and a shuffling gait.

Degeneration of the cartilage in the joints is a common problem that results in **osteoarthritis** (see Chapter 22). In this condition, the **articular cartilage** becomes thin and erosions occur, impairing joint movement and causing pain, particularly in the large weight-bearing joints such as the knees and hips. In some cases, bone spurs or overgrowths develop at points of stress, further restricting movement. The fibrocartilage in the **intervertebral discs** degenerates and may result in herniation of the disc, causing pressure on the spinal nerves and severe back pain (see Chapter 20). The intervertebral discs also become thin, contributing to loss of height.

Skeletal muscle mass declines with aging due to both **atrophy** and a decreased number of fibers. Skeletal muscle fibers cannot be replaced. Loss of muscle and subcutaneous tissue leads to an increased susceptibility to skin breakdown and pressure-related ulcers because of the reduced cushion between skin and bone. There is some decrease in the strength of muscle contractions, but this also depends on the activity level of the individual. Flexibility is reduced as elastic fibers degenerate throughout the body. Often movements become slower, stiffness becomes evident, and coordination and balance are reduced; these changes are associated with changes in the musculoskeletal structures as well as the neurologic components. Dressing, walking, food preparation, and many other daily activities require a long time to complete. Regular moderate exercise helps to delay the onset of degenerative changes, both by increasing the efficiency and activity of muscle and bone and by improving the circulation of blood to the tissues. Good nutrition, particularly protein, minerals, and vitamins, is also important in maintaining the integrity of the basic structures in older people.

Respiratory Changes

In aging individuals **compliance** in the lungs is decreased for several reasons. Elasticity in the tissues is reduced. The costal cartilage between the ribs and the

Thinkabout 10–4

a. Using your knowledge of normal physiology, suggest how improved circulation with exercise could slow the onset of degenerative changes in the musculoskeletal system.

b. Why would severe trauma to skeletal muscle such as a crush injury have permanently disabling effects?

sternum calcifies, reducing rib movement. Skeletal muscle atrophies, and any skeletal change may reduce thoracic movement. Decreased compliance leads to decreased expansion for deep breathing and coughing and a decreased expiratory volume. Vital capacity is therefore reduced, and residual volume is increased. The intercostal muscles also tend to be weaker, further reducing cough effort. When the capability for initiating an effective cough is impaired, secretions tend to accumulate, and the risk of pneumonia increases.

Vascular degeneration in the lungs leads to decreased perfusion and reduced gas exchange in the alveoli. There tends to be a reduced oxygen level rather than an increased carbon dioxide level. Oxygen therapy may be helpful in assisting respiratory function and supporting physical activity.

Neurologic Changes

Because neurons are not replaced after birth, a natural reduction in brain mass occurs with aging. Loss may occur in different areas of the brain and to varying degrees, and in many cases it does not have a significant effect on function because there is a considerable reserve of neurons. Maintenance of high activity levels and stimulation of the nervous system in the later years appear to assist in maintaining brain function.

Some of the degenerative changes observed in the brain tissue include lipid accumulations in the neurons, loss of the myelin sheath, and development of abnormal **neurofibrils** (masses of tiny, tangled fibrils) and **plaques** on the cells. Vascular impairment such as arteriosclerosis hastens the degenerative process. Neurofibrils and plaques are present in much higher numbers in those who become mentally incompetent through organic brain syndrome, a condition that includes senile dementia and Alzheimer's disease (see Chapter 20). There also appears to be a decreased cellular response in the brain to **neurotransmitter** chemicals such as norepinephrine, leading to delays in synaptic transmission.

General changes in function commonly noticed in older persons include slower response time, decreased reflexes, and short-term memory lapses. The elderly can learn new information and skills. Sometimes the learning process is slower because the individual incorporates past experiences and uses more functions of the brain rather than learning by rote. The autonomic nervous system does not always provide adequate adaptation, resulting in decreased tolerance to extreme hot or cold temperatures. The elderly feel chilled owing to poor blood circulation, decreased metabolism, and decreased activity levels. Often there is reduced temperature sensitivity in the skin when touching hot or cold surfaces.

Changes usually occur in the special senses as well. In the eye, the iris and its associated muscles degenerate, resulting in decreased adaptation by the pupil to light and possible obstruction of flow of aqueous humor, leading to increased intraocular pressure and **glaucoma** (see Chapter 20). The lens becomes yellow and less transparent, interfering with color perception, especially blue hues. Night vision is impaired, and many elderly people are unable to drive safely at night. The lens eventually may become opaque as **cataracts** develop. If vision is lost, surgery may be required to remove the cataract. The lens also becomes larger and less elastic, causing **presbyopia** (far-sightedness) and possibly cataracts. Vascular degeneration may affect the **retina** of the eye, which contains the nerve cells for receiving images, and this condition causes permanent visual loss.

Hearing loss associated with aging is usually due to degenerative changes in the inner ear in either the nerve cells of the cochlea or the nerve fibers supplying the ear. In noisy surroundings it may become difficult to discriminate between sounds, impairing communication and deterring socialization.

The senses of taste and smell often diminish with aging. Taste may be altered by reduced salivary secretions or by decreased perception within the central nervous system. There is a reduced ability to discriminate among odors. Diminished powers of taste and smell may impair appetite and nutrition.

Thinkabout 10–5

Describe four neurologic changes that can be expected to occur in an older individual.

Gastrointestinal Changes and Nutrition

Maintenance of good nutrition is a concern in the elderly. In the mouth, loss of teeth due to **periodontal disease** (inflammation and infection in the tissue surrounding the teeth) and decreased salivary secretions frequently restrict dietary choices as the older person experiences difficulty in chewing many foods. Often dentures are not satisfactory for chewing as the gums and bone recede. The fragile tissues are easily irritated by ill-fitting dentures or accumulated food particles. **Xerostomia** or dry mouth is common because the amount of saliva is reduced. Decreased saliva may also result from use of certain drugs or from the mouth-breathing associated with many respiratory problems. Swallowing difficulties due to neurologic causes or mechanical obstructions such as scar tissue or hiatal hernia may develop (see Chapter 18). The need for a soft diet and other factors such as lack of socialization, fatigue, restricted mobility, or financial concerns may also limit food choices and interfere with nutritional status.

Obesity is common in some older individuals who lead **sedentary** lives. In some cases, excessive carbohydrate and fat intake may mask the signs of protein, fiber, or vitamin deficits. Obesity increases cardiac workload as well as the likelihood of atherosclerosis. Gallstones are also a complication of obesity, as is osteoarthritis in the weight-bearing joints.

Atrophy of the mucosa and glands of the digestive tract frequently reduces digestive secretions and absorption of essential nutrients. Absorption of vitamin B_{12}, calcium, and iron may be impaired. Decreased mucus secretion predisposes the older person to peptic ulcer development. Unfortunately, signs of ulcers are vague or may be masked by self-medication in the early stages.

Older individuals are predisposed to malignancies in the digestive tract, particularly in the stomach and colon, that may be related to hereditary factors as well as dietary intake. **Carcinogenic** substances in the diet are more hazardous when they are associated with con-

Thinkabout 10–6

a. Using your knowledge of normal physiology, list the factors that lead to constipation.

b. Describe several possible pathologic conditions involving the digestive tract in older people.

c. Explain why obesity is undesirable in the elderly.

stipation because of the prolonged exposure of the tissues to these substances during transit through the gut. Constipation is common in the elderly. Many factors contribute to it, including decreased activity, low fiber and fluid intake, and excessive use of laxatives. Chronic constipation frequently leads to hemorrhoids.

Urinary System Changes

Kidney function is reduced with aging owing to loss of glomeruli and degeneration of the tubules and blood vessels. The kidneys have a diminished ability to compensate for rapid changes in electrolyte and acid levels and may have a reduced capacity to secrete drugs into the urine, resulting in excessively high blood levels.

A major complication of aging is reduced control of bladder function as the muscles of the urethra and bladder become weaker. Reduced bladder capacity and incomplete bladder emptying result in frequency, **nocturia** and infection. In women the pelvic floor muscles have often been stretched and weakened by childbirth, reducing the ability of the external sphincter to restrict urinary outflow. Also, decreased estrogen levels may decrease smooth muscle tone. Sensory perception of a full bladder is reduced, and this problem, combined with a weakened urethral sphincter, often results in **incontinence** (involuntary voiding of urine). Incontinence usually results in incomplete emptying of the bladder, which leads to residual urine and frequent urinary tract and bladder infections (cystitis) (see Chapter 19).

OTHER FACTORS

Infections are common in the elderly, in whom poor circulation impairs the normal defense mechanisms, and tissue healing is delayed owing to the reduced rate of mitosis. Although the antibody pool is large, the immune response to new microbes is less effective because lymphocytes are slower to respond to antigens and are less active in the later years. Skin breakdown and ulcers may predispose those with immune deficient states to infection.

Cancer is more common because the immune system becomes a less effective surveillance unit and older people have had a higher cumulative exposure to carcinogens (see Chapter 5). There are more *autoimmune* disorders and more *degenerative* pathologies related to wear-and-tear, many of which are *chronic* progressive disorders. Adaptation to *stressors* is slower and more difficult because the tissues may be unable to respond to the increased demands. Many elderly people take a large number of *medications*, both prescribed drugs and over-the-counter agents. These combinations increase the possibility of undesirable drug interactions. Other problems with medications in the elderly include a higher risk of idiosyncratic or unexpected reactions, toxic effects due to unpredictable absorption, distribution, and elimination of drugs, and impaired function such as lethargy or lack of coordination. As the tissue receptors and body mass change in the elderly, it is often necessary to adjust the dosage and combinations of medications.

STUDY QUESTIONS

1. Describe appropriate guidelines for a healthy diet for an older individual.

2. Explain the different ways in which regular moderate exercise can benefit an older person.

3. Suggest some reasons why the aging process varies among different individuals.

MUSCULOSKELETAL EFFECTS
CUTANEOUS EFFECTS
CARDIOVASCULAR EFFECTS
RESPIRATORY EFFECTS

GASTROINTESTINAL EFFECTS
URINARY EFFECTS
EFFECTS ON CHILDREN
STUDY QUESTIONS

KEY TERMS

atelectasis	decubitus ulcer	gravity	paraplegia
atrophy	edema	hemiplegia	peristalsis
basic metabolic rate	embolus	hypercalcemia	pneumonia
(BMR)	extensor	orthostatic hypotension	stasis
constipation	flaccidity	osteoblastic	supine
contracture	flexor	osteoclastic	thrombus

Immobility, or lack of movement, may involve only one part of the body, such as a fractured arm, the lower part of the body, as in people with **paraplegia,** one side of the body (**hemiplegia),** or the entire body as in a person in a coma or with an acute illness. The effects depend on the extent of the immobilization and on its duration. The amount of physiotherapy or passive exercise imposed on the involved area of the body can minimize the effects of lack of movement.

When the body is **supine,** the loss of the force of **gravity** affects many of its natural functions. Noticeable effects result from the lack of stress normally exerted on bone by skeletal muscle and on the decreased circulation of blood. Also affected are respiratory function, metabolism, and renal function.

MUSCULOSKELETAL EFFECTS

Inactive muscle loses strength, endurance, and mass very quickly. Perhaps you have seen an arm or a leg with *atrophied* muscle (often called disuse **atrophy**) after it has been confined to a cast for several weeks. Correct positioning and reduction of abnormal stress on immobilized muscles and joints are important because these

structures may stretch or shorten, resulting in abnormal fixation of a joint; for example, an ankle may develop "foot-drop" when a tight heavy blanket or improper positioning puts excessive and inappropriate pressure on the foot (Fig. 11–1). Generally, **flexor** muscles are stronger than the opposing **extensor** muscles, and this imbalance may allow an inactive joint to slip into an abnormal position if flexibility is not maintained by range-of-motion exercises. With inactivity, tendons and ligaments shorten and lose elasticity. With prolonged immobility, fibrous tissue replaces muscle cells, leading to muscle wasting and weakening and causing decreased flexibility, further deformity (**contracture**), and loss of function.

The lack of muscular activity impairs venous return, which causes pooling of blood in dependent areas of the body, development of dependent **edema**, and a decrease in cardiac output, which may cause dizziness or fainting.

Bone deteriorates with inactivity. It is a "living" tissue in which new bone is constantly forming (**osteoblastic** activity) and other bone is being resorbed (**osteoclastic** activity). Bone demineralization occurs because the lack of weight-bearing and muscle action reduces osteoblastic activity or bone formation; however osteoclastic ac-

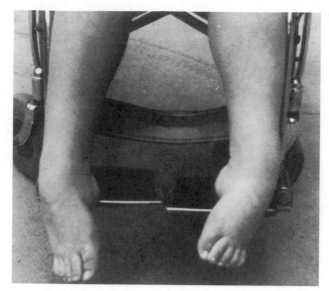

FIGURE 11–1. Contracture of the feet in a patient with muscular dystrophy. (From Jahss MH: Disorders of the Foot and Ankle, 2d ed. Vol. 1. Philadelphia, WB Saunders, 1991.)

tivity continues. This process leads to *osteoporosis* and the potential for spontaneous fractures if undue stress is placed on the bones.

The breakdown of muscle and bone tissue results in elevated serum levels of nitrogen wastes such as creatinine and elevated serum calcium. **Hypercalcemia** may cause renal calculi or kidney stones if fluid intake is inadequate and the urine is too concentrated (see Chapter 19). Also, high serum calcium levels can further impede muscle activity because it decreases muscle tone and leads to **flaccidity**.

Thinkabout 11–1

Briefly describe three effects of immobility on musculoskeletal structures.

CUTANEOUS EFFECTS

The skin breaks down easily when its circulation is impaired and cell regeneration is reduced. Blood supply is often reduced in places where bony projections are close to the skin and there is little fatty or muscular tissue to cushion the weight of the body. Areas that are particularly vulnerable to poor blood perfusion include the ischial tuberosities and sacrum on the trunk, the

heels, and the elbows. Pressure at these points causes ischemia and necrosis of tissue. Other factors that promote skin breakdown and development of **decubitus ulcers** (pressure sores) include generally poor circulation, edema, mechanical irritation or friction by clothing, braces, or other equipment, excessive moisture from perspiration or urine, poor hygiene, anemia, and inadequate nutrition or hydration. The skin is easily traumatized by clothing or sheets if a patient is moved without due care or slides down in bed, or if skeletal muscle spasms occur. Adhesive tape may irritate the skin directly or indirectly when it is removed. Elderly people, who have less subcutaneous tissue and more fragile skin, are more prone to ulcer development.

The risk of skin breakdown can be reduced if sensitive areas are protected by sheepskin pads or flotation devices and the patient's position is changed frequently to avoid prolonged pressure in certain areas, thereby maintaining adequate circulation. Tissue ischemia and impending skin breakdown can be expected when redness persists after any pressure is relieved or when the area appears edematous or purple. The ulceration often extends into the deeper tissues and is very slow to heal because the predisposing factors often remain.

Thinkabout 11–2

a. Explain why frequent changes of position are helpful in maintaining skin integrity.

b. List some specific factors that have caused you discomfort when you have been resting for a long time.

c. Suggest several specific ways of reducing the risk of skin breakdown and ulceration.

CARDIOVASCULAR EFFECTS

When a person is first immobilized, the horizontal body position leads to more blood pooling in the trunk, especially the lungs, rather than the legs and more blood returning easily to the heart. Initially, this added blood volume leads to an increased work load for the heart, which increases the heart rate and stroke volume. With *prolonged* immobility and bed rest, venous return and cardiac output are reduced, and the client is subject to **orthostatic hypotension** with periods of dizziness or fainting, pallor and sweating, and rapid pulse whenever the body position is changed. Normally, skeletal muscle contractions assist in returning the venous blood to the heart, and, when the body position changes from supine to upright, reflex vasoconstriction occurs in the skin and viscera to promote venous return. Adequate venous return ensures sufficient cardiac output to supply the brain and prevent a drop in blood pressure and fainting. When a patient first becomes mobile after a prolonged period of bed rest, it may take several weeks for the reflex controls to return to normal, ensuring adequate circulation.

Other problems occur when the blood pools in dependent areas. The increased volume of blood in these areas leads to increased capillary pressure and edema (see Chapter 6). A persistent increase in interstitial fluid (edema) leads to reduced arterial flow and capillary exchange of nutrients, thus predisposing the person to tissue necrosis, ulcers, and infection in the area.

The **stasis** of blood associated with immobility promotes **thrombus** formation in the veins, particularly in the legs. In addition to sluggish blood flow, blood clots may be encouraged by compression or damage to blood vessels resulting from pressure related to the body position in bed or a wheelchair. Blood clotting is also encouraged in patients with dehydration or cancer by the increased coagulability of the blood associated with these conditions. Thrombi are a threat because they may break away with movement or massage, resulting in pulmonary **emboli,** which have serious consequences for respiratory and cardiovascular function (see Chapter 17).

RESPIRATORY EFFECTS

Initially, when a person is immobilized there is less demand for oxygen because metabolism is decreased, unless some factor such as infection is increasing the **basic metabolic rate (BMR),** and therefore the respiratory system can easily meet the body's requirements. Usually, respirations become slow and shallow.

Deep breathing and coughing become more difficult because chest expansion is restricted by body weight when the person is supine in bed and by the upward pressure of the abdominal contents against the diaphragm. Gas exchange is decreased as thoracic capacity is reduced and air flow is diminished. Any muscle weakness will impair the effectiveness of respiratory efforts. Many drugs, including sedatives (to promote sleep and reduce anxiety) and analgesics (to control pain), depress neuromuscular activity and the respiratory control center, leading to slow shallow respirations.

When a person is immobilized, secretions build up in the airways and are difficult to remove because the cough mechanism is less effective. Ciliary action may be reduced if nutrition is impaired or if the patient is a smoker. Other factors leading to increased secretions in the lungs include more viscous mucus due to dehydration and inflammation due to instrumentation. Increased fluids further impair lung expansion. Stasis of secretions predisposes the patient to serious respiratory complications. The increased mucous secretions frequently lead to infection (hypostatic **pneumonia**) or obstruction of the airway and collapse of the lung (**atelectasis**). Pneumonia and atelectasis may also result from aspiration of food or water intake, which occur more easily when the patient is immobilized or in a supine position. Normally, in the upright position, gravity assists the rapid movement of food down the esophagus.

Thinkabout 11–3

Explain why pneumonia is a common occurrence in immobilized persons.

GASTROINTESTINAL EFFECTS

The major problem associated with immobility and the gastrointestinal tract is **constipation**. Elimination is affected by the slower passage of feces through the intestine due to muscle inactivity and body position, both of which result in a harder stool. In ill people the intake of food, fiber, and fluid is often reduced, leading to reduced **peristalsis** in the intestine and more water absorption. Weakened muscles make defecation more difficult, as does the awkwardness of using a bedpan in a supine position.

With immobility, appetite is often reduced, leading to decreased dietary intake. This may result in a negative nitrogen balance (protein deficit), especially when muscle tissue is breaking down. The protein imbalance contributes to a low hemoglobin level and delays in healing. Unfortunately, the decreased food intake usually aggravates fatigue and depression, which further decrease appetite and ultimately may cause malnutrition and further delays in healing and recovery. If normal nutrition cannot be maintained orally, it may be necessary to use total parenteral nutrition (TPN), in which the required nutrient solution is administered directly into a vein.

URINARY EFFECTS

Stasis of urine in the kidneys or bladder frequently causes infection or renal calculi (stones) to develop in the urinary tract (see Chapter 19). A supine position leads to residual urine in the renal calices because normal drainage by gravity into the ureter is impeded. It is also difficult to empty the bladder completely into a bedpan when one is supine or when the muscles are weakened. Renal calculi are more likely to develop in people with hypercalcemia due to prolonged immobility or with reduced fluid intake. Bladder infection (cystitis) is common in immobilized people if calculi form or if catheters are used to drain the urine.

EFFECTS OF IMMOBILITY ON CHILDREN

When children are immobilized for an extended period of time, a delay in growth often occurs because the stimulus for bone and muscle development is lost. Depending on the underlying condition, deformities involving the hips, spine, hands, and feet may develop. Other developmental delays are common when sensory and experiential stimulation is decreased.

STUDY QUESTIONS

1. Explain how immobility affects the circulation.

2. Give several reasons why healing may be delayed during a period of immobility.

3. Explain how frequent changes of position would affect
   a. the amount of interstitial fluid in an area,
   b. respiratory function, and
   c. the skin.

CHAPTER
12
The Influence of Stress

KEY TERMS

• •

adaptation	endorphins	lipolysis	physiologic
bronchodilation	exacerbating factors	maladaptive	ulcers
catabolism	homeostasis	necrosis	vasoconstriction

REVIEW OF THE STRESS RESPONSE

The stress response is a generalized or systemic response to a change (stressor), internal or external, and may be modified in specific situations. The role of stress in disease has become more firmly established in the twentieth century, particularly since Hans Selye, in 1946, defined his general **adaptation** syndrome (GAS), or "fight or flight" concept. His work revealed that the body constantly responds to minor changes in its needs or environment, such as altered food intake or activity level, and thus maintains **homeostasis**. The body has built-in mechanisms that compensate for **physiologic** changes in fluid balance or blood pressure. Minor fluctuations in the body are normal. A *stressor* is any factor that creates a significant change in the body or the environment. It may be physical or psychological or a combination of the two. A stressor may be a real or anticipated, or a short- or long-term factor. Possible stressors include pain, exposure to cold temperatures, trauma, anxiety or fear, a new job, infection, or a joyous occasion. *Stress* is considered to occur when an individual's status is altered by his or her reaction to a stressor. The stress response is the basic but complex response made by the body to any stressor. The body's physiologic response to different stressors is the same, although it may vary in intensity and effects in a given situation or

person. An additional specific response may occur with certain stressors; for example, infection may initiate a fever.

Each person may perceive stressors differently. A certain stressor for one individual may be exciting or stimulating, but for someone else the same stressor may be depressing. It may even cause illness in another person. If the individual can cope with the stressor, the body returns to its normal status, but if the person cannot adapt, harmful effects may result from the stress.

Stressors are a normal component of life and can be a positive influence on the body when appropriate coping mechanisms function well. Stressors may stimulate growth and development in many ways. Without any changes or stressors in life, a person would merely exist in a dull inert form. But if a stressor is severe or is perceived as a negative influence, or when multiple factors effect change at one time, the body's adaptive mechanisms may not suffice. Then the body systems become more disrupted, **maladaptive** behavior can occur, and homeostasis for that person is not possible. Factors such as aging or pathologic disorders may interfere with an individual's ability to respond to a stressor. A vicious cycle may develop when the original stressor remains, and the effects of this stressor prevent the body from coping with new stressors. More damage results, adding to the stress and lessening the person's coping capabilities even further, thereby decreasing the probability of a return to normal status. In the same way, maladaptive behaviors such as ignoring the stressor or eating unwisely are likely to add additional problems without removing the original stressful factor.

Thinkabout 12–1

a. Name two stressors present in your life at this time and two others that you have found difficult to cope with in the past.

b. Describe several coping mechanisms that you have found to be successful.

c. Describe several unsuccessful coping mechanisms you have tried.

d. Students usually find test-writing stressful. Suggest two ways to make the stress response helpful in this situation.

Selye originally defined three stages in the stress response (GAS). In the alarm stage, the body's defenses were mobilized by activation of the hypothalamus, sympathetic nervous system, and adrenal glands. In the second, or resistance stage, hormonal levels were elevated, and essential body systems operated at peak performance. The final stage, or stage of exhaustion, occurred when the body was unable to respond further or was damaged by the increased demands. Extensive research into various aspects of stress has followed Selye's work. It has been found that the stress response involves an integrated series of actions involving the hypothalamus and the hypophysis, the sympathetic nervous system, the adrenal medulla, and the adrenal cortex. The major actions are summarized in Figure 12–1. Significant effects of the stress response include elevated blood pressure and increased heart rate, **bronchodilation** and increased ventilation, increased blood glucose levels (resulting from glycogenolysis and gluconeogenesis in the liver and protein **catabolism** in muscle as well as **lipolysis**), arousal of the central nervous system, and decreased inflammatory and immune responses. These activities increase the general level of function in critical areas of the body such as the brain, heart, and skeletal muscle by such mechanisms as increasing oxygen levels, increasing circulation, and increasing the rate of cell metabolism. The stress response also results in an increased release of endorphins, which act as pain-blocking agents (see Chapter 13).

Thinkabout 12–2

a. Using your knowledge of normal physiology, explain the probable source of the increased glucose level in the blood with stress.

b. Name the organs in which vasoconstriction occurs and blood flow diminishes during a stress response. Name the areas that have increased blood flow.

c. State two ways by which oxygen supplies to the brain are increased.

d. List the hormones released during the stress response and two significant actions for each.

STRESS AND DISEASE

In most cases the body responds positively, the stressor is dealt with, the stress response diminishes, and body activity returns to normal. Sometimes, however, the stress response becomes a negative influence or a "distress" situation. In such cases the state of stress is severe or prolonged, or the individual's adaptive mechanisms are impaired for some reason. It may be noticed that when an illness requires additional treatment such as hospitalization or physiotherapy, extra stressors are added that may overwhelm the patient. For example, hospitalization may give rise to fear and pain, or to anxiety associated with separation from the family, change in routine and diet, and loss of privacy and control over one's life. In other cases, hospitalization may offer positive relief from the burden of illness.

A stress response may cause minor discomfort such as a headache, mouth **ulcers,** or nausea. More severe complications may arise if prolonged **vasoconstriction** in an area reduces function or causes tissue **necrosis**. In some patients who have preexisting pathologic conditions, a stress response may create an acute complication. For example, elevation of blood pressure due to a stress response may seriously aggravate the condition of an individual with a damaged heart.

Stress has been shown to be a precipitating or **exacerbating factor** in some disorders. The onset of cancer may follow a serious life crisis, which suggests that the immune system has been depressed. Many chronic diseases such as multiple sclerosis or rheumatoid arthritis are often aggravated by stress.

PROCESS

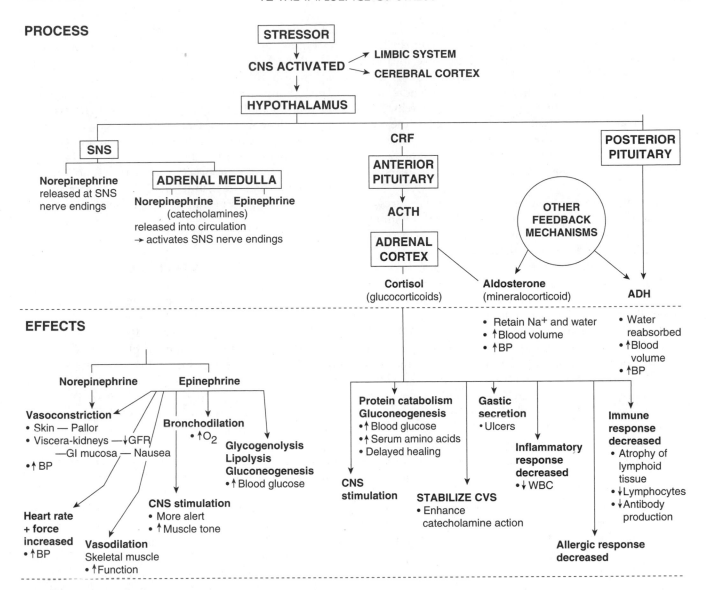

FIGURE 12-1. The stress response. CNS, Central nervous system; SNS, sympathetic nervous system; CRF, corticotropin releasing factor; ACTH, adrenocorticotropic hormone; ADH, antidiuretic hormone, GFR, glomerular filtration rate; GI, gastrointestinal; BP, blood pressure; WBC, white blood cell; CVS, cardiovascular system.

Potential Effects of Prolonged or Severe Stress

Severe stress may lead to a variety of serious complications such as renal failure or stress ulcers. *Acute renal failure* results from severe vasoconstriction and reduced blood supply to the kidney. Reduced blood supply causes tubule necrosis, obstruction of filtrate flow, and cessation of glomerular filtration (see Chapter 19).

Stress ulcers may develop with severe trauma, a good example being Curling's ulcers, which are associated with burns. Stress ulcers are multiple gastric ulcers, often asymptomatic, which frequently become manifest with gastric hemorrhage (see Chapter 18). Several factors in the stress response contribute to ulcer formation. Intense vasoconstriction in the gastric mucosa decreases mucosal regeneration and mucus production, decreased motility causes stasis of chyme in the stomach, and the catabolic effects of glucocorticoids delay tissue regeneration—all of which contribute to ulcer formation. When possible, preventive measures are taken to reduce the risk of complications from severe stress. For example, caregivers promote fluid flow through the kidney by encouraging increased hydration, and physicians order drugs that dilate the renal arterioles and thus protect renal function. Medications may be administered to protect the gastric mucosa and reduce acid secretions, thereby preventing ulcer development.

Another potential complication of severe stress is *infection*, which is related to depression of the inflammatory response and the immune system by increased cortisol secretion. Because these body defense mechanisms are reduced, opportunistic infections may develop, and the person becomes susceptible to infection by unusual organisms that are not normally pathogenic (see Chapter 3). The lack of an inflammatory response may mask the signs of infection until it is well established. In time, lymphoid tissue atrophies, and the circulating leukocytes are reduced in number and function. The increased incidence and growth of malignant tumors associated with severe stress has also been linked with the decreased efficiency of the surveillance function of the immune system.

Continued stress may impede the *healing* of tissue following trauma or surgery. Two major factors are involved. First, the increased amounts of cortisol reduce protein synthesis and tissue regeneration, and second, the increased catecholamine levels lead to vasoconstriction, reduced blood supply, and reduced delivery of nutrients to the area. In some cases, these effects lead to an increased risk of infection and increased amounts of scar tissue at the site.

Thinkabout 12-3

Explain how reduced blood flow in an area can interfere with healing and increase the risk of infection.

Stress-Related Disorders

In many chronic disorders stress is an exacerbating factor. The stressor may be physical or emotional. For example, rheumatoid arthritis, systemic lupus erythe-matosus, asthma, acne, herpes simplex (cold sores), ulcerative colitis, and eczema are some conditions that usually become more acute when a stressor is present. It is important for a person with a chronic illness to develop improved coping mechanisms for stress and an adequate support system to delay exacerbations or progressive degeneration in chronic illness.

In some diseases such as hypertension and coronary artery disease, stress is thought to be a developmental factor. It has been noted that serum cholesterol is elevated during stress, and the reactive vasoconstriction affects blood pressure and blood vessels when stress is sustained.

Coping with Stress

To prevent stress from becoming a negative influence on the body, it is important for each individual to recognize stress-inducing factors. People must take appropriate action to solve the problem or develop improved coping mechanisms if the stressor cannot be removed. For many people, this is easier to say than to do, especially when a stressor becomes overwhelming or when multiple stressors develop. A support system is essential to minimize the risk of development of pathologic effects due to stress. Strategies may include use of antianxiety medications (minor tranquilizers such as lorazepam) for a short term, or counseling and support services for a longer term. A change in life style may be necessary for some people to adapt to the new situation.

Many individuals benefit from learning relaxation techniques to maximize their coping abilities. Others find that regular moderate exercise assists in controlling stress, particularly if it is undertaken at midday. Aerobic exercise such as cycling, swimming, or running is useful to release muscle tension and improve circulation as well as to provide a distraction. During aerobic exercise the body uses more fats for energy, and therefore blood sugar levels remain more stable. A relatively constant blood supply to the brain prevents mood swings and reduces irritability. Other people prefer to engage in distracting activities for a time and then assess the problem more objectively. Some individuals deal with stressors methodically, assessing options or goals and making immediate decisions. Just as each person perceives stressors differently, each must develop an individualized set of coping mechanisms, and these skills will probably have to be modified periodically.

It is well to recognize any tendency toward maladaptive behavior at an early stage in the response to stress. Avoiding sleep, eating junk food, drinking too much coffee, and smoking constantly are behaviors that are more likely to add stress than to alleviate it.

STUDY QUESTIONS

1. List the factors or mechanisms in the stress response that contribute to increased oxygen supplies for the cells and explain how each factor contributes.

2. Describe a recent stressor in your life and the stress response that followed it.

3. List some disorders that are stress related.

4. Describe two potential complications of severe stress.

CHAPTER
13
Pain

KEY TERMS

afferent fibers
analgesic
anesthesia
bradykinin
cordotomy
dermatome
efferent

endogenous
histamine
hypothalamus
intractable
ischemia
lateral spinothalamic
    tract

neurotransmitter
nociceptors
opioids
parenterally
prostaglandins
reticular activating system
    (RAS)

reticular formation
rhizotomy
sedative
tachycardia
thalamus

Pain is difficult to define because it can have many variable characteristics. It is an unpleasant sensation, a feeling of discomfort resulting from stimulation of nociceptors when tissue damage occurs or is about to occur. Pain is a body defense mechanism and is a warning of a problem, particularly when it is acute. In cases of trauma, the danger may be obvious, but in other situations the cause may be hidden.

CAUSES OF PAIN

Pain may be caused by inflammation, infection, **ischemia** and tissue necrosis, stretching of tissue, chemicals, or burns. In skeletal muscle, pain may result from ischemia or hemorrhage. Viscera such as the liver or kidney become painful when the covering capsule is stretched by inflammation. In the digestive tract, pain may result from inflammation of the mucosa or from distention or muscle spasm.

PAIN PATHWAYS

Pain receptors or **nociceptors** are sensory free nerve endings that are present in most tissues of the body. These sensory nerves may be stimulated by thermal, chemical, or physical means. Thermal means refer to extremes of temperature, mechanical means could refer to pressure, and chemical sources could include acids or compounds produced in the body such as bradykinin, histamine or prostaglandins.

The *pain threshold* refers to the level of stimulation required to activate the nerve ending sufficiently for the individual to perceive pain. The associated nerve fibers then transmit the pain signal to the spinal cord and brain. There are two types of **afferent fibers** that conduct pain impulses: the small myelinated A delta fibers that transmit impulses very rapidly, and the large unmyelinated C fibers that transmit impulses slowly. Acute pain—the sudden, sharp pain related to thermal and physical stimuli—is transmitted by the A delta fibers, whereas chronic pain, often experienced as a dull burning or aching sensation, is transmitted by C fibers. C fibers receive thermal, physical, and chemical stimuli.

The peripheral nerves transmit the afferent pain impulse to the dorsal root ganglia and then into the spinal cord through the dorsal horn or substantia gelatinosa (see Chapter 20). Here at the synapse, a reflex response to sudden pain results in a motor, or efferent impulse back to the muscles that initiates an involuntary jerk away from the source of pain. After the impulse reaches the synapse, it crosses the spinal cord and ascends to the brain in the **lateral spinothalamic tract** (Fig. 13–1). This tract provides connections with the **reticular formation** in the brainstem, the **hypothalamus,** and the **thalamus** as it ascends to the somatic sensory area in the cerebral cortex of the parietal lobe of the brain. It is here that the location and characteristics of the pain are perceived. Each spinal nerve conducts impulses from a specific area of the skin called a **dermatome** (see Fig. 20–17), and the somatosensory cortex is "mapped" to correspond to areas of the body so that the source of the pain can be interpreted in the brain (see Fig. 20–1). The dermatomes can be used to test for areas of sensory loss and determine the site of damage following spinal cord injuries. The many branching connections from the ascending tracts provide information to other parts of the brain, forming the basis for an integrated response to pain.

Thinkabout 13–1

Trace the pathway of a pain impulse originating from touching a hot object by drawing a simple diagram and labeling the parts.

The arousal state of the **reticular activating system (RAS)** in the **reticular formation** in the pons and medulla influences the brain's awareness of the incoming pain stimuli. In clinical practice, many drugs depress the RAS, thereby decreasing the pain experienced. The hypothalamus plays a role in the response to pain through its connections with the pituitary gland and the sympathetic nervous system. Response to pain usually involves a stress response (see Chapter 12) as well as an emotional response such as crying, moaning, or angry words. There may be a physical response, perhaps rigidity, splinting, or guarding of an area of the body. The thalamus processes many types of sensory stimuli as they enter the brain and is important in the emotional response to pain through the limbic system.

Thinkabout 13–2

a. Describe your response to a sudden pain in your own experience, for example, an injury. Describe your physical response and your emotional reactions.
b. Using your knowledge of normal physiology, list the effects of increased sympathetic nervous system stimulation.

THEORY OF PAIN AND PAIN CONTROL

Pain is not an easily understood phenomenon. There are many variables in its source and perception and in the response to it. The *gate-control theory* is a useful explanation that can be related to many concepts of pain and pain control. According to this theory, control systems or "gates" are built into the normal pain pathways in the body that can modify the entry of pain stimuli into the spinal cord and brain. These gates at the nerve synapses in the spinal cord and brain can be open, thus permitting the pain impulses to pass from the peripheral nerves to the lateral spinothalamic tract and ascend to the brain (Fig. 13–2). Or they may be closed, reducing or modifying the passage of pain impulses. Gate closure can occur in response to other sensory stimuli that may diminish the pain sensations or modulate or inhibit impulses from the brain. For example, application of ice to a painful site may reduce pain because one is more aware of the cold than of the pain. Transcutaneous electrical nerve stimulation (TENS) is a therapeutic intervention that increases sensory stimulation at a site, thus blocking pain transmission. The brain can inhibit or modify incoming pain stimuli by producing efferent or outgoing transmissions through the reticular formation. Many factors can activate this control system, including prior conditioning, the emotional state of the affected person, or distraction away from the pain by other events. This last phenomenon has been observed in many individuals who feel no pain when injured suddenly but do experience delayed onset of pain.

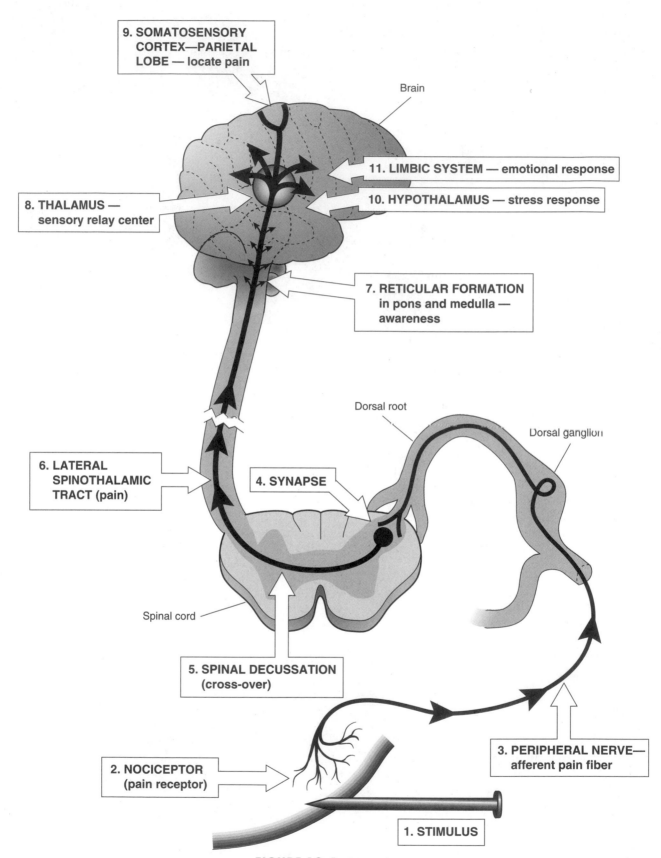

FIGURE 13–1. Pain pathway.

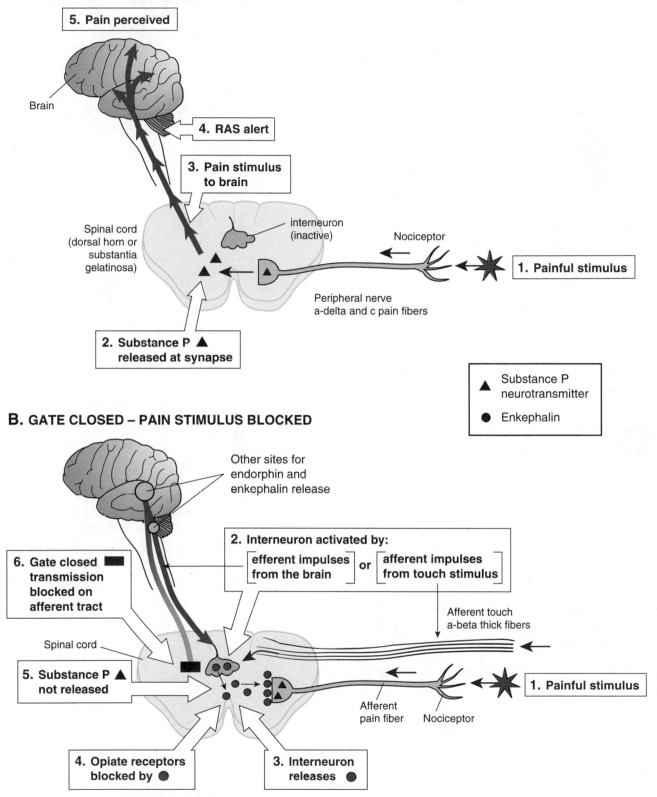

FIGURE 13-2. A schematic representation of the gate-control theory in pain control.

The key to blocking the transmission of pain impulses to the brain is the release of opiatelike chemicals (**opioids**) secreted by interneurons within the central nervous system. These substances block the conduction of pain impulses into the central nervous system. They resemble the drug morphine, which is derived from opium and is used as an **analgesic**, and they are called *endorphins* or **endogenous** morphine. Endorphins include enkephalin, dynorphin, and beta-lipotropin. Figure 13–2 illustrates how enkephalin is released and is attached to opiate receptors on the afferent neuron, thus blocking release of the **neurotransmitter** substance P at the synapse. This process prevents transmission of the pain stimulus into the spinal cord. *Serotonin* is another chemical released in the spinal cord that acts on other neurons in the spinal cord to increase the release of enkephalins. In addition, natural *opiate receptors* are found in many areas of the brain, as are secretions of endorphins, which can block pain impulses at that level. The body has its own endogenous analgesic or pain control system that explains some of the variables in pain perception experienced by individuals and can be used to assist in pain control.

Thinkabout 13–3

Briefly describe three methods of "closing the gate" and reducing pain.

CHARACTERISTICS OF PAIN

The *pain threshold* is the level of stimulation of a nociceptor that is perceived as pain. *Pain tolerance* is the degree of pain, either its intensity or its duration, that is endured before an individual takes some action. Tolerance may be increased by endorphin release or may be reduced by other factors such as fatigue. Tolerance does not necessarily depend on the severity of the pain. Rather, it varies among people and in different situations.

Signs and Symptoms

Pain is a real sensation, a subjective symptom perceived by an individual, who can describe it in some detail. The location of the pain can be pointed out. In addition to a verbal report, the patient may demonstrate a stress response with physical signs such as pallor and sweating or **tachycardia.** Sometimes nausea and vomiting or fainting and dizziness occur with acute pain. Anxiety and fear are frequently evident in people with chest pain but may be present in other situations as well. Individuals may be restless and may move constantly, or they may be immobilized by pain. There are many variations in the clinical picture of pain.

Many descriptive terms are used for pain, such as aching, burning, sharp, throbbing, and cramping. A description may be helpful in diagnosing the cause of the pain. Other important characteristics are the timing of the pain or its association with an activity such as food intake or movement, or with pressure applied at the site. Pain often leads to immobilization and protection, or "guarding," of the affected area.

Sometimes the source of pain stimuli can be localized to a specific area. In other cases the pain is generalized, and the source is difficult to determine. Sometimes the pain is perceived at a site distant from the source. This is called *referred* pain. Generalized and referred pain are characteristic of visceral damage such as occurs in the abdominal organs. In some conditions, such as acute appendicitis, the characteristics of the pain may change as pathologic changes occur.

Referred Pain

Referred pain occurs when the sensations of pain are identified in an area some distance from the actual source (Fig. 13–3). Usually the pain originates in a deep organ or muscle and is perceived on the surface of the body in a different area. For example, pain in the left neck and arm is characteristic of a heart attack or ischemia in the heart. Multiple sensory fibers from different sources connecting at a single level of the spinal cord make it difficult for the brain to discern the actual origin of the pain.

Factors Affecting Pain Perception and Response

Pain perception and response are subjective to a large extent and depend on the conditioning of the individual. Factors such as age, culture, family traditions, and prior experience shape one's perception and response to pain. For example, in certain groups it is customary to approach pain with stoic acceptance, whereas in other groups the proper response would include loud crying and wailing. Prior unpleasant experiences and anticipatory fear or anxiety can lower pain tolerance, magnifying the extent of the pain and the victim's response.

An individual's temperament and personality can influence his or her response to pain, and the circum-

A. LOCATIONS OF REFERRED PAIN

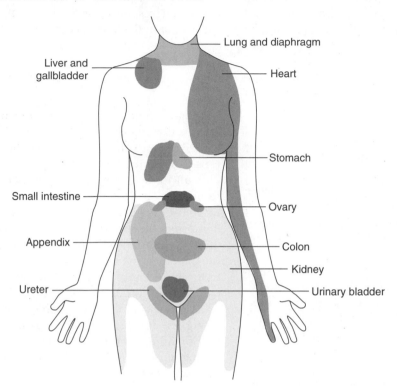

B. PROPOSED MECHANISM FOR REFERRED PAIN

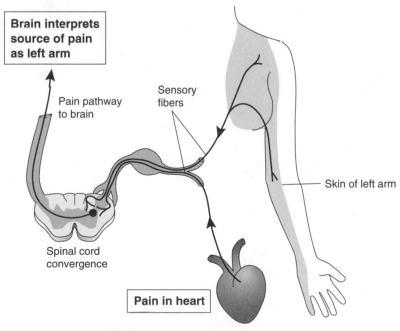

FIGURE 13–3. Referred pain.

stances existing at the time of the incident may affect his perception of it. Anxiety, fear, and stress can increase the severity of pain because in these circumstances the central nervous system is at a higher level of awareness. Fatigue, hunger, and the presence of other pathologies or problems may magnify a person's response. Likewise, the specific cause of the pain and its implications for the family or employment responsibilities might alter the person's perception of pain and his or her response to it.

Young Children and Pain

For many years it was thought that newborn infants, because of their immature nervous systems, did not sense pain. This notion has been discarded, and it has now been established that a young infant does perceive pain and responds to it physiologically, with tachycardia and increased blood pressure as well as characteristic facial expressions. Infants with their eyes tightly closed, their eyebrows low and drawn together, and their mouths open and squarish are probably in pain. Children may find it difficult to describe their pain verbally. A range of behavior that may not accurately reflect the severity of pain should be expected. There is great variation in the developmental stages and coping mechanisms of children. However, drawings of happy or sad faces or mechanical scales or multicolored symbols can be used by children to describe their feelings. Older children may flail their legs and arms and resist comfort measures, or they may become physically rigid.

Thinkabout 13-4

a. From your own experience, describe a sharp pain, an aching pain, and a cramping pain.
b. List factors that make pain seem more severe.
c. Differentiate pain threshold from pain tolerance.

ACUTE PAIN

Acute pain is usually sudden and severe but short-term. It indicates tissue damage and decreases once the cause has been treated. It may be localized or generalized. Acute pain usually initiates a physiologic stress response with increased blood pressure and heart rate,

cool, pale, moist skin, increased respiratory rate, and increased skeletal muscle tension (see Chapter 12). Vomiting may occur. In addition, there may be an emotional response, as indicated by facial or verbal expression and a high anxiety level.

CHRONIC PAIN

Long-term pain leads to different and often negative effects. Chronic pain is usually more difficult to treat effectively, and the outcome may be less hopeful. Because a specific cause is less apparent, the pain is more difficult to deal with. It is impossible to sustain a stress response over a long period of time, and the individual with chronic pain frequently is fatigued, irritable, and depressed. Sleep disturbances are common, and appetites may be affected. Chronic pain is often perceived by the patient as being more generalized. Long-term pain reduces tolerance to any additional injury. Constant pain frequently affects daily activities and may become a primary focus in the life of the individual, thus complicating any measures to effect pain control by medication or other methods. Periods of acute pain may accompany exacerbations of chronic disease, adding to the distress of the patient.

Thinkabout 13-5

Compare the characteristics of acute and chronic pain.

HEADACHE

Headache is a very common type of pain. There are many types of headaches associated with different causes, and some have specific locations and characteristics.

Headaches associated with congested sinuses, nasal congestion, and eyestrain are located in the eye and forehead area. Headaches associated with muscle spasm and tension result from emotional stress and cause the neck muscles to contract to a greater degree, pulling on the scalp. Sometimes when people work for long periods of time in one position, contraction and spasm of the neck muscles also result, causing a dull, constant ache usually in the occipital area. Headache in the temporal area is often associated with temporomandibular joint (TMJ) syndrome, in which the underlying cause is a malocclusion involving the jaw or inflammation of the joint (arthritis).

Migraine headaches are related to abnormal changes in blood flow and metabolism in the brain, but the exact mechanism is not yet fully understood. There are many precipitating factors, including atmospheric changes, stress, menstruation, and hunger. Migraine clinics are researching the hereditary factors as well as individual exacerbating factors. The pain is usually throbbing and severe and is sometimes incapacitating. Characteristically, migraine headaches begin unilaterally in the temple area but often spread to involve the entire head. In many cases there is a prodromal period with an aura or brief hallucinations or nausea, followed by the headache. The pain is often accompanied by visual disturbances and dizziness, nausea and abdominal discomfort, and fatigue. These headaches may last up to 24 hours, and there is often a prolonged recovery period. Treatment is difficult, although ergotamine may be effective if it is administered immediately after the onset of the headache.

Intracranial headaches result from increased pressure inside the skull. Any space-occupying mass stretches the cerebral vascular walls or the meninges covering the brain. Causes of increased pressure include trauma with edema or hemorrhage, tumors, infection such as meningitis, or inflammation resulting from toxins such as alcohol. Headaches may be occipital or frontal in location depending on the site of the problem. Usually other indicators of increased intracranial pressure accompany the headache (see Chapter 20).

Thinkabout 13–6

Compare the signs of a migraine headache with those of a tension headache.

PAIN CONTROL

Methods of Managing Pain

There are a number of ways of managing pain in addition to removing the cause as soon as possible. The most common method is the use of analgesic medications to relieve pain. These drugs may be administered in a variety of ways, including orally and **parenterally** (by injection). New drugs are constantly being developed to improve the efficacy of treatment and to reduce the side effects. Analgesics are classified by their ability to relieve mild pain, moderate pain, or severe pain. Mild pain is usually managed by acetaminophen or acetylsalicylic acid (ASA, aspirin), which acts primarily at the peripheral site. The latter is particularly useful when inflammation is present, whereas the former is popular because it has fewer side effects. These drugs are not effective even in high doses for severe pain. Nonsteroidal anti-inflammatory agents, such as naproxen and ibuprofen, are used to treat both acute and chronic pain due to inflammatory conditions (see Chapter 2).

For moderate pain, codeine is commonly used, and for severe pain, meperidine, morphine, or other narcotics are favored. These drugs block the pain pathways in the spinal cord and brain and also alter the perception of pain in a positive manner. Narcotics have a number of adverse effects, and concern is often expressed about addiction with long-term use. **Sedatives** and antianxiety drugs (minor tranquilizers such as lorazepam) are popular adjuncts to analgesic therapy because they promote rest and relaxation and reduce the dosage requirement for the analgesic.

In patients with chronic and increasing pain, such as occurs in some cases of cancer, pain management requires a judicious choice of drugs used successively to maximize the reduction of pain. Usually, tolerance develops in time to narcotic drugs, requiring an increase in dosage to be effective. Eventually, a new drug is required. Many patients with severe pain administer their own medications as needed using *patient-controlled analgesia (PCA)*. Small pumps are attached to vascular access sites, and the patient either receives a dose of analgesic such as morphine when needed or maintains a continuous infusion. This has been a highly successful approach and has been found to lessen the overall consumption of narcotic needed.

Other pain control methods may accompany the use of medications. Such measures include stress reduction and relaxation therapy, distracters, applications of heat and cold, massage, physiotherapy modalities, exercise, therapeutic touch, hypnosis imaging, and acupuncture. These measures may act in the spinal cord at the "gate" or may modify pain perception and response in the brain. Many of these strategies are believed to increase the levels of circulating endorphins that elevate the pain threshold. Specialized clinics deal with certain types of pain such as chronic back pain. Also, maintenance of basic nutrition and activity levels as well as adequate rest assist people in coping with pain.

For **intractable** pain that cannot be controlled with medications, surgical intervention is a choice. Procedures such as **rhizotomy** or **cordotomy** to sever the nerve pathway may be required. Injections can be given with similar effects. These procedures carry a risk of interference with other nerve fibers and functions, particularly when the spinal cord is involved.

Anesthesia

Local anesthesia may be used topically on the skin or mucosa. Local anesthetics may be used to block transmission of pain stimuli from a certain site. For example, an injection of lidocaine may be given prior to performing a tooth extraction, removal of a lesion, or a diagnostic procedure that is likely to be painful.

Spinal or *regional anesthesia* may be administered to block pain impulses from the legs or abdomen. Spinal anesthesia involves administering a local anesthetic into the epidural space or into the cerebrospinal fluid in the subarachnoid space at an appropriate level, blocking all nerve conduction at and below that level. *General anesthesia* involves administering a gas to be inhaled such as nitrous oxide or injecting a barbiturate such as sodium pentothal intravenously. Loss of consciousness accompanies general anesthesia. *Neuroleptanesthesia* is a type of general anesthesia in which the patient can respond to commands but is relatively unaware of the procedure or of any discomfort. For example, diazepam can be administered intravenously in combination with a narcotic analgesic such as meperidine or morphine. Innovar is a popular combination of droperidol (a neuroleptic) and fentanyl (a narcotic analgesic) that is administered by intravenous or intramuscular injection.

STUDY QUESTIONS

1. Describe the characteristics and role of each of the following in the pain pathway:
   a. nociceptor
   b. C fibers
   c. lateral spinothalamic tract
   d. parietal lobe
   e. reticular formation
   f. endorphins and enkephalins

2. Define and give an example of referred pain.

3. Differentiate the characteristics of acute, chronic, and intractable pain.

4. List several factors that can alter the perception of pain and the response to pain.

5. Briefly describe six possible methods of pain control.

CHAPTER
14
Substance Abuse

KEY TERMS

• •

depressant	hallucinogens	perception	synergism
euphoria	hepatotoxin	stimulant	

Substance abuse, or chemical dependency, is a term used to cover the older concepts of addiction and alcoholism. It is a matter of concern to all health care workers. Complications can easily arise in the care of such individuals because diagnostic tests may be distorted, unwanted drug interactions may occur, and pathologic processes may be initiated or aggravated by the inappropriate use of drugs. Substance abuse has implications for the family and employer of the individual as well as for society. Because access to drugs may be facilitated in the work environment, health care workers themselves may be directly involved in substance abuse. Early recognition of dependency can lead to more successful treatment of the problem. This chapter provides a brief overview of the topic.

TERMINOLOGY

Terminology frequently changes in the area of substance abuse, and there is also overlap or lack of clarity in the definitions. *Substance abuse,* or *chemical dependency,* is a broad term that refers to the inappropriate or unnecessary (nonmedical) use of drugs or chemicals that impairs a person's function in some way to some

extent. The substance is desired by the individual because it may cause **euphoria**, a sense of pleasure ("high"), or may alter one's perception of reality, or decrease one's awareness of people and the environment. Substance abuse is not limited to illegal or street drugs but may include prescribed drugs or other readily available substances. *Habit* means a practice, often involuntary, of using drugs or other substances at regular and frequent intervals. Habit may be associated with either common customs such as constant coffee drinking or cigarette smoking or with the use of illegal or street drugs. These terms do not apply to the occasional use of a substance such as alcohol on social occasions when the user feels no need to consume a large amount or to have a drink at regular short intervals.

Dependence includes both physiologic and psychological aspects. *Physiologic* dependence means that the body has adapted to the presence of the drug or chemical so that discontinuing the drug results in *withdrawal* signs such as tremors or abdominal cramps. *Psychological* dependence refers to a continuing desire to take the drug to be able to function. *Tolerance* implies that because the body adapts to the substance in time the amount of the substance taken must be increased to achieve the same effect. *Addiction* is an older term but is still in common use. It is used for the most serious form of substance abuse—the uncontrollable compulsion to use a substance, often with serious consequences for the individual, the family, and society. Frequently criminal activity is involved with abuse at this level, and others are affected when a person whose judgment is impaired by substance abuse causes automobile accidents or commits robberies or other acts of violence.

Thinkabout 14–1

Define the terms tolerance and physiologic dependence.

There are many ways of classifying abused substances, including mode of action and source. Under mode of action, commonly abused substances include alcohol and other nervous system *depressants* or tranquilizers; *narcotics* or pain-killers, which cause euphoria and drowsiness; *stimulants* such as coffee or amphetamines; *psychedelics* or **hallucinogens**, which alter a person's **perception** and awareness and produce illusions; and inhalants, which affect mood and perception. Some chemicals manifest both **stimulant** and **depressant** effects. For example, alcohol is really a central nervous system (CNS) depressant, although initially it appears to be a stimulant because it first depresses the higher brain centers used for judgment or the inhibitory neurons. A more recently developed category of abused substances involves the synthetic anabolic steroids, taken by some athletes and bodybuilders and some individuals with eating disorders.

Abused drugs are also classified by source. They include legally prescribed medications, often tranquilizers or sedatives that are continued long after the need for them has passed, medications shared with another person, prescriptions acquired from several sources, or medications combined with other substances such as alcohol or nonprescription drugs to achieve the desired effect. Prescribed drugs that are considered more addictive or dangerous are restricted by government agencies and are available only for research or with a written prescription without refill provisions. Heroin is so regulated. However, many psychoactive substances that are readily available without prescription, such as sleep-inducing or wake-up pills, hair lotions, glues, nail polish removers, aerosols, and solvents, are frequently misused, particularly by young people. These give a short

"high" followed by depression and disorientation. Illegal or street drugs are widely available now and are both costly and more dangerous for the user because their content is unpredictable. Such usage often leads to overdose or toxic effects due to adulterating substances. Many street drugs are better known by their common names than by their medical or chemical names. For example, "speed" or "uppers" is the term used for amphetamines, "angel dust" for PCP, and "snow" or "crack" for cocaine. The market for illegal drugs has become a matter of concern both economically and socially because of the criminal activity and violence associated with drug trafficking.

Thinkabout 14–2

Differentiate the effects of stimulants from those of psychedelic drugs.

PREDISPOSING FACTORS

Theories regarding the etiology or cause of substance abuse focus on psychological imbalances, personality deficits, biologic abnormalities, dysfunctional interpersonal relationships, or a combination of these factors. Substance abuse has been attributed to heredity, to disease, to the ready availability of drugs, to increased medical use of antianxiety agents, and to increased acceptance of alcohol or marijuana as a recreational tool in all age groups. The public receives mixed messages about substance abuse from the media. In many publications, both advertising and articles on drug use by high-profile personalities lend a glamorous facade to the abuse. This influences young people, who respond to peer pressure and the need to express independence among their contemporaries. Drug use among athletes in competitive sports has been well publicized. The rapid changes and increased complexity of current society as well as the increase in family breakdown have also contributed to the increase in abuse. Some individuals use drugs to cope with stress because drugs do alter one's mood or perception of reality. Unfortunately, the onset of abuse is becoming more common in adolescents. Educational measures to reduce substance abuse have not been very effective, and the "curiosity" factor remains a problem in young people. People who take narcotic analgesics for prolonged periods of time risk becoming dependent because the drugs are addictive, creating a state of euphoria as well as offering pain relief. Narcotics are helpful when dealing medically with severe pain, but they can present serious disadvantages. Heroin is rarely used medically because of its very strong tendency to produce dependency. Research on substance abuse continues in an effort to find not only its cause but also factors related to it and improved methods of prevention and treatment.

RECOGNITION OF ABUSE

Recognition of substance abuse is very difficult because the pattern of consumption can vary. A substance may be taken consistently and frequently or in large amounts periodically (for example, binge drinkers). Some individuals are affected by relatively small amounts, whereas others can function quite well with a high intake. Combinations of chemicals usually exert a more marked effect than does one substance.

The effects of individual drugs depend on the classification of the drug. Depressants usually decrease the level of CNS function, whereas stimulants increase CNS activity. Generally, drugs impair neurologic function in some way, for example, by slowing the reflexes, reducing coordination and judgment, or impairing sensitivity and perception. Information about specific drugs can be found in reference texts on substance abuse or pharmacology. The method of administration may also indicate drug abuse in some people, in whom, for example, intravenous use leaves injection marks on the arm.

General indications of substance abuse include changes in behavior, appearance (e.g., eyes), personality, daily living patterns, or work habits. Frequently, the person may be defensive, angry, or embarrassed if he or she is questioned about drug intake. Any stress will immediately require a pill or a drink. Often a cycle develops in which the person takes a depressant to relax or sleep and then needs a stimulant to wake up. As the need for drug support increases, more secretive behavior may ensue, there may be less personal care of clothes and appearance, more excuses for time and performance lapses, stronger efforts to acquire substitute drugs, and eventually thefts. Some individuals may become malnourished or may develop anemia or infection and require medical care.

It is important for any health care worker to be sensitive to the issue of substance abuse. Caution is advisable when strangers request specific drugs for pain relief, for example, in a dental office. Drugs, including samples and prescription order forms, should not be visible or readily available to the public.

POTENTIAL COMPLICATIONS OF SUBSTANCE ABUSE

Overdose

Overdose is a common acute problem. Some drugs have a relatively small safety margin, and an increased dose may cause toxic effects or death. Street drugs may be contaminated by other substances, thereby causing unanticipated effects. A common emergency situation develops when a combination of drugs, often including alcohol, results in a stronger reaction (**synergism**) than the individual components would suggest. Many hospital emergency rooms list alcohol-drug combinations as their major overdose situation and the primary cause of brain damage and death. The barbiturates, which induce sleep, and the narcotics morphine and heroin depress the CNS and compromise respiratory function. These substances may depress respiratory effort to a critical level (very slow and shallow respirations), leading to respiratory failure or cardiac arrest. Antidotes such as naloxone, which is given for narcotic overdose, can stimulate respiratory drive. Combinations of any depressant substance, other drugs, or alcohol can lead to excessive respiratory depression and coma because of the synergistic effect. Although the antianxiety drugs such as diazepam do not cause respiratory depression when used alone, they may cause brain damage and coma when combined with alcohol.

Withdrawal

Discontinuing a drug on which the body has become physically dependent results in withdrawal sickness. The signs of withdrawal may be mild or severe depending on the specific drug used and the amount of drug the body cells have adapted to. Common signs of withdrawal include irritability, tremors, nausea, vomiting and stomach cramps, high blood pressure, psychotic episodes, and convulsions. It is safer to experience withdrawal under medical supervision in a hospital or detoxification center.

Thinkabout 14–3

Differentiate between overdose and withdrawal, and include the cause and effects.

Pregnancy

Many chemical substances, including alcohol, can affect the fetus, resulting in congenital defects. Fetal alcohol syndrome is a tragic example of fetal damage. The newborn child of an alcoholic mother has characteristic physical and facial abnormalities and is mentally retarded. Heavy cigarette smoking can lead not only to low-birthweight babies that have a high risk of complications but also to an increase in the incidence of stillbirths and miscarriages. Some drugs such as cocaine and the barbiturates lead to addiction in the newborn, who must undergo withdrawal therapy.

Cardiovascular Problems

Cocaine and other stimulants such as amphetamines affect the cardiovascular system, causing irregular heart beats and increased blood pressure. This may lead to heart attacks, strokes, or heart failure at a young age.

Psychedelic Experiences

Hallucinogenic or psychedelic drugs such as lysergic acid diethylamide (LSD) and phencyclidine (PCP) lead to increased but unreal and distorted interpretation of sensory input into the brain with little control over the experience. The user hopes for a pleasant, euphoric experience (a "high") but may have an unpleasant episode with a combination of acute fear, panic, and depression, increasing the risk of suicide. Many hallucinogens also have physical effects, including increased blood pressure, nausea, and tremors. These drugs also impair the memory and distort the perceptions and judgment, presenting a high risk to those who operate machinery or drive an automobile while under the influence of the drug.

Infection

Infections such as hepatitis B and human immune deficiency virus (HIV) are common in drug abusers who share needles and other materials when injecting drugs.

Alcohol

CIRRHOSIS (LAËNNEC'S CIRRHOSIS)

Alcoholic liver disease or Laënnec's cirrhosis develops in persons with chronic alcoholism or long-term excessive alcohol intake. Alcohol is a **hepatotoxin**, an irritant that causes metabolic changes in the liver, leading first to lipid accumulation in the cells (fatty liver), then to inflammation and necrosis (alcoholic hepatitis), and finally to fibrosis or scar tissue formation (see Chapter 18 for a discussion of cirrhosis). Destruction of the liver takes place insidiously, with only mild signs and symptoms until the condition is well advanced and irreversible.

NERVOUS SYSTEM DAMAGE

Chronic alcoholism may cause serious nerve damage in the brain owing to a combination of neurotoxicity and malnutrition. A combination of Wernicke's syndrome, manifested by confusion, disorientation, and loss of motor coordination, and Korsakoff's psychosis, which involves altered personality and amnesia, is common.

ASSISTANCE WITH SUBSTANCE ABUSE

Overdose or withdrawal from an abused substance should be handled in a medical facility, preferably one with experience in dealing with this problem (e.g., a drug detoxification center). Supportive care is required to prevent complications or perhaps the use of narcotic antagonist drugs for a person with an overdose. Some clients may need psychiatric intervention. Secondary medical problems such as cirrhosis or pregnancy also require medical supervision.

Long-term therapy and support are usually required to maintain abstinence or a significant decrease in use. Such therapy may include methadone maintenance programs for heroin dependency. Methadone is a synthetic opioid that prevents withdrawal symptoms, improves function, and lessens the craving for narcotics in dependent persons who are unsuccessful in their efforts to be drug free. Methadone is administered in a controlled situation, and the patient is tested for any misuse of drugs. A different approach is needed when administering disulfiram (Antabuse) as a deterrent for the alcoholic. The drug is taken on a daily basis and causes a most unpleasant reaction (severe headache, vomiting, difficulty in breathing, and visual problems) when the patient ingests even a small amount of alcohol. In many persons requiring treatment for substance abuse malnutrition, particularly for protein and vitamin B deficits, is a problem and requires treatment. Counseling and behavior modification therapy are ongoing requirements. Some corporations have developed rehabilitation programs to assist employees with drug dependency, and some of the health professions have established "help" groups for their own members. Support groups such as Alcoholics Anonymous (AA) are available for those with dependency problems, as are groups for families of affected persons (such as Al-Anon). In addition, many community agencies can provide direction and resources.

STUDY QUESTIONS

1. List several factors that are considered to predispose a person to substance abuse.

2. Describe several signs that may indicate the presence of substance abuse.

3. Describe two potential health problems resulting from substance abuse.

CHAPTER

15

Environmental Hazards

KEY TERMS

. . . .

anaphylactic reaction	hemolytic anemia	occlusion	syncope
carcinogenic	hypersensitivity	paralysis	tinnitus
demyelination	lcukemia	particulate	toxicology
detoxification	mitosis	pathogenic	tympanic membrane
ecosystem	mutation	pica	vector
encephalopathy	necrosis	seizures	
gangrene	neuritis	solvents	

Many agents in the environment can cause damage to cells and organs in the human body. Frequently the damage occurs silently as the agent accumulates in the body. Sufficient documentation may have been gathered to enable researchers to discern the correct cause only years later, after signs and symptoms have become apparent. Only in recent years have additional safety procedures been instituted in the workplace and in the environment to protect individuals from some of these hazards. For example, improved ventilation systems may be required in factories, or soil in certain areas may be tested for contaminants before new housing is constructed. In many places, safety monitoring groups have been established, and workers are required to attend training programs that provide information about the standard symbols used for hazardous materials and the precautions recommended for handling them. To increase awareness of the role of these agents in pathologic processes, a few examples of disease arising from

environmental hazards are presented here. Additional information can be found in **toxicology** texts or environmental references. Anyone should feel free to question potential risk factors in the workplace or in the environment.

CHEMICALS

Unwanted chemicals may be ingested in contaminated food or water, inhaled into the lungs, or absorbed through the skin. Exposure may occur in the workplace or at home. Food and water may have been contaminated by industrial wastes; for example, fresh-water fish may absorb mercury in lakes and rivers. It is not unusual for chemical wastes to remain in the original dangerous form; alternatively, they may undergo transformation into more toxic materials or break down into harmless substances. For example, although pesticides may remain in the environment for a long time, some, such as DDT, do not break down into harmless chemicals, and therefore high levels gradually accumulate in the environment. Many **ecosystems** are disturbed by the use of pesticides, including those of microorganisms, some of which may become **pathogenic** or disease causing.

Tissue damage may result from a large dose in a single incident, or, more often, damage results from repeated exposure to small amounts of the unwanted material. The chemical may cause damage at the site of entry, or it may enter the blood and circulate to other sites in the body. Frequently, this process occurs without the knowledge of the individual. Normally, the liver is responsible for **detoxification** or inactivation and removal of foreign chemicals from the body. In many cases, however, these chemicals bypass the liver and are stored in certain tissues, gradually accumulating to dangerous levels over years of exposure. Usually there are no obvious signs of this accumulation. For example, hexachlorophene was widely used in hospitals and in the home as an antiseptic in soaps and powders until it was discovered that it was absorbed through the skin, particularly broken skin. Heavy use eventually caused brain damage. Now the use of hexachlorophene is somewhat restricted.

Chemicals may affect the body in different ways. Chemical substances often injure cells directly by damaging the cell membrane and causing swelling and eventual rupture of the cell. This results in inflammation and **necrosis** in the tissue. Some chemicals alter the metabolic pathways in the cell, leading to degenerative changes. Many chemicals are **carcinogenic**, that is, they cause **mutations** of the cell and lead to the onset of cancer such as **leukemia**. A few examples of dangerous chemicals are described in the following section.

Heavy Metals

Lead and mercury are examples of heavy metals that can accumulate in the tissues with long-term exposure. *Lead* can be ingested in food or water or inhaled and is then stored in the bone. Lead is heavily used in industry and is also a common childhood poison because children tend to chew not only on wood items such as pencils but also on older toys, furniture, and other items covered with lead-based paint.

Individuals who practice **pica** (the craving for nonfood substances such as clay) also develop high blood levels of lead. The toxic effects of lead include **hemolytic anemia** (destruction of erythrocytes leading to low hemoglobin levels), inflammation and ulceration of the digestive tract (lead colic), and inflammation of the kidney tubules. The most serious effects of chronic lead poisoning, however, involve damage to the nervous system such as **neuritis** (**demyelination** of peripheral nerves) and **encephalopathy** (edema and degeneration of neurons in the brain). Children manifest lead toxicity with **seizures** or convulsions, delayed development, and intellectual impairment. Even low doses of lead can cause irreversible brain damage. Lead poisoning can be detected by bone defects or "lead lines" in the bone as well as on the gingiva or gums adjacent to the teeth.

Inhalants

Inhalants can be classified as **particulate**, such as asbestos and silica, or gaseous, such as sulfur dioxide and ozone, or they may arise from **solvents** such as carbon tetrachloride. Sources of toxic inhalants include factories, laboratories, mines, insecticides, and aerosols. "Smog" is visible air pollution that contains both noxious gases such as hydrogen sulfide and particles from dust and smoke. Although local irritation of the eyes and nose is noticeable when exposure occurs, the inflammation of the respiratory tract and the effect on the central nervous system are not immediately apparent. Some solvents such as carbon tetrachloride diffuse into the circulation and eventually cause inflammation of the liver cells and irreversible hepatic damage.

Asbestos, iron oxide, and silica are examples of inhaled particles that frequently cause lung damage in workers in mines or other industries using these substances. These chemicals can cause episodes of acute inflammation, or they may lead to low-grade chronic inflammation resulting in fibrosis in the lung (chronic lung disease—see Chapter 17). Also, chronic cough and frequent infections result from the irritation and inflammation of the respiratory mucosa and may lead to additional damage. Many of these particles are carcinogenic and increase the risk of lung cancer.

Many gases such as sulfur dioxide also cause inflammation in the lungs. Carbon monoxide, which results from incomplete combustion (e.g., automobile exhaust), is not a threat in small amounts for healthy people. But because it displaces oxygen from hemoglobin, it can be dangerous for individuals with cardiovascular or respiratory disease because it leads to a further decrease in oxygen supply for these people. A current concern is the presence of second-hand or "passive" smoke in the air from cigarette smoking and its effects on nearby individuals. Cigarette smoking predisposes the smoker to lung disease including emphysema, bronchitis, and lung cancer and also to bladder cancer, peptic ulcers, and cardiovascular disease. Smoking during pregnancy also affects fetal development, leading to low-birthweight infants and an increased risk of complications. These concerns have led to social and political issues concerning cigarette smoking.

Thinkabout 15–1

a. Explain why chronic lung disease such as bronchitis occurs more frequently in highly industrialized regions.

b. Describe two possible effects of chemical toxicity in the body, giving an example of each.

PHYSICAL AGENTS

Hyperthermia

Although the body has mechanisms such as vasodilation and diaphoresis for adapting to temperature extremes, hyperthermia, an excessive elevation in core body temperature, can occur when the environmental temperature is unusually high, preventing effective cooling of the body. Also, strenuous activity that generates excessive body heat on a hot day or inadequate replacement for the fluid and salt lost in perspiration may lead to hyperthermia. Older people, infants, and cardiac patients are most at risk for overheating, as demonstrated in Chicago during the summer of 1995. Syndromes associated with hyperthermia include heat cramps with skeletal muscle spasms, heat exhaustion with nausea and **syncope** (fainting), or heat stroke with shock and coma. Prompt cooling and fluid replacement in persons with these syndromes are essential to prevent brain damage or cardiac failure.

Hypothermia

Exposure to cold temperatures may have localized or systemic effects. *Localized* frostbite usually affects the fingers, toes, or exposed parts of the face. Wet clothing increases the danger. In these areas, vascular **occlusion** occurs quickly and may lead to necrosis and **gangrene**. Usually sensation is lost early, and the individual may not be aware of the danger. Close observation of exposed areas for color changes, particularly whitish spots, is important.

Systemic exposure to cold temperature may occur with submersion in cold water or lack of adequate clothing in cold weather or wet clothing on a windy day, particularly if body movement is reduced. Low temperatures can affect many body tissues, depending on the length of time of the exposure and the actual temperature. Reflex vasoconstriction and increased blood viscosity lead to ischemia and reduced metabolism. When the core body temperature drops, the capillaries and cell membranes are damaged. This leads to abnormal shifts of fluid and sodium and ultimately to hypovolemic shock (low blood pressure) and cell necrosis. Shivering occurs initially in an effort to generate more body heat, then the muscles become rigid, and lethargy ensues. The pulse and respirations become slower, and the person becomes unresponsive. Rewarming must be done slowly and cautiously and must be accompanied by fluid replacement to maintain adequate circulation and minimize cell damage.

Thinkabout 15–2

a. Compare the effects of hypothermia and hyperthermia on the circulation.

b. Suggest some reasons why it would be difficult for a person submerged in an icy lake to continue swimming.

Radiation

Ionizing radiation includes x-rays and gamma rays as well as particles such as protons and neutrons. These rays and particles differ both in energy level and in their ability to penetrate body tissue, clothing, or lead. Radiation emissions are measured in roentgens. The amount of radiation absorbed by the body is measured in *rads*, or radiation-absorbed doses. Ionizing radiation, much of it arising from natural sources such as the sun and radioactive minerals in the soil, is a continuing hazard. However, the expanded use of radiation in homes (e.g., radon gas), in industry and defense systems, in nuclear reactors for generation of electricity, and in medicine for diagnostic procedures, such as x-ray and tracer studies, as well as for treatment present the primary risk of exposure for workers and clients.

Radiation damage may occur with a single large exposure, usually accidental, or it may accumulate with repeated small exposures. Cumulative damage is manifested by the development of skin cancers resulting from sun exposure, as seen frequently in older individuals. Routine use of skin lotions that block damaging sun rays is now recommended to reduce the risk of skin cancer. Health care workers who are at risk of exposure to radiation must use lead shields and wear monitoring devices to check individual exposure. Radiation primarily affects cells that undergo rapid **mitosis**, such as epithelial tissue, bone marrow, and the gonads (ovaries and testes). With small doses of radiation, cells can sometimes repair the ruptured DNA strands. With larger doses, DNA is altered, leading to mutations in the cell and development of cancer. Often the cells are destroyed (see Chapter 5). Exposure to large amounts of radiation leads to radiation sickness, resulting in damage to the bone marrow, digestive tract, and central nervous system.

Thinkabout 15-3

a. Epithelial tissue is very sensitive to radiation. List specific structures that include epithelial tissue likely to be damaged by radiation.

b. Give several specific examples of radiation sources.

Noise

Hearing impairment may result from excessive noise, for example, a single loud noise such as a gunshot or a variety of noise intensities that cause cumulative damage. A single loud noise may rupture the **tympanic membrane** (eardrum) or damage the nerve cells in the inner ear. Inner ear damage is usually irreversible. Cumulative damage due to noise may result directly from noise in the workplace but is often associated with higher noise levels in urban areas and with recreational sources such as rock music. Ear protection (e.g., plugs) is now required in most noisy work environments. Because only soft or high-pitched sounds are lost initially, the effects of such trauma are often gradual and go unnoticed until they are well advanced. In some cases, the individual may notice **tinnitus**, or ringing in the ears, which is a more obvious warning of the problem.

BIOLOGIC AGENTS

Bites and Stings

Bites and stings may cause disease (1) by direct injection of animal toxin into the human body, (2) by transmission of infectious agents through animal or insect **vectors** to humans, or (3) by an allergic reaction to the insect's secretion. Examples of toxins involved in bites include the neurotoxins produced by poisonous snakes or spiders that affect the nervous system, causing **paralysis** and respiratory failure or seizures. An example of an infection transmitted by an animal bite is rabies or hydrophobia, which is caused by an RNA virus. Rabies is caused primarily by the bites of wild animals, such as raccoons or skunks, but also occasionally by bites from domesticated animals (cats or dogs) who have been bitten by infected wild animals. Following any bite, the animal is usually impounded and monitored for infection. Rabies leads to nerve paralysis and death if it is not treated quickly. In certain regions, ticks and mosquitoes are a threat because they transmit infections such as rickettsial Rocky Mountain spotted fever. An example of an allergic reaction is the response of some individuals to bee or wasp stings: an **anaphylactic reaction**—a sudden and severe life-threatening **hypersensitivity** or circulatory allergic reaction. Anaphylaxis is identifiable by respiratory difficulty and shock in someone who has just been bitten (see Chapter 3).

Food Poisoning

Contaminated food and water are common sources of gastroenteritis, or vomiting and diarrhea. This topic is covered in Chapter 18. Infection can be spread in many ways. Organisms such as *Escherichia coli* are transmitted by the oral-fecal route when personal hygiene or community sanitation is not up to standard. So-called traveler's diarrhea is an example of this type of infection. In some regions a high risk of infection is associated with swimming in areas where adequate sewage treatment is not maintained or where water run-off drains through cattle pastures. Institutions frequently have outbreaks of *Salmonella* infection associated with contaminated poultry products or with food handlers who are *carriers* (a person who is a reservoir for the organism and can spread it but shows no clinical signs of infection). Widespread infection may also occur in nurseries or day care centers when careful handwashing and child management techniques have not been maintained. Stool cultures can be used to identify the responsible organism. In many cases such infections are self-limiting, but infants and the elderly are at increased risk and may become dehydrated very quickly.

STUDY QUESTIONS

1. Explain the potential benefits of reducing the use of pesticides and insecticides.

2. List examples of the dangerous gaseous and particulate components of chemical inhalants.

3. Describe the potential effects of chemicals on the respiratory tissues.

4. Explain how skin cancer is linked with sun exposure.

5. Give several examples of excessive noise in your environment.

6. Name a biologic agent and the associated problem for each of the following:
   a. transmission of an infection through a bite
   b. hypersensitivity reaction
   c. injection of a toxin

7. Define a carrier.

8. Define oral-fecal transmission of infection and give an example.

PATHOPHYSIOLOGY OF THE SYSTEMS

CHAPTER
16
Cardiovascular and Lymphatic Disorders

KEY TERMS

• •

achlorhydria	diaphoresis	hemostasis	orthopnea
adrenergic	dyspnea	hepatomegaly	oxyhemoglobin
agglutination	dysrhythmia	hypochromic	pallor
anastomoses	ecchymosis	infarction	pancytopenia
angiography	ectopic	interleukin	petechiae
angioplasty	electrode	leukocytosis	phagocytosis
auscultation	endarterectomy	leukopenia	phlebotomy
autoregulation	erythrocytosis	leukopoiesis	plasma
baroreceptors	erythropoietin	lymphadenopathy	plethoric
bilirubin	ferritin	macrocytic	reticulocyte
bradycardia	gastrectomy	macrophage	serum
cardiomegaly	glossitis	malabsorption	splenomegaly
chemoreceptors	hemarthrosis	megaloblast	stomatitis
cyanotic	hematocrit	microcirculation	sulcus
demyelination	hematopoiesis	microcytic	syncope
deoxyhemoglobin	hemolysis	murmurs	synergistic
depolarization	hemoptysis	myelotoxin	tachycardia
diapedesis	hemosiderin	neutropenia	thrombocytopenia

REVIEW OF THE NORMAL CARDIOVASCULAR SYSTEM

Blood

Blood provides the major transport system of the body for essentials such as oxygen, glucose and other nutrients, hormones, and wastes. It serves as a critical part of the body defenses, carrying antibodies and white blood cells for the removal of foreign material. As a vehicle promoting homeostasis, blood provides a mechanism for controlling body temperature by distributing core heat to the peripheral tissues. Blood is the medium through which body fluid levels and blood pressure are adjusted by various means. Clotting factors in the circulating blood are used for **hemostasis**. Blood buffers maintain a stable pH of 7.35 to 7.45 (see Chapter 6).

The adult body contains approximately 5 liters of blood. Blood consists of water and its dissolved solutes, which make up about 55 percent of the whole blood volume; the remaining 45 percent is composed of the cells or formed elements, the erythrocytes, leukocytes, and thrombocytes or platelets. **Hematocrit** refers to the proportion of red blood cells in blood and indicates the viscosity of the blood. The components of blood and their functions are summarized in Figure 16–1. Normal values for blood components are found inside the front cover of this book. **Plasma** is the clear yellowish fluid remaining after the cells have been removed, and **serum** is the fluid and solutes remaining after the cells and fibrinogen have been removed. The plasma proteins include albumin, which maintains osmotic pressure in the blood, globulins or antibodies, and fibrinogen, which is essential for the formation of blood clots.

BLOOD CELLS

All blood cells originate from the red bone marrow. They differentiate from a single stem cell, the hemocytoblast, during the process of *hemopoiesis* or **hematopoiesis** (Fig. 16–2). *Erythrocytes* or *red blood cells* (RBCs) are biconcave flexible discs (like doughnuts but with thin centers rather than holes) that are non-nucleated when mature and contain hemoglobin. The hormone **erythropoietin**, originating from the kidney, stimulates erythrocyte production in the red bone marrow in response to tissue *hypoxia*, or insufficient oxygen available to cells. Adequate RBC production and maturation depend on the availability of raw materials including amino acids, iron, vitamin B_{12}, and folic acid. Hemoglobin consists of the globin portion, two pairs of amino acid chains, and four heme groups, each containing a ferrous iron atom, to which the oxygen (O_2) can attach (see Fig. 16–7A). **Oxyhemoglobin** is a bright red color, which distinguishes arterial blood from venous blood. Deoxygenated hemoglobin (**deoxyhemoglobin** or reduced hemoglobn), is dark or bluish-red in color and is found in

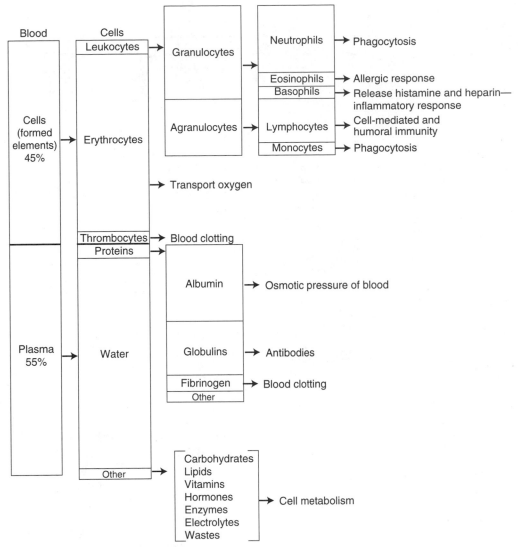

FIGURE 16-1. Components of blood and their functions.

venous blood. Only a small proportion of the carbon dioxide (CO_2) in blood is carried on hemoglobin, at a different site from that for oxygen. Most carbon dioxide is transported in blood as bicarbonate ion (in the buffer).

The life span of a normal RBC is approximately 120 days. As it ages, the cell becomes rigid and fragile and finally succumbs to **phagocytosis** in the spleen or liver and is broken down into globin and heme (see Fig. 16–8). Globin is broken down into amino acids, which can be recycled in the amino acid pool, and the iron can be returned to the bone marrow and liver to be reused in the synthesis of more hemoglobin. Excess iron can be stored as **ferritin** or **hemosiderin** in the liver and other body tissues. The balance of the heme component is converted to **bilirubin** and transported by the blood to the liver, where it is conjugated (or combined) with glucuronide to make it more soluble and then excreted

in the bile. Excessive **hemolysis** or destruction of RBCs may cause elevated serum bilirubin levels, which result in *jaundice*, the yellow color in the sclera of the eye and skin.

The five types of *leukocytes* vary in physical characteristics and functions. **Leukopoiesis** or production of white blood cells (WBCs) is stimulated by colony-stimulating factors or CSFs produced by cells such as **macrophage**s and T lymphocytes. For example, granulocyte CSF or multi-CSF (**interleukin**-3 [IL-3]) may be produced to increase certain types of WBCs during an inflammatory response (see Chapter 2). The roles of B and T lymphocytes are reviewed in Chapter 3. A *differential count* indicates the proportions of specific cell types in the blood and frequently assists in making a diagnosis. WBCs may leave the capillaries and enter the tissues by **diapedesis** or *ameboid* action when they are needed for defensive purposes.

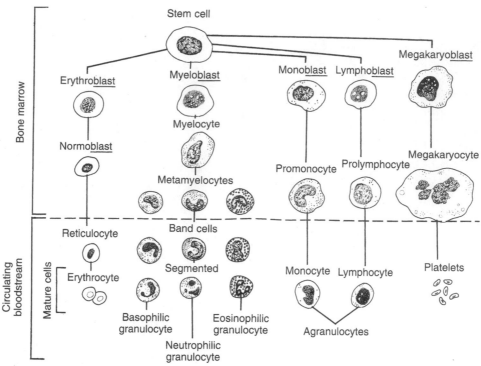

FIGURE 16–2. Hematopoiesis. (From Chabner DE: The Language of Medicine, 5th ed. Philadelphia, W.B. Saunders, 1996, p. 433.)

BLOOD CLOTTING

Thrombocytes, also called platelets, are an essential part of the blood-clotting process or hemostasis, which can be reviewed in Figure 16–10. There are three steps in hemostasis. The immediate response of a blood vessel to injury is vasoconstriction or vascular spasm. Second, thrombocytes tend to adhere at the site and, if the blood vessel is small, can form a platelet plug in the vessel. In larger vessels, the blood-clotting or coagulation mechanism is required, whereby the clotting factors that are present in inactive forms in the circulating blood are activated through a sequence of reactions ending in the formation of a fibrin mesh. These clotting factors are produced primarily in the liver. *Vitamin K*, a fat-soluble vitamin, is required for the synthesis of most clotting factors. *Calcium* ions are also essential for the clotting process.

BLOOD TYPES

An individual's blood type (e.g., ABO and Rh groups) is determined by the presence of specific antigens on the cell membrane of that person's erythrocytes. *ABO* groups are an inherited characteristic that depends on the presence of type A or B *antigens* or agglutinogens (Table 16–1). Shortly after birth, antibodies that can react with different antigens on another person's RBCs form in the blood of the newborn. Such an antigen-antibody reaction would occur with, for example, an incompatible blood transfusion, resulting in **agglutination** and hemolysis of the recipient's RBCs. Usually blood types of both donor and recipient are carefully checked prior to transfusion. Persons with type O blood lack A and B antigens and therefore are considered universal donors. Persons with type AB blood are universal recipients. Signs of a transfusion reaction include a feeling of warmth in the involved vein, flushed face, headache, fever and chills, pain in the chest and abdomen, decreased blood pressure, and rapid pulse. Plasma or colloidal volume-expanding solutions can be administered without risk of a reaction because they are free of antigens and antibodies. Another inherited factor in blood is the Rh factor, which may cause blood incompatibility if the mother is Rh negative and the fetus is Rh positive. Rh blood incompatibility between maternal and fetal blood is reviewed in Chapter 9.

TABLE 16–1	ABO Blood Groups and Transfusions Compatibilities		
Blood Group	RBC Antigens	Antibodies in Plasma	For Transfusion, Can Receive Donor Blood Group
O	None	Anti-A and Anti-B	O
A	A	Anti-B	O or A
B	B	Anti-A	O or B
AB	A and B	None	O, A, B, or AB

DIAGNOSTIC TESTS

Common diagnostic tests for blood include total RBCs, WBCs, and platelet counts and a differential count for WBCs, which provides the percentage of each type of WBC (see normal values inside the front cover of this book). These tests are useful screening tools. For example, **leukocytosis**, an increase in WBCs in the circulation, is often associated with inflammation or infection. **Leukopenia**, a decrease in leukocytes, occurs with some viral infections. An increase in eosinophils is common with allergic responses. The characteristics of the individual cells observed in a blood smear, including size and shape, uniformity, maturity, and amount of hemoglobin, are very important. A summary of the most common diagnostic tests is provided in Ready Reference 4. The hematocrit shows the percentage of blood volume composed of RBCs and indicates fluid and cell content; for example, loss of water from the blood leads to a high hematocrit. Hemoglobin is measured, and the amount of hemoglobin per cell is shown by the mean corpuscular volume (MCV). MCV indicates the oxygen-carrying capacity of the blood. Bone marrow function can be assessed by the **reticulocyte** (immature non-nucleated RBC) count plus a bone marrow aspiration and biopsy. In addition, analysis of the blood can determine the serum levels of iron, the vitamin B_{12} and folic acid levels, and the bilirubin values.

Blood-clotting disorders can be differentiated by tests such as bleeding time, prothrombin time (PT), and partial thromboplastin time (PTT), which measure the function of various components in the coagulation process.

Thinkabout 16–1

a. State the function of each type of cell in the blood.
b. State three functions of plasma proteins and list the component responsible for each.
c. What is the normal pH of blood?
d. Describe the three stages of hemostasis.

Heart

ANATOMY

The heart functions as the pump for the circulating blood in both the pulmonary and systemic circulations.

The path of a specific component of the blood such as an RBC through the heart and circulation is illustrated in Figure 16–3. The heart is located in the *mediastinum* between the lungs and is enclosed in the double-walled *pericardial* sac (see Fig. 16–25). The outer fibrous pericardium anchors the heart to the diaphragm. The visceral pericardium, also called the epicardium, consists of a serous membrane that provides a small amount of lubricating fluid within the pericardial cavity between the two pericardial membranes to facilitate heart movements. The middle layer of the heart is the myocardium—the cardiac muscle with its continuous powerful and rhythmic contractions that pump the blood efficiently through the body. The left ventricular wall is

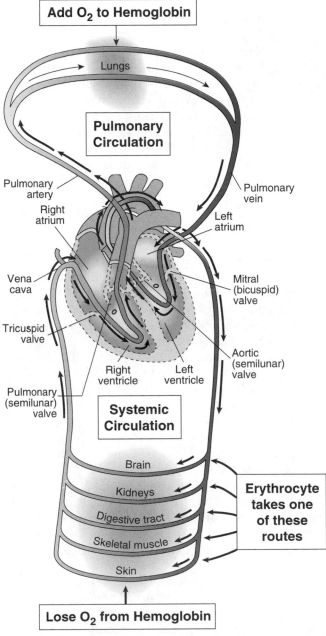

FIGURE 16–3. Path of erythrocyte in the circulation.

thicker because it must eject blood into the extensive systemic circulation. The inner layer of the heart is the *endocardium,* which also forms the four heart *valves* that separate the chambers of the heart and ensure the *one-way flow* of blood. The atrioventricular (AV) valves separate the atria from the ventricles; they comprise, on the right side, the tricuspid valve with three leaflets or cusps, and on the left side, the mitral or bicuspid valve with two leaflets. The semilunar valves, each with three cusps, include the aortic and pulmonary valves located at the exits to the large arteries from the ventricles. The interventricular *septum* separates the left and right sides of the heart.

CONDUCTION SYSTEM

Impulses to initiate cardiac contractions are conducted along specialized myocardial (cardiac muscle) fibers. No nerves are present in the cardiac muscle. The unique characteristics of cardiac muscle include the presence of intercalated discs at the junctions between fibers; these provide rapid transmission of impulses, allowing all muscle fibers of the atria or ventricles to contract together. This coordinated effort results in a rhythmic and efficient filling and emptying of the atria and ventricles that has sufficient force to sustain the flow of blood through the body. All cardiac muscle cells can initiate impulses, but normally the conduction pathway originates at the sinoatrial (SA) node, often called the *pacemaker,* in the right atrium. The SA node automatically generates impulses at the basic rate, called the *sinus rhythm* (approximately 70 beats per minute), but this can be altered by autonomic nervous system fibers that innervate the SA node and by circulating hormones such as epinephrine. From the SA node, impulses then spread through the atrial conduction pathways, resulting in contraction of both atria (see Fig. 16–18). The impulses then collect at the AV node, located in the floor of the right atrium near the septum. There is a slight delay in conduction at the AV node to allow for complete ventricular filling; then the impulses continue into the ventricle through the bundle of His (AV bundle), the right and left bundle branches, and the Purkinje network of fibers, stimulating the simultaneous contraction of the two ventricles.

Conduction of impulses produces an electric current that can be picked up by **electrodes** attached to the skin at various points on the body surface, producing the *electrocardiogram (ECG)* (see Figs. 16–18 and 16–19). The atrial contraction is represented by the **depolarization** in the P wave, and the ventricular contraction is shown by the large wave of depolarization in the ventricles (QRS). The third wave (T wave) represents the repolarization of the ventricles or recovery phase. Variations in the ECG known as *arrhythmias* may indicate acute problems such as an infarction or systemic problems such as

electrolyte imbalances (for example, potassium deficiency [see Fig. 6–6]).

CONTROL OF THE HEART

Heart rate and force of contraction are controlled by the *cardiac control center* in the medulla of the brain. The **baroreceptors** in the walls of the aorta and internal carotid arteries detect changes in blood pressure and alert the cardiac center, which then responds through stimulation of the sympathetic or parasympathetic nervous system to alter the rate and force of cardiac contractions appropriately. Sympathetic innervation increases heart rate (**tachycardia**) and contractility, whereas parasympathetic or vagus nerve stimulation slows the heart rate (**bradycardia).** The sympathetic or beta$_1$-**adrenergic** receptors in the heart (see Chapter 20) are an important site of action for some drugs (e.g., beta blockers). Because beta blockers fit the receptors and prevent normal sympathetic nervous system (SNS) stimulation, they are used to block any increases in rate and force of contractions after the heart has been damaged. Other factors, such as emotional responses, increased secretion of epinephrine, fever, and serum pH (detected by **chemoreceptors**), can also alter heart rate. Any stimulation of the SNS, as with stress, increases the secretion of epinephrine, which in turn stimulates beta receptors and increases the heart rate and contractility.

Thinkabout 16–2

a. Where is the mitral valve located? How many cusps does this valve have? Describe the direction and type of blood (oxygenated or nonoxygenated) that flows through this valve.
b. List two functions of the AV node.
c. Describe the control of heart rate.

CORONARY CIRCULATION

Cardiac muscle requires a constant supply of oxygen and nutrients to conduct impulses and contract efficiently, but it has very little storage capacity for oxygen. The coronary circulation arises from two major arteries, the right and left coronary arteries, branching immediately above the aortic valve, which receive blood from the aorta (see Fig. 16–16). The left coronary artery soon divides into the *left anterior descending* or *interventricular artery,* which follows the anterior interventricular **sulcus** or groove downward over the surface of the heart, and the *left circumflex artery,* which circles the exterior of the heart in the left atrioventricular sulcus. The passage of arteries over the surface of the heart in these grooves is helpful because it permits surgical replacement of obstructed arteries with "bypasses," usually veins from the legs. Similarly, the *right coronary artery* follows the right atrioventricular sulcus on the posterior surface of the heart, branches into the right marginal artery and the posterior interventricular artery, and then descends in the posterior interventricular groove toward the apex of the heart, where it comes close to the terminal point of

the left anterior descending artery. Many small branches extend inward from these large arteries to supply the myocardium and endocardium. Blood flow through the myocardium is greatest during diastole or relaxation and is reduced during systole or contraction as the contracting muscle compresses the arteries. Thus, very rapid or prolonged contractions can interfere with the blood supply to the muscle cells. **Anastomoses** or direct connections exist between small branches of the left and right coronary arteries near the apex as well as in other areas in which branches are nearby (Fig. 16–4). These junctions have the potential

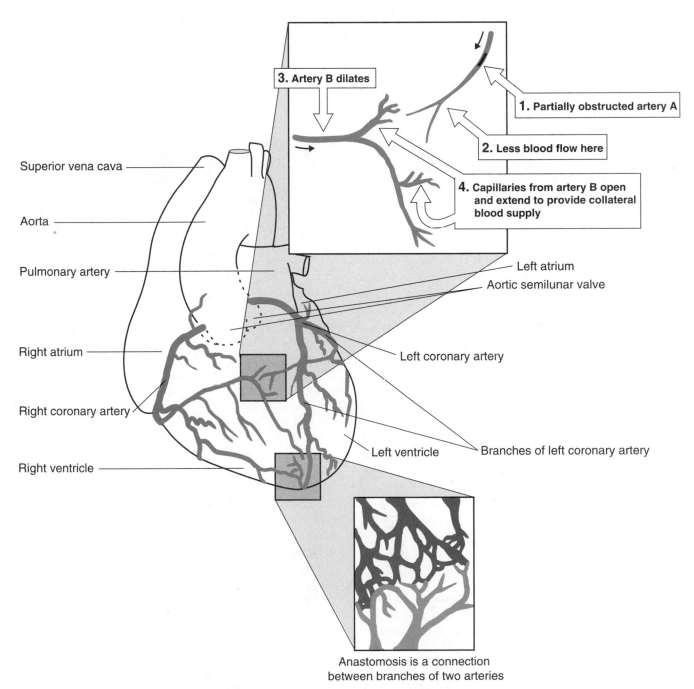

3. Artery B dilates

1. Partially obstructed artery A

2. Less blood flow here

4. Capillaries from artery B open and extend to provide collateral blood supply

Superior vena cava

Aorta

Pulmonary artery

Right atrium

Right coronary artery

Right ventricle

Left atrium
Aortic semilunar valve

Left coronary artery

Left ventricle

Branches of left coronary artery

Anastomosis is a connection between branches of two arteries

FIGURE 16–4. Collateral circulation in the heart.

to open up and provide another source of blood to an area. *Collateral* circulation (alternative source of blood and nutrients) is important if an artery becomes obstructed. When obstruction develops gradually, more capillaries from nearby arteries tend to enlarge or extend into adjacent tissues to meet the metabolic needs of the cells. Regular aerobic exercise contributes to cardiovascular fitness by stimulating the development of collateral channels.

Any interference with blood flow will affect heart function depending on the specific area supplied by that artery. The distribution of blood vessels varies among individuals. Generally, the right coronary artery supplies the right side of the heart and the inferior portion of the left ventricle as well as the posterior interventricular septum. The left anterior descending artery brings blood to the anterior wall of the ventricles, the anterior septum, and the bundle branches, and the circumflex artery nourishes the left atrium and the lateral and posterior walls of the left ventricle. The source of blood for the SA node depends on the specific position of the arteries, which varies in individuals. The SA node is supplied by the right coronary artery in slightly more than half the population and by the left circumflex artery in the remainder. The AV node is nourished primarily by the right coronary artery. This information implies that blockage of the right coronary artery is likely to result in conduction disturbances of the AV node (arrhythmias), whereas interference with the blood supply to the left coronary artery will probably impair the pumping capability of the left ventricle (congestive heart failure).

The course of the coronary or cardiac veins generally parallels that of the arteries, the majority of the blood returning to the coronary sinus and emptying directly into the right atrium.

CARDIAC CYCLE

The cardiac cycle refers to the alternating sequence of *diastole,* the relaxation phase of cardiac activity, and *systole,* or cardiac contraction, which is coordinated by the conduction system for maximum efficiency. Starting with the two atria relaxed and filling with blood from the inferior and superior venae cavae, the AV valves open as the pressure of blood in the atria increases and the ventricles are relaxed. Blood flows into the ventricles. The conduction system causes the atrial muscle to contract, forcing any remaining blood into the ventricles (Fig. 16–5), and then the atria relax. Once filled with blood, the two ventricles begin to contract, and as pressure increases in the ventricles, the AV valves close, and the semilunar valves open, forcing blood into the pulmonary artery and aorta. Note that the muscle contraction must be strong enough to overcome the opposing pressure in the artery to force the valve open,

particularly in the left ventricle, in which the pressure must be greater than the diastolic pressure in the aorta. Because the pulmonary circulation is a low-pressure system, the right ventricle does not have to exert as much pressure to pump blood into the pulmonary circulation. At the end of the cycle, the atria have begun to fill again, the ventricles relax, the aortic and pulmonary valves close to prevent backflow of blood, and the cycle begins again. The same volume of blood is pumped from the right and left sides of the heart during each cycle. This is important to ensure that blood flow through the systemic and pulmonary circulations is consistently balanced.

Thinkabout 16–3

a. Define collateral circulation and state its purpose.

b. Why is there a pause after the atrial contraction and before the ventricular contraction?

c. Predict the outcome if more blood is pumped into the pulmonary circulation than into the systemic circulation during each cardiac cycle.

The *heart sounds,* lubb-dupp, which can be heard with a stethoscope, result from vibrations due to closure of the valves. Closure of the AV valves at the beginning of ventricular systole causes a long, low "lubb" sound, followed by a "dupp" sound as the semilunar valves close with ventricular diastole. Defective valves that leak or do not open completely cause unusual turbulence in the blood flow, resulting in abnormal sounds or **murmurs.**

The *pulse* indicates the heart rate. The pulse can be felt by the fingers (not the thumb) placed over an artery that passes over bone or firm tissue, most commonly at the wrist (see Fig. 16–28). During ventricular systole the surge of blood expands the arteries. The characteristics of the pulse, such as weakness or irregularity in a peripheral pulse (e.g., the radial pulse in the wrist), often indicate a problem. The *apical* pulse refers to the rate measured at the heart itself. A *pulse deficit* is a difference in rate between the apical pulse and the radial pulse.

Cardiac function can be measured in a number of ways. *Cardiac output* (CO) is the volume of blood ejected by a ventricle in 1 minute and depends on heart rate (IIR) and *stroke volume* (SV, the volume pumped from one ventricle in one contraction).

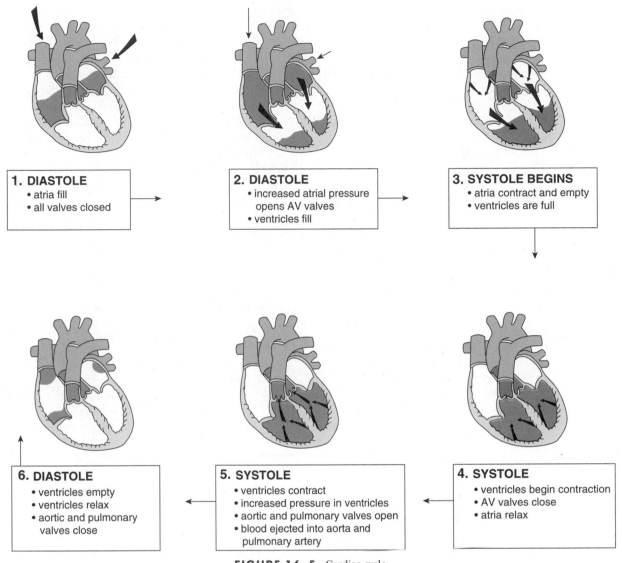

1. DIASTOLE
• atria fill
• all valves closed

2. DIASTOLE
• increased atrial pressure
  opens AV valves
• ventricles fill

3. SYSTOLE BEGINS
• atria contract and empty
• ventricles are full

6. DIASTOLE
• ventricles empty
• ventricles relax
• aortic and pulmonary
  valves close

5. SYSTOLE
• ventricles contract
• increased pressure in ventricles
• aortic and pulmonary valves open
• blood ejected into aorta and
  pulmonary artery

4. SYSTOLE
• ventricles begin contraction
• AV valves close
• atria relax

FIGURE 16–5. Cardiac cycle.

$$CO = SV \times HR = 70 \times 70 = 4900 \text{ mL}$$
or approximately 5 liters/minute

This means that at rest, the heart pumps into the system an amount equal to the total blood volume in the body every minute, which is a remarkable feat. During exercise, stress, or infection, cardiac output increases considerably. Stroke volume varies with sympathetic stimulation and venous return. When an increased amount of blood returns to the heart, as during exercise, the heart is stretched more, and the force of the contraction increases proportionately. Venous return may be referred to as *preload. Afterload* is determined by the *peripheral resistance* to the opening of the semilunar valves. For example, afterload is increased by a high diastolic pressure resulting from excessive vasoconstriction. *Cardiac reserve* refers to the ability of the heart to increase output in response to increased demand.

When necessary, the normal heart can increase its usual output by four or five times the minimum volume.

Thinkabout 16–4

a. List factors that can increase heart rate.

b. On the ECG, what does the QRS wave represent?

c. List the areas of the heart supplied by the left coronary artery.

d. Describe the effect if the atria were to contract at the same time as the ventricles, or if the ventricles should contract slightly before the atria.

Blood Vessels

The arteries, capillaries, and veins constitute a closed system for the distribution of blood throughout the body. Major blood vessels, most of which are paired left and right, are shown in Figures 16–27 and 16–30. There are two separate circulations—the pulmonary circulation allows the exchange of oxygen and carbon dioxide in the lungs, and the systemic circulation provides for the exchange of nutrients and wastes between the blood and the cells throughout the body. Arteries and veins are made up of three layers. The tunica intima, an endothelial layer, is the inner layer. The tunica media, a layer of smooth muscle that controls the diameter and lumen size of the blood vessel, is the middle layer. The tunica adventitia or externa is the outer connective tissue layer and contains elastic and collagen fibers. The vasa vasorum consists of tiny blood vessels that supply the tissues of the wall itself. Normally the large arteries are highly elastic in order to adjust to the changes in blood volume that occur during the cardiac cycle. For example, the aorta must expand during systole to prevent systolic pressure from rising too high, and during diastole the walls must recoil to maintain adequate diastolic pressure. Arteries transport blood away from the heart into the lungs or to body tissues. Arterioles are the smaller branches of arteries that control the amount of blood flowing into specific areas through the degree of contraction of smooth muscle in the vessel walls (vasoconstriction or dilation). Localized vasodilation or vasoconstriction is controlled by **autoregulation,** a local reflex adjustment, which varies depending on the needs of the cells in the area. For example, a decrease in pH, an increase in carbon dioxide, or a decrease in oxygen leads to local vasodilation. Release of chemical mediators such as histamine or an increase in temperature at a specific area can also cause vasodilation. These local changes do not affect the systemic blood pressure. Norepinephrine and epinephrine increase systemic vasoconstriction by stimulating alpha$_1$-adrenergic receptors in the arteriolar walls. Angiotensin is another powerful systemic vasoconstrictor. At all times, even at rest, vascular or vasomotor tone is maintained by constant input from the SNS that results in partial vasoconstriction throughout the body to ensure continued circulation of blood.

Capillaries are very small vessels organized in numerous networks that form the **microcirculation.** They consist of a single endothelial layer to facilitate the exchange of fluid, oxygen, carbon dioxide, electrolytes, glucose and other nutrients, and wastes between the blood and the interstitial fluid. Capillary exchange and abnormal electrolyte shifts are covered in Chapter 6. Blood flows very slowly through capillaries, and precapillary sphincters determine the amount of blood flowing from the arterioles into the various capillaries de-

pending on the metabolic needs of the tissues. From the capillary beds, blood finally returns to the heart through small venules that drain into the larger veins. Normally, a high percentage of the blood (approximately 70 percent) is located in the veins at any one time; hence, the veins are called capacitance vessels. Veins have thinner walls than arteries and less smooth muscle. Blood flow in the veins depends on skeletal muscle action, respiratory movements, and gravity. Valves in the larger veins in the arms and legs have an important role in keeping the blood flowing toward the heart.

Thinkabout 16–5

a. Explain why a high elastic content is required in the wall of the aorta.

b. Explain the purpose of smooth muscle in the arterioles.

c. Explain why there is an extensive network of capillaries in skeletal muscle and in the liver.

d. Explain why venous return increases with exercise.

Blood Pressure

Blood pressure commonly refers to the pressure of blood against the systemic arterial walls, a normal pressure commonly being in the range of 120/75 mm Hg at rest. *Systolic pressure,* the higher number, is the pressure exerted by the blood when ejected from the left ventricle. *Diastolic pressure,* the lower value, is the pressure that occurs when the ventricles are relaxed. Blood pressure is measured using the brachial artery in the arm, using a sphygmomanometer and an inflatable blood pressure cuff. *Pulse pressure* is the difference between the systolic and diastolic pressures.

Blood pressure depends on cardiac output and peripheral resistance. Specific variables include blood volume and viscosity, venous return, the rate and force of heart contractions, and the elasticity of the arteries. Peripheral resistance is the force opposing blood flow or the amount of friction with the vessel walls encountered by the blood. Decreasing the diameter (or lumen) of the blood vessel increases the resistance to blood flow. Any obstruction in the blood vessel also increases resistance. Normally, peripheral resistance can be altered by the constriction or dilation of the arterioles. Local vasoconstriction or dilation usually does *not* affect the systemic blood pressure. Systemic or widespread vasoconstriction occurs in response to sympathetic stimulation and increases blood pressure. Systemic vasodilation leading to decreased blood pressure results from decreased SNS stimulation (there is no parasympathetic nervous system innervation in the blood vessels).

Changes in blood pressure are sensed by the baroreceptors, relayed to the vasomotor control center in the medulla which adjusts the distribution of blood to maintain normal blood pressure. For example, when one arises from a supine position, blood pressure drops momentarily owing to gravitational forces until the reflex vasoconstriction mechanism in the body ensures that more blood flows to the brain. Blood pressure is elevated by SNS stimulation in two ways. First, SNS and epinephrine act at the beta$_1$-adrenergic receptors in the heart to increase both the rate and force of contraction. Second, SNS, epinephrine, and norepinephrine increase vasoconstriction by affecting the alpha$_1$ receptors in the arterioles of the skin and viscera. Other hormones also contribute to the control of blood pressure. Antidiuretic hormone (ADH) and aldosterone increase blood volume, thus elevating blood pressure. The renin-angiotensin-aldosterone system in the kidneys is an important control and compensation mechanism that is initiated when a decrease in blood flow stimulates the release of renin, which in turn activates angiotensin (vasoconstrictor) and stimulates aldosterone secretion (see Chapter 19).

Thinkabout 16-6

a. List four factors that can increase blood pressure.

b. List the compensatory mechanisms (in the correct sequence) that can help to return the blood pressure to normal levels following a slight drop.

c. Differentiate local vasoconstriction from systemic vasoconstriction by: (1) causes, (2) area involved, (3) effect on local tissue, and (4) effect on systemic blood pressure.

d. Describe the effect of a hot compress or pad on the tissues to which it is applied.

e. How does vasoconstriction in the skin and viscera increase venous return to the heart?

The Lymphatic System

The lymphatic system consists of vessels, lymph nodes, and lymphoid tissue, which includes the palatine and pharyngeal tonsils, the spleen, and the thymus gland (see Fig. 3–2). It functions to return excess interstitial fluid and protein to the blood. The lymph nodes and lymphoid tissue act as a defense system, filtering foreign or unwanted material from the lymph fluid before it enters the general circulation. The lymph nodes are essential to the immune response and the sensitization of B and T lymphocytes (see Chapter 3). Lymphatic capillaries in the intestinal villi absorb and transport lipids to the liver.

Lymph fluid is similar to plasma but may contain more lymphocytes. The lymphatic systemic begins with blind-ending capillaries containing minivalves at the terminus, into which excess interstitial fluid flows as pressure builds up in the tissues (see Fig. 6–2). The capillaries join to form larger vessels with valves to ensure a one-way flow of fluid. The vessels of the upper right quadrant of the body empty into the right lymphatic duct, which passes the lymph into the right subclavian vein. The remainder of the lymphatic vessels drain into the thoracic duct in the upper abdomen and thoracic cavity. This duct drains into the left subclavian vein. Lymph nodes containing many lymphocytes and macrophages are situated along all lymphatic and blood vessels, ensuring constant surveillance and filtration of body fluid.

Thinkabout 16-7

a. State two purposes of the lymphatic system and explain each.

b. Describe the result of destruction of the lymph nodes in a specific region.

BLOOD DYSCRASIAS

The Anemias

Anemias cause a reduction in oxygen transport in the blood owing to a decrease in hemoglobin production, a decrease in erythrocytes, or a combination of these factors. Reduced oxygen leads to less energy production in all cells and reduced cell metabolism and reproduction. Compensation mechanisms to improve the oxygen supply include tachycardia and peripheral vasoconstriction. These changes lead to the general signs of anemia, which include fatigue, **pallor**, **dyspnea**, and tachycardia. Severe anemia may lead to angina during stressful situations if the oxygen supply to the heart is sufficiently reduced. Chronic severe anemia may cause congestive heart failure. The digestive tract tends to become inflamed and ulcerated in people with anemia, and **stomatitis** and dysphagia may develop; the hair and skin may show degenerative changes.

Anemias may occur when there is a deficiency of a required nutrient, when bone marrow production is impaired, or when blood loss or excessive destruction of erythrocytes occurs (hemolytic anemias). Hemolytic anemias have many causes, including genetic defects, deficits of enzymes that protect RBCs from metabolic damage, immune reactions, changes in blood chemistry, the presence of toxins in the blood, and blood incompatibility in the newborn (erythroblastosis fetalis). This section of the chapter covers a few examples of different types of anemias.

IRON DEFICIENCY ANEMIA

PATHOPHYSIOLOGY

Iron deficiency anemia is very common; it ranges from mild to severe and occurs in all age groups. Because iron deficiency anemia is frequently a sign of an underlying problem, it is important to determine the cause of the deficit. Insufficient iron impedes the synthesis of hemoglobin, thereby reducing the amount of oxygen transported in the blood (see Fig. 16–7). This results in **microcytic** (small cell), **hypochromic** (less color) erythrocytes owing to a low concentration of hemoglobin in each cell. There is a decrease in stored iron, as indicated by decreased serum ferritin, decreased hemosiderin, and decreased iron-containing histiocytes in the bone marrow.

ETIOLOGY

An iron deficit can occur for many reasons. Dietary intake of iron-containing vegetables or meat may be below the minimum requirement, particularly during the adolescent growth spurt or during pregnancy, when needs increase. A common cause of iron deficiency is a slow and chronic blood loss from a bleeding ulcer, hemorrhoids, cancer, or excessive menstrual flow. Continuous blood loss, even small amounts of blood, means that less iron is recycled to maintain an adequate production of hemoglobin. Duodenal absorption of iron may be impaired by many disorders, including **malabsorption** syndromes and **achlorhydria**. Normally, only 5 to 10 percent of ingested iron is absorbed, but this can increase to 20 percent when there is a deficit. Severe liver disease may affect both iron absorption and iron storage. In the form of iron deficiency anemia associated with some infections and cancers iron is present but is not well used, leading to low hemoglobin levels but high storage iron levels.

SIGNS AND SYMPTOMS

Mild anemias are frequently asymptomatic. As the hemoglobin value drops, the general signs of anemias become apparent: pallor of the skin and mucous membranes related to cutaneous vasoconstriction; fatigue, lethargy, and cold intolerance as cell metabolism decreases; irritability, a central nervous system response to hypoxia; and degenerative changes such as brittle hair, spoon-shaped (concave) and ridged nails, and stomatitis and **glossitis,** inflammation in the oral mucosa and tongue, respectively. Females may develop menstrual irregularities. As anemia becomes more severe, it leads to tachycardia, palpitations, and dyspnea, and perhaps **syncope** as well as delayed healing.

DIAGNOSTIC TESTS

Laboratory tests demonstrate low values for hemoglobin, hematocrit, mean corpuscular volume and mean corpuscular hemoglobin, serum ferritin and serum iron, and transferrin saturation. On microscopic examination the erythrocytes appear hypochromic and microcytic.

TREATMENT

The underlying cause must be established and resolved if possible. Iron-rich foods or iron supplements in the least irritating and easily absorbable forms for the individual may be given. It is advisable to take iron with food to reduce gastric irritation and nausea. Iron supplements may lead to constipation. Liquid iron stains teeth and dentures, and therefore a straw should be used for drinking the medication.

Thinkabout 16–8

> a. Explain why chronic bleeding leads to iron deficiency anemia.
> b. State the signs of anemia that indicate compensation for hypoxia.

PERNICIOUS ANEMIA—VITAMIN B_{12} DEFICIENCY (MEGALOBLASTIC ANEMIA)

Megaloblastic anemia is characterized by very large, nucleated, immature erythrocytes. This type of anemia usually results from a deficit of folic acid or vitamin B_{12}. There is now an increased interest in the folic acid deficiency that may occur during the first 2 months of pregnancy, resulting in an increased risk of spina bifida in the child.

PATHOPHYSIOLOGY

A deficit of vitamin B_{12} (cyanocobalamin) leads to impaired maturation of erythrocytes due to interference with DNA synthesis. The RBCs are very large (**megaloblasts** or **macrocytes**) and contain nuclei.

These large erythrocytes are destroyed prematurely, resulting in a low erythrocyte count or anemia. The hemoglobin in these cells is normal and is capable of transporting oxygen. Often the maturation of granulocytes is also affected, resulting in development of abnormally large neutrophils.

Pernicious anemia is the common form of megaloblastic anemia that results from the malabsorption of vitamin B_{12} owing to a lack of intrinsic factor (IF) produced in the glands of the gastric mucosa (Fig. 16–6). Lack of IF has resulted from the formation of autoantibodies against IF or the parietal cells that produce IF in the gastric mucosa (see Chapter 18). The subsequent immune reaction leads to atrophy of the gastric mucosa and glands. Intrinsic factor must bind with vitamin B_{12} to enable absorption of the vitamin in the lower ileum. An additional problem occurs with the atrophy of the mucosa because the parietal cells can no longer produce hydrochloric acid. Achlorhydria interferes with the early digestion of protein in the stomach and with the absorption of iron; thus, an iron-deficiency anemia may be present as well.

Lack of vitamin B_{12} is a direct cause of **demyelination** of the peripheral nerves and eventually of the spinal cord. Loss of myelin interferes with conduction of nerve impulses and may be irreversible. Sensory fibers are affected first, followed by motor fibers.

ETIOLOGY

Dietary insufficiency is rarely a cause of this anemia because very small amounts of vitamin B_{12} are required. Because the source of the vitamin is animal foods, vegetarians occasionally have a deficit. The most common cause of vitamin B_{12} deficiency is malabsorption, which may result from an autoimmune reaction as mentioned earlier, particularly in older individuals, from chronic gastritis, which is common in alcoholics and causes atrophy of the gastric mucosa, or from inflammatory conditions such as regional ileitis. The condition may also be an outcome of such surgical procedures as **gastrectomy**, in which the parietal cells are removed, or resection of the ileum, which is the site of absorption.

SIGNS AND SYMPTOMS

In addition to the basic manifestations of anemia, the tongue is typically enlarged, red, and shiny. The neurologic effects include tingling or burning sensations (paresthesia) in the extremities or loss of coordination and ataxia. The decrease in gastric acid leads to digestive discomfort, often with nausea and diarrhea.

DIAGNOSTIC TESTS

The erythrocytes appear macrocytic or megaloblastic on microscopic examination and are reduced in number in the peripheral blood. The bone marrow is hyperactive with increased numbers of megaloblasts. Granulocytes are hypersegmented and are decreased in number. The serum vitamin B_{12} level is below normal.

In Schilling's test radioactive vitamin B_{12} is used to measure absorption following oral administration. The presence of hypochlorhydria or achlorhydria confirms the presence of gastric atrophy.

TREATMENT

Oral supplements are recommended as prophylaxis for pregnant women and vegetarians. Vitamin B_{12} can be administered by injection as replacement therapy for people with pernicious anemia.

Thinkabout 16–9

a. Explain why individuals with pernicious anemia have a low hemoglobin level.

b. Briefly describe the additional manifestations of pernicious anemia.

c. Why is oral administration of vitamin B_{12} not effective as a treatment for pernicious anemia?

APLASTIC ANEMIA

PATHOPHYSIOLOGY

Aplastic anemia results from depression of bone marrow function, leading to loss of stem cells. **Pancytopenia**, or decreased numbers of erythrocytes, leukocytes, and platelets, leads to many complications. In a few cases only one type of cell is suppressed. The bone marrow is hypocellular with increased fatty tissue.

ETIOLOGY

In approximately half the cases the patients are middle-aged, and the cause is unknown or idiopathic. In many other cases **myelotoxins**, such as radiation, chemicals (e.g., benzene), and drugs (e.g., chloramphenicol, gold salts, phenylbutazone, phenytoin, and antineoplastic drugs) may damage the bone marrow. In these cases it is important to detect and remove the causative factor quickly to allow the marrow to recover. When severe aplastic anemia due to cancer treatment is a risk, the patient's stem cells may be harvested prior to treatment and then transfused later when needed. Viruses, particularly hepatitis C (non A–non B hepatitis) may cause aplastic anemia.

SIGNS AND SYMPTOMS

In the majority of cases, the onset is insidious. Manifestations include those of anemia (pallor, weakness, and dyspnea), those of leukopenia, such as recurrent or multiple infections, and those related to **thrombocytopenia** (**petechiae**—flat, red, pinpoint hemorrhages on the skin—and a tendency to bleed excessively, particularly in the mouth).

A. Normal Erythropoiesis

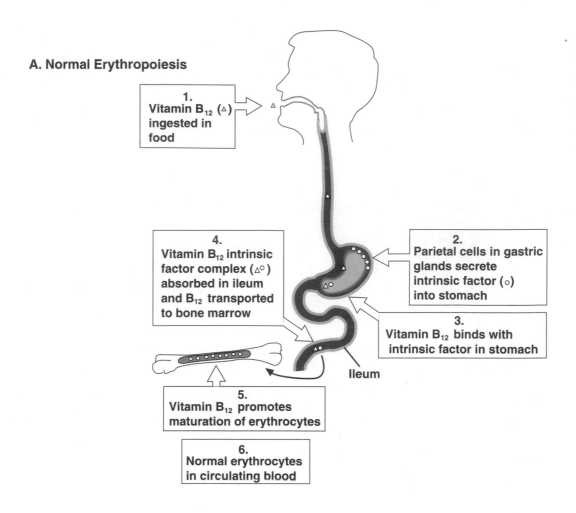

1.
Vitamin B$_{12}$ ($\triangle$) ingested in food

2.
Parietal cells in gastric glands secrete intrinsic factor ($\circ$) into stomach

3.
Vitamin B$_{12}$ binds with intrinsic factor in stomach

4.
Vitamin B$_{12}$ intrinsic factor complex ($\triangle\circ$) absorbed in ileum and B$_{12}$ transported to bone marrow

Ileum

5.
Vitamin B$_{12}$ promotes maturation of erythrocytes

6.
Normal erythrocytes in circulating blood

B. Vitamin B$_{12}$ Deficit

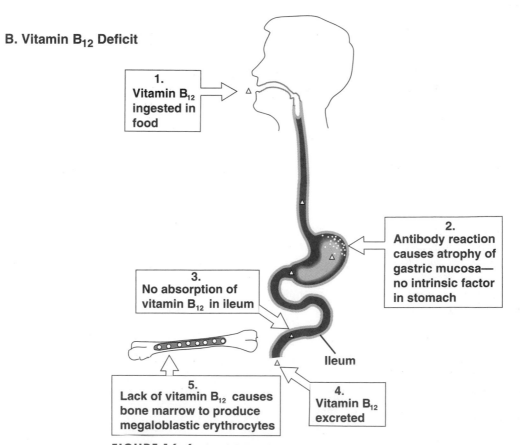

1.
Vitamin B$_{12}$ ingested in food

2.
Antibody reaction causes atrophy of gastric mucosa— no intrinsic factor in stomach

3.
No absorption of vitamin B$_{12}$ in ileum

Ileum

4.
Vitamin B$_{12}$ excreted

5.
Lack of vitamin B$_{12}$ causes bone marrow to produce megaloblastic erythrocytes

FIGURE 16–6. *A* and *B*, Development of pernicious anemia.

DIAGNOSTIC TESTS

Blood counts indicate pancytopenia. A bone marrow biopsy may be required to confirm the cause of the pancytopenia. The erythrocytes are often normal in appearance.

TREATMENT

Prompt treatment of the underlying cause and removal of any bone marrow suppressants are essential. Blood transfusion may be necessary if stem cell levels are very low. Bone marrow transplantation may be helpful in younger patients; its success depends on the accuracy of the tissue match using human leukocyte antigen (HLA). Chemotherapy and radiation are used to prepare the recipient's bone marrow for transplantation of stem cells (taken from the marrow of the pelvic bone of a suitable donor). New techniques allow physicians to harvest stem cells from the peripheral blood, not the marrow. The donor stem cells are infused intravenously into the blood of the recipient; they migrate to the bone marrow and provide a new source of blood cells after several weeks. Antirejection drugs are required for a year, but unlike the situation with other transplants, these drugs can then be discontinued. Common complications include damage to the digestive tract from the preparatory treatment, infection resulting from immune suppression, and rejection.

Thinkabout 16-10

Explain why excessive bleeding occurs with aplastic anemia.

SICKLE CELL ANEMIA (HEMOLYTIC ANEMIA)

PATHOPHYSIOLOGY

Sickle cell anemia is representative of a large number of hemoglobinopathies. In this anemia, an inherited characteristic leads to the formation of an abnormal hemoglobin, hemoglobin S (HbS). In HbS one amino acid in the pair of beta-globin chains has been changed from the normal glutamic acid to valine (Fig. 16–7). When this altered hemoglobin is deoxygenated, it crystallizes and changes the shape of the RBC from a disc to a crescent or "sickle" shape. The cell membrane is damaged, leading to hemolysis, and the cells have a shorter life span than normal, perhaps only 20 days. In addition to the basic anemia the high rate of hemolysis

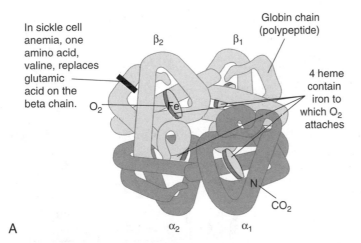

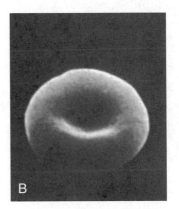

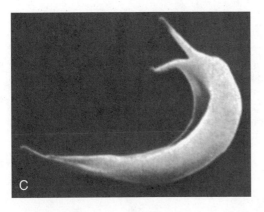

FIGURE 16–7. *A*, Structure of hemoglobin. *B*, An oxygenated sickle-cell erythrocyte. *C*, A deoxygenated sickle cell erythrocyte. (*B* and *C* courtesy of Dr. James White.)

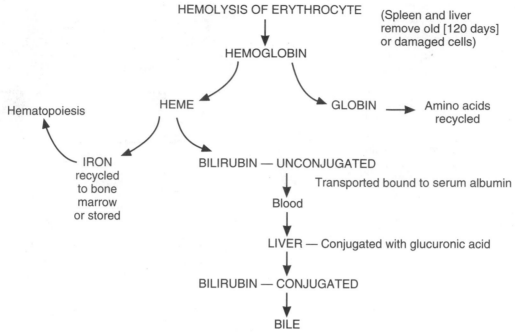

HEMOLYSIS OF ERYTHROCYTE   (Spleen and liver remove old [120 days] or damaged cells)

HEMOGLOBIN

HEME   GLOBIN → Amino acids recycled

Hematopoiesis

IRON recycled to bone marrow or stored

BILIRUBIN — UNCONJUGATED

Transported bound to serum albumin

Blood

LIVER — Conjugated with glucuronic acid

BILIRUBIN — CONJUGATED

BILE

FIGURE 16–8. Breakdown of hemoglobin.

leads to hyperbilirubinemia and jaundice (Fig. 16–8 and Chapter 18). The bone marrow is hyperplastic, and more reticulocytes (immature RBCs) are released into the circulation. HbS can transport oxygen in the normal fashion, but the erythrocyte count is very low. Also, the sickled cells cause obstruction of the small blood vessels, resulting in repeated multiple **infarctions** or areas of tissue necrosis throughout the body. The deoxygenation of hemoglobin may occur in the peripheral circulation as the oxygen content of the blood is gradu-

ally reduced, or a "crisis" may occur in people with lung infection or dehydration when basic oxygen levels are reduced.

ETIOLOGY

The gene for HbS is recessive and is very common in the black population. In homozygotes most of the normal hemoglobin (hemoglobin A [HbA]) is replaced by HbS, resulting in clinical signs of sickle cell anemia (Fig. 16–9). In heterozygotes less than half the hemoglobin is the abnormal HbS, and therefore clinical signs occur

A. PARENT WITH SICKLE CELL TRAIT

	s	a	Probability
a	sa trait	aa normal	50% for child with sickle cell trait
a	sa trait	aa normal	

NORMAL PARENT

B. PARENT WITH SICKLE CELL TRAIT

	s	a	Probability
S	ss anemia	sa trait	25% normal 25% with sickle cell anemia 50% with sickle cell trait
a	sa trait	aa normal	

PARENT WITH SICKLE CELL TRAIT

C. PARENT WITH SICKLE CELL ANEMIA

	s	s	Probability
a	sa trait	sa trait	100% with sickle cell trait
a	sa trait	sa trait	

NORMAL PARENT

KEY
aa = normal: HbA
ss = sickle cell anemia: HbS
sa = sickle cell trait: mixed HbA and HbS

FIGURE 16–9. Inheritance of sickle cell anemia.

only with severe hypoxia under unusual circumstances; this condition is termed the sickle cell trait. Interestingly, the carrier population in Africa is very high, evidently owing to a protective effect of the gene against malaria.

SIGNS AND SYMPTOMS

Clinical signs do not appear until the child is about 6 months of age, when fetal hemoglobin (HbF) has been replaced by HbS. Severe anemia causes pallor, weakness, tachycardia, and dyspnea. Hyperbilirubinemia (high serum levels of unconjugated bilirubin) is indicated by jaundice, the yellowish color being most obvious in the sclerae of the eye. The high bilirubin concentration in the bile may cause the development of gallstones (see Chapter 18). **Splenomegaly** is common in young people because sickled cells cause congestion, but in adults the spleen is usually small and fibrotic owing to recurrent infarction.

Vascular occlusions and infarctions lead to periodic painful crises and permanent damage to organs and tissues. Such damage may be manifest as ulcers on the legs and feet, areas of necrosis in the bone or kidneys, or seizures or hemiplegia resulting from cerebral infarctions (strokes).

DIAGNOSTIC TESTS

Carriers of the defective gene can be detected by a simple blood test. This identification is useful in helping to prevent severe hypoxia and sickling episodes as well as in assisting the parents in decision making about the risk of having an affected child (see Chapter 7). Prenatal diagnosis can be checked by DNA analysis of the fetal blood. The diagnosis can be confirmed by the presence of sickled cells in peripheral blood and the presence of HbS.

TREATMENT

The search continues for effective drugs to reduce sickling. Other supportive measures are used to prevent dehydration, acidosis, infection, or exposure to cold, all of which increase the sickling tendency.

Thinkabout 16-11

a. Why is a person with sickle cell anemia considered anemic?

b. Explain why vascular occlusions are common in patients with sickle cell disease.

c. Compare sickle cell trait and sickle cell anemia in terms of the genetic factor involved, the amount of HbS present, and the presence of clinical signs.

d. Prepare a chart comparing iron deficiency anemia, pernicious anemia, aplastic anemia, and sickle cell anemia with regard to cause and major effects, and list one treatment measure for each.

Polycythemia

PATHOPHYSIOLOGY

Primary polycythemia or polycythemia vera is a condition in which there is an increased production of erythrocytes and other cells in the bone marrow; it is considered a neoplastic disorder. Serum erythropoietin levels are low.

Secondary polycythemia or erythrocytosis is an increase in RBCs that occurs in response to increased erythropoietin secretion. It may be a compensation mechanism intended to provide increased oxygen transport in the presence of chronic lung disease or heart disease. Some cases result from erythropoietin-secreting tumors such as renal carcinoma or from living at high altitudes. Usually the increase in RBCs is not as marked in secondary polycythemia, and more reticulocytes appear in the peripheral blood.

In polycythemia vera there is a marked increase in erythrocytes and often in granulocytes and thrombocytes as well, resulting in increased blood volume and viscosity. Blood vessels are distended, and blood flow is sluggish, leading to frequent thromboses and infarctions throughout the body, especially when platelet counts are high. Hemorrhage is frequent in places where the blood vessels are distended. The spleen and liver are congested and enlarged, and the bone marrow is hypercellular.

In some patients the bone marrow eventually becomes fibrotic, hematopoiesis develops in the spleen, and anemia follows. In a few patients, acute myeloblastic leukemia develops in the later stages, especially if treatment has involved chemotherapy.

ETIOLOGY

Primary polycythemia is a neoplastic disorder of unknown origin that commonly develops between the ages of 40 and 60.

SIGNS AND SYMPTOMS

The patient appears **plethoric** and **cyanotic**, the deep bluish-red tone of the skin and mucosa resulting from the engorged blood vessels and sluggish blood flow. **Hepatomegaly** and splenomegaly are present. Pruritus is common. Blood pressure increases, the pulse is full and bounding, and dyspnea, headaches, or visual disturbances are common. Thromboses and infarctions may affect the extremities, liver, or kidneys as well as the brain or the heart. Congestive heart failure frequently develops because of the increased work load resulting from the increased volume and viscosity of blood.

DIAGNOSTIC TESTS

Blood cell counts and hematocrit are markedly elevated. Hyperuricemia is present because of the high cell destruction rate. Bone marrow is hypercellular, with the red marrow replacing some fatty marrow.

TREATMENT

Drugs or radiation may be used to suppress the activity of the bone marrow. There is more risk that fibrosis or leukemia may develop with this method. Periodic **phlebotomy** or removal of blood may be used to minimize the possibility of thromboses or hemorrhages.

Thinkabout 16–12

Compare the general effects of anemia and polycythemia in terms of hemoglobin level, hematocrit, and general appearance.

Blood-Clotting Disorders

Spontaneous bleeding or excessive bleeding following minor tissue trauma indicates a blood-clotting disorder (Fig. 16–10). In some cases, the blood vessels are more fragile secondary to severe vitamin C deficits or certain infections. Fragility is indicated by the presence of petechiae or **ecchymoses** (bruises) in the skin or mucous membranes and normal coagulation test results.

A second group of blood-clotting disorders results from thrombocytopenia or defective function of the thrombocytes (platelets). Thrombocytopenia may be caused by autoimmune reactions (idiopathic thrombocytopenic purpura), viral infections such as human immunodeficiency virus (HIV), and certain drugs. Defective platelet function is associated with uremia (end-stage kidney failure) and ingestion of aspirin (ASA). Anyone with a bleeding disorder should avoid ASA or ASA-containing drugs as well as nonsteroidal anti-inflammatory drugs (NSAIDs) because all of these interfere with platelet adhesion. Petechiae, ecchymoses, and bleeding in the mouth are common, and excessive bleeding occurs with trauma. Bleeding time, the duration of bleeding from a small skin puncture, assesses platelet function and vascular integrity and therefore is prolonged in these two groups of patients. Coagulation or whole blood clotting time, the time for fresh blood to clot in a tube (in vitro), measures the intrinsic mechanism and so is normal in these cases. PT,

also normal, is a better more specific test. Tests and factors are summarized in Ready Reference 4.

Vitamin K deficiency may cause a decrease in prothrombin and fibrinogen levels. Vitamin K is a fat-soluble vitamin produced by the intestinal bacteria and is present in some foods as well. A deficiency of vitamin K may occur in patients with liver disease accompanied by a decrease in bile production and in those with malabsorption problems. However, vitamin K is a useful antidote when an excess of warfarin, an oral anticoagulant, causes bleeding.

Other bleeding disorders result from a deficiency of one of the clotting factors, often due to an inherited defect. Serum factor analysis and more specific tests are useful here. These include PT to measure the extrinsic pathway, activated partial thromboplastin time (APTT) to measure the intrinsic pathway, and thrombin time for the final stage, fibrinogen to fibrin.

When a patient with any bleeding disorder is at risk for hemorrhage because of an invasive procedure, it is best to be prepared by using laboratory tests to check the current blood-clotting status and to administer prophylactic medications if needed. Personnel should be ready and supplies should be available for any emergency, including the application of pressure, cold dressings, and absorbable hemostatic packing agents such as Gelfoam or Oxycel and styptics.

HEMOPHILIA A

PATHOPHYSIOLOGY

Hemophilia A or classic hemophilia is a deficit or abnormality of clotting factor VIII and is the most common inherited clotting disorder (Fig. 16–11). Hemophilia B (Christmas disease) is similar and involves a deficit of factor IX, and hemophilia C (Rosenthal's hemophilia) is a milder form resulting from a decrease in factor XI. The defect causing hemophilia A is transmitted as an X-linked recessive trait, and therefore it is manifest in males but is carried by females, who are asymptomatic (see Chapter 7). With improved treatment and a longer life span for males, this pattern could change. An affected male and a carrier female could produce a female child who inherits the gene from both parents. Some cases of hemophilia result from a spontaneous gene mutation in a person with no previous family history of the disease. There are varying degrees of severity of hemophilia depending on the percentage of deficit of the factor involved. In mild forms (more than 5 percent factor VIII activity) excessive bleeding occurs only after trauma, whereas frequent spontaneous bleeding is common in people with severe deficiencies (less than 1 percent factor VIII activity).

SIGNS AND SYMPTOMS

Prolonged or severe hemorrhage occurs following tissue trauma. Prolonged oozing of blood after minor

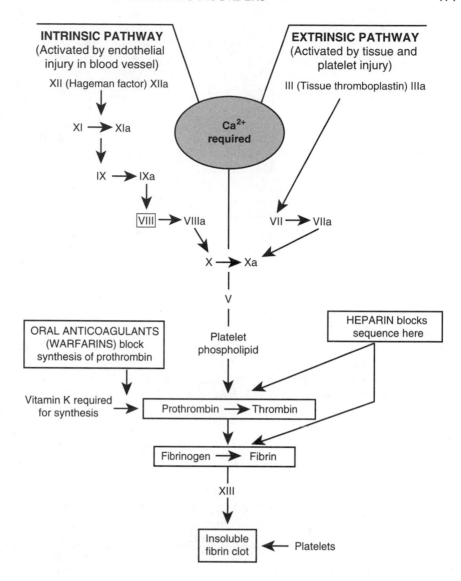

FIGURE 16-10. Hemostasis and anticoagulant drugs.

injuries and hematomas is common. Spontaneous hemorrhage into joints (**hemarthroses**) may occur, eventually causing painful and crippling deformities resulting from recurrent inflammation. Blood may appear in the urine (hematuria) or feces because of bleeding in the kidneys or digestive tract.

DIAGNOSTIC TESTS

Bleeding time is normal, but the PTT, APTT, and coagulation time are prolonged. Serum levels of factor VIII are low. Thromboplastin generation time differentiates between deficits of factor VIII and IX.

TREATMENT

All precautions mentioned earlier should be followed. Replacement therapy for factor VIII, for example, cryoprecipitate, is available and should be administered periodically and especially prior to any surgical or dental procedure. Unfortunately, hepatitis and HIV have been transmitted through these prod-

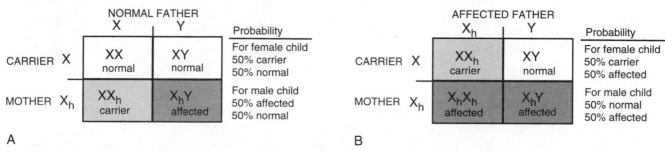

FIGURE 16-11. Inheritance of hemophilia A.

ucts. Although blood is now treated to destroy known viruses, there remains a risk that some unknown infection may be acquired by such treatment.

DISSEMINATED INTRAVASCULAR COAGULATION

PATHOPHYSIOLOGY

Disseminated intravascular coagulation (DIC) is a disorder that involves both excessive bleeding and excessive clotting. It occurs as a complication of the primary problem, which activates the clotting process in the microcirculation throughout the body. Clotting may be induced by the release of tissue thromboplastin or by injury to the endothelial cells, causing platelet adhesion. The process causes multiple thromboses and infarctions but also uses up the clotting factors and platelets and stimulates fibrinolysis. This consumption of clotting factors and fibrinolysis then leads to hemorrhage and eventually to hypotension or shock.

ETIOLOGY

A variety of disorders can initiate DIC. It may result from an obstetric complication such as toxemia, amniotic fluid embolus, or abruptio placentae, in which tissue thromboplastin is released from the placenta. Infection, particularly gram-negative infection, leads to endotoxins that cause endothelial damage or stimulate the release of thromboplastin from monocytes. Many carcinomas release substances that trigger coagulation. Major trauma such as burns or crush injuries and widespread deposits of antigen-antibody complexes result in endothelial damage, releasing thromboplastin and initiating the process.

SIGNS AND SYMPTOMS

Whether hemorrhage or thrombosis dominates the clinical effects depends somewhat on the underlying cause. Obstetric patients usually manifest increased bleeding, whereas cancer patients tend to have more thromboses. More often, hemorrhage is the critical problem. This is indicated by low plasma fibrinogen level, thrombocytopenia, and prolonged bleeding time, PT, APTT, and thrombin time. Accompanying hemorrhage are the effects of low blood pressure or shock. Petechiae or ecchymoses may be present on the skin or mucosa, and hematuria may develop. Vascular occlusions are frequently present in small blood vessels but occasionally affect the large vessels as well, causing infarcts in the brain or other organs.

TREATMENT

The underlying cause, such as infection, must be treated successfully, as well as the major current problem, whether it be excessive clotting or hemorrhage. A fine balance is required to treat the coagulation imbalance, particularly in severe cases.

Thinkabout 16–13

a. State the probability that a child with a carrier mother will have hemophilia A.
b. Describe briefly three other causes of excessive bleeding.

The Leukemias

PATHOPHYSIOLOGY

The leukemias are a group of neoplastic disorders involving the white blood cells. One or more of the leukocyte types are present as undifferentiated, immature, nonfunctional cells that multiply uncontrollably and are released as such into the general circulation. As the numbers of leukemic cells increase, they infiltrate the spleen, liver, and other organs. Leukemias are classified and named according to the cell type involved, the maturity of the cell, and the severity of the problem (Table 16–2). Acute leukemias are characterized by a high proportion of very immature, nonfunctional cells (blast cells) in the bone marrow and circulation; it usually has an abrupt onset with marked signs and complications. Chronic leukemias have a higher proportion of mature cells, an insidious onset, and mild signs and thus a better prognosis. Both acute and chronic leukemias can be further differentiated according to the cell type involved, for example, lymphocytic leukemia (see Table 16–2). The major groups are then further differentiated, for example, acute monoblastic leukemia, which is a type of myelogenous leukemia. In some severe forms of acute leukemias only undifferentiated stem cells can be identified. When the cells are primitive, the term blast is used in the name.

The proliferation of leukemic cells in the bone marrow suppresses the production of other normal cells,

TABLE 16-2 Types of Leukemias	
Type	**Malignant Cells**
Acute lymphoblastic leukemia (ALL)	Lymphocytes
Acute myeloblastic (or myelocytic) leukemia (AML)	Granulocytes (neutrophils, eosinophils, and basophils)
Acute monocytic leukemia	Monocytes
Chronic lymphocytic leukemia (CLL)	B Lymphocytes
Chronic myeloid leukemia (CML)	Granulocytes
Hairy cell leukemia	Lymphocytes and monocytes

leading to anemia, thrombocytopenia, and a lack of normal functional leukocytes. The rapid turnover of cells leads to hyperuricemia and a risk of kidney stones and kidney failure, especially in patients who are receiving chemotherapy. The crowding of the bone marrow also causes bone pain due to pressure on the nerves in the rigid bone and the stretching of the periosteum. As the malignancy progresses, the increased numbers of leukemic cells cause congestion and enlargement of lymphoid tissue, **lymphadenopathy**, splenomegaly, and hepatomegaly. Death usually results from a complication such as overwhelming infection.

ETIOLOGY

Chronic leukemias are more common in older people, whereas acute leukemias occur primarily in children and young adults. Leukemia, the most common childhood cancer, usually begins between the ages of 2 and 6. The cause in children has not been established. A number of factors have been shown to be associated with leukemia in adults, including exposure to radiation, chemicals such as benzene, and certain viruses. There also appears to be an association with chromosomal abnormalities, particularly translocations; this factor is evident in the increased incidence of leukemia in children with Down's syndrome. Of interest is the fact that many adults with chronic myeloblastic leukemia have the Philadelphia chromosome, a specific abnormal chromosomal translocation that serves as a marker in the diagnosis of chronic myeloblastic leukemia.

SIGNS AND SYMPTOMS

The onset of acute leukemia is usually marked by infection that is unresponsive to treatment or by excessive bleeding, and these problems persist through the active stages. Multiple infections often develop because of the nonfunctional WBCs, and severe hemorrhage occurs because of thrombocytopenia; either of these are life threatening. The signs of anemia develop as the erythrocyte count drops. Bone pain is severe and steady, continuing during rest. Weight loss and fatigue result from the hypermetabolism associated with neoplastic growth, from anorexia due to infection, from pain, and from the effects of chemotherapy. Fever may result from hypermetabolism or infection. The lymph nodes, spleen, and liver are often enlarged and may cause discomfort. If leukemic cells infiltrate the central nervous system, headache, visual disturbances, drowsiness, or vomiting follows.

Chronic leukemia tends to have more insidious signs and may be diagnosed on a routine blood check. Early signs include fatigue, weakness, and frequent infections.

DIAGNOSTIC TESTS

Peripheral blood smears show the immature leukocytes and the altered numbers of WBCs, which are usually greatly increased. A high percentage of the WBCs are immature and appear abnormal. Numbers of RBCs and platelets are decreased. Bone marrow aspiration confirms the diagnosis.

TREATMENT

Chemotherapy is administered (see Chapter 5). Some types of leukemia such as acute lymphoblastic leukemia (ALL) in children respond well to drugs, and remissions or cures may ensue. Chemotherapy is less successful in adults. It is important to try to maintain the proper level of nutrition and hydration, particularly if high uric acid levels develop. Alkalinizing the urine by ingesting antacids may help to prevent the formation of kidney stones. The prognosis is often related to the WBC count and the proportion of blast cells present. Chemotherapy may have to be temporarily discontinued if the blood cell counts drop too low, for example, in marked thrombocytopenia or **neutropenia.** Transfusions of platelets or blood cells may be required. Bone marrow transplantation may be tried when chemotherapy is ineffective. Any tumor cells must be eradicated in the recipient, and a suitable donor must be located before transplantation is attempted (see earlier section on Aplastic Anemia).

Thinkabout 16–14

a. Prepare a chart comparing the characteristics of acute and chronic leukemias, including the age groups involved, onset, and typical blood cell characteristics.

b. Why are multiple opportunistic infections common in patients with leukemia?

c. Explain why it is best to defer (if possible) any invasive procedures in leukemic patients, including dental treatment, until the blood counts become more normal.

d. The mouth and mucosa of the digestive tract are usually inflamed and ulcerated because of anemia, the effects of chemotherapy, and the presence of infections, such as *Candida.* Explain how this situation would affect food and fluid intake and list some possible subsequent effects on the client.

HEART DISORDERS

Heart disease is ranked as a major cause of morbidity and mortality in North America. Heart disease includes congenital heart defects, hypertensive heart disease, angina and heart attacks, cardiac arrhythmias, and congestive heart failure.

Diagnostic Tests for Cardiovascular Function

Because many of the same tests are used in the diagnosis and monitoring of a variety of cardiovascular disorders, a few of the common tests are summarized here. Other specific tests are mentioned under the appropriate topic and in Ready Reference 4.

An ECG is useful in the initial diagnosis and monitoring of arrhythmias, myocardial infarction, infection, and pericarditis (see Figs. 16–18 and 16–19). It is a noninvasive procedure and can illustrate the conduction activity of the heart as well as the effects of systemic abnormalities such as serum electrolyte imbalance. A portable *Holter monitor* may be worn by an individual to record ECG changes while he or she pursues daily activities. A normal baseline ECG recording is recommended for everyone; it can be used for comparison if cardiovascular disease ever develops.

Valvular abnormalities or abnormal shunts of blood cause *murmurs* that may be detected by **auscultation** of heart sounds using a stethoscope. A recording of heart sounds may be made using a phonocardiogram. *In echocardiography* ultrasound is used to record the image of the heart and valve movements.

Exercise stress tests (bicycle, step, or treadmill) are useful in assessing general cardiovascular function and in checking for exercise-induced problems such as arrhythmias. They may be used in health clubs before setting up an individualized fitness program or by insurance companies in the evaluation of an individual's health risks as well as in cardiac rehabilitation programs following heart attacks or cardiovascular surgery.

Chest x-ray films can be used to show the shape and size of the heart as well as any evidence of pulmonary congestion associated with heart failure. *Nuclear imaging* with radioactive substances is used to assess the size of an infarct in the heart, the extent of myocardial perfusion, and the function of the ventricles.

Blood flow in the coronary arteries can be visualized with coronary **angiography** using cardiac catheterization and a contrast dye. Blood flow in the peripheral vessels can be assessed using *Doppler* studies, which are essentially a microphone placed over the blood vessel that records the sounds of blood flow or obstruction. Invasive procedures, involving insertion of a catheter into a large blood vessel such as the pulmonary artery, may be used to provide information on *central venous pressure* and *pulmonary capillary wedge pressure,* which indicate blood flow to and from the heart. *Cardiac catheterization* may also be used to visualize the inside of the heart and its function.

Blood tests are used to assess serum triglyceride and cholesterol levels and the levels of sodium, potassium, calcium, and other electrolytes. Hemoglobin, hematocrit, blood cell counts, and the differential count for white cells are also routine aspects of blood tests. Arterial blood gas determination is essential in patients with shock or myocardial infarction to check the oxygen level and acid-base balance.

General Treatment Measures for Cardiac Disorders

Because some treatment measures apply to many disorders, a number of common therapies are covered here. Additional specific treatment modalities are mentioned with the disorder to which they apply.

Dietary modifications usually include reducing total fat intake and intake of saturated (hydrogenated or animal) fat. General weight reduction may be recommended for some persons. Salt (sodium) intake is decreased as well.

A regular exercise program is suggested to improve overall cardiovascular function and circulation to all areas of the body. Exercise assists in lowering serum lipid levels, increasing HDL levels, and reducing stress levels, which in turn lessen peripheral resistance and blood pressure.

Cessation of cigarette smoking decreases the risk of coronary disease because smoking appears to increase vasoconstriction and heart rate, thus increasing the work load on the heart. Smoking increases platelet adhesion and serum lipid levels. Also, carbon monoxide, a product of smoking, displaces oxygen from hemoglobin. In a compromised patient, this decrease in oxygen can be dangerous.

Drug therapy is an important component in the maintenance of cardiac patients. Many individuals take several drugs. *Vasodilators* such as nitroglycerin or long-acting isosorbide reduce peripheral resistance and act as coronary vasodilators. These actions decrease the work of the heart and provide a better balance of oxygen supply and demand in the heart muscle. Vasodilators may cause a decrease in blood pressure, resulting in dizziness or syncope and a flushed face. A person should sit quietly for a few minutes after taking nitroglycerin sublingually.

Beta-blockers such as propranolol, metoprolol, or atenolol are used to treat angina, hypertension, and arrhythmias. These drugs block the beta$_1$-adrenergic receptors in the heart and prevent the SNS from increasing heart activity.

A newer group of effective cardiovascular drugs is the *calcium channel blockers,* which block the movement of calcium ions into the cardiac and smooth muscle fibers. Members of the group may be used as agents to decrease cardiac contractility, as an antiarrhythmic particularly for excessive atrial activity, or as an antihypertensive and vasodilator. Some drugs such as diltiazem are more selective for the myocardium and reduce both conduction and contractility. Verapamil slows the heart rate by depressing the action of the SA and AV nodes, preventing tachycardia and fibrillation. Others, like nifedipine, are more effective as peripheral vasodilators. Note that these drugs do not affect skeletal muscle because more calcium is stored in skeletal muscle cells.

Digoxin, a cardiac glycoside, has been used for many years as a treatment for heart failure and as an antiarrhythmic drug for atrial dysrhythmias. It slows conduction of impulses and heart rate. Digoxin improves the efficiency of the heart because it also is inotropic and increases the contractility of the heart. The contractions are less frequent but stronger. Because the effective dose is close to the toxic dose, patients must be observed for signs of toxicity.

Antihypertensive drugs may be used to lower blood pressure to more normal levels. In addition to the groups previously mentioned, the beta-blockers and calcium blockers, which may be used as antihypertensives, the diuretics and angiotensin-converting enzyme inhibitors that are mentioned later in this section may be included in the treatment of high blood pressure. The basic antihypertensive drugs may act on the SNS centrally (brain), may block peripheral (arteriolar) alpha$_1$-adrenergic receptors, or may act as direct vasodilators. Combinations of drugs from various classifications are frequently prescribed to achieve a lower blood pressure with minimal side effects. These drugs may be used for treatment of essential hypertension or congestive heart failure or after myocardial infarction. Many antihypertensive agents cause orthostatic hypotension because the normal SNS reflex for controlling blood pressure with position change is lost.

Diuretics remove excess sodium and water from the body through the kidneys by blocking the reabsorption of sodium or water (see Chapter 19). Patients often refer to them as "water pills." They are useful drugs in the treatment of high blood pressure and congestive heart failure because they increase urine output, reducing blood volume and edema. Examples are hydrochlorothiazide, a mild diuretic, and furosemide, a more potent drug. These diuretics may also remove excessive potassium from the body, requiring supplements to prevent hypokalemia. Spironolactone is an example of a "potassium-sparing" diuretic.

Angiotensin-converting enzyme inhibitors (ACE inhibitors) are useful adjuncts in the treatment of patients with hypertension and CHF, by blocking the conversion of angiotensin I to angiotensin II in the renin mechanism. These drugs, such as captopril, reduce peripheral resistance (vasoconstriction) and aldosterone secretion (thus decreasing sodium and water retention).

Anticoagulants may be used to reduce the risk of blood clot formation in coronary or systemic arteries or on damaged or prosthetic heart valves. In many cases, a small daily dose of ASA decreases platelet adhesion. Oral anticoagulants such as warfarin may be taken by individuals in high-risk groups. These drugs block the coagulation process (see Fig. 16–10). It is essential to monitor clotting ability, using PT or APTT closely in these patients to prevent hemorrhage.

Coronary Artery Disease or Ischemic Heart Disease

Sometimes also called coronary heart disease (CHD), coronary artery disease includes angina pectoris or temporary cardiac ischemia and myocardial infarction or heart attack, in which part of the heart muscle is damaged. A common cause of disability and death, CHD may ultimately lead to heart failure, serious arrhythmias, or sudden death. The basic problem is insufficient oxygen for the needs of the heart muscle.

ARTERIOSCLEROSIS AND ATHEROSCLEROSIS

PATHOPHYSIOLOGY

Arteriosclerosis may be used as a general term for all types of arterial changes. It is best applied to degenerative changes in the small arteries and arterioles, commonly occurring in older individuals and diabetics. Elasticity is lost, the walls become thick and hard, and the lumen gradually narrows and may become obscured. This leads to diffuse ischemia and necrosis in various tissues such as the kidneys, brain, or heart.

Atherosclerosis is characterized by *atheromas,* plaques consisting of lipids, cells, fibrin, and cell debris, often with attached thrombus, which form inside the walls of large arteries (Fig. 16–12). The process appears to begin

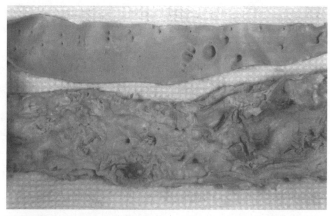

FIGURE 16-12. Comparison of a normal aorta *(top)* with an atherosclerotic aorta *(bottom).* (Courtesy of Paul Emmerson and Seneca College of Applied Arts and Technology, Toronto.)

with endothelial injury in the artery, often at a very young age. When endothelial injury occurs, white blood cells, particularly monocytes and macrophages, and lipids accumulate in the intima or inner lining of the artery and in the media or muscle layer, and smooth muscle cells multiply because of this irritation. Thus, a plaque forms. Platelets adhere to the rough, damaged surface of the arterial wall, forming a thrombus.

Lipids, which are transported in various combinations with proteins, are constantly present in the blood. Lipids, including cholesterol and triglycerides, are essential elements in the body and are synthesized in the liver; therefore, they can never be totally eliminated

from the body. Elevated serum levels of lipids and cholesterol, particularly low-density lipoprotein (LDL), which has a high cholesterol content and transports cholesterol from the liver to cells, is the other major factor contributing to atheroma formation (Fig. 16–13). LDL binds to receptors, for example, on the membranes of vascular smooth muscle cells, and enters them; it is considered the "bad" lipoprotein that promotes atheroma formation. High-density lipoprotein (HDL) is the "good" lipoprotein; it has a low cholesterol content and is used to transport cholesterol away from the peripheral cells to the liver, where it undergoes catabolism and excretion. It has been demon-

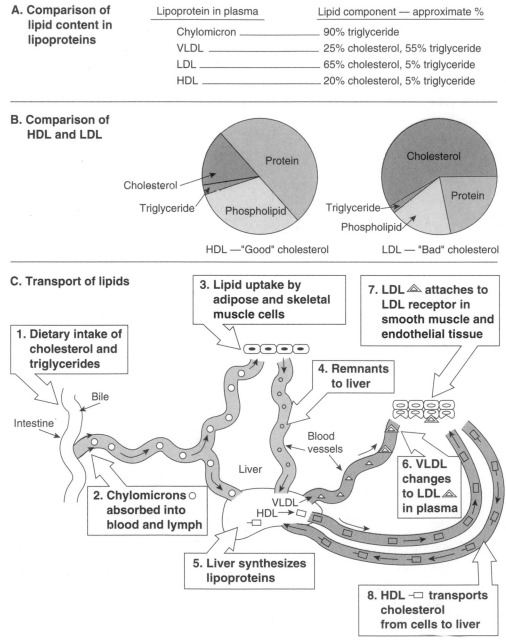

FIGURE 16–13. Composition of lipoproteins and transport of lipoproteins in blood.

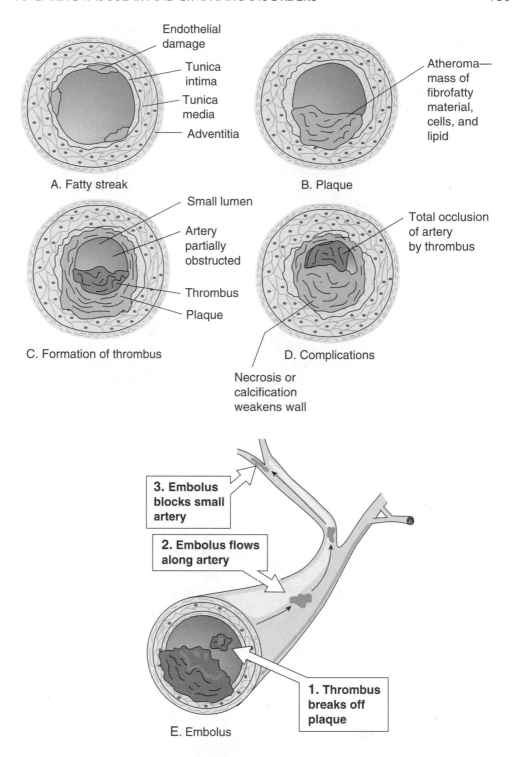

FIGURE 16-14. Development of an atheroma leading to arterial occlusion.

strated that excessive amounts of cholesterol, present either as LDL or as very low-density lipoprotein (VLDL), do predispose to atheroma formation. Lipids continue to build up at the site of arterial injury along with fibrous tissue. Platelets may adhere and release prostaglandins, which may precipitate vasospasm and encourage more platelets to aggregate at the site (Fig. 16–14), forming thrombus. Arterial flow becomes progressively smaller as the lumen narrows. The atheroma also damages the arterial wall, weakening the structure and decreasing its elasticity. In time, the atheroma may calcify, causing further rigidity of the wall. This process may lead to aneurysm, a bulge in the arterial wall, or to rupture and hemorrhage in the wall.

Initially, the atheroma presents as a yellowish fatty streak on the wall. It becomes progressively larger, eventually becoming a large, firm projecting mass with an irregular surface on which thrombus forms. As the atheroma increases in size and the coronary arteries are partially obstructed, angina may occur; a total obstruction leads to myocardial infarction. Atheromas form primarily in the large arteries, such as the aorta and iliac arteries, the coronary arteries, and the carotid arteries, particularly at points of bifurcation, where turbulent blood flow may encourage the development of atheroma. Thus, atheromas are also a common cause of strokes, causing brain damage and peripheral vascular disease, which affects the legs and feet.

ETIOLOGY

The cause of arteriosclerosis appears to be multifactorial, and some of the factors are **synergistic**, enhancing the total effect. There are two groups of risk factors for atherosclerosis, one group of which can be modified to some extent and the other cannot. The factors that cannot be changed include age, gender, and genetic factors. Atherosclerosis is more common after age 40, particularly in males. Females are protected by higher HDL levels until after menopause, when estrogen levels decrease. Genetic or familial factors seem to have a strong influence on serum lipid levels, metabolism, and cell receptors for lipids. Some conditions are inherited, such as familial hypercholesterolemia, but family life style factors may also have a role.

The other group of predisposing factors may be modifiable. These include factors that elevate serum lipid levels, especially LDL, such as obesity and diets high in cholesterol and animal fat, cigarette smoking, sedentary life style, and the presence of diabetes mellitus or hypertension. In diabetics, especially those whose disease is not well controlled, serum lipid levels are increased and there is a tendency toward endothelial degeneration. The risk associated with smoking is directly related to the number of packs of cigarettes smoked per day. Smoking decreases HDL, increases LDL, promotes platelet adhesion, and increases fibrinogen and clot formation as well as vasoconstriction. Uncontrolled hypertension eventually causes endothelial damage. When oral contraceptives contained high doses of hormones, they were associated with an increased risk, particularly in women who also smoked. However, the newer forms of oral contraceptives are much less hazardous.

DIAGNOSTIC TESTS

Serum lipid levels, including those of LDL and HDL, should be checked to identify the patient's risk and to monitor the efficacy of treatment. Exercise stress testing can be used for screening or to assess the degree of obstruction in arteries. Radioisotopic studies can be used to determine the degree of tissue perfusion, the presence of collateral circulation, and the degree of local cell metabolism.

TREATMENT

Lowering serum cholesterol and LDL levels by reducing the intake of saturated or animal fats and using unsaturated or vegetable oils has been well promoted as an effective means of slowing the progress of atherosclerosis. Sodium intake should be minimized as well. High dietary fiber intake and the use of fish oils appear to decrease LDL levels. General weight reduction decreases the work load on the heart. Lipid-reducing drugs such as probucol, clofibrate, and lovastatin may help in resistant cases. These measures may slow the progress of previously formed lesions and also prevent new ones. Control of primary disorders such as diabetes or hypertension is important. If thrombus formation is a concern, oral anticoagulant therapy may be required; this may include a small daily dose of ASA or warfarin-type drugs.

When atheromas are advanced, surgical intervention (**angioplasty**) may be required to reduce obstruction using invasive procedures requiring cardiac catheterization. The catheter contains an inflatable balloon that flattens the atheroma. Newer techniques use laser angioplasty, a laser beam and fiberoptic technology with a catheter. The high energy laser causes the obstruction to disintegrate into microscopic particles that are removed by macrophages. There appears to be less risk of recurrence with this method. Vein grafts may be used to bypass an obstructed artery when angioplasty is not recommended. Bypass surgery for coronary artery obstruction using the left internal mammary artery for a graft appears to have an improved long-term prognosis.

Thinkabout 16–15

a. List three ways of reducing the risk of atherosclerosis.

b. Give three common locations of atheromas.

c. Describe two ways in which an artery can become totally obstructed.

ANGINA PECTORIS

PATHOPHYSIOLOGY

Angina or chest pain occurs when there is a deficit of oxygen for the heart muscle. This can occur when the blood or oxygen supply to the myocardium is impaired, when the heart is working harder than usual and needs more oxygen, or when a combination of these factors is present (Fig. 16–15). Usually the heart can meet its own needs by vasodilation (autoregulation) unless the vessel wall is hard and cannot relax. The blood supply may be decreased owing to partial obstruction by atherosclerosis or spasm in the coronary arteries. When the supply

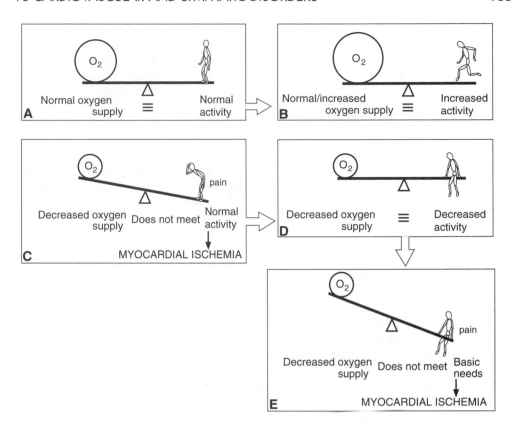

FIGURE 16–15. Angina—balance between oxygen supply and activity.

and demand for oxygen are marginally balanced, an increase in demand with any physical or emotional exertion can cause a relative deficit of oxygen in the heart. Chest pain may occur in a variety of patterns: classic or exertional angina, variant angina, in which vasospasm occurs at rest, and unstable angina, a more serious form. Most commonly, an episode of anginal pain occurs when the demand for oxygen increases suddenly. Angina can be classified in subgroups depending on the cause. In most cases, no permanent damage to the heart results from angina unless the episodes are frequent, prolonged, and severe.

ETIOLOGY

Insufficient myocardial blood supply is associated with atherosclerosis, arteriosclerosis, vasospasm (a localized contraction of arteriolar smooth muscle), and myocardial hypertrophy, in which the heart has outgrown its blood supply. Severe anemias and respiratory disease can also cause an oxygen deficit. Increased demands for oxygen can arise in circumstances such as tachycardia associated with hyperthyroidism or the increased force of contractions associated with hypertension.

When precipitating factors play a role they are related to activities that increase the demands on the heart such as running upstairs, getting angry, respiratory infection with fever, exposure to cold weather, or eating a large meal.

SIGNS AND SYMPTOMS

Angina occurs as recurrent, intermittent brief episodes of substernal chest pain, usually triggered by a physical or emotional stress that increases the demand by the heart for oxygen. Pain is described as a tightness or pressure in the chest and may radiate to the neck and left arm. Often pallor, **diaphoresis**, and nausea are also present. Attacks vary in severity and last a few seconds or minutes.

TREATMENT

It is important to determine the factors predisposing to attacks to minimize their frequency and severity. Avoidance of sudden physical exertion, especially in cold or hot weather, marked fatigue, or strong emotional incidents is recommended. Antianxiety and stress reduction techniques may be necessary in certain situations.

Anginal pain is usually quickly relieved by rest and the administration of vasodilators such as nitroglycerin. The drug may relieve vasospasm in the coronary arteries but primarily acts to reduce systemic resistance, thus decreasing the demand for oxygen. Many patients carry nitroglycerin with them at all times to be administered sublingually (the tablet is not swallowed but dissolves under the tongue) in an emergency. Some clients use a topical ointment, a skin patch, a nasal spray, or oral tablets (isosorbide) on a regular basis as prophylaxis to reduce the number of attacks.

If chest pain persists following treatment, it is important to seek hospital care because the pain may indicate the presence of a myocardial infarction.

Thinkabout 16–16

a. Describe the characteristics of anginal pain.

b. When reviewing the tasks that you perform in your professional area, list any factors that could precipitate anginal pain in a patient. Suggest ways to reduce the risk of angina occurring.

MYOCARDIAL INFARCTION

PATHOPHYSIOLOGY

A myocardial infarction (MI) or heart attack occurs when a coronary artery is totally obstructed, leading to prolonged ischemia (over 20 minutes), cell death, or infarction of the myocardium (Fig. 16–16). The most common cause is atherosclerosis, usually with thrombus attached (see earlier discussion under Coronary Artery Disease). Infarction may develop in three ways. The thrombus may build up to occlude the artery, or vasospasm may occur in the presence of a partial occlusion by an atheroma leading to total obstruction, or part of the thrombus may break away, forming an embolus that flows through the coronary artery until it lodges in a smaller branch, occluding that vessel (see Fig. 16–14). Most infarctions are transmural—that is, all three layers of the heart are involved. The majority involve the critical left ventricle. The size and location of the infarct determine the severity of the damage.

At the point of obstruction, the heart tissue becomes necrotic, and an area of injury and inflammation develops around the necrotic zone. With cell necrosis, specific enzymes are released into tissue fluid and blood that can assist in the diagnosis. The functions of myocardial contractility and conduction are lost quickly as oxygen supplies are depleted. If the blood supply can be restored in the first 30 minutes, irreversible damage may be prevented. After 48 hours, the inflammation begins to subside. If sufficient blood supply has been maintained in the area of inflammation, function can resume. On the other hand, if treatment has not been instituted quickly, or is not effective, the area of infarction may increase. Because the myocardium does not regenerate, the area of necrosis is gradually replaced by fibrous (nonfunctional) tissue, beginning around the seventh day. It may take 6 to 8 weeks to form the scar, depending on the size of the lesion.

The presence of collateral circulation may reduce the size of the infarct (see earlier in this chapter under Review of the Normal Cardiovascular System). The effectiveness of a collateral circulation depends on the location of the obstruction, the presence or absence of anastomoses, and whether collateral circulation was established before infarction in response to the gradual partial occlusion. Also, if the atheroma has developed gradually, there may have been several warning episodes of chest pain with exertion. If the infarction has resulted from an embolus, there has been no opportunity for collateral channels to develop, and therefore the infarct will be larger.

SIGNS AND SYMPTOMS

Sudden substernal chest pain that radiates to the left arm and neck is the hallmark of myocardial infarction. The pain is usually described as severe, steady, and crushing, and no relief occurs with rest or vasodilators. In some cases, pain is not present (silent myocardial infarction) or is interpreted as gastric discomfort. Fear and anxiety are marked. Other signs are pallor and sweating (diaphoresis), nausea, dizziness and weakness, and dyspnea. Hypotension is common, and the pulse is rapid and weak as cardiac output decreases. Low-grade fever develops.

DIAGNOSTIC TESTS

Typical changes occur in the ECG during the course of a myocardial infarction that confirm the diagnosis and assist in monitoring progress. It is well to monitor serum electrolytes, particularly potassium and sodium. Serum enzymes and isoenzymes released from necrotic cells also follow a typical pattern with elevations of lactic dehydrogenase (LDH-1), aspartate aminotransferase

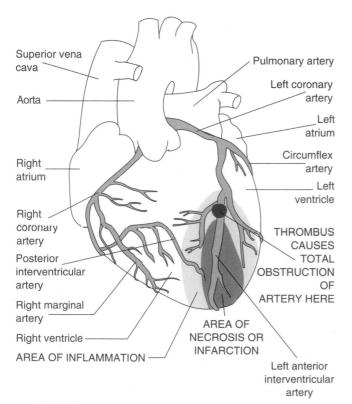

FIGURE 16–16. Damage caused by myocardial infarction.

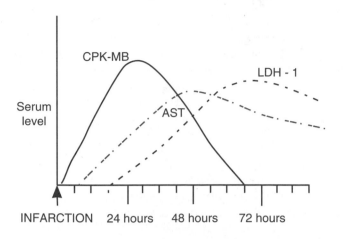

FIGURE 16–17. Serum enzyme and isoenzyme levels with myocardial infarction. CPK-MB; creatine phosphokinase; AST, aspartate aminotransferase, LDH-1; lactate dehydrogenase.

(AST, formerly SGOT), and creatine-phosphokinase (CK-MB or CPK-2) (Fig. 16–17). These particular isoenzymes, LDH-1 and CK-MB, are more specific for heart tissue. Leukocytosis and an elevated erythrocyte sedimentation rate are common. Arterial blood gases are helpful, particularly if shock is pronounced. Pulmonary artery pressure measurements are helpful in determining ventricular function.

COMPLICATIONS

Complications are common. Sudden death shortly after myocardial infarction occurs frequently, usually due to ventricular arrhythmias and fibrillation (see next section, Cardiac Dysrhythmias). One type of **dysrhythmia,** heart block, may occur when the conduction fibers are located in the infarcted area. Second, an area of necrosis and inflammation outside the conduction pathway may stimulate additional spontaneous impulses at an **ectopic** site, causing, for example, *premature ventricular contractions* (PVCs) that lead to ventricular fibrillation. In some cases, arrhythmias occur later as inflammation spreads to the conduction pathways, leading to heart block. Conduction irregularities may also be precipitated by hypoxia, by increased potassium released from necrotic cells, by acidosis, and by drug toxicities.

Cardiogenic shock may develop if the pumping capability of the left ventricle is greatly impaired. Also, *congestive heart failure* is a common occurrence when the contractility of the ventricle is reduced and stroke volume declines. Less frequent complications include *rupture* of the necrotic heart tissue, particularly in hypertensive patients, pericarditis, and ventricular aneurysm. *Thromboembolism* may result from thrombus that develops over the infarcted surface inside the heart (mural thrombus) and eventually breaks off as well as thrombus that may form in the leg veins because of immobility

and poor circulation (phlebothrombosis). The latter leads to pulmonary embolus (see Chapter 17).

TREATMENT

Rest, oxygen therapy, and analgesics such as morphine for pain relief are the usual treatment modalities. Anticoagulants such as heparin or warfarin may be used, or thrombolytic agents including streptokinase, urokinase, or tissue plasminogen activator may be administered to dissolve the clot in the first hours. Depending on the individual circumstances, medication to reduce arrhythmias or a pacemaker (which may be temporary) may be required. Specific measures may be required if shock or congestive heart failure develop.

Cardiac rehabilitation programs that offer individual plans for regular exercise, dietary modifications, and stress reduction as needed are useful following recovery. A schedule for the resumption of normal activities such as climbing stairs, returning to work, and resuming sexual relationships can be established.

Thinkabout 16–17

a. Compare the cause of the chest pain that occurs with angina and with myocardial infarction.
b. Explain why an embolus may cause a larger infarction than an atheroma with thrombus.
c. List the tests that confirm a diagnosis of myocardial infarction.
d. Explain why part of the myocardium is nonfunctional following myocardial infarction.
e. Suggest several treatment measures that may minimize the area of infarction.

Cardiac Arrhythmias (Dysrhythmias)

Alterations in cardiac rate or rhythm may result from damage to the heart's conduction system or from systemic causes such as electrolyte abnormalities (see Chapter 6 for the effects of potassium imbalance), fever, hypoxia, stress, infection, and drug toxicity. Interference with the conduction system may result from inflammation or from scar tissue associated with rheumatic fever or myocardial infarction. Arrhythmias reduce the efficiency of the heart's pumping cycle. A slight increase in heart rate increases cardiac output, but a very rapid heart rate prevents adequate filling during diastole, and a very slow rate reduces output to the tissues, including the brain and the heart itself. Irregular contractions are inefficient because they interfere with the normal filling and emptying cycle. The ECG provides a method of monitoring the conduction system. Holter monitors, which can be worn by outpatients, record the ECG that results from the patient's normal daily activities. Among the many types of abnormal conduction patterns that exist, only a few examples are considered here.

SINUS NODE ABNORMALITIES

The SA node is the pacemaker for the heart, and its rate can be altered (Fig. 16–18). *Bradycardia* refers to a regular but slow heart rate, less than 60 beats per minute; it often results from vagal nerve or parasympathetic nervous system stimulation. An exception is athletes at rest who may have a slow heart rate because they are conditioned to produce a large stroke volume. A regular rapid heart rate, 100 to 160 beats per minute, is referred to as *tachycardia* (Fig. 16–19*B*). This may be a normal response to sympathetic stimulation, exercise, fever, or stress, or it may be compensation for decreased blood volume. *Sick sinus syndrome* is a heart condition marked by alternating bradycardia and tachycardia and often requires a mechanical pacemaker.

ATRIAL CONDUCTION ABNORMALITIES

Premature atrial contractions or *beats* (PAC/PAB) are extra contractions or *ectopic* beats of the atria that usually arise from a focus of irritable atrial muscle cells outside the conduction pathway. They tend to interfere with the timing of the next beat. Ectopic beats may also

develop from *reentry* of an impulse that has been delayed in damaged tissue and then completes a circuit to reexcite the same area before the next regular stimulus arrives. Sometimes people feel *palpitations,* which are rapid or irregular heart contractions that often arise from excessive caffeine intake, smoking, or stress. Atrial *flutter* refers to a heart rate of 160 to 350 beats per minute, and atrial *fibrillation* is a rate over 350 beats per minute. With flutter, the AV node delays conduction, and therefore the ventricular rate is slower. A pulse deficit may occur because a reduced stroke volume is not felt at the radial pulse. Ventricular filling is not totally dependent on atrial contraction, and therefore these atrial arrhythmias are not always noticed unless they spread to the ventricular conduction pathways.

ATRIOVENTRICULAR NODE ABNORMALITIES—HEART BLOCKS

Heart block occurs when conduction is excessively delayed or stopped at the AV node or bundle of His. Partial blocks may be first degree, in which the conduction delay prolongs the PR interval, the time between the atrial and ventricular contractions, or second degree, in which a longer delay leads to a missed ventricular contraction periodically. In total or third-degree heart block, there is no transmission of impulses from the atria to the ventricles. The ventricles contract spontaneously at a slow rate of 30 to 45 beats per minute, totally independent of the atrial contraction, which continues normally (see Fig. 16–19*C*). In this case, cardiac output is greatly reduced, sometimes to the point

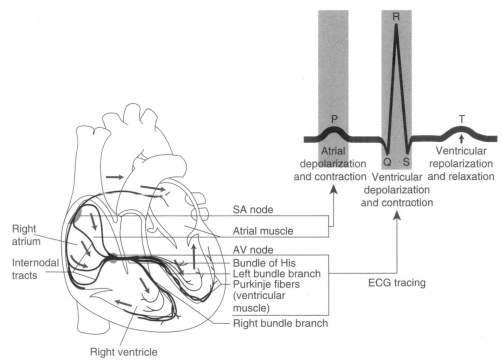

FIGURE 16–18. Conduction system in the heart and its relationship to the ECG.

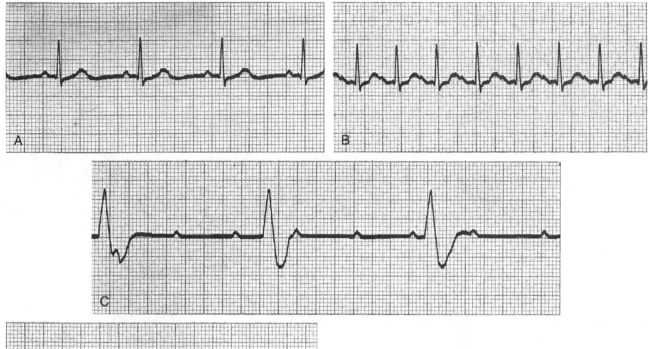

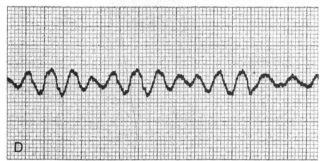

FIGURE 16-19. Arrhythmias on electrocardiogram. *A*, Normal sinus rhythm. *B*, Sinus tachycardia. *C*, Third-degree atrioventricular (AV) heart block. *D*, Ventricular fibrillation. (From Copstead LC: Perspectives on Pathophysiology. Philadelphia, W.B. Saunders, 1995, pp. 414, 419, 420.)

of fainting (syncope), causing a *Stokes-Adams* attack or cardiac arrest.

VENTRICULAR CONDUCTION ABNORMALITIES

Bundle branch block refers to interference with conduction in one of the bundle branches. This usually does not alter cardiac output but does appear on the ECG as a wide QRS wave. Ventricular *tachycardia* is likely to reduce cardiac output because the filling time is reduced. In ventricular *fibrillation* the muscle fibers contract independently and rapidly (uncoordinated quivering) and therefore are ineffective in ejecting blood (see Fig. 16–19D). Cardiac output ceases, and the heart ceases to beat (standstill or cardiac arrest) because of severe hypoxia. *Premature ventricular contractions (PVCs)* are additional beats arising from a ventricular muscle cell or ectopic pacemaker. Occasional PVCs do not interfere with heart function, but increasing frequency, multiple ectopic sites, or paired beats are of concern because ventricular fibrillation often develops from these, leading to arrest.

TREATMENT OF CARDIAC ARRHYTHMIAS

The cause of the arrhythmia should be determined and treated. Easily correctable problems include those caused by drugs, such as digitalis toxicity, bradycardia due to beta blockers, or potassium imbalance related to diuretics. In these examples, a change in dosage or drug may eliminate the arrhythmia. Antiarrhythmic drugs are effective in many cases of heart damage. Beta-adrenergic blockers and calcium channel blockers were discussed earlier in this chapter. Atrial dysrhythmias often respond to digoxin, which slows AV node conduction and strengthens the contraction, thus increasing efficiency.

SA nodal problems or total heart block require a pacemaker, either a temporary attachment or a device that is permanently implanted in the chest; such a device provides electrical stimulation · through electrodes directly to the heart muscle. Caution is required with the use of some electronic equipment when a pacemaker is in place. Serious life-threatening arrhythmias may require the use of defibrillators and cardioversion devices that transmit electrical currents to the heart to interrupt the disorganized electrical activity that occurs with fibrillation, for example, and then allows the SA node to take control again.

CARDIAC ARREST OR STANDSTILL

Cardiac arrest is the cessation of all activity in the heart. There is no conduction of impulses, and the ECG shows a flat line. Lack of contractions means that no cardiac output occurs, and there is no pulse at any site including the apical and carotid sites (see Fig. 16–28). Loss of consciousness takes place immediately, and respiration ceases.

Arrest may occur for many reasons; for example, excessive vagal nerve stimulation may slow the heart, or there may be insufficient oxygen to maintain the heart tissue due to severe shock or ventricular fibrillation. When attempting to resuscitate the patient with cardiopulmonary resuscitation (CPR), it is important to ensure that blood and oxygen reach the heart as well as the brain.

Thinkabout 16–18

a. Define PVCs, atrial flutter, and total heart block.

b. Using one type of arrhythmia as an example, explain how cardiac output may be reduced.

c. Why are no pulses present with ventricular fibrillation?

Congestive Heart Failure

PATHOPHYSIOLOGY

Congestive heart failure (CHF) occurs when the heart is unable to pump sufficient blood to meet the metabolic needs of the body. CHF usually occurs as a complication secondary to another condition. It may present as an acute episode but usually is a chronic condition. CHF may result from a problem in the heart itself such as infarction or a valve defect, or it may arise from increased demands on the heart such as those imposed by hypertension or lung disease, or it may involve a combination of factors. Depending on the cause, one side of the heart usually fails first, followed by the other side. For example, an infarction in the left ventricle or essential hypertension (high blood pressure) affects the left ventricle first, whereas pulmonary valve stenosis or pulmonary disease affects the right

ventricle first. It is helpful in the early stages to refer to this problem as left-sided CHF or right-sided CHF.

Initially, various compensation mechanisms maintain cardiac output (Fig. 16–20). Unfortunately, these mechanisms often aggravate the condition instead of providing assistance. The reduced blood flow into the systemic circulation and thus the kidneys leads to increased renin and aldosterone secretion. The resulting vasoconstriction (increased afterload) and increased blood volume (increased preload) add to the heart's work load. The SNS response also increases heart rate and peripheral resistance. The heart tends to dilate and become hypertrophied (**cardiomegaly**), but this process demands increased blood supply in the heart itself. Increased heart rate may decrease the efficiency of the heart and impede filling.

There are two basic effects when the heart cannot maintain its pumping capability. Cardiac output or stroke volume decreases, resulting in less blood reaching the various organs and tissues, a "forward" effect. This leads to decreased cell function, creating fatigue and lethargy. Mild acidosis develops, which is compensated by increased respirations (see Chapter 6). Because the affected ventricle cannot pump its load adequately, the return of blood to that side of the heart is impeded, and there is a "backup" effect in the circulation behind the affected ventricle (Fig. 16–21). The output from the ventricle is less than the inflow of blood. For example, if the left ventricle cannot pump all of its blood into the systemic circulation, the normal volume of blood returning from the lungs cannot enter the left side of the heart. This eventually causes congestion in the pulmonary circulation, increased capillary pressure, and possible pulmonary edema, in which fluid is forced into the alveoli. This situation is termed left-sided CHF.

In right-sided CHF the right ventricle cannot maintain its output, so less blood proceeds to the left side of the heart and the systemic circulation (forward effect). The backup effect or congestion is apparent in the systemic circulation, as shown by increased blood volume and congestion in the legs and feet and eventually also in the portal circulation (liver and digestive tract) and neck veins. Right- and left-sided failure are compared in Table 16–3.

ETIOLOGY

Infarction that impairs the pumping ability or efficiency of the conducting system, valve defects, or congenital heart defects may cause failure of the affected side. Increased demands on the heart cause heart failure that may take various forms depending on the ventricle most adversely affected. For example, essential hypertension increases diastolic blood pressure, requiring the left ventricle to contract with more force to open the aortic valve and eject blood into the aorta. Eventually the left ventricle fails. Pulmonary disease, which damages the lung capillaries and increases pulmonary

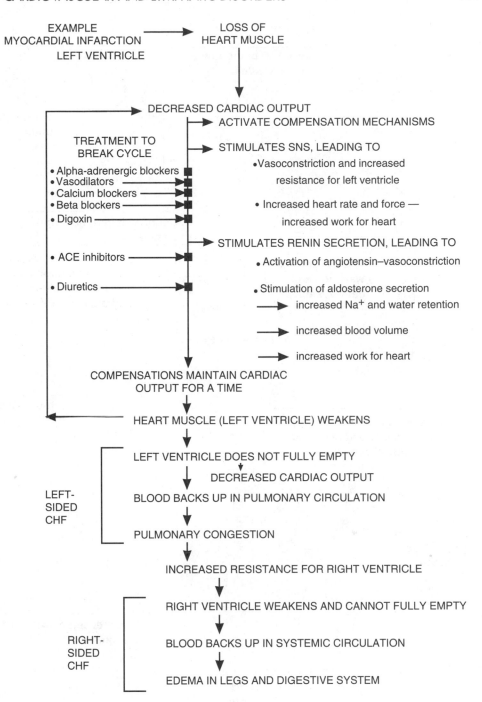

FIGURE 16-20. Course of congestive heart failure.

resistance, increases the work load for the right ventricle, and eventually the right ventricle fails. Right-sided CHF due to pulmonary disease is referred to as *cor pulmonale.*

SIGNS AND SYMPTOMS

With failure of either side, the forward effects are similar: decreased blood supply to the tissues and general hypoxia. The signs and symptoms become more severe as the condition progresses. Fatigue and weakness, dyspnea (breathlessness) and shortness of breath, especially with exertion, exercise intolerance, cold intolerance, and dizziness occur. Compensation mecha-

nisms are indicated by tachycardia, pallor, and daytime oliguria. The backup effects of left-sided failure are related to pulmonary congestion and include dyspnea and **orthopnea** or difficulty in breathing when lying down as increased fluid accumulates in the lungs in the recumbent position. The lungs become a dependent area when the body is recumbent. As well, in this position, excess interstitial fluid returns to the blood, reducing edema, but increasing blood volume and pooled fluid in the lungs. Cough is commonly associated with the fluid irritating the respiratory passages. *Paroxysmal nocturnal dyspnea* indicates the presence of

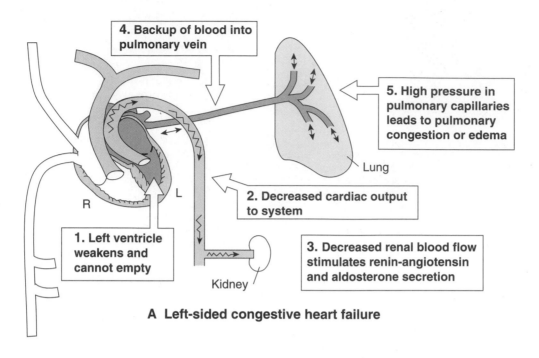

4. Backup of blood into pulmonary vein

5. High pressure in pulmonary capillaries leads to pulmonary congestion or edema

Lung

2. Decreased cardiac output to system

R   L

1. Left ventricle weakens and cannot empty

3. Decreased renal blood flow stimulates renin-angiotensin and aldosterone secretion

Kidney

A Left-sided congestive heart failure

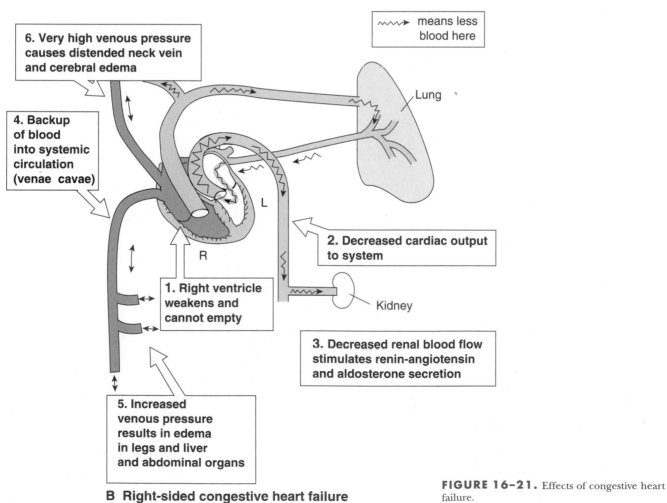

6. Very high venous pressure causes distended neck vein and cerebral edema

~~~→ means less blood here

Lung

4. Backup of blood into systemic circulation (venae cavae)

L

2. Decreased cardiac output to system

R

1. Right ventricle weakens and cannot empty

Kidney

3. Decreased renal blood flow stimulates renin-angiotensin and aldosterone secretion

5. Increased venous pressure results in edema in legs and liver and abdominal organs

B Right-sided congestive heart failure

FIGURE 16–21. Effects of congestive heart failure.

TABLE 16-3 Congestive Heart Failure (CHF)

	Left-Sided CHF	Right-Sided CHF
Causes	Infarction of left ventricle	Infarction of right ventricle
	Aortic valve stenosis	Pulmonary valve stenosis
	Hypertension	Pulmonary disease (cor pulmonale)
	Hyperthyroidism	
Basic effects	Decreased cardiac output, pulmonary congestion	Decreased cardiac output, systemic congestion and edema of legs and abdomen
Signs & symptoms		
Forward effects (decreased output)	Fatigue, weakness, dyspnea, exercise intolerance, cold intolerance	
Compensations	Tachycardia and pallor, secondary polycythemia, daytime oliguria	
Backup effects	Orthopnea, cough, shortness of breath, paroxysmal nocturnal dyspnea, hemoptysis, rales	Dependent edema in feet, hepatomegaly and splenomegaly, ascites, distended neck veins, headache, flushed face

acute pulmonary edema. This usually develops during sleep, when the increased blood volume in the lungs leads to increased fluid in the alveoli and interferes with oxygen diffusion and lung expansion. The individual awakes in a panic, struggling for air and coughing, sometimes producing a frothy blood-stained sputum (**hemoptysis**) if capillaries have ruptured with the pressure. Rusty-colored sputum may be present with recurrent pulmonary edema, indicating the presence of hemosiderin-containing macrophages in the lungs. Rales (bubbly sounds of fluid in the lungs) and a rapid, weak pulse together with cool, moist skin are usually present. Sleeping with the upper body elevated may prevent this complication. Excess fluid in the lungs frequently leads to infections such as pneumonia.

Signs of right-sided failure and systemic backup include dependent edema in the feet or legs or areas such as buttocks, hepatomegaly and splenomegaly, and eventually digestive disturbances as the wall of the digestive tract becomes edematous. *Ascites* is a complication that occurs when fluid accumulates in the peritoneal cavity, leading to marked abdominal distention. Hepatomegaly and ascites may impair respiration if upward pressure on the diaphragm impedes lung expansion. Acute right-sided failure is indicated by increased pressure in the superior vena cava, resulting in flushed face, distended neck veins, headache, and visual disturbances. This condition requires prompt treatment to prevent brain damage.

YOUNG CHILDREN WITH CHF

Infants and young children manifest heart failure somewhat differently. Heart failure is often secondary to congenital heart disease (see next section, Congenital Heart Defects). Feeding difficulties are often the first sign, with failure to gain weight or meet developmental guidelines. Sleep periods are short because the baby falls asleep while feeding and is irritable when awake. There may be a cough, rapid grunting respirations, flared nostrils, and wheezing. With right-sided failure, hepatomegaly and ascites are common. Often a third heart sound is present (gallop rhythm).

DIAGNOSTIC TESTS

Radiographs show cardiomegaly and any fluid in the lungs. Catheters can be used to monitor the hemodynamics or pressures in the circulation. Arterial blood gases are used to measure hypoxia.

TREATMENT

The underlying problem should be treated if possible. Reducing the work load on the heart by avoiding excessive fatigue, stress, and sudden exertion is important in preventing acute episodes. Prophylactic measures such as influenza vaccine are important in preventing respiratory infections. Other common treatment measures have been outlined earlier in this chapter. Maintaining an appropriate diet with a low sodium intake, adequate protein and iron, and sufficient fluids is essential. Antianxiety drugs or sedatives may be useful. Depending on the underlying problem, cardiac support is provided by drugs previously mentioned. Medications such as ACE inhibitors can reduce renin secretion and vasoconstriction, antihypertensives and vasodilators reduce blood pressure, and diuretics decrease sodium and water accumulations. Because patients often take a number of medications on a long-term basis, it is important to check all of them for effectiveness, cumulative toxicities, and interactions.

Thinkabout 16-19

a. Define cor pulmonale.

b. Give two causes of left-sided heart failure, one related to the heart and one systemic.

c. How should a patient with left-sided heart failure be positioned in a reclining chair or bed for treatment?

d. Explain why it is important to maintain an up-to-date medical and drug history for a patient with CHF.

Congenital Heart Defects

PATHOPHYSIOLOGY

Cardiac *anomalies* are developmental defects that arise during the first 8 weeks of embryonic life. A structure may be altered or missing. Several specific examples are described following this introduction. Heart defects are the major cause of death in the first year of life. Both genetic and environmental factors contribute to the errors. Frequently, cardiac anomalies are associated with congenital problems elsewhere in the body. Congenital heart disease may include valvular

A. NORMAL VALVE

Blood flows freely forward   No backflow of blood

B. STENOSIS

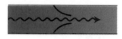 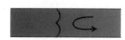

Less blood flows through   No backflow of blood
narrowed opening

C. INCOMPETENT VALVE

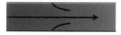 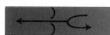

Blood flows freely forward   Blood regurgitates backward through "leaky" valve

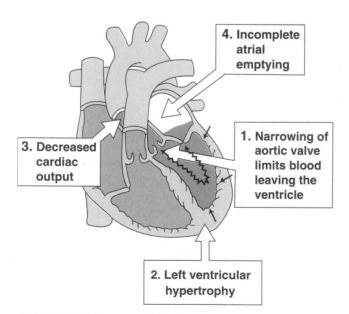

4. Incomplete atrial emptying

1. Narrowing of aortic valve limits blood leaving the ventricle

3. Decreased cardiac output

2. Left ventricular hypertrophy

D. EFFECT OF AORTIC STENOSIS

FIGURE 16–22. Effects of heart valve defects.

defects that interfere with the normal flow of blood (Fig. 16–22), septal defects that allow mixing of oxygenated blood from the pulmonary circulation with unoxygenated blood from the systemic circulation, shunts, or abnormalities in position or shape of the large vessels (aorta and pulmonary artery), or combinations of these (Fig. 16–23). Most defects can be detected by the presence of heart murmurs. All significant defects result in a decreased oxygen supply to the tissues unless adequate compensations are available. If untreated, the child may develop heart failure.

Many variations and degrees of severity are possible with these defects, but if the basic cardiac cycle is understood, the effects of a change in blood flow in each situation can be predicted. Various methods of classifying the defects are possible, using either the type of defect or the presence of *cyanosis*. When an abnormal communication permits mixing of blood, the fluid always flows from a high-pressure area to a low-pressure area, and flow occurs only in one direction. For example, a left-to-right shunt means that blood from the left side of the heart is recycled to the right side and to the lungs, resulting in an increased volume in the pulmonary circulation, a decreased cardiac output, and an inefficient system. On the other hand, a right-to-left shunt means that unoxygenated blood from the right side of the heart bypasses the lungs directly and enters the left side of the heart. The *direction* and *amount* of the abnormal blood flow determine the effects on the individual. *Acyanotic* conditions are disorders in which systemic blood flow consists of oxygenated blood, although the amount may be reduced. In *cyanotic* disorders significant amounts of unoxygenated hemoglobin in the blood bypass the lungs and enter the systemic circulation. The high proportion of unoxygenated blood produces a bluish color (characteristic of cyanosis) in the skin and mucous membranes, particularly the lips and nails. Death occurs in infancy in some severe cases, but many anomalies can be treated relatively easily and successfully.

ETIOLOGY

Most defects appear to be multifactorial and reflect a combination of genetic and environmental influences. These defects are often associated with chromosomal abnormalities such as Down's syndrome. Environmental factors include viral infections such as rubella, maternal alcoholism (fetal alcohol syndrome), and maternal diabetes.

COMPENSATION MECHANISMS

Through a sympathetic response, the heart increases its rate and force of contraction in an effort to increase cardiac output. This response increases the oxygen demand in the heart, restricts coronary perfusion, and increases peripheral resistance. The heart dilates and becomes hypertrophied. However, this response is ineffective because of the defect in the heart itself. Respira-

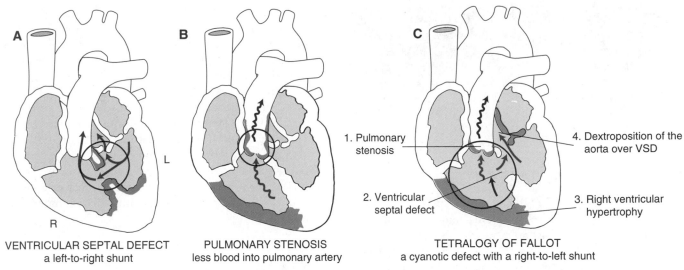

A

VENTRICULAR SEPTAL DEFECT
a left-to-right shunt

B

PULMONARY STENOSIS
less blood into pulmonary artery

C

1. Pulmonary stenosis

2. Ventricular septal defect

4. Dextroposition of the aorta over VSD

3. Right ventricular hypertrophy

TETRALOGY OF FALLOT
a cyanotic defect with a right-to-left shunt

FIGURE 16–23. Congenital heart defects.

tory rate increases if the oxygen deficit results in acidosis due to increased lactic acid in the body, but oxygen levels must drop considerably before this factor influences respiratory rate (see Chapter 17). Secondary polycythemia develops with chronic hypoxia as erythropoietin secretion increases as a compensation.

SIGNS AND SYMPTOMS

Small defects are asymptomatic other than the presence of a heart murmur. Large defects lead to tachycardia, with a very rapid sleeping pulse and frequently a pulse deficit. Dyspnea on exertion, tachypnea, diaphoresis, and the signs of heart failure are often present. Toddlers and older children frequently assume a squatting position, which appears to modify blood flow and be more comfortable. Clubbed fingers (thick, bulbous fingertips) develop, and the child frequently shows a marked intolerance for exercise and exposure to cold weather.

DIAGNOSTIC TESTS

Congenital defects, particularly severe ones, may be diagnosed at birth, but others may not be detected for some time. There are many techniques and modalities, both invasive and noninvasive, that can be used. Cardiomegaly can be observed on radiograph. These include cardiac catheterization, echocardiograms, and ECG.

TREATMENT

Surgical repair is often needed to close abnormal openings or replace valves or parts of vessels. Palliative surgery may take place immediately and then is followed up several years later by additional surgery. The timing of surgery depends on the individual situation, the severity of the defect, the ability of the individual to withstand surgery, and the impact of surgery on growth. In some cases, septal defects close spontaneously with time. Supportive measures and drug therapy are similar to those used for CHF.

VENTRICULAR SEPTAL DEFECT

Ventricular septal defect (VSD) is the most common congenital heart defect and is commonly called a "hole in the heart." Septal defects may also occur in the atrial septum. VSD is an opening in the interventricular septum, which may vary in size and location. Small defects do not affect cardiac function significantly but are susceptible to infective endocarditis. Large lesions permit a *left-to-right shunt* of blood (see Fig. 16–23). *Blood can flow in only one direction from the high-pressure area to the low-pressure area.* In this case, the *left* ventricle is the high-pressure area, and therefore blood flows through the septal defect from the left ventricle to the right ventricle. The effect of this altered flow is that less blood leaves the left ventricle, reducing stroke volume and cardiac output to the systemic circulation. More blood enters the pulmonary circulation, some of which is already oxygenated; this reduces the efficiency of the system and in time overloads and irreversibly damages the pulmonary blood vessels, causing pulmonary hypertension. This complication, which may occur in untreated VSD, would lead to an abnormally high pressure in the right ventricle and a reversal of the shunt to a right-to-left shunt, leading to cyanosis.

Thinkabout 16–20

a. Describe the altered blood flow in the presence of an atrial septal defect. Include the direction of flow and the type and amount of blood present in each circulation.

b. Patent ductus arteriosus (PDA) results when the ductus arteriosus, a vessel between the aorta and the pulmonary artery that is present during fetal development, fails to close after birth. Using your knowledge of normal anatomy, draw a sketch of the defect and describe the abnormal pattern of blood flow, including the rationale for it. Would a heart murmur be present?

VALVULAR DEFECTS

Malformations affect the aortic and pulmonary valves most commonly. Valve problems may be classified as *stenosis* or narrowing of a valve, which restricts the forward flow of blood, or valvular *incompetence*, which is a valve that fails to close completely, allowing blood to regurgitate or leak backward (see Fig. 16–22). Mitral valve *prolapse* is a common occurrence; it refers to abnormally enlarged and floppy valve leaflets that balloon backward with pressure or to posterior displacement of the cusp, which permits regurgitation of blood. An effect similar to stenosis arises from abnormalities of the large vessels near the heart, for example, coarctation (constriction) of the aorta.

Valvular defects reduce the efficiency of the heart "pump" and reduce stroke volume. If the opening is narrow, the myocardium must contract with more force to push the blood through. In time, that heart chamber will hypertrophy and may eventually fail. If a valve leaks and blood regurgitates backward, the heart must also increase its efforts to maintain cardiac output.

Thinkabout 16–21

a. Explain why an incompetent valve reduces the efficiency of the heart contraction.
b. Would a case of mitral valve prolapse cause a cyanotic or acyanotic condition? Explain your reasoning.

TETRALOGY OF FALLOT

Tetralogy of Fallot is the most common congenital cyanotic heart condition. It is more complex and more serious than the others described so far because it includes four (Greek, *tetra*) abnormalities and is a cyanotic disorder (patients are sometimes called "blue babies"). The four defects are pulmonary valve stenosis, ventricular septal defect, dextroposition of the aorta (to

the right over the VSD), and right ventricular hypertrophy (see Fig. 16–23). The restricted outflow from the right ventricle leads to right ventricular hypertrophy and high pressure in the right ventricle. This pressure, now higher than the pressure in the left ventricle, leads to a right-to-left shunt of blood through the VSD. The flow of unoxygenated blood from the right ventricle directly into the systemic circulation is promoted by the aorta, which is positioned over the septum or VSD. The end result is that the pulmonary circulation receives a small amount of unoxygenated blood from the right ventricle, and the systemic circulation receives a larger amount of blood consisting of mixed oxygenated and unoxygenated blood.

Thinkabout 16–22

a. List the four defects present in tetralogy of Fallot and state the effect each has on blood flow. Describe the ultimate path of blood flow.
b. State three specific effects of the oxygen deficit on cell and tissue function.
c. Why is this called a cyanotic condition?
d. Describe three signs of CHF in infants.

Inflammation and Infection in the Heart

RHEUMATIC FEVER AND RHEUMATIC HEART DISEASE

PATHOPHYSIOLOGY

Rheumatic fever is an acute inflammatory condition that usually occurs in children 5 to 15 years of age. Although rheumatic fever occurs less frequently now in many areas, it remains a threat because new strains of *Streptococcus* continue to appear, and the long-term effects, seen as rheumatic heart disease, may be complicated by infective endocarditis and heart failure.

The inflammation appears to result from an abnormal immune reaction that occurs a few weeks after an untreated infection, usually caused by certain strains of group A beta-hemolytic *Streptococcus* (often appearing as an upper respiratory infection, tonsillitis, or strep throat). Antibodies to the streptococcus organisms form as usual and then react with connective tissue (collagen) in the skin, joints, brain, and heart, causing inflammation (Fig. 16–24). The heart is the only site where scar tissue may form, leading to rheumatic heart disease.

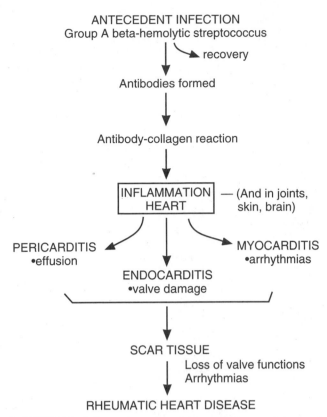

ANTECEDENT INFECTION
Group A beta-hemolytic streptococcus

↘ recovery

Antibodies formed

↓

Antibody-collagen reaction

↓

INFLAMMATION HEART — (And in joints, skin, brain)

PERICARDITIS
•effusion

MYOCARDITIS
•arrhythmias

ENDOCARDITIS
•valve damage

↓

SCAR TISSUE

Loss of valve functions
Arrhythmias

↓

RHEUMATIC HEART DISEASE

FIGURE 16-24. Development of rheumatic fever and rheumatic heart disease.

During the acute stage, the inflammation in the heart may involve one or more layers of the heart. Pericarditis, inflammation of the outer layer, may include effusion (excessive fluid accumulation), which impairs filling. Myocarditis, in which the inflammation develops as localized lesions in the heart muscle called Aschoff bodies, may interfere with conduction. Endocarditis, the most common problem, affects the valves, which become edematous, and verrucae form, rows of small wartlike vegetations along the outer edge of the valve cusps. The mitral valve is affected most frequently, disrupting the flow of blood and the effectiveness of the left ventricle. Eventually, the valve may be scarred, leading to stenosis if the cusps fuse together or incompetence if fibrous tissue shrinks, or a combination of these, and leading to rheumatic heart disease (see Fig. 16-22). In some cases the chordae tendineae are involved in the inflammatory reaction and fibrosis ensues, leading to a shortened chordae and malfunctioning valve. Recurrent inflammation is likely to cause more damage to the valves, which are also at risk for infective endocarditis.

Other sites of inflammation in patients with rheumatic fever include the large joints, which may be involved with synovitis in a migratory polyarthritis, and the skin, which may show a nonpruritic rash known as erythema marginatum (red macules or papules that enlarge and have white centers), or small nontender subcutaneous nodules that usually form on the extensor surfaces at the wrists, elbows, knees, or ankles. Occurring more frequently in girls, the basal nuclei in the brain may be involved, causing involuntary jerky movements of the face, arms, and legs (Sydenham's chorea or St. Vitus dance). Not all areas are necessarily affected in a single individual.

Rheumatic heart disease develops years later in some individuals, when scarred valves or arrhythmias compromise heart function. Congestive heart failure may occur in either the acute or chronic stage.

SIGNS AND SYMPTOMS

The general indications of a systemic inflammation are usually present— low-grade fever, leukocytosis, malaise, anorexia, and fatigue. Tachycardia, even at rest, is common. Heart murmurs indicate the site of inflammation. Epistaxis and abdominal pain may be present. Acute heart failure may develop from the arrhythmias or severe valve distortion. Recovery often requires a prolonged period of rest and treatment.

DIAGNOSTIC TESTS

Elevated serum antibody levels remain after the infection has been eradicated (antistreptolysin O [ASO] titer). Leukocytosis and anemia are common. Heart function tests, as previously mentioned, may be required.

TREATMENT

Antibacterial agents such as penicillin may be administered to eradicate any residual infection. Specific treatment is required for arrhythmias or heart failure, as previously described.

Following the acute episode, it is important to prevent recurrences by promptly treating any streptococcal infections with antibacterial drugs. When valve damage has occurred, precautionary measures such as prophylactic penicillin prior to invasive procedures or dental treatment is recommended to prevent bacteremia and infective endocarditis. Potential complications, such as heart failure resulting from severe valve damage, are similar to those mentioned earlier under congenital heart defects.

Thinkabout 16-23

a. Describe the stages of development of acute rheumatic fever
b. Explain how the mitral heart valve can become stenotic, and describe the effect of this stenosis on blood flow.

INFECTIVE ENDOCARDITIS

PATHOPHYSIOLOGY

There are two forms of infective endocarditis, the subacute type, in which the defective heart valves are invaded by organisms of low virulence such as *Streptococcus viridans,* which is part of the normal flora of the mouth, and the acute type, in which normal heart valves are attacked by highly virulent organisms such as *Staphylococcus aureus,* which tend to cause severe damage and may be difficult to treat successfully. Formerly called bacterial endocarditis, it is now recognized that many different types of organisms can cause endocarditis, and it is important to identify and treat the specific organism promptly. The basic effects are the same.

Microorganisms in the general circulation attach to the endocardium and invade the heart valves, causing inflammation and formation of vegetations on the cusps. Vegetations are large fragile masses made up of fibrin strands, platelets and other blood cells, and microbes. In the acute stage, these may interfere with the opening and closing of the valves. Pieces may break away, forming infective or septic emboli that then cause infarction and infection in other tissues. This process causes additional destruction and scarring of the valve and the chordae tendinae.

ETIOLOGY

There are many predisposing conditions in which abnormal valves increase the risk of subacute infective endocarditis. These include congenital defects, rheumatic fever, mitral prolapse, and artificial or replacement valves. Persons with septal defects, catheters, or other artificial implants are also susceptible to infection. Such individuals should be premedicated with penicillin or another antibacterial drug prior to any instrumentation or invasive procedure such as scaling of the teeth, in which a transient bacteremia could occur. Intravenous drug users have an increased incidence of acute endocarditis. Anyone in whom the immune system is suppressed, such as those taking corticosteroids or those with acquired immune deficiency syndrome (AIDS), is vulnerable. Endocarditis, both bacterial and fungal, is also a risk with cardiac surgery.

Subacute infective endocarditis is most frequently caused by alpha streptococci but may occur with many other bacteria, fungi, or other unusual organisms.

Thinkabout 16–24

Explain why a tooth extraction or scaling procedure could predispose a client with an artificial heart valve to infective endocarditis.

SIGNS AND SYMPTOMS

Subacute infective endocarditis is frequently insidious in onset, manifesting only an intermittent low-grade fever or fatigue. Anorexia, splenomegaly, and Osler's nodes (painful red nodules on the fingers) are common signs. Initially, it may be difficult to detect any change in the heart murmur from the predisposing condition. Congestive heart failure develops in severe cases.

Acute endocarditis has a sudden, marked onset with spiking fever, chills, and drowsiness. Septic emboli may cause infarctions or abscesses in organs, resulting in appropriate signs related to location.

TREATMENT

Following a blood culture to identify the causative agent, antimicrobial drugs are given, usually for a minimum of 4 weeks, to completely eradicate the infection.

Thinkabout 16–25

a. Explain how acute infective endocarditis can develop.

b. Describe the possible destination of an embolus from the mitral valve.

PERICARDITIS

PATHOPHYSIOLOGY

Pericarditis may be acute or chronic and is usually secondary to another condition either in the heart or surrounding structures. Pericarditis can be classified by cause or by the type of exudate associated with the inflammation. Acute pericarditis may involve a simple inflammation of the pericardium, in which the rough swollen surfaces cause chest pain and a friction rub (a grating sound heard on the chest with a stethoscope). In some cases, an *effusion* may develop with excess fluid accumulating in the pericardial sac (Fig. 16–25). This fluid may be serous as with inflammation, fibrinous and purulent, as with infection, or hemorrhagic, as with injury or cancer. Small volumes of fluid have little effect on heart function, but a large amount of fluid that accumulates rapidly may compress the heart and impair its expansion and filling, thus decreasing cardiac output (*cardiac tamponade*). The right side (low-pressure side) of the heart is affected first, causing increased pressure in the systemic veins and, if acute, distended neck veins. If fluid accumulates slowly, the heart adjusts, and a very large amount can build up before signs appear.

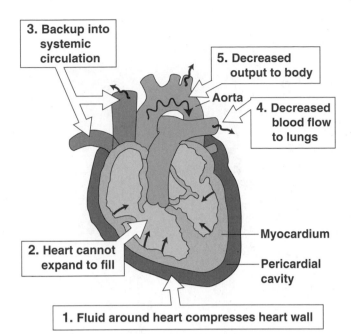

FIGURE 16–25. Effects of pericardial effusion.

Chronic pericarditis results in formation of adhesions between the pericardial membranes, or scar tissue may become constrictive, causing the pericardium to become a tight fibrous enclosure, thus limiting movement of the heart.

ETIOLOGY

Acute pericarditis may be secondary to open heart surgery, myocardial infarction, rheumatic fever, systemic lupus erythematosus, cancer, trauma, or viral infection. The fibrous tissue of chronic pericarditis often results from tuberculosis or radiation to the mediastinum. Effusion may be secondary to hypoproteinemia resulting from liver or kidney disease.

SIGNS AND SYMPTOMS

Signs vary with the underlying problem and its effects on the pericardium. Tachycardia is present, and chest pain, dyspnea, and cough are common signs. ECG changes and a friction rub may be present.

Effusion and cardiac tamponade lead to distended neck veins, faint heart sounds, and pulsus paradoxus, in which systolic pressure drops 10 mm Hg during inspiration.

Chronic pericarditis causes fatigue, weakness, and abdominal discomfort due to systemic venous congestion.

TREATMENT

First, the primary problem must be treated successfully. Fluid may be aspirated from the cavity (paracentesis) and analyzed to determine the cause. If effusion is severe, immediate aspiration of the excess fluid may be required to prevent tamponade and shock.

Thinkabout 16–26

Explain why a large volume of fluid in the pericardial cavity decreases cardiac output.

VASCULAR DISORDERS

Arterial Diseases

HYPERTENSION

PATHOPHYSIOLOGY

Hypertension, or high blood pressure, in both its primary and secondary forms is a very common problem. Because of the insidious onset and mild signs, it is often undiagnosed until complications arise. Also, patient compliance with treatment measures may be poor until the problem is severe. There are three major categories of hypertension. Primary or *essential* hypertension is idiopathic and is the form discussed in this section. *Secondary* hypertension results from renal (e.g., chronic glomerulonephritis) or endocrine disease (e.g., hyperaldosteronism), or pheochromocytoma, a benign tumor of the adrenal medulla or SNS chain of ganglia. In this type of hypertension, the underlying problem must be resolved. The third type is *malignant* hypertension, which is an uncontrollable, severe, and rapidly progressive form with many complications. Sometimes hypertension is classified as systolic or diastolic depending on the measurement that is elevated. For example, elderly persons with loss of elasticity in the arteries frequently have a high systolic pressure and low diastolic value.

Essential hypertension develops when the blood pressure is consistently above 140/90. This figure may be adjusted for the individual's age. The diastolic pressure is important because it indicates the degree of peripheral resistance and the increased work load of the left ventricle. The condition may be mild, moderate, or severe. In essential hypertension there is an increase in arteriolar vasoconstriction, which is attributed variously to increased susceptibility to stimuli or increased stimulation. A very slight decrease in the diameter of the arterioles causes a major increase in peripheral resistance, reduces the capacity of the system, and increases the diastolic pressure or afterload substantially. Frequently, vasoconstriction leads to decreased blood flow through the kidneys, leading to increased renin, angiotensin, and aldosterone secretion. These substances increase vasoconstriction and blood volume, further

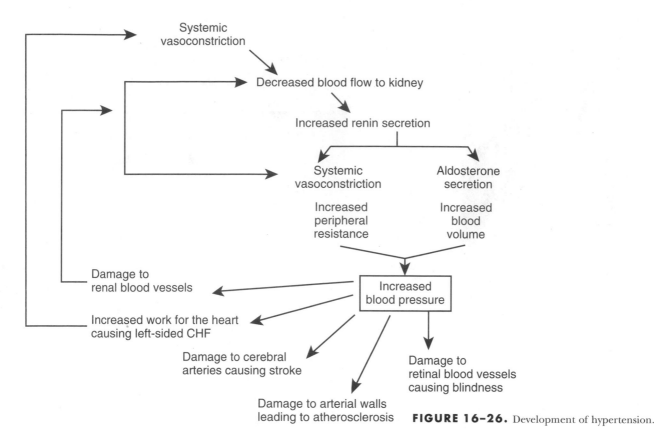

FIGURE 16-26. Development of hypertension.

increasing blood pressure (Fig. 16–26). If this cycle is not broken, blood pressure can continue to increase.

Over a long period of time, the increased blood pressure causes damage to the arterial wall. It becomes hard and thick (*sclerotic*), narrowing the lumen, and may dilate or tear, forming an aneurysm, or encourage atheroma formation. Blood supply to the involved area is reduced, leading to ischemia and necrosis with loss of function. The areas most frequently damaged are the kidneys, brain, and retina of the eye. In many cases, the progressive changes are asymptomatic until they are well advanced. One area that is easily checked through the pupil of the eye is the retina, where the blood vessels can easily be observed for sclerotic changes and rupture. The end result of poorly controlled hypertension can be chronic renal failure, stroke due to hemorrhage, loss of vision, and congestive heart failure. The lifespan may be considerably shorter, particularly in males, when hypertension is not controlled.

ETIOLOGY

Even in idiopathic hypertension, the form discussed here, many factors appear to predispose to the condition. The incidence increases with age, although hypertension does occur in children. Males are affected more frequently and more severely, but the incidence in females increases after middle age. Genetic factors are involved because blacks have a higher incidence than whites and experience a more severe form of hypertension. There are also familial trends, but these may reflect lifestyle characteristics also.

Other factors implicated in the development of essential hypertension include high sodium intake, excessive alcohol intake (small amounts of alcohol appear to decrease blood pressure), obesity, and prolonged or recurrent stress.

SIGNS AND SYMPTOMS

Hypertension is frequently asymptomatic in the early stages, and the initial signs are often vague and nonspecific. They include fatigue, malaise, and sometimes morning headache. Consistently elevated blood pressure under various conditions is the key sign. The complications are also asymptomatic until they are well advanced.

TREATMENT

Essential hypertension is usually treated in a sequence of steps, beginning with life style changes as needed to reduce salt intake, reduce body weight and stress, and generally increase cardiovascular fitness. Mild diuretics such as the thiazide diuretics, which also have an antihypertensive action, are suggested for the next stage. Subsequently, one or more drugs may be added to the regimen until blood pressure responds.

Combinations of drugs with different actions are quite effective and reduce the side effects. The choice of drug also depends on the individual situation. For example, a patient with a high serum sodium level needs a stronger diuretic such as furosemide, and a patient with high renin levels may take an ACE inhibitor. Other antihypertensive agents block the sympathetic stimulation in various ways, alpha$_1$-blockers causing vasodilation, calcium blockers reducing heart activity and peripheral resistance, and beta blockers reducing heart action and sometimes renin release. Patient compliance can be difficult when no obvious signs of illness are present. Also, many of the drugs do have significant side effects, such as orthostatic hypotension, nausea, and impotence. The lack of reflex vasoconstriction when rising from a supine position can cause a decrease in blood flow to the brain. This causes dizziness and fainting and can result in falls if the patient rises too quickly or lacks assistance and support when rising to a standing position. Diuretics may cause increased urinary frequency in the morning and generalized weakness. Beta blockers may prevent the heart rate from increasing with exercise. This interference with normal responses can lead to misinterpretation of the results of exercise stress testing.

Thinkabout 16–27

  a. State the cause of elevated blood pressure in essential hypertension.
  b. Describe the long-term effects of uncontrolled hypertension.
  c. Explain why orthostatic (postural) hypotension may occur with vasodilator drugs.
  d. Explain how compensation by renin aggravates hypertension.

PERIPHERAL VASCULAR DISEASE AND ATHEROSCLEROSIS

PATHOPHYSIOLOGY

Peripheral vascular disease refers to any abnormality in the arteries or veins outside the heart. The cause, development, and effects of atheromas have been discussed previously in this chapter (see Figs. 16–12 to 16–14). The most common sites of atheromas in the peripheral circulation are the abdominal aorta and the femoral and iliac arteries (Fig. 16–27), where partial occlusions may impair both muscle activity and sensory function in the legs. Total occlusions may result from a thrombus obstructing the lumen or breaking off (an embolus) and eventually obstructing a smaller artery. Loss of blood supply in a limb leads to necrosis, ulcers, and gangrene, which is a bacterial infection of necrotic tissue.

SIGNS AND SYMPTOMS

Atheromas develop gradually, leading to increasing fatigue and weakness as blood flow decreases. *Intermittent claudication,* or leg pain associated with exercise due to muscle ischemia, develops. Initially, pain subsides with rest. As the obstruction advances, pain becomes more severe and may be present at rest, particularly in the distal areas such as the feet and toes. Sensory impairment may also be noted as paresthesias, or tingling, burning, and numbness. Peripheral pulses distal to the occlusion (e.g., the popliteal and pedal pulses) become weak or absent (Fig. 16–28). The appearance of the skin in the feet and legs changes, with marked pallor or cyanosis becoming evident when the legs areelevated, and rubor or redness when they are dangling. The skin is dry and hairless, the toenails are thick and hard, and poorly perfused areas in the legs or feet feel cold.

DIAGNOSTIC TESTS

Blood flow can be assessed by Doppler studies (ultrasonography) and arteriography. Plethysmography, measures the size of limbs and blood volume in organs or tissues.

TREATMENT

Maintenance of a dependent position for the legs can improve arterial perfusion. Reduction of serum cholesterol levels is recommended. Thrombus formation can be reduced by platelet inhibitors or anticoagulant medications and cessation of smoking, which promotes platelet adhesion. In addition, an exercise program can be helpful in preserving existing circulation. Care should be taken to avoid any skin trauma, and regular examination of the feet is important to avoid pressure from shoes, especially if there is sensory impairment. Specially fitted shoes may be required. Peripheral vasodilators such as calcium blockers may be helpful because they may enhance the collateral circulation. Gangrenous ulcers can be treated with antibiotics and débridement. Amputation of a gangrenous toe or foot is often required to prevent spread of the infection into the systemic circulation and to relieve the severe pain of ischemia. In many cases, multiple amputations are required, beginning with a toe, then a foot, lower leg, and so on. Vascular disease is the primary reason for amputation. Healing is very slow because of the poor blood supply, and a prosthesis may be difficult to fit and maintain. Surgical procedures to restore blood flow include bypass grafts using a vein or synthetic material, angioplasty to reduce plaques, or **endarterectomy** (removal of the intima and obstructive material).

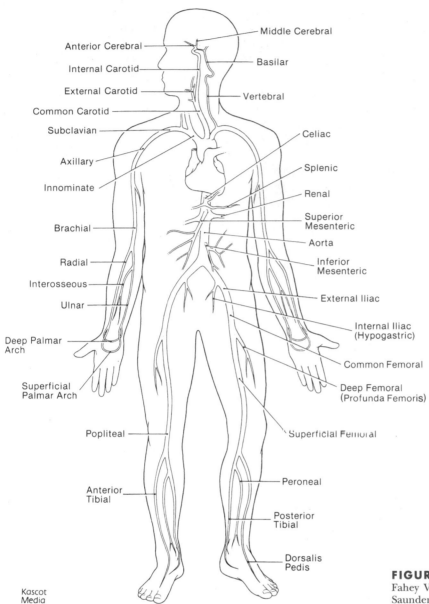

Middle Cerebral

Anterior Cerebral

Internal Carotid

External Carotid

Common Carotid

Subclavian

Axillary

Innominate

Brachial

Radial

Interosseous

Ulnar

Deep Palmar Arch

Superficial Palmar Arch

Popliteal

Anterior Tibial

Basilar

Vertebral

Celiac

Splenic

Renal

Superior Mesenteric

Aorta

Inferior Mesenteric

External Iliac

Internal Iliac (Hypogastric)

Common Femoral

Deep Femoral (Profunda Femoris)

Superficial Femoral

Peroneal

Posterior Tibial

Dorsalis Pedis

Kascot Media

FIGURE 16–27. Anatomy of major arteries. (From Fahey VA: Vascular Nursing, 2nd ed. Philadelphia, W.B. Saunders, 1994, p. 5.)

Thinkabout 16–28

a. Why are the peripheral pulses weak when the iliac artery is blocked?

b. Why should the feet be carefully inspected on a daily basis?

c. Why may amputation be required?

d. Why may healing and fitting of a prosthesis be difficult?

THROMBOANGIITIS OBLITERANS (BUERGER'S DISEASE)

Buerger's disease is an inflammatory condition of medium-sized and small arteries, most commonly in the legs. Sometimes the veins are involved. It occurs commonly in young males. Thrombus formation and fibrosis lead to vascular occlusion similar to that seen with atheromas. Because it affects the small blood vessels, surgical intervention is not feasible. In addition to its vasoconstricting effects, cigarette smoking plays a direct role in the inflammatory process, perhaps because of an autoimmune process, and must cease before any improvement occurs.

RAYNAUD'S SYNDROME

Primary Raynaud's syndrome or disease is common in young women and is considered idiopathic. Secondary Raynaud's syndrome is associated with many conditions such as systemic lupus erythematosus (SLE). It is an example of a vasospastic condition, in which periodic temporary but severe vasoconstriction occurs in the arterioles and small arteries in the superficial tissues of the fingers and toes. Vasospasm causes a temporary ischemia with pallor, numbness, and cyanosis, followed by vasodilation, redness, and throbbing pain. Episodes

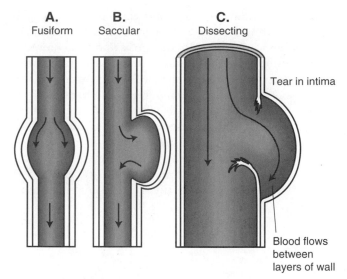

FIGURE 16-29. Types of aortic aneurysms.

are triggered by exposure to cold, stress, or smoking. Patients should always protect their hands from touching cold objects. Permanent damage is rare because ischemia is temporary. If frequent severe attacks do occur, paresthesias and ulcerations may develop on the fingertips. Paresthesias can affect manual dexterity.

ANEURYSMS

PATHOPHYSIOLOGY

An aneurysm is a localized dilatation in an arterial wall. The most common location is the aorta, either the abdominal or thoracic aorta. The aneurysm may take different shapes, a saccular shape, which is a bulging wall on one side, or a *fusiform* shape, which is a circumferential dilatation along a section of artery (Fig. 16–29). *Dissecting* aneurysms develop when there is a tear in the intima, allowing blood to flow along the length of the vessel between the layers of the arterial wall. Aneurysms also occur in the cerebral circulation and are discussed in Chapter 20.

The aneurysm develops from a defect in the medial layer, often associated with turbulent blood flow at the site, from a bifurcation, or from an atheroma. Over time the dilatation enlarges, particularly if hypertension develops. Frequently, thrombus forms in the dilated area, obstructing branching arteries such as the renal arteries, or becoming a source of embolus. Many aneurysms eventually rupture, causing massive hemorrhage.

ETIOLOGY

Common causes are atherosclerosis, trauma (particularly car accidents), syphilis, and congenital defects.

SIGNS AND SYMPTOMS

Aneurysms are frequently asymptomatic for a long period of time until they become very large or rupture.

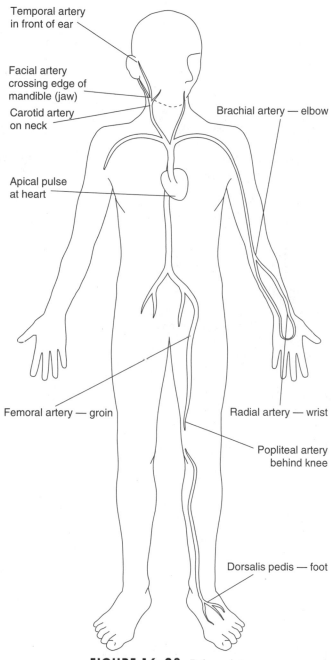

FIGURE 16-28. Pulse points.

Abdominal aneurysms are sometimes detected as palpable pulsating masses with bruits (abnormal sounds). In certain locations, earlier diagnosis may be achieved if a large aneurysm compresses the nearby structures, causing signs such as dysphagia from pressure on the esophagus or pain if a spinal nerve is compressed.

Rupture occasionally leads to moderate hemorrhage but more often causes severe bleeding and death. Signs include severe pain and indications of shock. A dissecting aneurysm causes obstruction of the aorta and its branches as the intima peels back and blood flow is diverted between the layers. The dissection tends to progress down the aorta and sometimes back toward the heart as well. Dissection causes severe pain, loss of pulses, and organ dysfunction as normal blood flow is lost. Many dissecting aneurysms ultimately rupture.

DIAGNOSTIC TESTS

Radiography, ultrasound, and CT scans confirm the problem.

TREATMENT

Pending surgery, it is of critical importance to maintain blood pressure at a normal level, preventing sudden elevations due to exertion, stress, coughing, or

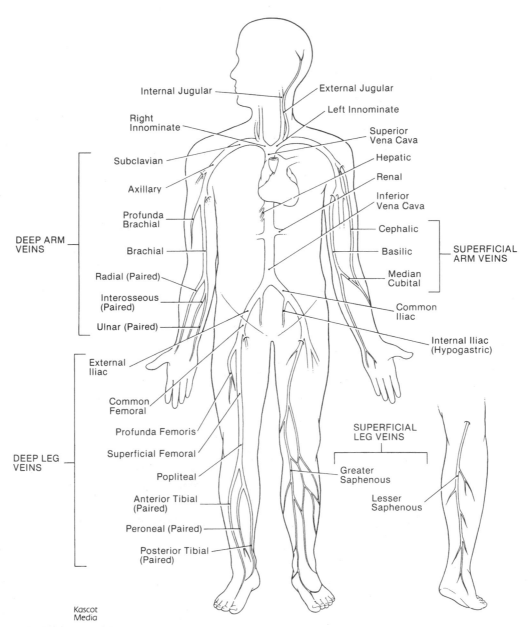

Kascot
Media

FIGURE 16–30. Anatomy of major veins. (From Fahey VA: Vascular Nursing, 2nd ed. Philadelphia, W.B. Saunders, 1994, p. 23.)

A.

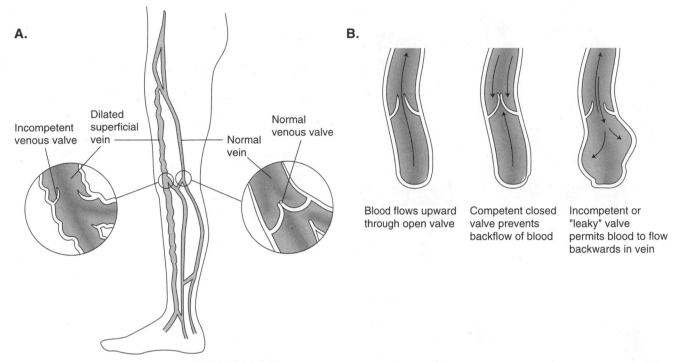

Incompetent venous valve

Dilated superficial vein

Normal vein

Normal venous valve

B.

Blood flows upward through open valve

Competent closed valve prevents backflow of blood

Incompetent or "leaky" valve permits blood to flow backwards in vein

FIGURE 16-31. *A* and *B*, Development of varicosities in legs.

constipation. In some cases, small tears may occur before a major rupture; these need immediate surgical repair. Surgery with resection and grafting can prevent rupture.

Venous Disorders

VARICOSE VEINS

PATHOPHYSIOLOGY

Varicosities are irregular dilated and tortuous areas of the superficial or deep veins (Fig. 16–30). The most common location is the legs, but varicosities are also found in the esophagus (esophageal varices) and in the rectum (hemorrhoids). Varicose veins in the legs may develop from a defect or weakness in the vein walls or in the valves (Fig. 16–31). If a section of vein wall is weak, eventually the excessive hydrostatic pressure of blood under the influence of gravity causes the wall to stretch or dilate. The weight of blood then damages the valve below, leading to back flow of blood into the section distal to the starting point. If the basic problem is a defective valve, reflux of blood into the section of vein distal to the valve occurs, the overload distending and stretching the walls. The continued back pressure of blood in the leg veins leads to progressive damage down the vein. Some blood may be diverted into other veins such as blood flowing from the deep veins through connecting veins into the superficial veins, further ex-

tending the damage. Varicosities can predispose to thrombus formation in the presence of other contributing factors such as immobility.

ETIOLOGY

There is a familial tendency, probably related to an inherent weakness in the vein walls. The superficial leg veins are frequently involved because there is less muscle support for these veins. Valves may be damaged by trauma, intravenous administration of fluids, or thrombophlebitis. Many factors can increase pressure in the leg veins, such as standing for long periods of time, crossing the legs, wearing tight clothing, and pregnancy.

SIGNS AND SYMPTOMS

Superficial varicosities on the legs appear as irregular, purplish, bulging structures. There may be edema in the feet as the venous pressure rises. Fatigue and aching are common as the increased interstitial fluid interferes with arterial flow and nutrient supply (see Chapter 2). Increased interstitial fluid or edema also leads to a shiny, pigmented, and hairless skin, and varicose ulcers may develop as arterial blood flow continues to diminish and the skin breaks down.

TREATMENT

Treatment is directed toward keeping the legs elevated and using support stockings to encourage venous return and relieve discomfort. Restrictive clothing should be avoided, and the patient should refrain from crossing the legs. When standing for long periods, intermittent voluntary muscle contractions or position changes are helpful. For more severe varicosities, sclerosing agents that obliterate the veins or vein stripping may be tried, rerouting the blood to functional veins.

Thinkabout 16–29

a. Compare the ideal position in a chair for a client with arterial obstruction with that for a client with varicose veins.

b. Explain how leg ulcers develop in people with varicose veins.

THROMBOPHLEBITIS AND PHLEBOTHROMBOSIS

PATHOPHYSIOLOGY

The terms thrombophlebitis and phlebothrombosis as well as phlebitis and thromboembolic disease are often used interchangeably. It can be difficult to differentiate the two conditions, but sometimes there is a significant difference in the predisposing factors, early signs, and risks of emboli. Thrombophlebitis refers to the development of thrombus in a vein in which inflammation is present. The platelets adhere to the inflamed site, and thrombus develops. In phlebothrombosis, thrombus forms spontaneously in a vein without prior inflammation, although inflammation may develop secondarily in response to thrombosis. The clot is less firmly attached in this case, and its development is asymptomatic or silent.

Several factors usually predispose to thrombus development. The first group of factors involves stasis of blood or sluggish blood flow, which is often present in people who are immobile. Endothelial injury, which may have arisen from trauma, chemical injury, intravenous injection, or inflammation, is another factor. The third factor involves increased blood coagulability, which may result from dehydration, cancer, pregnancy, or increased platelet adhesion.

The critical problem is that venous thrombosis may lead to pulmonary embolism (see Chapter 17). A piece of thrombus (often the tail) breaks off, usually because of some activity, and flows in the venous blood returning to the heart. The first smaller blood vessels along the route are those of the lungs, where the clot lodges, obstructing the pulmonary circulation and causing both respiratory and cardiovascular complications. Sudden chest pain and shock are indicators of pulmonary embolus.

Thinkabout 16–30

Draw and label a simple diagram of the pathway of an embolus from the greater saphenous vein to its destination.

SIGNS AND SYMPTOMS

Often thrombus formation is unnoticed until pulmonary embolus occurs, with severe chest pain and shock. Thrombophlebitis in the superficial veins may present with aching or burning and tenderness in the affected leg. The leg may be warm and red in the area of the inflamed vein.

Thrombus in the deep veins may cause aching pain, tenderness, and edema in the affected leg as the blood pools distal to the obstructing thrombus. A positive Homans' sign (pain in the calf muscle when the foot is dorsiflexed) is common. Systemic signs such as fever, malaise, and leukocytosis may be present.

TREATMENT

Preventive measures, such as exercise, elevating the legs, and minimizing the effects of primary conditions, are important. Depending on the particular situation, compression or elastic stockings may be needed as well as exercise to reduce stasis. Anticoagulant therapy, in-

TABLE 16–4 Types of Shock		
Type	**Mechanism**	**Specific Causes**
Hypovolemic	Loss of blood or plasma	Hemorrhage, burns, dehydration, peritonitis pancreatitis
Cardiogenic	Decreased pumping capability of the heart	Myocardial infarction of left ventricle, cardiac arrhythmia, pulmonary embolus, cardiac tamponade
Anaphylactic	Systemic vasodilation and increased permeability due to severe allergic reaction	Insect stings, drugs, nuts, shellfish
Neurogenic (vasogenic)	Vasodilation due to loss of sympathetic and vasomotor tone	Pain and fear, spinal cord injury
Septic (endotoxic)	Vasodilation due to severe infection, often with gram-negative bacteria	Virulent microorganisms or multiple infections

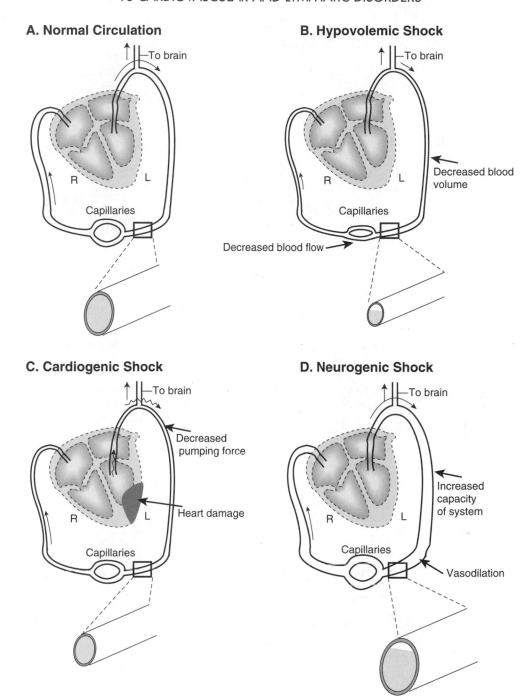

A. Normal Circulation

To brain

R   L

Capillaries

B. Hypovolemic Shock

To brain

R   L

Decreased blood volume

Capillaries

Decreased blood flow

C. Cardiogenic Shock

To brain

Decreased pumping force

R   L

Heart damage

Capillaries

D. Neurogenic Shock

To brain

Increased capacity of system

R   L

Capillaries

Vasodilation

FIGURE 16-32. *A–D*, Causes of shock.

cluding heparin, fibrinolytic therapy, and surgical interventions such as thrombectomy may be used to reduce or remove the clot and prevent embolization.

SHOCK

Shock or hypotension leads to decreased tissue perfusion and general hypoxia. In most cases, cardiac output is low. Shock is most easily classified by the cause, which also indicates the basic pathophysiology and treatment

(Table 16-4). It may be caused by a loss of blood volume (hypovolemic shock), inability of the heart to pump the blood through the circulation (cardiogenic shock), and its subcategory, interference with blood flow through the heart (obstructive shock), or changes in peripheral resistance leading to pooling of blood in the periphery (distributive, vasogenic, neurogenic, septic, or anaphylactic shock).

PATHOPHYSIOLOGY

Blood pressure is determined by blood volume, heart contraction, and peripheral resistance (Fig. 16–32).

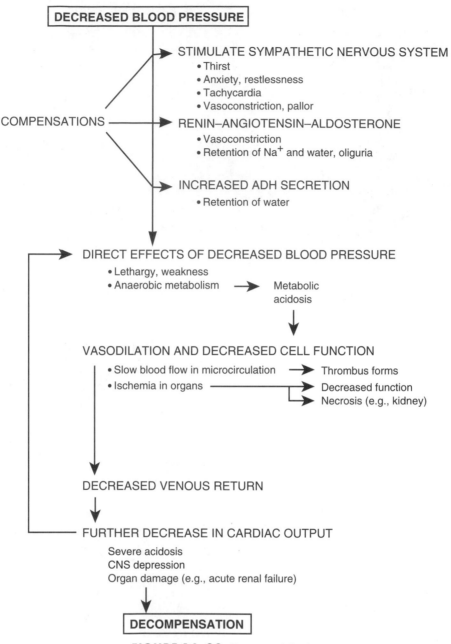

FIGURE 16-33. Progress of shock.

When blood volume is decreased, it is difficult to maintain pressure within the distribution system. If the force of the pump declines, blood flow slows, and venous return is reduced. The third factor, peripheral resistance, is altered by general vasodilatation, which increases the capacity of the vascular system, leading to a lower pressure within the system and sluggish flow. In patients with shock there is usually less cardiac output, and blood flow through the *microcirculation* is decreased. The decreased blood flow leads to reduced oxygen and nutrients for the cells, resulting in *anaerobic* metabolism and increased lactic acid levels. If shock is prolonged,

cell metabolism is diminished. Cell wastes are not removed, leading to lower pH or *acidosis*, which further impairs cell enzyme function. Acidosis also tends to cause vasodilation, and relaxes precapillary sphincters first, contributing further to the pooling of blood in the periphery and decreasing venous return to the heart (Fig. 16-33).

If shock is not reversed quickly, it becomes even more difficult to do so because the compensations and effects of shock tend to aggravate the problem. Vasoconstriction reduces arterial blood flow into tissues and organs, causing ischemia and eventually necrosis. Thrombus forms in the microcirculation, further reducing venous return and cardiac output. Fluid shifts from the blood to the interstitial fluid. Organs and tissues can no longer function or undergo mitosis. Eventually the cells degenerate and may die. When organ damage occurs, shock may be irreversible. Complications of shock include acute renal failure owing to tubular necrosis, shock lung, or adult respiratory distress syndrome (ARDS) due to alveolar damage, hepatic failure due to cell necrosis, paralytic ileus, hemorrhagic ulcers, and infection or sepsis resulting from digestive tract ischemia. Cardiac function is depressed by the oxygen deficit, by acidosis and hyperkalemia, and by myocardial depressant factor released from the ischemic pancreas. Eventually cardiac arrhythmias and ischemia develop, perhaps resulting in cardiac arrest. Of concern is the occurrence of multiple organ failure after the patient appears stabilized.

Compensation mechanisms are initiated as soon as blood pressure decreases. The SNS and adrenal medulla are stimulated to increase the heart rate, the force of contractions, and systemic vasoconstriction. Renin is secreted to activate angiotensin, a vasoconstrictor, and aldosterone to increase blood volume. Increased secretion of ADH also promotes reabsorption of water from the kidneys to increase blood volume. Glucocorticoids are secreted that help to stabilize the vascular system. Acidosis stimulates respirations, increasing oxygen supplies and reducing carbon dioxide levels.

ETIOLOGY

There are a multitude of causes for shock, and only a few can be mentioned here. *Hypovolemic shock* results from loss of blood or loss of plasma as occurs in patients with burns, dehydration, or peritonitis. *Cardiogenic shock* is associated with cardiac impairment such as acute infarction of the left ventricle, or arrhythmias. A subcategory, *obstructive shock,* is caused by cardiac tamponade or a pulmonary embolus that blocks blood flow through the heart. The causes of vasogenic shock (distributive shock) may be classified in a variety of ways. *Anaphylactic shock* results from general vasodilation due to the release of large amounts of histamine. *Neurogenic* or *vasogenic shock* may develop from pain, fear, drugs, or loss of SNS stimuli with spinal cord injury. Metabolic dysfunction such as hypoglycemia or severe acidosis may lead to shock. Last, *septic shock* may develop in persons with severe infection, particularly infections with gram-negative endotoxins. Initial circulatory changes vary with the causative organism, but eventually systemic vasodilation develops. In some cases, the organism affects the heart as well.

SIGNS AND SYMPTOMS

Often missed, the first signs of shock are thirst and agitation or restlessness because the SNS is quickly stimulated by hypotension. This is followed by the char-

acteristic signs of compensation, cool, moist, pale skin, tachycardia, and oliguria. Vasoconstriction shunts blood from the viscera and skin to the vital areas. Then the direct effects of a decrease in blood pressure and blood flow become manifest by lethargy, weakness, dizziness, and a weak, thready pulse. Acidosis or low serum pH due to anaerobic metabolism is compensated for by increased respirations. Initially, hypoxemia and respiratory alkalosis are present as respirations increase. As shock progresses, metabolic acidosis dominates. Manifestations of shock are summarized in Table 16–5.

If shock is prolonged, the body's responsiveness decreases as oxygen supplies dwindle and wastes accumulate in the body. Compensated metabolic acidosis progresses to a decompensated acidosis when serum pH drops below 7.35 (see Chapter 6), leading to central nervous system depression and loss of cell metabolism and reducing the effectiveness of medications. Acute renal failure, indicated by increasing serum urea and creatinine, due to tubular ischemia and necrosis is a common occurrence.

When shock is severe and prolonged, monitoring may include the use of arterial catheters to assess blood pressure, ventricular filling, and cardiac output. Constant monitoring of arterial blood gases is essential (see Chapter 6).

TABLE 16–5 Manifestations of Shock

	Manifestations	Rationale
Early signs	Anxiety and restlessness	Hypotension stimulates SNS
Compensation	Tachycardia	SNS response stimulates heart
	Cool pale, moist skin	Peripheral vasoconstriction
	Oliguria	Renal vasoconstriction and renin mechanism
	Thirst	Osmoreceptors stimulated
	Rapid respirations	Anaerobic metabolism increases lactic acid secretion, which leads to increased respiratory rate
Progressive	Lethargy, weakness, faintness	Decreased blood flow and cardiac output
	Metabolic acidosis	Anaerobic metabolism increases lactic acid secretion
		Decreased renal excretion of acids and production of bicarbonate due to decreased glomerular filtration rate

TREATMENT

The primary problem must be treated. In patients with hypovolemic shock, whole blood, plasma, or fluid is required. When the cause is anaphylaxis, antihistamines and corticosteroids are given as well. Antimicrobials are necessary to control infection. General supportive measures include maintaining body warmth and ensuring blood flow to the brain and heart by keeping the person in a supine position. Oxygen supply should be maximized. Fluid, electrolytes, and bicarbonate may be given in any type of shock. The use of vasoconstrictors and vasodilators depends on the specific situation. Epinephrine acts both to reinforce heart action and constrict blood vessels. Dopamine and dobutamine increase heart function and, in low doses, dilate renal blood vessels, which may prevent acute renal failure.

Thinkabout 16–31

a. List and explain the signs indicating that compensation is occurring in patients with shock.

b. Give two reasons why acidosis develops in shock.

c. Give the arterial blood gas measurements with rationale for compensated acidosis with shock (see Chapter 6).

d. Give several reasons why shock tends to become progressively more serious.

LYMPHATIC DISORDERS

Lymphomas

Lymphomas are malignant neoplasms involving lymphocytes and their precursors. There are two main types, Hodgkin's and non-Hodgkin's lymphoma. Non-Hodgkin's lymphoma involves diffuse multiple lymph nodes and other extranodal tissues such as liver or bone and primarily affects the B lymphocytes.

HODGKIN'S LYMPHOMA

PATHOPHYSIOLOGY

Usually the malignancy involves a single lymph node initially. Later the cancer spreads to adjacent nodes and organs via the lymphatics. The T lymphocytes appear to be defective, and the lymphocyte count is de-creased. The typical cell used for diagnosis is the Reed-Sternberg cell, a giant cell. Staging for Hodgkin's disease uses the diaphragm as the differential. The Ann Arbor staging system generally defines a stage I cancer as affecting a single lymph node or region and stage II as affecting two or more lymph node regions on the same side of the diaphragm or in a relatively localized area. Stage III cancer involves nodes on both sides of the diaphragm and the spleen. Stage IV represents diffuse extralymphatic involvement such as bone, lung, or liver. Extensive testing is required to stage lymphomas.

SIGNS AND SYMPTOMS

Initially, the affected lymph node, often cervical, is large, painless, and nontender. Later, splenomegaly and enlarged lymph nodes at other locations may cause pressure effects; for example, enlarged mediastinal nodes may compress the esophagus. General signs of cancer such as weight loss, anemia, low-grade fever, and fatigue may develop. Generalized pruritus is common. Recurrent infection is common because the abnormal lymphocytes interfere with the immune response. In advanced stages, the liver, lungs, and digestive tract are usually involved.

TREATMENT

Surgery, radiation, and particularly chemotherapy are used with much greater success now than formerly. The prognosis for patients in the early stages of disease, when the malignancy is localized, is excellent.

MULTIPLE MYELOMA OR PLASMA CELL MYELOMA

PATHOPHYSIOLOGY

Multiple myeloma is a neoplastic disease involving the plasma cells that damages the bone marrow and bone. An increased number of mature and immature plasma cells replace the bone marrow and erode the bone. Blood cell production is impaired. Multiple tumors develop in the vertebrae, ribs, pelvis, and skull. Pathologic or spontaneous fractures at weakened sites in the bone are common. Hypercalcemia develops as bone is broken down.

SIGNS AND SYMPTOMS

Pain, related to bone involvement, is common in the back and is present at rest because blood cell production is affected. Anemia and abnormal immunoglobulins develop, leading to recurrent infection. Proteinuria and renal failure are common complications because the abnormal plasma cells produce a protein that is toxic to the renal tubules.

TREATMENT

Chemotherapy is the most common treatment. Blood transfusions are required in the late stage.

Thinkabout 16–32

a. Explain why infections occur frequently in patients with lymphomas.

b. State the prognosis for a person with a stage 1 and a stage 4 Hodgkin's lymphoma and explain your reasoning.

CASE STUDIES

CASE STUDY A
Myocardial Infarction

Mr. X, aged 55, arrives at the emergency department with severe chest pain. He appears very anxious, and his face is cool and clammy. The blood pressure is 90/60, and the pulse around 90, weak and irregular. He is given oxygen, an intravenous line is opened, and ECG is attached. Blood is taken for determination of serum enzymes and electrolytes. Tentative diagnosis is myocardial infarction involving the left ventricle. His wife arrives and, in response to questions, indicates that her husband is a heavy cigarette smoker, prefers a diet of fried foods and meat (he is obese), and had complained periodically of indigestion, with brief episodes of epigastric pain. He also seemed to be more fatigued at night recently but was very busy at work. He was fearful of heart disease because his father had died of a heart attack. He had also noticed more fatigue and intermittent leg pain when playing golf recently. Generalized atherosclerosis is suspected.

Thinkabout 16–33

a. List the high-risk factors for atherosclerosis in this patient's history.

b. Describe how atherosclerosis causes myocardial infarction.

c. It is suspected that the indigestion reported in the history was really angina. Explain how this pain may have occurred.

d. Explain why Mr. X had a rapid but weak pulse on admission.

e. Explain each of the admitting signs.

f. Why are serum enzyme and electrolyte levels important?

g. What purpose does the ECG serve?

It is determined that Mr. X has a large infarct in the anterior left ventricle.

h. Mr. X is showing increasing PVCs on the ECG. State the cause and describe the effect if they continue to increase in frequency.

i. Explain why Mr. X is at risk of venous thrombosis.

j. Describe how Mr. X's heart will heal and how its function is likely to be affected.

k. Blood tests show hyperlipidemia with high LDL levels. Estimate the risk of recurrence of myocardial infarction based on these levels.

l. Suggest several measures that can reduce the risk of recurrence.

m. Mr. X is at risk of congestive heart failure. List the significant signs of this if it develops.

n. During Mr. X's recovery, extensive tests are administered. They show generalized atherosclerosis, including lesions in the abdominal aorta and iliac arteries. How are these lesions probably connected to the fatigue and leg pain experienced while playing golf?

o. Suggest some precautions in regard to foot care that Mr. X can take.

CASE STUDY B
Acute Lymphocytic Leukemia

PM, aged 6 years, has returned to the family doctor because of a recurrent sore throat and cough. Her mother mentions unusual listlessness and anorexia. The physician notices several bruises on her legs and arms and one on her back. The doctor orders blood tests and a course of antibacterial drugs. Test results indicate a low hemoglobin level, thrombocytopenia, and a high lymphocyte count with abnormally high numbers of blast cells. Following a bone marrow aspiration, a diagnosis of ALL is confirmed.

Thinkabout 16–34

a. Describe the pathophysiology of ALL.

b. State the rationale for each of PM's signs.

c. Explain the significance of blast cells in the peripheral blood.

d. Describe the effects of hypermetabolism in leukemia.

e. Explain how chemotherapy aggravates the effects of leukemia.

f. Describe the possible effects if leukemic cells infiltrate the brain.

g. Describe the pain associated with leukemia and explain the reason for it.

CASE STUDY C
Essential Hypertension

Ms. SJ, aged 48, has essential hypertension, diagnosed 4 years ago. She has not been taking her medication during the past 6 months because she has been feeling fine. Now she has a new job and has been too busy to enjoy her usual swimming and golf. She has decided to have a checkup because she is feeling tired and dyspneic and has had several bouts of dizziness, blurred vision, and epistaxis (nosebleeds) lately. On examination, her blood pressure is found to be 190/120, some rales are present in the lungs, and the retina of her eyes shows some sclerosis and several arteriolar ruptures. The physician orders rest and medication to lower the blood pressure as well as an appointment with a nutritionist and urinary tests to check kidney function.

Thinkabout 16–35

a. Describe the pathophysiology of essential hypertension.

b. Explain the possible problems associated with the high diastolic pressure.

c. Explain the significance of the retinal changes.

d. The doctor suspects mild congestive heart failure. Explain how this can develop from hypertension. Give two other possible signs of CHF.

e. List two medications that are helpful in treating hypertension and describe their actions.

STUDY QUESTIONS

1. Name six substances that are transported in the blood and the function of each.

2. Explain the cause of incompatible blood transfusion.

3. List three types of clotting problems.

4. Name three mechanisms that can increase cardiac output.

5. Explain the effect on blood flow of mitral valve incompetence.

6. Explain the reason for each of the following:
   a. high elastic fiber content in the aorta
   b. smooth muscle in the arterioles
   c. extensive capillaries in the liver and lungs
   d. valves in the leg veins

7. Explain why vasodilator drugs are of limited value in arterial disease.

8. Explain how aortic stenosis may develop following rheumatic fever.

9. Explain how pernicious anemia may develop from chronic gastritis.

10. For which conditions could secondary polycythemia develop as a compensation: VSD, CHF, chronic lung disease, aplastic anemia, multiple myeloma.

11. Explain how DIC develops and state two signs of its development.

12. Explain why bone pain occurs with leukemia.

13. Define and explain the term intermittent claudication.

14. Describe three early signs of shock and the rationale for each.

15. Differentiate angina from myocardial infarction with regard to its cause and the characteristics of pain associated with it.

16. Choose one aspect of CHF that might apply in your field of work and explain your concern.

17. If you had a client with persistent chest pain following rest and administration of nitroglycerin, what action would you take?

18. Why would you recommend avoidance of prolonged stress for a patient with congenital heart disease?

19. List and explain briefly three possible causes of cardiac dysrhythmias.

20. Differentiate heart blocks from PVCs with regard to causes and effects on heart action.

CHAPTER
17
Respiratory Disorders

KEY TERMS

●●

apnea	dyspnea	inhaler	pulsus paradoxus
bifurcation	embolus	malaise	rales
bronchodilation	empyema	necrosis	rhonchi
carbaminoglobin	eupnea	orthopnea	sputum
caseation	expectorant	oxyhemoglobin	steatorrhea
chemoreceptors	hemoptysis	paroxysmal nocturnal	stridor
clubbing	hypercapnia	dyspnea	surface tension
cohesion	hypoxemia	perfusion	thrombus
cyanosis	hypoxic	protease	wheezing
diffusion	infarction		

REVIEW OF NORMAL STRUCTURES IN THE RESPIRATORY SYSTEM

Purpose and General Organization

The respiratory system provides a mechanism for transporting oxygen from the air into the blood and for removing carbon dioxide from the blood. Oxygen is essential for cell metabolism. Carbon dioxide is a waste material resulting from cell metabolism and influences acid-base balance in body fluids.

There are two anatomic areas in the respiratory system. The *upper respiratory* tract is made up of the passageways that conduct air between the atmosphere and the lungs, and the *lower respiratory* tract consists of the trachea and the lungs, where gas exchange takes place. In addition, the pulmonary circulation, the muscles required for ventilation, and the nervous system, which plays a role in controlling respiratory function, are integral to the function of the respiratory system.

Structures in the Respiratory System

THE UPPER RESPIRATORY TRACT

When air is inhaled into the respiratory system, it first enters the *nasal* passages, passing over the conchae or turbinates, where it is warmed and moistened by the highly vascular mucosa and foreign material is filtered out by the mucous secretions and hairs before the air enters the delicate lung tissue. Opening off the nasal cavity through small canals are four pairs of *paranasal sinuses*, which are small cavities in the skull bones (Fig. 17–1). The sinuses reduce the weight of the facial bones and add resonance to the voice. They are named by the bones in which they are located—the frontal, ethmoid, sphenoid, and maxillary sinuses. The sinuses are lined by a continuation of the respiratory mucosa. The *respiratory mucosa* consists of pseudostratified columnar epithelium, which includes mucus-secreting goblet cells and cilia. The resultant mucous blanket "traps" foreign particles, and the cilia "sweep" the mucus and debris up and out of the respiratory tract. Excessive amounts of mucus or particles stimulate a sneeze or a cough, which assists in expelling unwanted material away from the lungs. Smoking impairs the function of the cilia, and the irritation caused by smoke leads to replacement of ciliated epithelium by squamous cells, removing this protective mechanism.

The air flow continues through the *nasopharynx* and larynx into the trachea. On the posterior wall of the nasopharynx are located the *pharyngeal tonsils* or adenoids, which consist of lymphoid tissue, another defense mechanism. If these tonsils become enlarged owing to infection, they can obstruct the flow of air

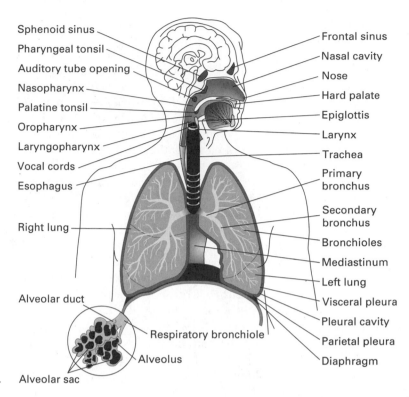

FIGURE 17-1. Anatomy of the respiratory system.

through the nasopharynx, leading to "mouth breathing." When air passes through the mouth to the respiratory tract, it is not warmed, moistened, and filtered properly before it reaches the delicate lung tissue. Also, the tissues of the mouth become dry and irritated, and there is a risk of increased dental caries as normal salivary cleansing function is lost. The *palatine tonsils*, popularly called "the tonsils," are located in the posterior portion of the oral cavity (see Fig. 18–2 in Chapter 18). Also opening off the nasopharynx are the two *auditory* (eustachian) tubes, which connect to the middle ear cavities. The continuous mucosa into the sinuses and middle ear creates a predisposition to the spread of infection from the upper respiratory tract. The upper respiratory tract has a *resident flora*, whereas the lungs are sterile, containing no microorganisms.

The *pharynx* serves as a common passage for air and food where the nasopharynx joins the oropharynx and descends to the point of separation of the esophagus and trachea. In the airway, the cartilaginous *epiglottis* protects the opening into the larynx or voice box by flipping up or down with swallowing or ventilation. The larynx consists of various cartilages and their associated muscles. The largest is the thyroid cartilage, which forms the "Adam's apple," a structure that may protrude in the anterior neck area. There are two pairs of vocal cords, which are infoldings of the mucous membrane: the upper, or "false," pair and the lower pair comprising the *true vocal cords*. The *glottis* refers to the true vocal cords and the space between them. When air is expired through the larynx, the true vocal cords

vibrate, producing the sound of the voice. Other structures affect the characteristics of this sound, including the mouth, tongue, pharynx, and sinuses. The vocal cords, when approximated, prevent food from entering the trachea and lungs. As inspired air is tracked downward through the larynx, it flows into the *trachea* or windpipe. The trachea is composed of smooth muscle and elastic tissue in which are located C-shaped rings of cartilage, whose open side is on the posterior surface to allow for esophageal expansion. This cartilage supports the wall of the airway, preventing its collapse.

Thinkabout 17–1

a. Name and locate the lymphoid structures in the upper respiratory tract.

b. Describe the structure and function of the paranasal sinuses.

c. Describe how inhaled air may be altered as it passes through the nasal passages and pharynx.

THE LOWER RESPIRATORY TRACT

At the lower end of the trachea, inhaled air proceeds into the right or left *bronchus*. The right bronchus is larger and straighter and therefore is the more likely destination for any aspirated material. The point at which the bronchus enters the lung is the hilum. Each major or primary bronchus then branches into many smaller (secondary) bronchi and then into bronchioles, forming an inverted bronchial "tree." As the bronchi become smaller, the cartilaginous rings diminish in size, and smooth muscle increases. This smooth muscle contracts or relaxes to adjust the diameter of the bronchioles. **Bronchodilation** results when sympathetic stimulation relaxes the smooth muscle, dilating or enlarging the bronchioles. Many elastic fibers are present in the lung tissue, enabling the expansion and recoil of the lungs during ventilation. The respiratory mucosa is continuous throughout all branches of the bronchi and bronchioles. Air in the bronchioles then flows into the *alveolar* ducts and *alveoli,* or air sacs, which resemble a cluster of grapes. The alveoli are formed by a single layer of simple squamous epithelial tissue, which promotes the **diffusion** of gases into the blood, the endpoint for inspired air (see Fig. 17–4). The respiratory membrane is the combined alveolar and capillary wall, a very thin membrane, through which gas exchange takes place. There are millions of alveoli, and the capillaries of the pulmonary circulation are in close contact, providing a very large surface area for the diffusion of gases. The alveoli contain macrophages, which can remove any foreign material that penetrates to this level. The inside surfaces of the alveoli are coated with a very small amount of fluid containing *surfactant,* produced by specialized cells in the alveolar wall. Surfactant has a detergent action that reduces **surface tension,** facilitating inspiration and preventing total collapse of the alveoli during expiration. When inspiration is complete, the process of expiration reverses air flow in the passageways, forcing air out of the alveoli and up the bronchi, trachea, and nose.

The *lungs* are cone-shaped structures positioned on either side of the heart. The *mediastinum* is the region in the center of the chest, which contains the heart, the major blood vessels, the esophagus, and the trachea. The dome-shaped muscular diaphragm forms the inferior boundary. The right lung is divided into three lobes and the left lung into two lobes because of the position of the heart, and each lobe is then divided into segments. The lung tissue (lungs, bronchi, and pleurae) is nourished by the bronchial arteries, which branch from the thoracic aorta. Each lung is covered by a separate double-walled sac, the *pleural membrane.* The *visceral pleura* is attached to the outer surface of the lung and then doubles back to form the *parietal pleura,* which lines the inside of the thoracic cavity, adhering to the chest wall and the diaphragm. The visceral pleura lies closely against the parietal pleura, separated only by very small amounts of fluid in the pleural cavity or space, which is considered only a *potential* space. The slightly negative (less than atmospheric pressure) pressure in the pleural cavity also assists in holding the pleura in close approximation and promoting lung expansion. The pleural fluid provides lubrication during respiratory movements and a **cohesive** force (high surface tension) between the two pleural layers during inspiration. The *thorax,* consisting of ribs, vertebrae, and sternum (breastbone) provides a rigid protective wall for the lungs. The upper seven pairs of ribs (true ribs) articulate with the vertebrae and are attached to the sternum by costal cartilage. The next three pairs of ribs are "false" ribs, which are connected to the costal cartilage of the seventh rib, not directly to the sternum. The last two ribs (also false), the eleventh and twelfth pairs, are not attached and are therefore called floating ribs. Between the ribs are located the intercostal muscles, external and internal, which move the thoracic structures during ventilation.

Ventilation

THE PROCESS OF INSPIRATION AND EXPIRATION

Air flow during expiration and inspiration depends on a *pressure* gradient, with air always moving from a *high pressure* area to a *low pressure* area. If atmospheric pressure is higher than air pressure inside the lungs, air will move from the atmosphere into the lungs (inspiration). For expiration to occur, pressure must be higher in the lungs than in the atmosphere. These pressure changes in the lungs result from alterations in the size of the thoracic cavity. *As the size of the thoracic cavity decreases, the pressure inside the cavity increases* (Boyle's law). A sequence of events is responsible for the change in size of the thorax and the changes in air flow with inspiration and expiration.

Normal *quiet inspiration* begins with contraction of the diaphragm and the external intercostal muscles. The diaphragm flattens and descends, increasing the length of the thoracic cavity (Fig. 17–2). The external intercostal muscles raise the ribs and sternum up and outward, increasing the transverse and anteroposterior diameters of the thorax. The increased size of the thoracic cavity results in decreased pressure in the pleural cavity and in the alveoli and airways. As the ribs and diaphragm move, the attached parietal pleura pulls the adhering visceral pleura and lungs along with it. As the visceral pleura moves outward, the elastic lungs expand with it, resulting in a decrease in air pressure inside the lungs. At this point, atmospheric pressure is greater than intra-alveolar pressure, so air flows from the atmosphere down the airways into the alveoli. Note that the thorax and lungs must expand *before* more air can enter the lungs; it is not the air entering the lungs that makes them expand. During *normal expiration* the diaphragm and external intercostal muscles must then relax, lead-

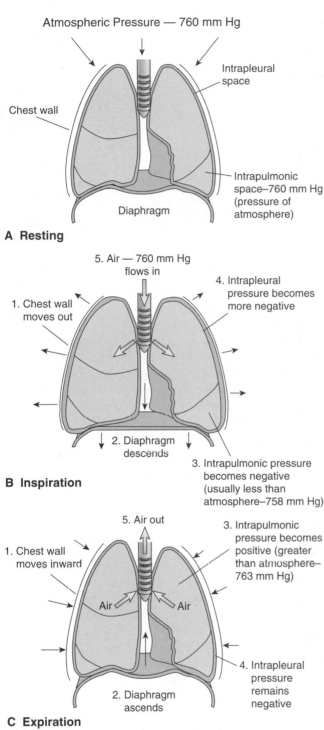

A Resting

Atmospheric Pressure — 760 mm Hg

Chest wall

Intrapleural space

Intrapulmonic space–760 mm Hg (pressure of atmosphere)

Diaphragm

B Inspiration

5. Air — 760 mm Hg flows in

1. Chest wall moves out

4. Intrapleural pressure becomes more negative

2. Diaphragm descends

3. Intrapulmonic pressure becomes negative (usually less than atmosphere–758 mm Hg)

C Expiration

5. Air out

1. Chest wall moves inward

3. Intrapulmonic pressure becomes positive (greater than atmosphere–763 mm Hg)

Air   Air

2. Diaphragm ascends

4. Intrapleural pressure remains negative

FIGURE 17-2. Ventilation: changes in pressure with inspiration and expiration.

ing to a decrease in thoracic size. This decrease, combined with the natural elastic recoil of the alveoli, results in increased intra-alveolar pressure (greater than atmospheric pressure), and therefore air flows out of the alveoli into the atmosphere. Quiet expiration is a *passive* process and does not require energy. *Forced* inspiration or expiration requires additional energy and muscular activity. In forced inspiration the sternoclei-

domastoid, scalene, pectoralis minor, and serratus muscles increase the elevation of the ribs and sternum. During forceful expiration the abdominal muscles and the internal intercostal muscles contract to increase upward pressure on the diaphragm, pulling the ribs and sternum down and inward, respectively. *Compliance* is the term used to refer to the ability of the lungs to expand. Compliance depends largely on the elasticity of the tissues but can also be affected by other factors such as the shape, size, and flexibility of the thorax.

Thinkabout 17–2

a. Describe the purpose of (1) surfactant, (2) the ribs, (3) the respiratory membrane, (4) the diaphragm, (5) alveolar macrophages, and (6) the bronchial artery.

b. Describe the sequence of events that takes place during inspiration.

c. Explain why frequent forced expirations are fatiguing.

PULMONARY VOLUMES

Pulmonary volumes are a measure of ventilatory capacity because they measure the air moving in and out of the lungs with normal or forced inspiration and expiration (Fig. 17–3). Some of the basic volumes are summarized in Table 17–1. *Residual volume* is the volume of air remaining in the lungs after expiration. This air continues to provide gas exchange and maintains partial inflation of the lungs. Pulmonary volumes can change with disease processes and are helpful in monitoring a patient's progress or response to treatment. For example, impaired expiration can cause an increase in residual volume and increased carbon dioxide levels. *Vital capacity* is another important measure that represents the maximal amount of air that can be moved in and out of the lungs. It can be altered by lung disease, size of the thorax, amount of blood in the lungs, or body position. *Dead space* refers to the passageways or areas where gas exchange cannot take place. Anatomic dead space includes areas such as the bronchi and bronchioles. Dead space can be increased by obstruction in the passageways or collapse of alveoli.

CONTROL OF RESPIRATION

The control center for breathing is located in the medulla and pons. The inspiratory center in

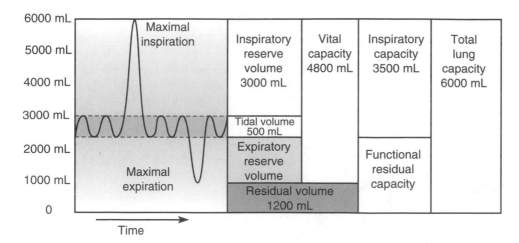

FIGURE 17–3. Pulmonary volumes.

the medulla stimulates the phrenic nerves to the diaphragm and the intercostal nerves to the external intercostal muscles. These stimuli occur spontaneously in a rhythmic fashion. The expiratory center in the medulla appears to function primarily when forced expiration is required because normal quiet expiration is a cessation of activity following each inspiration. Additional centers in the pons play a role in coordinating inspiration, expiration, and the intervals for each.

The rate and depth of breathing set by the medullary center can be modified by a number of factors. Any depression of central nervous system activity, for example, by drugs, can lead to slow, shallow breathing. Other factors include activity of the hypothalamus, perhaps in response to emotions; or the stretch receptors in the lungs or the Hering-Breuer reflex, which prevents excessive lung expansion; or voluntary control, as required when singing. However, voluntary control is limited by the levels of carbon dioxide in the blood. When the concentration or partial pressure of carbon

dioxide (Pa_{CO_2}) in the blood rises, breathing resumes automatically. For this reason, a child who intentionally holds his or her breath will eventually have to breathe spontaneously.

Chemical factors are most important in respiratory control. **Chemoreceptors** sense changes in the levels of carbon dioxide, hydrogen ions, and oxygen. The central chemoreceptors in the medulla respond quickly to slight elevations in P_{CO_2} (from a normal 40 mm Hg to 43 mm Hg) or to a decrease in pH of the cerebrospinal fluid. The peripheral chemoreceptors, located in the carotid bodies at the **bifurcation** of the common carotid arteries and the aortic body in the aortic arch, are sensitive to decreased oxygen levels in arterial blood as well as to low pH. A marked decrease in oxygen (from approximately 105 mm Hg to 60 mm Hg) is necessary before the chemoreceptors respond to **hypoxemia.** Normal oxygen levels provide a substantial reserve of oxygen in the venous blood. This control mechanism can be important when individuals with chronic lung disease adapt to a sustained elevation in P_{CO_2} and move to a *hypoxic drive.* Such individuals are dependent on low oxygen levels rather than the normal slight elevation in carbon dioxide to stimulate inspiration. Therefore, it is important for these people always to remain slightly **hypoxic** and not be given excessive amounts of oxygen at any time.

When carbon dioxide levels in the blood increase (**hypercapnia**), carbon dioxide easily diffuses into the cerebrospinal fluid, lowering pH and stimulating the respiratory center, resulting in an increased rate and depth of respirations (hyperventilation). Hypercapnia causes respiratory acidosis, and acidosis depresses the nervous system. Hypocapnia, or low P_{CO_2}, may be caused by hyperventilation when excessive amounts of carbon dioxide have been expired. Hypocapnia causes respiratory alkalosis. To review the conditions of respiratory acidosis and alkalosis and the role of arterial blood gases, refer to Chapter 6.

TABLE 17–1 Pulmonary Volumes		
Name	**Volume**	**Meaning**
Tidal volume (TV)	500 mL	Amount of air entering lungs with each normal breath
Residual volume (RV)	1200 mL	Amount of air remaining in the lungs after forced expiration
Inspiratory reserve (IRV)	3000 mL	Maximal volume of air inspired following maximal expiration
Expiratory reserve (ERV)	1100 mL	Maximal volume of air expired following a passive expiration
Vital capacity (VC)	4600 mL	Maximal amount of air expired following a maximal inspiration
Total lung capacity (TLC)	5800 mL	Total volume of air in the lungs after maximal inspiration

Thinkabout 17–3

a. Name the major stimulus for inspiration.

b. How do elevated carbon dioxide levels alter serum pH and respiratory pattern?

c. State the normal serum pH and describe how compensation for decreased serum pH due to a respiratory impairment is achieved.

d. Describe how acidosis affects the central nervous system and give two physiologic signs of this condition.

Gas Exchange

Gas exchange, or external respiration, is the flow of gases between the alveolar air and the blood in the pulmonary circulation. Diffusion of oxygen and carbon dioxide in the lungs depends on the relative concentrations or partial pressures of the gases, and movement always occurs from a high pressure area to a low pressure area. It is customary to refer to the concentration of a gas such as oxygen in a mixture as the partial pressure of that gas, e.g., Po_2. When the measurement refers specifically to the partial pressure of oxygen (or another gas) in arterial blood, it is expressed as Pao_2. Each gas in a mixture moves or diffuses according to its own partial pressure gradient and independent of other gases. For example, oxygen diffuses from alveolar air, an area with a high concentration of oxygen, to the blood in the pulmonary capillary, which has a low concentration of oxygen, until the concentrations become equal (Fig. 17–4). Meanwhile, carbon dioxide diffuses out of the pulmonary capillary into the alveolar air depending on its relative concentrations. Air contains oxygen, carbon dioxide, nitrogen, and water. Because the air is not totally expired from the alveoli during expiration and has been humidified during its passage into the lungs, alveolar air has different concentrations of gases than either atmospheric air or blood. The residual air in the alveoli allows continuing gas exchange between expiration and inspiration because blood continually flows through the pulmonary circulation.

The pulmonary circulation is composed of the pulmonary arteries, which bring venous blood (dark blue-red in color) from the right side of the heart to be oxygenated; the pulmonary capillaries, in which diffusion or gas exchange occurs; and the pulmonary veins, which return the oxygenated blood (bright red) to the

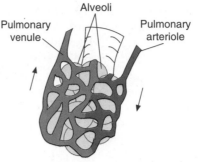

A Pulmonary capillaries around alveolus

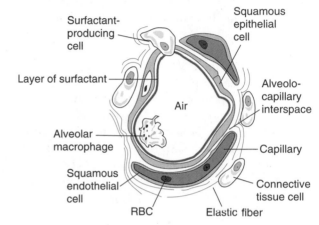

B Cross-section of an alveolus

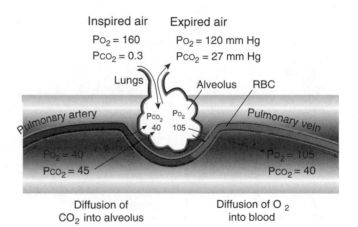

C Diffusion of gases
FIGURE 17–4. The alveolus.

left side of the heart, which then pumps it out into the systemic circulation.

FACTORS AFFECTING DIFFUSION

In addition to the partial pressure gradient, diffusion can be altered by other factors such as the thickness of the respiratory membrane. When fluid accumulates in the alveoli or interstitial tissue, diffusion, particularly diffusion of oxygen, is greatly impaired. Normally the pressure in the pulmonary circulation is very low, reducing the risk of excessive fluid in the interstitial space and alveoli. The presence of extra fluid may also impede blood flow through the pulmonary capillaries and increase surface tension in the alveoli, restricting expansion of the lung. Another major factor in gas exchange is the surface area available for diffusion. The alveoli are the only structures that provide such a surface area, and both ventilation and **perfusion** must be adequate for diffusion to occur (see Fig. 17–14). If part of the alveolar wall is destroyed, as in emphysema, or if fibrosis occurs in the lungs, the surface area is greatly reduced. If air flow into the alveoli is obstructed or if the capillaries are damaged, the involved surface area becomes nonfunctional. This imbalance is measured by the ventilation-perfusion ratio ($\dot{V}A/\dot{Q}$). An autoregulatory mechanism in the lungs can adjust ventilation and blood flow in an attempt to produce a good match. For example, if Po_2 is low because of poor ventilation in an area, vasoconstriction occurs in the pulmonary arterioles, shunting the blood to other areas of the lungs where ventilation may be better. If air flow is good, the pulmonary arterioles dilate to maximize gas exchange.

Thinkabout 17–4

a. Explain why oxygen diffuses from alveolar air into the blood.

b. Name the blood vessels bringing blood into the pulmonary circulation, and describe the blood in these vessels.

c. Describe the effect of a thickened respiratory membrane on blood levels of oxygen and carbon dioxide. Which gas is affected more?

TRANSPORT OF OXYGEN AND CARBON DIOXIDE

Only about 1 percent of total oxygen is dissolved in plasma because oxygen is relatively insoluble in water. The *dissolved* form of the gas is that which diffuses from the alveolar air into the blood in the pulmonary capillaries and also diffuses into the interstitial fluid and the cells during the process of internal respiration. Most

oxygen is transported reversibly bound to hemoglobin by the iron molecules and is called **oxyhemoglobin** (see Fig. 16–7 in Chapter 16). When all four heme molecules in hemoglobin have taken up oxygen, the hemoglobin is termed *fully saturated* (measurement expressed as SaO_2). As oxygen diffuses out of the blood into the interstitial fluid and the cells, hemoglobin releases oxygen to replace it, so dissolved oxygen is always available in the plasma, ready to diffuse into the cells. The rate at which hemoglobin binds or releases oxygen depends on factors such as Po_2 (the partial pressure of dissolved oxygen), temperature, and plasma pH. Normally, approximately 25 percent of the bound oxygen is released to the cells for metabolism during an erythrocyte's trip through the systemic circulation, leaving 75 percent of the hemoglobin in the venous blood still saturated with oxygen. This provides a good safety margin of oxygen that is available to meet cell needs.

Carbon dioxide, which results from cell metabolism, is transported in several forms. Approximately 7 percent is dissolved in the plasma and is capable of diffusion. Roughly 20 percent is loosely and reversibly bound to hemoglobin, attached to an amino group on the globin (not the heme) portion, and is termed **carbaminoglobin.** The majority of carbon dioxide resulting from cell metabolism diffuses into the red blood cells (RBCs), where it is converted under the influence of the enzyme carbonic anhydrase into bicarbonate ions or carbonic acid (see equation below). These bicarbonate ions can then diffuse back into the plasma to function in the buffer pair (see Chapter 6).

A ratio of 20 parts bicarbonate ion to 1 part carbonic acid maintains blood pH at 7.35. Thus, carbon dioxide plays a major role in control of blood pH through this buffer system.

Diagnostic Tests

Pulmonary volumes may be determined by spirometry, which can measure volume and air flow times. Arterial blood gas determinations are used to check oxygen, carbon dioxide, and bicarbonate levels as well as pH. Exercise testing is useful in patients with chronic pulmonary disease for diagnosis and monitoring of the patient's progress. Radiography may be helpful in evaluating tumors or infections such as pneumonia or tuberculosis. Bronchoscopy may be used in performing a biopsy or in checking for the site of a lesion or bleeding. Culture and sensitivity tests on exudates from the upper

$$CO_2 + H_2O \leftrightarrow H_2CO_3 \leftrightarrow H^+ + HCO_3^-$$
carbon dioxide + water $\leftrightarrow$ carbonic acid $\leftrightarrow$ hydrogen ion + bicarbonate ion

respiratory tract or **sputum** specimens can identify pathogens and assist in determining the appropriate therapy.

GENERAL MANIFESTATIONS OF RESPIRATORY DISEASE

A *sneeze or cough* is a reflex response to irritation in the respiratory tract and assists in removing the irritant. Sneezing is associated with inflammation or foreign material in the nasal passages. Coughing may result from irritation due to nasal discharge dripping into the oropharynx or from inflammation or foreign material in the lower tract. The cough reflex is controlled by a center in the medulla and consists of coordinated actions that inspire air and then close the glottis and vocal cords. This is followed by forceful expiration in which the glottis is opened and the unwanted material is blown upward and out of the mouth. In some cases the product of a cough is swallowed. The effectiveness of the cough depends on the strength of the muscle action in both inspiration and expiration. An occasional cough is considered a normal event in a healthy person, but a persistent cough may be evidence of a respiratory disease or chronic irritation. Aspiration of food or fluid may cause a spasm of coughing. A constant dry or unproductive cough can be fatiguing because it interferes with sleep and the respiratory muscles are used excessively. In such cases, a cough-suppressant medication (e.g., codeine or dextromethorphan) may be used at night. A productive cough usually occurs when secretions or exudate accumulate in the lungs, and removal of such fluids from the airways is beneficial. Excess secretions may become infected and tend to obstruct the airways. It is helpful in such cases to increase fluid intake to keep the secretions thin and easy to remove. An **expectorant** medication (e.g., guaifenesin) or a humidifier also may assist in removing secretions. Thick or sticky mucus is particularly difficult to raise from the lungs, especially in elderly or debilitated patients.

Sputum or mucoid discharge from the respiratory tract may have significant characteristics depending on the abnormality causing it. Normal secretions are relatively thin, clear, and colorless. Yellowish-green, cloudy, thick mucus is often an indication of a bacterial infection. Rusty or dark-colored sputum is usually a sign of pneumococcal pneumonia. Very large amounts of purulent (contains pus) sputum with a foul odor may be associated with bronchiectasis. Thick, tenacious mucus may occur in patients with asthma or cystic fibrosis. Blood-tinged secretions may result from a chronic cough and irritation that causes rupture of superficial capillaries, but it may also be a sign of a tumor or tuberculosis. **Hemoptysis** is blood-tinged (bright red) frothy sputum that is usually associated with pulmonary edema. It is important not to confuse hemoptysis with hematemesis, which is vomitus containing blood and is usually granular and dark in color (coffee-grounds vomitus).

Breath sounds may be abnormal or absent in respiratory disorders. **Rales** and **rhonchi** are abnormal sounds resulting from air mixing with excessive secretions in the lungs. Rales are light bubbly or crackling sounds associated with serous secretions, whereas *rhonchi* are deeper or harsher sounds resulting from thicker mucus. The *absence* of breath sounds indicates nonaeration or collapse of a lung (atelectasis).

Breathing patterns and characteristics may be altered with respiratory disease. The normal rate (**eupnea**) is 10 to 18 inspirations per minute, and the normal pattern is regular and effortless. Changes in the rate, rhythm, depth, and effort of ventilation are significant. Kussmaul respirations, deep rapid respirations or "air hunger," are typical of a state of acidosis or may follow strenuous exercise. Labored respirations or prolonged inspiration or expiration times are associated with obstruction of the airways. **Wheezing** or whistling sounds indicate obstruction in the small airways, whereas **stridor**, a high-pitched crowing noise, usually indicates upper airway obstruction.

Dyspnea is a subjective feeling of discomfort that occurs when a person feels unable to inhale enough air. It may be manifested as breathlessness or shortness of breath, either with exertion or at rest. In severe cases, dyspnea may be accompanied by *flaring* of the nostrils (nares), use of the accessory respiratory muscles, or *retraction* (pulling in) of the muscles between or above the ribs. For example, intercostal retractions between the ribs are visible to the observer.

Orthopnea is dyspnea that occurs when a person is lying down. Pulmonary congestion develops as more blood pools in the lungs as the person lies down and also as the abdominal contents push upward against the lungs. Raising the upper part of the body with pillows often facilitates breathing in persons with respiratory or cardiovascular disorders. **Paroxysmal nocturnal dyspnea** is a sudden acute type of dyspnea common in patients with left-sided congestive heart failure. During sleep the body fluid is redistributed, leading to pulmonary edema, and the individual wakes up gasping for air and coughing (see Chapter 16).

Cyanosis is the bluish coloring of the skin and mucous membranes that results from large amounts of unoxygenated hemoglobin in the blood. This may occur in patients with cardiovascular conditions as well as respiratory disease, and its presence must be considered in conjunction with other data. Cyanosis is not a reliable early indicator of hypoxia.

Pleural pain results from inflammation or infection of the parietal pleura. It is a cyclic pain that increases as the inflamed membrane is stretched with inspiration or coughing. A *friction rub* may be heard, a soft sound produced as the rough membranes move against each other. Pleural inflammation may be caused by lobar pneumonia or lung **infarction.**

Clubbed fingers and sometimes toes result from chronic hypoxia associated with respiratory or cardiovascular diseases. **Clubbing** is a painless, firm, fibrotic enlargement of the end of the digit.

Hypoxemia refers to inadequate oxygen in the blood (Pao_2). *Hypoxia,* or inadequate oxygen supply to the cells, may have many causes. One of these is a deficit of erythrocytes (RBCs) or hemoglobin levels that are too low for adequate oxygen transport. Another cause is circulatory impairment, which may lead to decreased cardiac output from the heart to the lungs or to the systemic circulation; or there may be excessive release of oxygen from RBCs if circulation is sluggish through the system or is partially obstructed by vascular disease. Impaired respiratory function, including inadequate ventilation, inhalation of oxygen-deficient air, or impaired diffusion also leads to hypoxia. One important cause of hypoxia is carbon monoxide poisoning, in which carbon monoxide binds tightly and preferentially to heme, displacing oxygen. Unfortunately, carbon monoxide does not cause obvious signs of hypoxia or affect ventilation, but it can be fatal very quickly and quietly.

Hypoxia affects cell metabolism, reducing cell function and leading to anaerobic metabolism and the development of metabolic acidosis. The brain is most susceptible to an oxygen deficit because it has little storage capacity for oxygen and yet has a constant demand. Cerebral hypoxia stimulates the sympathetic nervous system. Decreased cell function is indicated by fatigue, lethargy or stupor, and muscle weakness. Extreme or prolonged hypoxia can result in cell death. Compensation mechanisms for hypoxia due to respiratory impairment include increased cardiovascular activity such as tachycardia and increased blood pressure. In people with chronic hypoxia due to respiratory or circulatory impairment, erythropoietin secretion is increased, stimulating the bone marrow to produce additional red blood cells (secondary polycythemia).

Acid-base imbalance may develop from respiratory disorders (see Chapter 6). Respiratory acidosis due to excess carbon dioxide is more common and results from impaired expiration. Arterial blood gases in this situation indicate high Pco_2 and low serum pH. Respiratory alkalosis occurs when the respiratory rate is increased, usually because of acute anxiety or excessive intake of aspirin.

Thinkabout 17–5

a. Define the terms sputum, rales, orthopnea, and hemoptysis.

b. Differentiate a productive cough from an unproductive cough by general cause, signs, and possible complications.

c. List the signs indicating a possible obstruction in the airways.

INFECTIOUS DISEASES

Upper Respiratory Tract Infections

COMMON COLD (INFECTIOUS RHINITIS)

The common cold is caused by a viral infection of the upper respiratory tract. The most common pathogen is a rhinovirus, but it may also be an adenovirus or coronavirus. There are more than 100 possible causative organisms, so it is difficult for an individual to develop sufficient immunity to avoid all colds. Children do acquire more colds than adults, usually as a brief self-limiting infection, unless a secondary bacterial infection develops. The common cold is spread through respiratory droplets, which are either directly inhaled or are spread by secretions on hands or contaminated objects such as facial tissue. The infection is highly contagious because the virus is shed in large numbers from the infected nasal mucosa during the first few days of the infection and can survive for several hours outside the body.

Initially, the mucous membranes of the nose and pharynx are red and swollen with the increased secretions. The signs of a cold include nasal congestion and copious watery discharge, sneezing, and sometimes watery eyes. Mouth breathing is common, and a change in the tone of voice is noticeable. There may be sore throat, headache, slight fever, and **malaise.** Cough may develop from the irritation of the secretions dripping into the pharynx. Sometimes the feeling of stuffiness and irritation persists as the secretions become more viscous for a few days after the acute period has passed. Treatment is symptomatic, consisting of acetaminophen for fever and headache and decongestants (vasoconstrictors) to reduce the edema and congestion in the respiratory passages. Antihistamines reduce secretions but may cause excessive drying of tissues and cough. Humidifiers aid in keeping the secretions liquid

TABLE 17–2 General Comparison of Respiratory Infections in Children

	Laryngotracheobronchitis	**Epiglottitis**	**Bronchiolitis**
Age group	3 months to 3 years	3–7 years	2–12 months
Cause	Virus	*Haemophilus influenzae*	Virus—RSV
Pathology	Inflammation of mucosa of larynx and trachea obstructs airway	Supraglottic inflammation and swelling of epiglottis obstructs airway	Inflammation of mucosa of bronchioles obstructs small passages
Onset	Gradual	Rapid	Gradual
Signs	Hoarse, barking cough	Drooling, dysphagia	Increasing dyspnea
	Inspiratory stridor	High fever, appears ill	Paroxysmal cough, wheezing
	Restlessness	Rapid respirations and pulse	Chest retractions
		Tripod position	Flared nares

and easily drained. The role of vitamin C in prevention and therapy remains controversial. Antibiotics do not cure viral infections and are usually reserved for secondary bacterial infections such as sinusitis, otitis media (see Chapter 20), or tracheitis or for prophylactic use in high-risk patients (such as those with chronic illnesses). Proper handwashing and disposal of tissues reduces the risk of transmission to others.

SINUSITIS

Sinusitis is usually a bacterial infection secondary to a cold or an allergy that has obstructed the drainage of one or more of the paranasal sinuses into the nasal cavity (see Fig. 17–1). Common causative organisms include pneumococci, streptococci, or *Haemophilus influenzae*. As the exudate accumulates, pressure builds up inside the sinus cavity, causing severe pain at the site. The pain may be confused with headache (ethmoid sinus) or toothache (maxillary sinus). Other signs, such as nasal congestion, fever, or sore throat may already be present. Decongestants and analgesics are recommended until the sinuses are draining well, and a course of antibiotics is often required to eradicate the infection totally.

LARYNGOTRACHEOBRONCHITIS (CROUP)

Laryngotracheobronchitis is a common viral infection, particularly in children between 1 and 2 years old, although adults may also have laryngitis, tracheitis, or bronchitis. Common causative organisms are parainfluenza viruses and adenoviruses (Table 17–2). The infection begins as an upper respiratory condition with nasal congestion and cough. In the young child, the larynx and subglottic area become inflamed with swelling and exudate, leading to obstruction and a characteristic barking cough (croup), hoarse voice, and inspiratory stridor. The condition often becomes more severe at night. Cool, moisturized air from a humidifier or shower or croup tent often relieves the obstruction. The infection is usually self-limited, and full recovery occurs in several days. In some children with allergic tenden-

cies, smooth muscle spasm may exacerbate the obstruction, requiring additional medical treatment.

EPIGLOTTITIS

Epiglottitis is an acute infection usually caused by a bacterial organism, *H. influenzae* type B. It is common in children in the 3- to 7-year-old group, although the incidence has been increasing in adults. The infection causes swelling of the larynx, supraglottic area, and epiglottis, which appears as a round, red ball obstructing the airway. Onset is rapid, fever and sore throat develop, and the child refuses to swallow. Drooling of saliva is apparent, and inspiratory stridor is heard. The child appears anxious and pale and assumes a sitting position (tripod position) with the mouth open, struggling to breathe. Caution is required during laryngeal examination to prevent total obstruction of the airway. Treatment consists of oxygen and antibiotic therapy, with intubation or tracheotomy if necessary.

INFLUENZA (FLU)

Influenza is a viral infection that may affect both the upper and the lower respiratory tracts. Although the influenza infection itself may be mild, it is frequently complicated by secondary problems such as pneumonia. The mortality rate from complications can be high, particularly in those older than 65 years and in those with chronic cardiovascular or respiratory disease. Influenza may occur sporadically, in epidemics or pandemics, usually during colder weather. It is transmitted directly by respiratory droplet or indirectly by contact with a contaminated object. The influenza virus is difficult to control because it undergoes constant antigenic changes. This limits the ability of individuals to develop long-term immunity to the virus and requires the preparation of new vaccines annually to match the predicted new strains of the virus for the coming year. The constituents of each vaccine, often three in number, are specifically designated each year. For example, one antigen might be called A/Texas/36/91, which indicates the type, geographic origin, strain number, and year of isolation for a particular viral strain.

The influenza viruses are classified as RNA viruses of the myxovirus type. There are three groups of the influenza virus—type A, the most prevalent pathogen, and types B and C. They all essentially affect the respiratory mucosa in the same way, causing **necrosis** and inflammation of the tissue and shedding of the virus into the secretions. The widespread necrosis of the respiratory mucosa typical of influenza leaves the area vulnerable to secondary infection by bacteria, which are often resident flora of the upper tract. The infection may be limited to the upper respiratory area, nasal passages, pharynx, and trachea, or it may cause a viral pneumonia in the lungs. Influenza usually has a sudden, acute onset with fever and chills, marked malaise, headache, general muscle aching, sore throat, unproductive cough, and nasal congestion. The infection is often self-limiting, although fatigue may persist for several weeks afterward. Continued fever or other signs usually indicate complications, such as the development of bacterial pneumonia.

Treatment is symptomatic and supportive unless bacterial infection occurs. An antiviral drug, amantadine, may reduce the symptoms in some cases. Annual administration of the vaccine in the fall is recommended for those with chronic disease, those older than 65 years of age, those living in institutions, and health care workers.

Thinkabout 17–6

a. Compare the signs of the common cold, sinusitis, and epiglottitis.

b. Explain why secondary bacterial infections commonly follow viral infections in the respiratory tract.

c. Explain why frequent handwashing may reduce the transmission of influenza.

d. Explain why antibacterial drugs are not effective against virus infections (see Chapter 4).

Lower Respiratory Tract Infections

BRONCHIOLITIS (RSV INFECTION)

Bronchiolitis is a common infection in young children 2 to 12 months of age and is caused by the respiratory syncytial virus (RSV), a myxovirus. It is transmitted directly by oral droplet and occurs more frequently in the winter months. Predisposing factors in-

clude a familial history of asthma and the presence of cigarette smoke. Bronchiolitis varies in severity. The virus causes necrosis and inflammation in the bronchioles, with edema, increased secretions, and reflex bronchospasm leading to obstruction of the small airways. Signs include wheezing and dyspnea; rapid, shallow respirations; cough; rales; chest retractions; fever; and malaise. There may be areas of hyperinflation with air trapping due to partial obstruction (see Fig. 17–12C) or areas of atelectasis or nonaeration resulting from total obstruction (see Fig. 17–17). Treatment is supportive and symptomatic, with monitoring of blood gases in severe cases to ensure that oxygen levels are adequate.

PNEUMONIA

Pneumonia may develop as a primary acute infection in the lungs, or it may be secondary to another respiratory or systemic condition in which tissue resistance is reduced. Pneumonia is a risk following any aspiration or inflammation in the lung, when fluids pool or defense mechanisms such as cilia are reduced. In most cases the organisms enter the lungs directly by inhalation (virus) or by resident bacteria spreading along the mucosa or aspirated in secretions. Occasionally the infection is bloodborne.

Pneumonia may be classified by causative agent or by anatomic location of the infection. For example, the agent may produce viral pneumonia or bacterial pneumonia or may originate as aspiration or lipoid pneumonia. Anatomic distribution of lesions may be diffuse (patchy) or lobar (confined to one lobe). Usually lobar pneumonia is bacterial, the most common agent being a pneumococcus, but other causative organisms include *Staphylococcus aureus* and *Legionella* (Legionnaire's disease). Severe pneumococcal pneumonia is less common now because antibacterial medications are quickly administered, but it remains a major threat to those with chronic disease. In immune-suppressed individuals, other organisms such as *Candida* (fungus) or *Pneumocystis carinii* may cause pneumonia. *Nosocomial* (hospital-acquired) pneumonia often results from gram-negative organisms such as *Klebsiella pneumoniae* or *Pseudomonas aeruginosa*.

Lobar Pneumonia

Lobar pneumonia is caused by *Streptococcus pneumoniae* (pneumococcus), and the infection is localized in one or more lobes (Fig. 17–5). The first stage in its development is *congestion*, in which inflammation and vascular congestion develop in the alveolar wall, and exudate forms in the alveoli. This change interferes greatly with oxygen diffusion. Next, neutrophils, RBCs, and fibrin accumulate in the alveolar exudate, forming

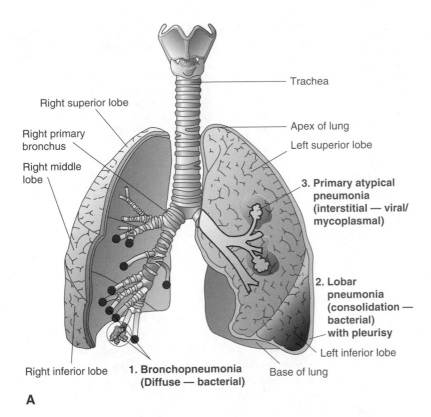

Trachea

Right superior lobe

Right primary bronchus

Right middle lobe

Apex of lung

Left superior lobe

3. Primary atypical pneumonia (interstitial — viral/ mycoplasmal)

2. Lobar pneumonia (consolidation — bacterial) with pleurisy

Left inferior lobe

Right inferior lobe

1. Bronchopneumonia (Diffuse — bacterial)

Base of lung

A

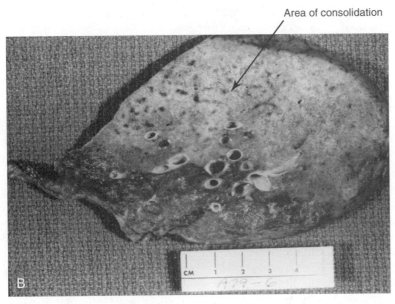

Area of consolidation

B

FIGURE 17–5. *A*, Types of pneumonia. *B*, Lobar pneumonia showing acute pneumococcal consolidation in area of left lung. (Courtesy of R.W. Shaw, M.D., North York General Hospital, Toronto, Ontario.)

a solid mass in the lobe, called *consolidation*. The presence of these erythrocytes in the exudate produces the typical rusty sputum associated with lobar pneumonia. Eventually, the RBCs break down, and as the infection resolves, macrophages break down the exudate to allow it to be expectorated or resorbed. Because a complete lobe is usually involved in the inflammatory process, the adjacent pleurae are frequently involved, producing pleuritic pain at the affected site. Chest radiographs confirm the typical distribution of the infection, and a sputum culture confirms the identity of the organism.

The filling of the alveoli with exudate reduces the diffusion of gases, particularly oxygen, and decreases blood flow through the affected lobe. Hypoxia results and is more marked because the demand for oxygen increases with the higher metabolic rate associated with the infection. The oxygen deficit also leads to metabolic acidosis. Dehydration may result from the high fever, hyperventilation, and inadequate fluid intake.

	Lobar Pneumonia	**Bronchopneumonia**	**Interstitial Pneumonia (Primary Atypical Pneumonia, PAP)**
Distribution	All of one or two lobes	Scattered small patches	Scattered small patches
Cause	*Streptococcus pneumoniae*	Multiple bacteria	Influenza virus *Mycoplasma*
Pathophysiology	Inflammation of alveolar wall and leakage of cells, fibrin, and fluid into alveoli causing consolidation Pleura may be inflamed	Inflammation and purulent exudate in alveoli often arising from prior pooled secretions or irritation	Interstitial inflammation around alveoli Necrosis of bronchial epithelium
Onset	Sudden and acute	Insidious	Variable
Signs	High fever and chills Rales progressing to no breath sounds in affected lobes Productive cough with rusty sputum	Mild fever Productive cough with yellow-green sputum Dyspnea	Variable fever, headache Aching muscles Nonproductive hacking cough

TABLE 17–3 Types of Pneumonia

Pneumococcal pneumonia is characterized by its sudden onset, with dyspnea, high fever, and chills. Pleuritic pain is indicated by splinting or restriction of respiratory expansion on the affected side. Initially, rales can be heard over the affected lobe, and then the breath sounds disappear as consolidation occurs. A productive cough develops with the typical rusty-colored sputum. Systemic responses such as leukocytosis are present. In severe cases, in which several lobes are involved, the patient may become quite lethargic and confused or disoriented. Treatment involves the administration of antibacterials such as penicillin in combination with supportive measures.

Bronchopneumonia

Bronchopneumonia occurs as a diffuse pattern of infection in both lungs, but it occurs often more in the lower lobes. One or several species of microorganisms may cause the infection. In many cases, pooled secretions in the lungs become infected by organisms draining from the upper passages, particularly in immobilized patients (hypostatic pneumonia). The inflammatory exudate forms in the alveoli, interfering with oxygen diffusion. Onset tends to be insidious, with moderate fever, cough, and rales. Congestion causes a productive cough with purulent sputum, usually yellow or green in color. Sputum culture and sensitivity tests indicate the appropriate choice of antibacterial treatment. Recovery usually occurs without residual lung damage.

Primary Atypical Pneumonia

Primary atypical pneumonia differs in both the causative organisms and the pathophysiology, which involves interstitial inflammation. Mycoplasma pneumonia is common in children and young adults. Viral pneumonia, also common, is often caused by influenza A or B, but other viruses are also found. The infection frequently begins with inflammation in the mucosa of the upper respiratory tract and then descends to involve the lungs. These organisms produce inflammation that is diffuse and interstitial, with little exudate forming in the alveoli. Therefore, cough is unproductive, and rales are not pronounced. A radiograph may show some poorly defined patches of congestion. The infection varies greatly in severity from mild cases that may not even be diagnosed to severe cases that may be complicated by secondary bacterial infection. The onset of primary atypical pneumonia is often vague, with nonproductive cough and sore throat, mild fever, and malaise. The infection is usually self-limiting. A brief comparison of the different types of pneumonia is found in Table 17–3.

TUBERCULOSIS

Pathophysiology

Tuberculosis (TB) is an infection that is usually caused by *Mycobacterium tuberculosis* and affects primarily the lungs, but the pathogen may invade other organs as well. There are two stages in the pathogenesis of tuberculosis—primary infection and secondary or reinfection (Fig. 17–6). Initially, the microorganisms enter the lungs, causing a local inflammatory reaction, usually on the periphery of the upper lobe. Some bacilli migrate to the lymph nodes, activating a type IV or cell-mediated hypersensitivity response (see Chapter 3). This *hypersensitivity* reaction apparently stimulates granuloma formation at the site of inflammation. The granuloma involves migration of macrophages and lymphocytes to the site, which wall off the bacilli, forming a *tubercle*. In the center of the tubercle, **caseation** necrosis, a core of cheese-like material, occurs. These lesions are very tiny and with time may become fibrotic or calcify. However, the bacilli may remain viable in a dormant state inside the tubercle for years. If calcified, the tubercle may be visible on a chest radiograph. As long as the individual's resistance and immune responses remain high, the bacilli remain walled off within the tubercle. The individual has been exposed to the bacillus and infected but does *not* have active disease. This is considered primary infection.

The hypersensitivity reaction initiated by *M. tuberculosis* is the basis for the tuberculin test (e.g., Mantoux test), which is used to detect exposure to the bacillus. Several weeks after exposure, the person has become hypersensitive and will produce a positive skin reaction (a large area of induration [a hard raised red area]) in response to administration of tuberculoprotein. A chest radiograph will determine whether active infection is present.

In people with low resistance, the primary infection may not be controlled but instead progresses to active infection, spreading through the lungs and to other organs, similar to secondary or reinfectious tuberculosis. Miliary tuberculosis is a rapidly progressive form that affects large areas of the lungs and rapidly disseminates into the circulation and other tissues such as bone or kidney.

Secondary tuberculosis is the active form of the disease. It often arises years later when the bacilli in the tubercles are reactivated, usually because of decreased host resistance. *Cavitation* or liquefaction necrosis occurs, with destruction of lung tissue and erosion into the bronchi and blood vessels (Fig. 17–7). Cavitation promotes spread of the organisms into other parts of the lung, and bacilli are present in the sputum, where they may be passed to others. Hemoptysis is common as blood vessels are eroded.

Etiology

M. tuberculosis is transmitted by oral droplets released from a person with active infection that are inhaled into the lungs. In some countries where milk is not pasteurized, tuberculosis may be caused by *Mycobacterium bovis*. *Mycobacterium* is an acid-fast, aerobic, slow-growing bacillus that is somewhat resistant to drying and to many disinfectants. Tuberculosis occurs more frequently in persons living in crowded conditions or in those whose resistance is lowered because of malnutrition, alcoholism, or chronic disease. There is probably a genetic susceptibility, and children are easily infected. Tuberculosis was declining in response to improved drug therapy until the 1980s, but since then the incidence has risen because of increased travel and immigration, the prevalence of the infection in patients with acquired immune deficiency syndrome (AIDS), and the development of drug-resistant strains of the organism.

Signs and Symptoms

Primary tuberculosis is asymptomatic. The onset of secondary or active tuberculosis is insidious. Systemic

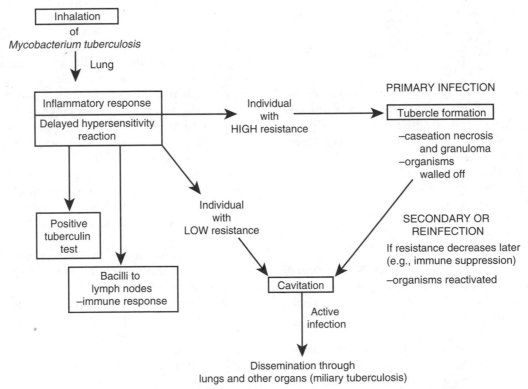

FIGURE 17–6. Development of tuberculosis.

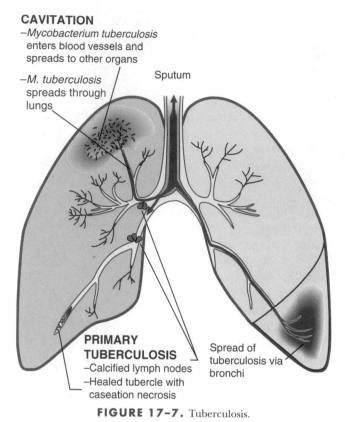

CAVITATION
–*Mycobacterium tuberculosis* enters blood vessels and spreads to other organs

–*M. tuberculosis* spreads through lungs

Sputum

PRIMARY TUBERCULOSIS
–Calcified lymph nodes
–Healed tubercle with caseation necrosis

Spread of tuberculosis via bronchi

FIGURE 17–7. Tuberculosis.

signs often appear first, with vague manifestations such as anorexia, malaise, fatigue, and weight loss. Afternoon low-grade fever and night sweats develop. Cough becomes increasingly severe and, as cavitation develops, more productive. Sputum becomes purulent and often contains blood.

Diagnosis

First exposure or primary infection is indicated by a positive tuberculin test result. This test is of no value (that is, it produces a false-positive result) if the person has previously received the bacillus Calmette-Guérin (BCG) vaccine for tuberculosis. Active infection can be confirmed by chest radiograph and sputum culture. New techniques involving the use of bacterial DNA provide faster confirmation.

Treatment

A person with active tuberculosis is now usually treated at home or in a general hospital. Long-term treatment with a combination of drugs is recommended. The length of treatment varies from 3 months to a year or longer depending on the situation. Drugs of choice include isoniazid (INH), rifampin, ethambutol, pyrazinamide, and streptomycin. Sputum culture usually is negative for tuberculosis organisms after 1 to 2 months of treatment, and the risk of transmission be-

comes much less. Patient compliance with the drug regimen is important in totally eradicating the infection and preventing the development of drug-resistant microbes. It is recommended that contacts of the patient be given prophylactic isoniazid for a year and receive tuberculin testing as well.

Thinkabout 17–7

a. Compare the causative organism and two significant signs of lobar pneumonia with those of bronchopneumonia.

b. What factors predispose to bronchopneumonia in immobilized persons?

c. Describe and explain the significance of a tubercle and cavitation in individuals with tuberculosis.

d. Describe several specific precautions that could be taken by affected individuals or by health professionals that would limit the spread of *M. tuberculosis*.

OBSTRUCTIVE LUNG DISEASES

Cystic Fibrosis

PATHOPHYSIOLOGY

Cystic fibrosis (CF), sometimes called mucoviscidosis, is a common genetic disorder. A defect in the exocrine glands causes abnormal secretions, such as thick, tenacious mucus. The basic cause of the altered secretions is related to a defect in chloride ion transport in the glands. The primary effects of cystic fibrosis are seen in the lungs and the pancreas, where the sticky mucus obstructs the passages; other tissues are affected less frequently (Fig. 17–8). The severity of the effects varies among individuals. In the *lungs*, the mucus obstructs air flow in the bronchioles and small bronchi, causing air trapping or atelectasis with permanent damage to the bronchial walls. Because stagnant mucus is an excellent medium for bacterial growth, infections are common and add to the progressive destruction of lung tissue. Organisms commonly causing infection in patients with cystic fibrosis include *P. aeruginosa* and *S. aureus*. Bronchiectasis and emphysematous changes are seen frequently as fibrosis and obstructions advance. Eventually, respiratory failure or cor pulmonale (right-sided congestive heart failure) develops. With improved treatment, the life span of many children with cystic fibrosis has been extended into adulthood.

Usually several areas in the body are affected in an individual. In the digestive tract, the first indication of abnormality may be *meconium ileus,* in which the small intestine of the neonate is blocked by mucus at birth, preventing the excretion of meconium shortly after birth. In the *pancreas,* the ducts of the exocrine glands become blocked, leading to a deficit of pancreatic digestive enzymes in the intestine. Malabsorption and malnutrition result. Also, the obstruction and backup of secretions eventually cause damage to the pancreatic tissue, including the islets of Langerhans, resulting in diabetes mellitus in some individuals. The *bile ducts* of the liver may be blocked by viscid mucus, preventing bile from reaching the duodenum and interfering with digestion and absorption of fats and fat-soluble vitamins. Ultimately, this abnormality also contributes to the general state of malabsorption, malnutrition, and

dehydration. If obstruction is severe, the backup of bile behind the obstruction may cause inflammation and permanent damage to the liver in the form of biliary cirrhosis.

The *salivary glands* are often mildly affected, with secretions that are abnormally high in sodium chloride and mucus plugs that cause patchy fibrosis of the submaxillary and sublingual glands. The *sweat glands* are also affected, producing sweat that is very high in sodium chloride content. This is usually not a serious problem unless hot weather or strenuous exercise lead to excessive loss of electrolytes in the sweat. The *reproductive system* may be affected, with thick mucus obstructing the vas deferens in males or the cervix in females, leading to sterility or infertility. In some males the testes and ducts do not develop normally.

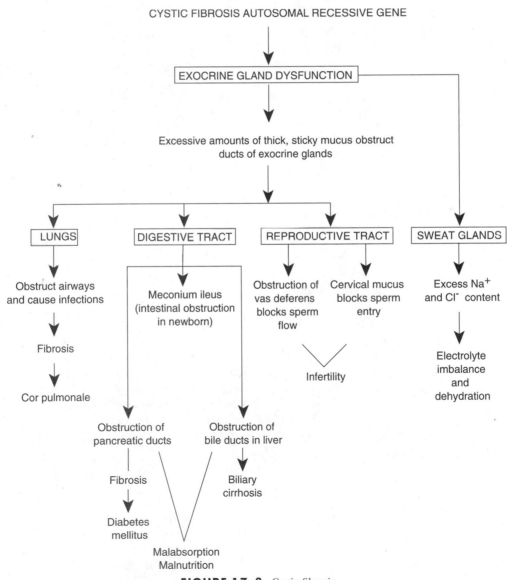

FIGURE 17–8. Cystic fibrosis.

ETIOLOGY

The gene for cystic fibrosis is located on the seventh chromosome, and the disease is transmitted as an autosomal recessive disorder (see Chapter 7). It is much more common in whites. When a family history of cystic fibrosis warrants testing, the defect can be diagnosed prenatally and in carriers with reliable results.

SIGNS AND SYMPTOMS

Signs such as meconium ileus may appear at birth or when a mother of a newborn with cystic fibrosis tastes salty skin when kissing the child. This may lead to a *sweat test* and the diagnosis of cystic fibrosis. In some cases, the diagnosis may be delayed a few months or several years. The signs of malabsorption may become apparent during the first year of life, with **steatorrhea** (bulky, fatty, foul stools), abdominal distention, and failure to gain weight. These signs indicate a lack of the pancreatic enzymes and bile needed to digest food and absorb nutrients. Fats and the fat-soluble vitamins (vitamins A, D, E, and K) are affected initially, but in turn protein and carbohydrate deficits develop. Pulmonary involvement results in chronic cough and frequent respiratory infections in the child. As lung damage proceeds, hypoxia, fatigue, and exercise intolerance develop. The chest may be overinflated owing to air trapping, and rhonchi are audible. The child may not meet the normal growth milestones, usually because of chronic respiratory problems.

DIAGNOSTIC TESTS

Sweat is analyzed for abnormal electrolyte content. Stools may be checked for fat content and trypsin content (pancreatic enzyme). Lung involvement can be assessed with radiographs, pulmonary function tests, and blood gas analysis.

TREATMENT

Treatment of a child with cystic fibrosis requires a team or interdisciplinary approach because there is multisystemic involvement with numerous complications and implications for the child's growth and development. Replacement therapy for pancreatic enzymes, for example, pancrelipase (Cotazym), and, if necessary, bile salt replacement can be administered with meals and snacks to improve digestion and absorption and promote general health and resistance to infection. A well-balanced diet, with high protein, low fat, and vitamin supplements, is recommended, but the suggested total dietary intake is much greater than is usually recommended to allow for some malabsorption. It is important to avoid dehydration resulting from excessive losses in the sweat or stool because a fluid deficit may result in thicker and more tenacious respiratory mucus. Intensive chest physiotherapy, including postural drainage, percussion, and coughing techniques, is a time-consuming but necessary daily exercise to ensure removal of the tenacious mucus. The use of bronchodilators and humidifiers also promotes drainage. Regular moderate aerobic exercise is helpful in removing secretions and promoting general health. Immediate aggressive treatment is required for infections and has extended the life span of patients. In patients with advanced lung disease, oxygen therapy as well as medication for congestive heart failure may be required (see Chapter 16). Heart-lung transplants have been performed in some individuals with cystic fibrosis (see Chapter 3).

Thinkabout 17–8

a. Describe how cystic fibrosis affects the lungs and the sweat glands.

b. Describe the potential complications of cystic fibrosis in the lungs and the pancreas.

c. Explain the probability of cystic fibrosis occurring in a child when one parent is a carrier.

Lung Cancer

The lungs are a common site of both secondary and primary lung cancer. Metastases develop in the lungs because the venous return and lymphatics bring tumor cells from many distant sites in the body to the heart and then into the pulmonary circulation, which provides the first small blood vessels and hospitable environment in which tumor cells can lodge (see Fig. 5–3 in Chapter 5). Primary lung cancer is a major cause of death, and much attention has been focused on it as the relationship between cigarette smoking and lung cancer has been documented. Also, the prognosis for lung cancer remains poor. Benign lung tumors are rare.

PATHOPHYSIOLOGY

Bronchogenic carcinoma, arising from the bronchial epithelium, is the most common type of malignant lung tumor. There are a number of subgroups. Squamous cell carcinoma usually develops from the epithelial lining of a bronchus near the hilum and projects into the airway (see Fig. 5–1). Sometimes tumors are preceded by dysplasia, metaplasia, or carcinoma in situ. Adenocarcinomas (from glands) and bronchioalveolar cell carcinomas are usually found on the periphery of the lung, making them less symptomatic and more difficult to detect in the early stages (Fig. 17–9A). The cells of adenocarcinomas may secrete mucin. Small-cell or "oat-cell" carcinomas are a rapidly growing type of lung cancer often located near a major bronchus in the central part of the lung. They tend to be invasive and metastasize very early in their development. This type of tumor cell frequently secretes hormones or hormone-like substances such as antidiuretic hormone (ADH) or adrenocorticotropic hormone (ACTH). The endocrine effects may complicate both diagnosis and treatment. Large-cell carcinomas are usually found in the periphery and consist of undifferentiated large cells that have a rapid growth rate and metastasize early. Lung cancer is staged at the time of diagnosis based on the tumor-node-metastases (TNM) classification (see Chapter 5). Stage I tumors are localized, whereas stage III lesions are disseminated. Common sites of metastases from the lungs include the brain, bone, and liver.

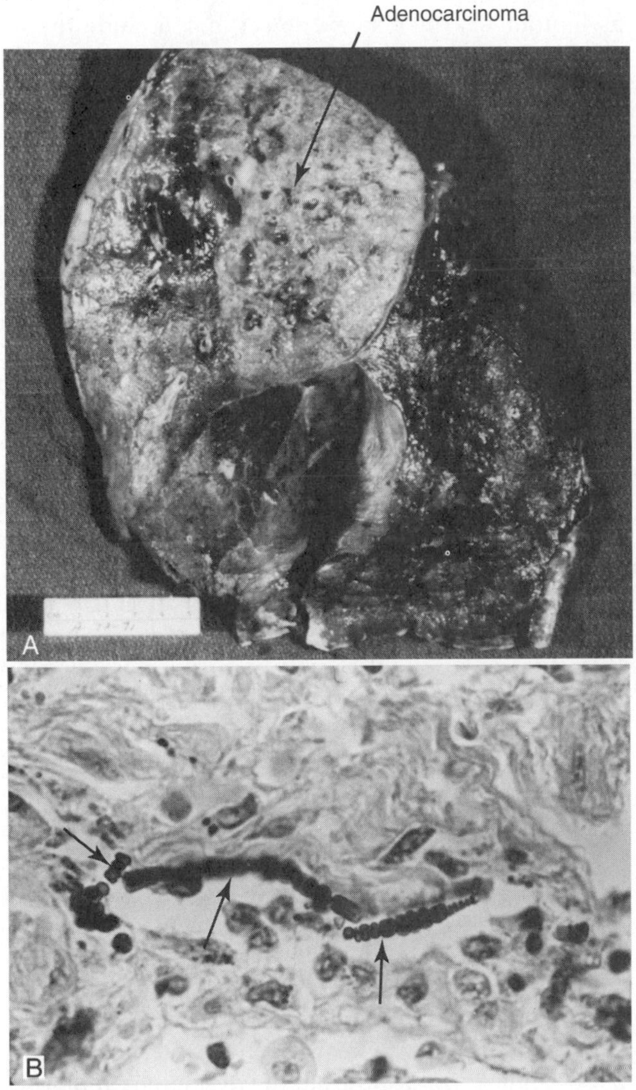

Tumors in the lungs have many effects. Malignant tumors that grow into a bronchus obstruct air flow, causing abnormal breath sounds and dyspnea. Surrounding the tumor is an area of inflammation that frequently stimulates a cough. Frequent infections may occur because secretions pool distal to the tumor. A mass located on the lung periphery may cause pleural effusion associated with the inflammation or a pneumothorax if it erodes the pleural membrane. Paraneoplastic syndrome may accompany bronchogenic carcinoma. This syndrome may include ectopic secretion of hormones or hormonelike substances, neuromuscular disturbances, or hematologic disorders such as disseminated intravascular coagulation (DIC) (see Chapter 16).

ETIOLOGY

The incidence of lung cancer continues to rise and is now very high in women as well as men. Cigarette smoking is the major factor in its development. "Second-hand smoke" in the environment has been implicated in a significant number of cases. The risk of developing cancer is higher in persons who begin smoking early, persist for many years, and are considered heavy smokers (i.e., they smoke more than a pack per day). Not all smokers develop lung cancer, and therefore there is probably a genetic factor involved that also influences the cellular changes (see Chapter 5). Occupational or industrial exposure to carcinogens such as silica, vinyl chloride, or asbestos (see Fig. 17–9B) is the other major cause of lung cancer, and the risk is greatly increased if a second factor such as cigarette smoking is also present in an occupationally exposed individual. In addition to the direct carcinogenic effect, any irritant such as smoke leads to chronic inflammation and frequent infections in the respiratory tract, which in turn cause cellular changes, for example, in the mucosa, where there is a change from ciliated columnar epithelium to squamous cell epithelium. The alterations in the respiratory mucosa as it changes through metaplasia to dysplasia demonstrate the cell mutations caused by carcinogens and could perhaps lead to earlier diagnosis.

SIGNS AND SYMPTOMS

There are four possible categories of signs of lung cancer: (1) those related to the direct effects of the tumor on the respiratory structures, (2) those resulting from metastatic tumors at other sites, (3) those representing the systemic effects of cancer, and (4) those

FIGURE 17–9. *A,* Cut surface of lung showing papillary adenocarcinoma. *B,* Photomicrograph of lung showing asbestos bodies. (Courtesy of R.W. Shaw, M.D., North York General Hospital, Toronto, Ontario.)

caused by associated paraneoplastic syndromes. The onset of lung cancer is insidious because the early signs of cancer are often masked by signs of the predisposing factor, such as a "smoker's cough." In many cases, the cancer has already metastasized before diagnosis, and the signs of a metastatic tumor lead to diagnosis. Early signs related to respiratory involvement include persistent productive cough, dyspnea, and wheezing. In some cases, tumors are detected on chest radiographs taken when an individual develops pneumonia or other complication. Large tumors or involved lymph nodes may cause hoarseness (laryngeal nerve compression), facial or arm edema and headache (compression of the superior vena cava), dysphagia (compression of the esophagus), or atelectasis. Infiltrating tumors may cause hemoptysis, pleural effusion, or pneumothorax. Chest pain occurs with advanced tumors that involve the pleura or mediastinum. Systemic signs of lung cancer include weight loss, anemia, and fatigue. Paraneoplastic syndrome is indicated by the signs of an endocrine disorder such as Cushing's syndrome due to excessive ACTH secretion or signs of a neurologic problem.

DIAGNOSTIC TESTS

Chest radiographs demonstrate the lesion and complications such as atelectasis or pleural effusion. Bronchoscopy provides secretions containing malignant cells from central lesions for definitive diagnosis, and biopsy may be required for less accessible lesions. Pulmonary function tests can clarify the effects of the tumor on air flow.

TREATMENT

Surgical resection may be performed on localized lesions. Chemotherapy and radiation are used in conjunction with surgery or as palliative treatment, although many tumors are not responsive to such therapy. The prognosis is poor unless the tumor is in an early stage of development.

Aspiration

Aspiration involves the passage of food or fluid, vomitus, drugs, or other foreign material into the trachea and lungs. The right lower lung is often the destination of aspirated material because the right branching bronchus tends to continue almost straight down, whereas the bronchus in the left lung branches at a sharper angle. Normally, a cough removes such material from the upper tract, and the vocal cords and epiglottis prevent entry into the lower tract. The characteristics of the aspirate determine the specific effects on respiratory function. For example, vomitus may contain solid objects as well as highly acidic gastric secretions, lipids, or alcohol. The common result is obstruction whether the aspirate is an irritating liquid causing inflammation or a solid object causing direct obstruction.

Aspiration is a common problem in young children but may also occur in individuals when the swallowing or gag reflex is depressed for any reason, for example, following anesthesia or stroke or in patients with coma or neurologic damage. Individuals who eat or drink or perhaps take medications when lying down also risk aspiration because the gravitational force is of no value in moving food quickly and completely down the esophagus. Residual liquid often remains in the mouth and oropharynx, to drip at a later time into the trachea.

PATHOPHYSIOLOGY

Solid objects lodge in a passageway and totally obstruct air flow at that point. A small obstruction may be asymptomatic, but a large object may occlude the trachea and block all air flow, a life-threatening situation. In such cases, no sound can be made to alert others to the problem, and consciousness is lost very quickly as oxygen supplies are depleted. Solid objects lodging in a bronchus lead to nonaeration and collapse of the area distal to the obstacle (see Fig. 17–17C). Sometimes such objects create a ball-valve effect, in which air is able to pass down the tract on inspiration, but the passageway totally closes on expiration, leading to a buildup of air distal to the obstruction. Some foods such as dried beans may swell after aspiration and become more firmly lodged. Sharp pointed objects, such as bone fragments, also lodge in a passageway. Although not totally occluding the airway by itself, such an object traumatizes the mucosa, causing an acute inflammatory response that adds to the barrier. The inflammatory response may stimulate bronchoconstriction. Also, an object that straddles the airway will collect any other material entering the area, increasing the obstruction. Fatty or irritating solids such as peanuts also cause inflammation around the area, creating edema and further impeding air flow. If not removed, a granuloma or fibrous tissue develops around such material (Fig. 17–10). Irritating liquids, particularly acids (vomitus), alcohol, or oils (milk), tend to disperse into several bronchi. These materials cause severe inflammation, leading to narrow airways, and increased secretions, which make the lungs more difficult to expand. In some cases, the alveoli are involved in the inflammation, and gas diffusion is impaired. Respiratory distress syndrome may develop if inflammation is widespread. This type of inflammation may be called chemical or aspiration pneumonia; it predisposes to the development of infection later. Certain materials such as solvents, if aspirated in large amounts, may be absorbed into the blood and cause systemic effects.

Meat

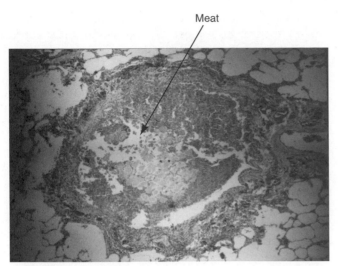

FIGURE 17-10. Photomicrograph of granuloma in the lung resulting from aspiration of meat in a patient with multiple sclerosis. (Courtesy of R.W. Shaw, M.D., North York General Hospital, Toronto, Ontario.)

ETIOLOGY

Aspiration can occur under many different circumstances. Young children are most prone to aspiration of solid objects. Smooth round objects are most dangerous. Common examples are chunks of hot dogs, candy, nuts, grapes, and raw carrots. Buttons or coins and balloons are frequent nonfood examples. Inhalation of substances such as baby powder can also cause inflammation in the delicate lung tissue. Children may aspirate toxic fluids such as cleaning materials or lighter fluid. Some fluids such as those containing hydrocarbons, for example, turpentine, have a low viscosity and a low surface tension and therefore tend to spread in a very thin film over a large area of the lung, causing extensive irritation and damage. Adults may aspirate food or fluid, especially when combining eating with talking at social events, particularly if the food is not well chewed and alcohol intake has depressed protective reflexes. Vomitus is frequently aspirated following a high alcohol intake or postoperatively from the effects of anesthetics or drugs. Normally a patient is not allowed to eat or drink preoperatively to reduce the risk of aspiration. Children with congenital anomalies such as a cleft palate or tracheoesophageal fistula are especially at risk for aspiration (see Chapter 18).

SIGNS AND SYMPTOMS

Coughing and choking with marked dyspnea are common. Stridor and hoarseness are characteristic of upper airway obstruction, and wheezing is common with aspiration of liquids into the lungs. Tachycardia and tachypnea are common. Nasal flaring, chest retractions, and marked hypoxia occur in individuals with severe respiratory distress. As mentioned earlier, total obstruction at the larynx or trachea prevents any sounds or cough from being produced. Cardiac arrest quickly ensues.

TREATMENT

Aspiration is frequently easier to prevent than to treat. In cases of severe obstruction by solid material, back blows or the Heimlich maneuver (an upward thrust of a fist into the abdomen) often can dislodge and eject the object. Sometimes an individual can use a finger probe successfully to access an object at the back of the tongue. Instrumentation may be necessary in some cases to remove the offending object. In case of total obstruction, an emergency tracheotomy is necessary. In patients with widespread inflammation, oxygen and supportive therapy may be required as well as prophylactic antibiotics.

Thinkabout 17–9

a. Describe the incidence of lung cancer.
b. Explain why (1) wheezing, (2) hemoptysis, and (3) pleural effusion may occur in patients with lung cancer.
c. Explain the result of aspirating a large object and why the problem may be difficult to identify.

Asthma

Asthma is a disease that involves periodic episodes of severe but reversible bronchial obstruction in persons with hyperresponsive airways. Frequent repeated attacks of acute asthma may lead to irreversible damage in the lungs and the development of chronic asthma (chronic obstructive lung disease). There are two basic types of asthma. The first is often called *extrinsic* asthma and involves acute episodes triggered by a type 1 hypersensitivity reaction to an inhaled antigen (see Chapter 3). Frequently, there is a familial history of other allergic conditions such as allergic rhinitis (hay fever) or eczema, and onset commonly occurs in children and young adults. The second type of asthma is *intrinsic* asthma. In this disease other types of stimuli initiate the acute attack. These stimuli include respiratory infections, exposure to cold, exercise, drugs such as aspirin, stress, and inhalation of irritants such as cigarette smoke. Many patients have a combination of the two types.

PATHOPHYSIOLOGY

The bronchi and bronchioles are excessively responsive to stimuli, leading to contraction of smooth muscle (bronchoconstriction), inflammation with edema, and increased secretion of thick mucus in the passages (Fig. 17–11). These changes obstruct the airways, partially or totally, and interfere with air flow and oxygen supply. In patients with extrinsic asthma, the antigen reacts with IgE on the sensitized mast cells in the respiratory mucosa, releasing histamine, leukotrienes, prostaglandins, and other chemical mediators, which then cause bronchospasm, edema, and increased mucus secretion. The reaction also stimulates branches of the vagus nerve, causing reflex bronchoconstriction. In the second stage of the allergic response, which occurs a few hours later, the increased leukocytes, particularly eosinophils, release additional chemical mediators and also cause epithelial cell damage. The precise mechanism whereby a similar response occurs in patients with intrinsic asthma has not been determined. The tissues are hyperresponsive, and an imbalance in autonomic innervation to the tissues is a suspected factor.

Partial obstruction of the small bronchi and bronchioles results in *air trapping* with hyperinflation of the lungs (Fig. 17–12*C*). Air passes into the areas distal to the obstruction and alveoli but is only partially expired. Because expiration is a passive process, less force is available to move air out, and forced expiration often collapses the bronchial wall, creating a further barrier to expiratory air flow. Residual volume increases. As a result, it becomes more difficult to inspire fresh air or to cough effectively to remove the mucus. To understand hyperinflation of the lungs, take several breaths but exhale only partially after each inspiration. Consider how your lungs feel and the position of your ribs. Can you take a deep breath? Can you cough?

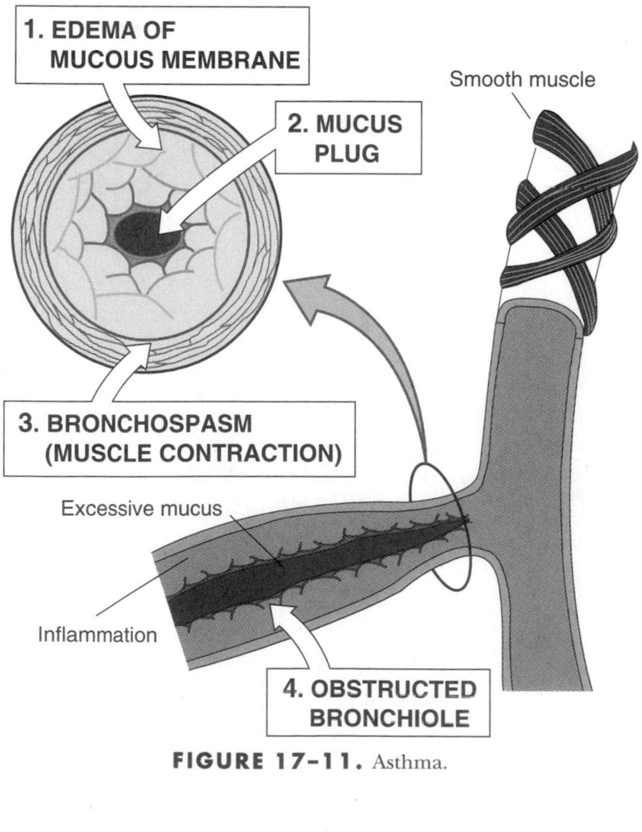

Total obstruction of the airway results when mucus plugs completely block the flow of air in the already narrowed passage. This leads to atelectasis or nonaeration of the tissue distal to the obstruction (see Fig. 17–17*C*). The air in the distal section diffuses out and is not replaced, resulting in collapse of that section of the lung. Both partial and total obstruction lead to marked hypoxia. Oxygen levels are further depleted by the increased demand for oxygen to supply increased muscle activity and by the stress response as the individual fights for air. Both respiratory and metabolic acidosis result from severe respiratory impairment. Hypoxemia causes vasoconstriction in the pulmonary blood vessels, reducing blood flow through the lungs and increasing the work load of the right side of the heart.

Status asthmaticus is a persistent severe attack of asthma that does not respond to therapy. It is often related to inadequate medical treatment. It may be fatal owing to severe hypoxia and acidosis leading to cardiac arrhythmias or central nervous system depression.

With repeated acute asthmatic attacks, irreversible damage takes place in the lungs. The bronchial walls become thickened, and fibrous tissue resulting from the frequent infections that follow attacks develops in atelectatic areas. Because it is impossible to remove all the tiny mucus plugs in the small passages, complications are common following frequent episodes of asthma.

SIGNS AND SYMPTOMS

Cough, marked dyspnea, a tight feeling in the chest, and agitation develop as airway obstruction increases. Wheezing is characteristic as air passes through the narrowed bronchioles. Thick and tenacious or sticky mucus is coughed up. Breathing is rapid and labored, and the use of accessory muscles and chest retractions is apparent. Tachycardia occurs and perhaps **pulsus paradoxus** when the pulse differs on inspiration and expiration. Paradoxical pulse is observed when a blood pressure measurement is taken during an asthma attack. The sounds registering systolic pressure are heard first during expiration, and there is a gap of 10 mm Hg or more before the sounds of both inspiration and expiration are heard. Initially, hyperventilation occurs, leading to respiratory alkalosis, but in time marked fatigue causes decreased respiratory effort and a weaker cough. Severe respiratory distress is evident. Hypoventilation leads to increasing hypoxemia and respiratory acidosis. Respiratory failure is indicated by decreasing responsiveness, cyanosis, and arterial blood gas measurements

1. EDEMA OF MUCOUS MEMBRANE

Smooth muscle

2. MUCUS PLUG

3. BRONCHOSPASM (MUSCLE CONTRACTION)

Excessive mucus

Inflammation

4. OBSTRUCTED BRONCHIOLE

FIGURE 17–11. Asthma.

A Normal Alveolus

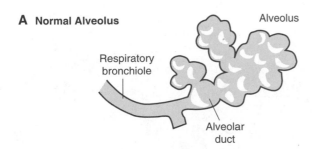

B Emphysema

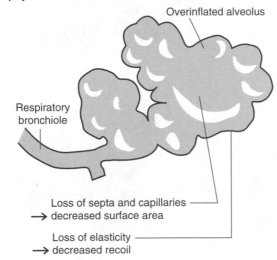

C Air Trapping

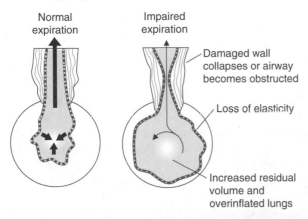

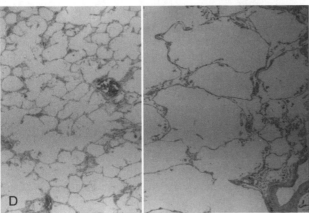

FIGURE 17-12. Emphysema. *A,* Normal alveolus. *B,* Emphysema. *C,* Air trapping. *D,* Left, normal lung; right, large spaces characteristic of emphysema. (Courtesy of R.W. Shaw, M.D., North York General Hospital, Toronto, Ontario.)

indicating a Pao₂ of below 50 mm Hg or a Paco₂ of above 50 mm Hg.

TREATMENT

Avoidance of triggering factors such as airborne irritants or drugs such as acetylsalicylic acid is recommended. Good ventilation in the home and workplace is recommended. When attacks occur, controlled breathing techniques and a reduction in anxiety often lessen the severity and extent of the attack because a feeling of panic frequently aggravates the condition. Regular swimming sessions are of great benefit, particularly to affected children, to strengthen chest muscles and improve cardiovascular fitness as well as to reduce stress. Many individuals carry **inhalers** so that they can self-administer a bronchodilator, usually a beta₂-adrenergic agent such as albuterol or terbutaline. These more specific drugs, which have largely replaced isoproterenol and epinephrine, act on receptors to relax bronchial smooth muscle but have minimal effects on the heart. These inhalers, when properly used, provide a measured dose of the medication and are most effective when used at the first indication of an attack. They may also be administered prior to exercise or exposure to a known stimulus. Glucocorticoids such as beclomethasone may be administered by inhalation also and are more effective in reducing the second stage of inflammation in the airways. Cromolyn sodium is a prophylactic medication that is administered by inhalation on a regular daily basis. The drug inhibits release of chemical mediators from sensitized mast cells in the respiratory passages and decreases the number of eosinophils, thus reducing the hyperresponsiveness of the tissues. It is particularly useful for athletes and sports enthusiasts. It is of no value during an acute attack.

Thinkabout 17-10

a. Which structures in the lungs contain a higher percentage of smooth muscle?

b. Explain how obstruction develops in an asthmatic patient following exposure to an inhaled allergen.

c. Compare the effects of partial and total obstruction of the airways on ventilation and on oxygen levels in the blood.

d. Explain the timing and development of respiratory alkalosis, respiratory acidosis, and metabolic acidosis during an asthma attack.

CHRONIC OBSTRUCTIVE PULMONARY DISEASE

Chronic obstructive pulmonary disease (COPD), sometimes also called chronic obstructive lung disease (COLD), is a group of common chronic respiratory disorders that lead to progressive tissue degeneration and obstruction in the airways of the lungs. They are debilitating conditions that affect the individual's ability to work and function independently. Examples of these disorders are emphysema, chronic bronchitis, and chronic asthma. In some patients, several primary diseases overlap, for example, asthma and bronchitis. Other conditions such as cystic fibrosis and bronchiectasis may lead to similar obstructive effects. In contrast, many occupational lung diseases such as silicosis, asbestosis, and farmer's lung are classified as *restrictive lung diseases* because the irritant causes *interstitial* inflammation and fibrosis, resulting in loss of compliance or "stiff lung" (see Fig. 17–19*C*).

COPD causes irreversible and progressive damage to the lungs. Eventually, respiratory failure may result because of severe hypoxia or hypercapnia. In many patients COPD leads to the development of *cor pulmonale*, right-sided congestive heart failure due to lung disease (see Chapter 16). As the pulmonary blood vessels are destroyed and hypoxia causes pulmonary vasoconstriction, pulmonary hypertension develops. The increased pressure in the pulmonary circulation increases resistance to the right ventricle, and eventually it fails. Many patients with respiratory disease manifest signs of heart failure. The signs of cor pulmonale are related to decreased cardiac output causing constant fatigue, increased renin secretion, and elevated blood pressure. Also, the backup effect of right-sided heart failure causes ascites and edema in dependent areas such as the legs. Acute heart failure is indicated by headache, flushed face, and distended neck veins.

Emphysema

PATHOPHYSIOLOGY

The significant change in emphysema is the destruction of the alveolar walls, which leads to large, permanently inflated alveolar air spaces (Fig. 17–12*B*). With advanced emphysema, the adjacent alveoli coalesce, and the lung appears full of large holes called blebs or bullae, indicating significant loss of tissue (Fig. 17–13). Emphysema may be further classified by the specific location of the changes—for example, in the distal alveoli (panacinar) or the bronchiolar (centrilobular) area. The breakdown of the alveolar wall means a loss of surface area and pulmonary capillaries, affecting perfusion and the diffusion of gases, and a loss of elastic fibers, affecting the ability of the lung to recoil on

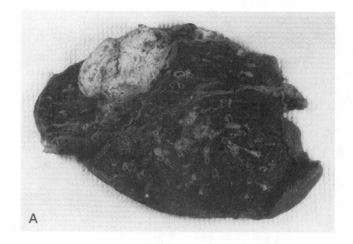

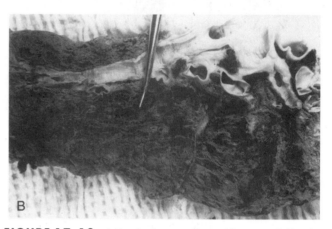

FIGURE 17–13. *A*, Emphysematous lung with tumor. *B*, Emphysematous blebs. (Courtesy of Paul Emmerson and Seneca College of Applied Arts and Technology, Toronto, Ontario.)

expiration. The ventilation-perfusion ratio may be altered as various changes occur in the alveoli (Fig. 17–14). The loss of tissue also decreases support for other structures such as the small bronchi, which often leads to collapse of the walls and additional obstruction of air flow during expiration.

Several factors contribute to the destruction of tissue in the alveoli. In some individuals there is a genetic deficiency of alpha$_1$-antitrypsin, a substance normally present in tissues and body fluids that inhibits the activity of **proteases**, which are destructive enzymes released by neutrophils during an inflammatory response. An example of a protease is elastase, which breaks down elastic fibers. This destructive process seems to be accelerated in persons with low alpha$_1$-antitrypsin levels. This genetic tendency is often found in individuals who develop emphysema relatively early in life. Cigarette smoking is a major predisposing factor in emphysema. Smoking increases both the number of neutrophils in the alveoli and the release and activity of elastase but decreases the effect of alpha$_1$-antitrypsin, thus greatly contributing to the breakdown of alveolar structures. Certain pathogenic bacteria present with infection also release proteases.

A Normal ventilation and perfusion

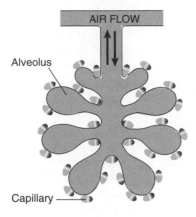

AIR FLOW

Alveolus

Capillary

B Destruction of alveolar wall and capillaries → Decreased ventilation and perfusion

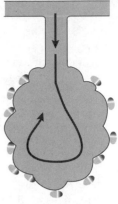

C Decreased ventilation

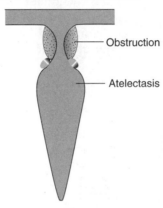

Obstruction

Atelectasis

D Good ventilation – Obstruction in pulmonary circulation → Decreased perfusion

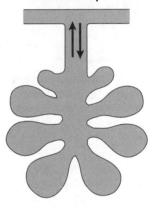

E Inflammation impairs ventilation, perfusion, and diffusion of O$_2$

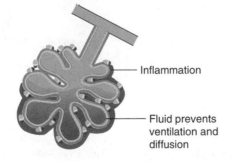

Inflammation

Fluid prevents ventilation and diffusion

FIGURE 17-14. Relationship between ventilation and perfusion.

In many cases of emphysema, fibrosis and thickening of the bronchial walls have resulted from chronic irritation and the frequent infections associated with smoking and increased mucus production. These conditions lead to narrowed airways and interference with expiratory air flow. Progressive difficulty with expiration leads to air trapping (see Fig. 17–12C), increased residual volume and overinflation of the lungs, fixation of the ribs in an inspiratory position, and an increased anterior-posterior diameter of the thorax. The diaphragm appears flattened on radiographs. As emphysema advances, hypoxia and hypercapnia become marked. In some cases, large blebs near the surface of the lung may rupture, resulting in pneumothorax. The patient's respiratory control adapts to a chronic elevation of carbon dioxide levels, and hypoxia becomes the driving force for respiration. Infections develop frequently because secretions are more difficult to remove past obstructions, and airway defenses are impaired.

ETIOLOGY

Cigarette smoking is implicated in most cases of emphysema. However, a genetic factor contributes to early development of the disease. Exposure to other air pollutants also predisposes to emphysematous changes, which may develop in conjunction with other chronic lung disorders such as cystic fibrosis and chronic bronchitis.

SIGNS AND SYMPTOMS

The onset of emphysema is insidious. Dyspnea occurs first on exertion and then progresses until it is marked even at rest. A prolonged expiratory phase, use of the accessory muscles, and hyperinflation leading to development of a "barrel chest" mark the ventilation difficulty. The chest is hyperresonant on percussion. Anorexia and fatigue contribute to weight loss. Chronic hypoxia results in clubbed fingers and secondary polycythemia. Pulmonary function tests indicate the presence of increased residual volume and total lung capacity as well as decreased forced expiratory volume and vital capacity.

TREATMENT

Avoidance of respiratory irritants and sources of respiratory infections, cessation of smoking, maintenance of adequate nutrition and hydration, and a moderate exercise program may slow the progress of emphysema. Learning appropriate breathing techniques such as pursed-lip breathing can maximize ventilation with less expenditure of energy. Bronchodilators, antibiotics, and oxygen therapy may be necessary as the condition advances.

Thinkabout 17–11

a. List the factors that interfere with oxygenation of the blood in patients with emphysema.

b. Explain why expiration is significantly impaired in patients with emphysema.

c. Explain why heart failure may develop in patients with emphysema.

d. Describe and explain how you would position a patient with COPD (e.g., one who is having dental treatment). Should the patient be relatively supine, upright, or otherwise positioned?

Chronic Bronchitis

PATHOPHYSIOLOGY

Although there may be some overlap in the basic conditions comprising COPD, chronic bronchitis is differentiated by significant changes in the *bronchi* resulting from constant irritation from smoking or exposure to industrial pollution. The mucosa is inflamed and swollen. There is hypertrophy and hyperplasia of the mucous glands, and increased secretions are produced. The number of goblet cells is increased, and there is decreased ciliated epithelium. There may be dysplasia or metaplasia in the epithelial lining (possibly precancerous changes). Chronic irritation and inflammation lead to fibrosis and thickening of the bronchial wall. Frequent infections occur because of the constant inflammation, excessive secretions, and loss of cilia. The effects are irreversible and progressive. Airway obstruction is the end result of the combination of edematous walls, increased mucus, and fibrosis. Severe dyspnea and fatigue interferes with nutrition, communication, and daily activities, leading to general debilitation.

ETIOLOGY

Individuals with chronic bronchitis usually have a history of cigarette smoking or living in an urban or industrial area, particularly in geographic locations where smog is common. Heavy exposure to inhaled irritants leads to inflammation and frequent infections, initiating the cycle. In some cases, asthma is an associated condition.

SIGNS AND SYMPTOMS

Constant productive cough is the significant indicator of chronic bronchitis, as is tachypnea and shortness of breath. Cough and rhonchi are usually more severe in the morning because the secretions have pooled during sleep. Airway obstruction leads to hypoxia and eventually cyanosis as well as hypercapnia. The term "blue bloater" was sometimes applied to the person with cyanosis and edema associated with chronic bronchitis, whereas "pink puffer" was used to describe the better oxygen status of the individual with emphysema. Secondary polycythemia, severe weight loss, and cor pulmonale often develop as the damage progresses.

TREATMENT

Reducing exposure to irritants and prompt treatment of infection slow the progress of the disease. Use of expectorants and bronchodilators and appropriate chest therapy, including postural drainage and percussion, assist in removing excessive mucus. Low-flow oxygen and nutritional supplements are helpful.

Bronchiectasis

Bronchiectasis is usually a secondary problem, not a primary one, that develops in patients with conditions such as cystic fibrosis or COPD. Some cases result from childhood infection, aspiration of foreign bodies, or a congenital weakness in the bronchial wall. Depending on the cause, the condition may be localized in one lobe, or it may be diffuse in both lungs. The incidence in North America has decreased owing to effective use of antibiotics in treatment of the predisposing disorders.

PATHOPHYSIOLOGY

Bronchiectasis is an irreversible abnormal dilation or widening, primarily of the medium-sized bronchi. These dilations may be saccular or elongated (fusiform) and result from obstruction in the airways or a weakening of the muscle and elastic fibers in the bronchial wall, or from a combination of these. In dilated or ballooning areas, large amounts of fluid collect and become infected. Infecting organisms are usually mixed and include streptococci, staphylococci, pneumococci, and *H. influenzae.* These infections then cause loss of cilia and metaplasia in the epithelium, additional fibrosis, and obstruction. The obstructions and loss of cilia interfere with the removal of the fluids, continuing the cycle of events.

SIGNS AND SYMPTOMS

The significant signs of bronchiectasis are chronic cough and production of copious amounts of purulent sputum (1 to 2 cups per day). Cough may be paroxysmal in the morning as the purulent sputum shifts in the lungs with changes in body position, stimulating the cough reflex. Other signs include rales and rhonchi in the lungs, foul breath, dyspnea, and hemoptysis. Systemic signs include weight loss, anemia, and fatigue.

TREATMENT

Antibiotics, bronchodilators, and chest physiotherapy as well as treatment of the primary condition reduce the severity of the infections and progressive damage to the lungs.

Thinkabout 17–12

a. Describe the conditions predisposing to chronic bronchitis and relate them to the pathologic changes occurring in the lungs.

b. Describe the factors contributing to recurrent infections in the lungs and relate them to your professional practice.

c. Explain why bronchiectasis tends to be progressive.

d. Prepare a chart comparing emphysema, chronic bronchitis, and bronchiectasis with regard to pathologic changes in the lungs, the significant signs that can be observed in a patient, and potential complications.

VASCULAR DISORDERS

Pulmonary Edema

PATHOPHYSIOLOGY

Pulmonary edema refers to fluid in the alveoli and interstitial area. Normally, pressure in the pulmonary capillaries is very low, and there is minimal fluid in the air passages and alveoli. Pulmonary edema commonly develops because of high hydrostatic pressure in the pulmonary capillaries, leading to a shift of fluid out of the capillaries (see Chapter 6). Excessive amounts of fluid in the interstitial areas and alveoli interfere with the diffusion of oxygen, causing severe hypoxemia, as well as with the action of surfactant, leading to difficulty in expanding the lungs, which ultimately collapse (Fig. 17–15). Capillaries may rupture, causing blood-streaked sputum.

ETIOLOGY

Pulmonary edema can result from many conditions. A common cause is left-sided congestive heart failure, in which the backup of blood from the left ventricle creates high pressure in the pulmonary circulation (see Chapter 16). Pulmonary edema also results from hypoproteinemia due to kidney or liver disease, in which low serum albumin levels cause low osmotic pressure in the blood, which in turn causes excessive amounts of fluid to shift out of the capillaries. Other causes include inflammation with increased capillary permeability due to inhalation of toxic gases or blocked lymphatics in the lungs due to tumors or fibrosis.

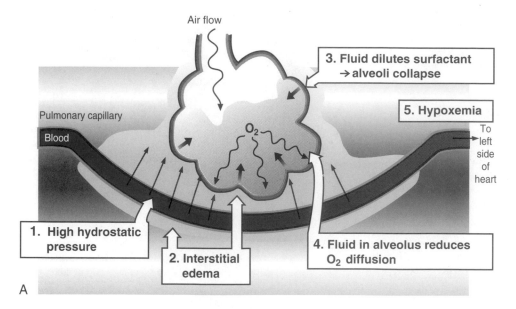

Air flow

**3. Fluid dilutes surfactant
→ alveoli collapse**

5. Hypoxemia

To
left
side
of
heart

Pulmonary capillary

Blood

O₂

**1. High hydrostatic
pressure**

**2. Interstitial
edema**

**4. Fluid in alveolus reduces
O₂ diffusion**

A

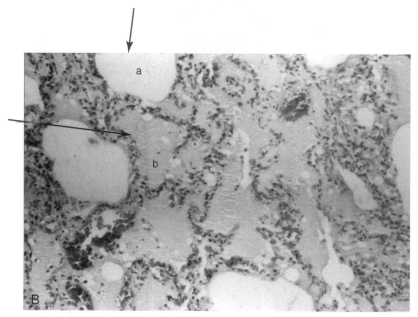

a

b

B

FIGURE 17-15. *A,* Pulmonary edema. *B,* Photomicrograph showing acute pulmonary edema due to congestive heart failure: a, alveolar air space; b, fluid-filled alveolus. (Courtesy of R.W. Shaw, M.D., North York General Hospital, Toronto, Ontario.)

SIGNS AND SYMPTOMS

Signs of mild pulmonary edema include cough, orthopnea, and rales. As congestion increases, hemoptysis occurs. Sputum is frothy due to air mixed with the secretions and blood-tinged due to ruptured capillaries in the lungs. Breathing becomes labored as it becomes more difficult to expand the lungs. The individual feels as if he or she is drowning. Hypoxemia increases, and cyanosis develops in the advanced stage. Acute congestive heart failure may cause such an episode, called paroxysmal nocturnal dyspnea, during a sleep period.

TREATMENT

The causative factors must be treated, and supportive care such as oxygen should be offered. In severe cases

positive-pressure mechanical ventilation may be necessary. There is an increased risk of pneumonia developing after an episode of pulmonary edema because of the residual secretions. Individuals with a tendency to pulmonary edema should be positioned with the upper body elevated.

Pulmonary Embolus

A pulmonary **embolus** is a blood clot or other material that obstructs the pulmonary artery or a branch of it, blocking the flow of blood through the lung tissue. Most pulmonary emboli are thrombi or blood clots originating from the leg veins. Any embolus to the lungs travels from its source through larger and larger veins until it reaches the heart and pulmonary artery. It then lodges as soon as it reaches a smaller artery in the lungs through which it cannot pass. Other types of pulmonary emboli include fat emboli from the bone marrow resulting from fracture of a large bone (e.g., the femur), vegetations resulting from endocarditis in the right side of the heart, amniotic fluid emboli from placental tears occurring during labor and delivery, tumor cell emboli that break away from a malignant mass, or air embolus injected into a vein.

PATHOPHYSIOLOGY

The effects of a pulmonary embolus depend largely on the size and therefore on the location of the obstruction in the pulmonary circulation (Fig. 17–16). Small pulmonary emboli are frequently "silent" or asymptomatic. Because lung tissue is supplied with oxygen and nutrients by the bronchial circulation, infarction does not follow obstruction of the pulmonary circulation unless the general circulation is compromised. Infarction usually involves a segment of the lung and the pleural membrane in the area. However, multiple small emboli (a "shower") often have an effect equal to that of a large embolus. Emboli that block moderate-sized arteries usually cause respiratory impairment because fluid and blood fill the alveoli of the involved area. Reflex vasoconstriction in the area further increases the pressure in the blood vessels. Large emboli (usually those involving more than 60 percent of the lung tissue) affect the cardiovascular system, causing right-sided heart failure and decreased cardiac output (shock). Sudden death often results in these cases, which involve greatly increased resistance in the pulmonary arteries because of the embolus plus reflex vasoconstriction due to released chemical mediators such as serotonin and histamine. This resistance to the output from the right ventricle causes acute cor pulmonale. Also, there is much less blood returning from the lungs to the left ventricle and then to the systemic circulation (decreased cardiac output). This can be appreciated by visualizing a large embolus lying across the bifurcation of the pulmonary artery and totally blocking the flow of blood from the right ventricle into the lungs.

ETIOLOGY

A high percentage of pulmonary emboli travel from the deep veins of the legs as a result of phlebo-

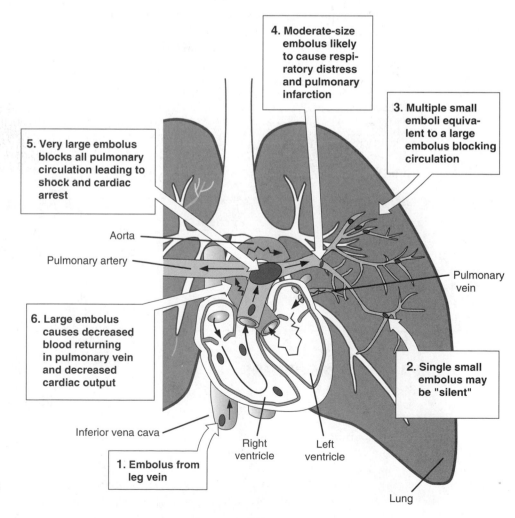

FIGURE 17-16. Pulmonary embolus.

thrombosis or thrombophlebitis (see Chapter 16). Risk factors for these emboli include immobility, trauma to the legs, childbirth, congestive heart failure, dehydration, increased coagulability of the blood, and cancer. Thrombi tend to break off with sudden muscle action or massage, trauma, or changes in blood flow.

SIGNS AND SYMPTOMS

Chest pain, tachypnea, and dyspnea develop suddenly. Later, hemoptysis and fever are present. Hypoxia stimulates a sympathetic response with anxiety and restlessness, pallor, and tachycardia. Massive emboli cause severe crushing chest pain, low blood pressure, rapid weak pulse, and loss of consciousness. Fat emboli are distinguished by development of acute respiratory distress, a petechial rash on the trunk, and neurologic signs such as confusion and disorientation.

TREATMENT

Assessment of risk factors in an individual and preventive measures are recommended. The underlying cause of the embolus must be considered. In patients with pulmonary embolus due to **thrombus**, oxygen is administered and usually intravenous heparin as well to prevent additional clots. Use of thrombolytic therapy depends on the particular situation. Mechanical ventilation may be necessary, and in some cases embolectomy is performed.

Thinkabout 17–13

a. List three possible causes of pulmonary edema and give the rationale for each.

b. Explain which is more likely to occur with acute pulmonary edema—hypoxemia, hypercapnia, or both equally.

c. Explain how a pulmonary embolus can cause immediate death.

EXPANSION DISORDERS

Atelectasis

Atelectasis is the nonaeration or collapse of a lung or part of a lung leading to decreased gas exchange and hypoxia. It occurs as a complication of many primary conditions. Treatment depends on the underlying cause, whether obstruction or compression.

PATHOPHYSIOLOGY

When the alveoli become airless, they shrivel up as the natural elasticity of the tissues dominates. This process also interferes with blood flow through the lung. Both ventilation and perfusion are altered, and this in turn primarily affects oxygen diffusion. Unless a very large proportion of the lungs is affected, the increased respiratory rate can control carbon dioxide levels because this gas diffuses easily. If the lungs are not reinflated quickly, the lung tissue can become necrotic and infected, and permanent lung damage results.

ETIOLOGY

A variety of mechanisms can result in atelectasis (Fig. 17–17). Total obstruction of the airway due to mucus or tumor leads to diffusion into the tissue of air distal to the obstruction; this air is not replaced. Compression atelectasis results when a mass such as a tumor exerts pressure on a part of the lung and prevents air from entering that section of lung. Alternatively, when the pressure in the pleural cavity is increased, as with increased fluid or air, and the adhesion of the pleural membranes is destroyed, the lung cannot expand. Another type of atelectasis occurs when surface tension increases in the alveoli as with pulmonary edema or respiratory distress syndrome, preventing expansion of the lung.

Postoperative atelectasis commonly occurs 24 to 72 hours following surgery, particularly abdominal surgery. A number of factors are implicated in this situation, including restricted ventilation due to pain, abdominal distention, slow shallow respirations due to anesthetics and analgesics, increased secretions due to the supine position, and decreased cough effort.

SIGNS AND SYMPTOMS

Small areas of atelectasis are asymptomatic. Large areas cause dyspnea, increased heart and respiratory rates, and chest pain. Chest expansion may appear abnormal or asymmetrical depending on the cause of the atelectasis. For example, obstructive atelectasis leads to a potential low pressure "gap" or space on the affected side, and therefore the other lung compensates by overinflating. The affected side often "lags" behind the unaffected side during ventilation.

Pleural Effusion

A pleural effusion is the presence of excessive fluid in the pleural cavity. Normally a very small amount of fluid is present to provide lubrication for the membranes. Effusions vary in type and mechanism according to the primary problem. Both lungs may be involved, but

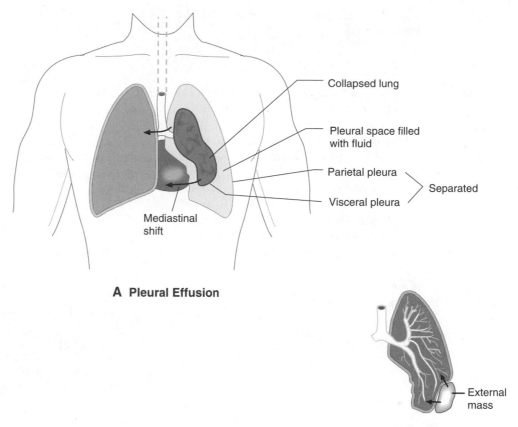

A Pleural Effusion

B Compression Atelectasis

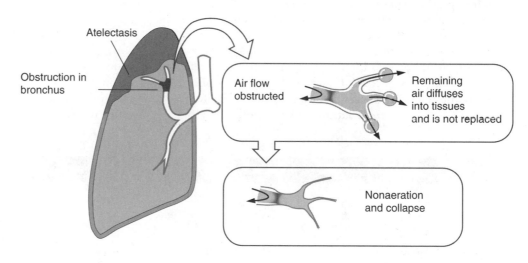

C Obstructive Atelectasis – Absorption Atelectasis

FIGURE 17–17. Atelectasis.

PATHOPHYSIOLOGY

more often only one lung is affected because each lung is enclosed in a separate pleural membrane. The effects of effusion depend on the amount, type, and rate of accumulation of the fluid.

Small amounts of fluid are drained from the pleural cavity by the lymphatics and have little effect on respiratory function. Large amounts of fluid first increase the pressure in the pleural cavity and then cause separation of the pleural membranes, preventing their cohesion during inspiration. These effects prevent expansion of the lung, leading to atelectasis, particularly when fluid accumulates rapidly (see Fig. 17–17A). A large amount of fluid causes atelectasis on the affected side and a shift of the mediastinal contents toward the unaffected lung, limiting its expansion also. A tracheal deviation indicates this shift. Venous return in the inferior vena cava and cardiac filling may be impaired because large effusions increase pressure in the mediastinum.

ETIOLOGY

Different types of fluid may collect in the pleural cavity. *Exudative* effusions are a response to inflammation, perhaps from a tumor, in which increased capillary permeability allows fluid containing protein and white blood cells to leak into the pleural cavity. *Transudates* are watery effusions, sometimes called *hydrothorax*, that result from increased hydrostatic pressure or decreased osmotic pressure in the blood vessels, leading to a shift of fluid out of the blood vessels into the potential space in the pleural cavity. These effusions may occur secondary to liver or kidney disease. **Empyema** occurs when the fluid is purulent due to infection, often related to pneumonia. *Hemothorax* is the term used when the fluid is blood resulting from trauma, cancer, or surgery. *Pleurisy* (pleuritis) is a condition in which the pleural membranes are inflamed, swollen, and rough, perhaps associated with lobar pneumonia. Pleurisy may precede or follow an effusion or may occur independently.

SIGNS AND SYMPTOMS

The general signs include dyspnea, chest pain, and increased respiratory and heart rates. Usually dullness to percussion and absence of breath sounds over the affected area are found because air no longer flows through the passages. Pleurisy is manifested by cyclic pleuritic pain and a friction rub as the rough swollen membranes move against each other during respiratory movements. Tracheal deviation and hypotension indi-cate a massive effusion that interferes with both respiratory and circulatory function.

TREATMENT

Measures are required to remove the underlying cause and to treat the respiratory impairment. The fluid may have to be analyzed to confirm the cause. Chest drainage tubes may be used to assist inflation. If a large quantity of fluid forms, thoracocentesis (needle aspiration) is required to remove the fluid and relieve the pressure.

Thinkabout 17–14

a. Compare the mechanisms involved in the development of atelectasis in a patient with cystic fibrosis and in one with pleural effusion.
b. Explain why a large pleural effusion may have more serious consequences than an obstruction in a major bronchus.
c. Describe the signs of atelectasis

Pneumothorax

Pneumothorax refers to air in the pleural cavity. The presence of air at atmospheric pressure in the pleural cavity and the separation of the pleural membranes by

	TABLE 17–4 Types of Pneumothorax		
	Closed	**Large Open**	**Tension**
Cause	Spontaneous, idiopathic Ruptured emphysematous bleb	Puncture wound	Open—puncture through thorax Closed—tear in lung surface Both with flap or one-way valve
Air entry	From inside lung through tear in visceral pleura	From outside body through opening in thorax and parietal pleura	
Effects	Atelectasis	Atelectasis	Atelectasis
	Leak seals as lung collapses	Air enters pleural cavity with each inspiration and leaves with each expiration	Air enters pleural cavity with each inspiration. Flap closes with expiration, and air pressure increases in pleural cavity
	One lung impaired	Unaffected lung compressed by mediastinal shift on inspiration	Unaffected lung is increasingly compressed by mediastinal shift
	No additional cardiovascular effects	Mediastinal flutter impairs venous return to heart	Mediastinal shift reduces venous return to heart
Signs	All three types: increased, labored respirations with dyspnea, tachycardia, pleural pain, and asymmetrical chest movements		
	Absent breath sounds	"Sucking" noise Tracheal swing Decreased blood pressure	Absent breath sounds on affected side Tracheal deviation to unaffected side Increasing respiratory distress Shock, distended neck veins, cyanosis
	Hypoxemia	Moderate hypoxemia	Severe hypoxemia

air prevent expansion of the lung, leading to atelectasis. When pneumothorax is caused by a malignant tumor or trauma, fluid or blood may also be present in the cavity. For example, with fluid in the more dependent area and air above it, the condition could be called hydropneumothorax. There are several different types of pneumothorax (Table 17–4). Chest radiographs can determine the type and extent of pneumothorax.

A *simple* or *spontaneous pneumothorax* occurs when a tear on the surface of the lung allows air to escape from inside the lung through a bronchus and the visceral pleura into the pleural cavity (Fig. 17–18). As the lung tissue collapses, it seals off the leak. Simple pneumothorax often occurs in young men who have no prior lung disease but perhaps an idiopathic bleb or defect on the lung surface. *Secondary pneumothorax* is associated with underlying respiratory disease resulting from rupture of an emphysematous bleb on the surface of the lung or erosion by a tumor or tubercular cavitation through the visceral pleura. Again, this condition lets inspired air pass into the pleural cavity.

A large *open pneumothorax* or "sucking wound" is caused by an injury that creates an opening in the chest wall. Air enters the pleural cavity through the opening in the chest wall and parietal pleura, causing immediate atelectasis on the affected side. Because more air enters the pleural cavity during inspiration, the mediastinum pushes against the unaffected lung, limiting its expansion. Subsequently, on expiration, as air is pushed out of the pleural cavity through the opening, the mediastinal contents shift back toward the affected side. These abnormal movements occur as the pressure changes with rib movements on inspiration and expiration. The sound of the air moving through the hole is often referred to as a sucking noise. This mediastinal flutter or "to and fro" motion impairs both ventilation in the unaffected lung and venous return through the inferior vena cava. (Recall that normal respiratory movements and pressure changes promote movement of venous blood upward to the heart.) This is the reason why it is suggested that penetrating objects not be removed from the chest wall until medical assistance is available and why first-aid measures include covering any openings in the chest wall to limit air flow in and out of the pleural cavity.

The most serious form of pneumothorax is a *tension pneumothorax*. This situation may result from an opening through the chest wall and parietal pleura (open pneumothorax) or from a tear in the lung tissue and visceral pleura (closed pneumothorax) that causes atelectasis (see Fig. 17–18). The particular pattern of damage creates a flap of tissue or a one-way valve effect, whereby the opening enlarges on inspiration, promoting air flow into the pleural cavity. However, on expiration, the opening is sealed off, preventing removal of air from the pleural cavity. Thus, with each inspiration this lesion leads to continual increases in the amount of air in the pleural cavity. Pressure increases on the affected side eventually push the mediastinal contents against the other lung, compressing the inferior vena cava. Severe hypoxia and respiratory distress develop quickly and can become life threatening if the source of the valve effect and increasing intrapleural pressure is not removed.

SIGNS AND SYMPTOMS

The general signs of pneumothorax include those of atelectasis, dyspnea, cough, and chest pain. Breath sounds are reduced over the atelectatic area. Other signs related to chest movements, unequal expansion, and mediastinal shift vary with the type of pneumothorax. Hypoxia develops and leads to a sympathetic response, including anxiety, tachycardia, and pallor. Interference with venous return leads to hypotension.

Flail Chest

Flail chest results from fractures of the thorax, usually fractures of three to six ribs in two places or fracture of the sternum and a number of consecutive ribs. Chest wall rigidity is lost, resulting in *paradoxical* (opposite) movement during inspiration and expiration (Fig. 17–19). During inspiration the flail or broken section of ribs moves inward rather than outward as intrathoracic pressure is decreased. This inward movement of the ribs prevents expansion of the affected lung. On expiration, the unstable flail section is pushed outward by the increasing intrathoracic pressure. If the flail section is large, the paradoxical movement of the ribs alters air flow. On inspiration, the inward motion of the ribs pushes the air over into the unaffected lung, along with newly inspired air. During expiration, air from the unaffected lung moves across into the affected lung as the outward movement of the ribs decreases pressure in the affected area. Note that a sequence of pressure changes occurs. For example, on inspiration, there is an immediate decrease in pressure inside the lungs, which permits the flail ribs to move inward. The inward motion of the ribs compresses the adjacent lung tissue, pushing the air out of that section and up the bronchus. Because air is flowing down the trachea and into the other lung, the air from the flail section crosses into the other lung. Hypoxia results from both the limited expansion and decreased inspiratory volume of the flail lung and from the shunting of "stale" air between lungs, which lowers the oxygen content of the air. The abnormal movement is obvious, and therefore first-aid measures include stabilizing the flail section with a flat heavy object, thus limiting the outward paradoxical movement of the thorax until surgical repair can be

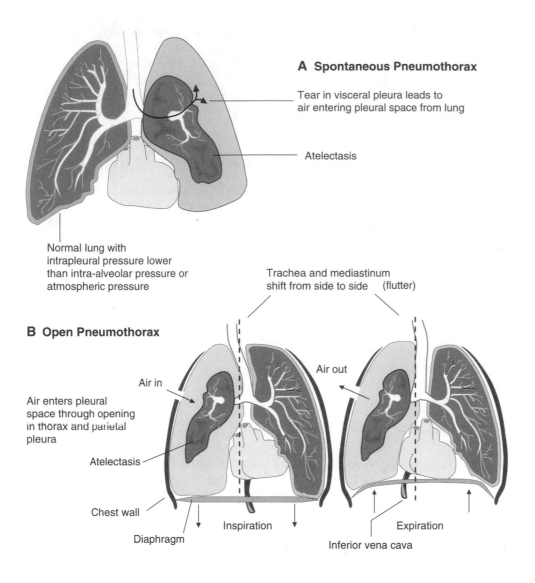

A Spontaneous Pneumothorax

Tear in visceral pleura leads to
air entering pleural space from lung

Atelectasis

Normal lung with
intrapleural pressure lower
than intra-alveolar pressure or
atmospheric pressure

Trachea and mediastinum
shift from side to side   (flutter)

B Open Pneumothorax

Air in

Air out

Air enters pleural
space through opening
in thorax and parietal
pleura

Atelectasis

Chest wall

Diaphragm

Inspiration

Expiration

Inferior vena cava

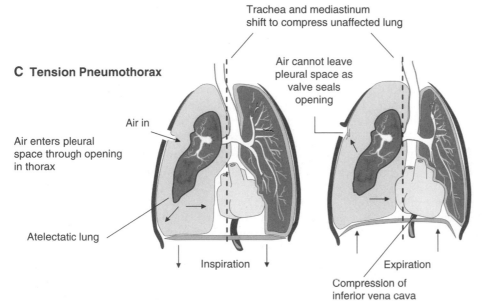

Trachea and mediastinum
shift to compress unaffected lung

C Tension Pneumothorax

Air in

Air cannot leave
pleural space as
valve seals
opening

Air enters pleural
space through opening
in thorax

Atelectatic lung

Inspiration

Expiration

Compression of
inferior vena cava

FIGURE 17-18. Types of pneumothorax.

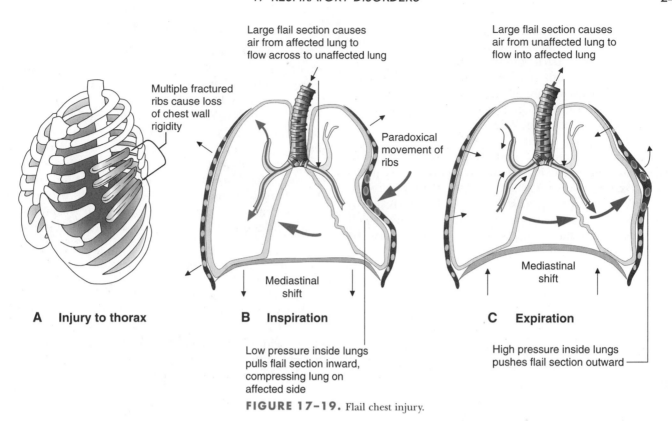

Large flail section causes air from affected lung to flow across to unaffected lung

Multiple fractured ribs cause loss of chest wall rigidity

Large flail section causes air from unaffected lung to flow into affected lung

Paradoxical movement of ribs

Mediastinal shift

Mediastinal shift

A   Injury to thorax

B   Inspiration

C   Expiration

Low pressure inside lungs pulls flail section inward, compressing lung on affected side

High pressure inside lungs pushes flail section outward

FIGURE 17–19. Flail chest injury.

performed. Atelectasis does not occur as a direct result of the trauma but may follow as a complication if a broken rib punctures the pleura.

Thinkabout   17–15

a. Describe two ways in which atmospheric air can enter the pleural cavity.

b. List in the proper sequence the changes in the structures and the pressures that occur during normal inspiration and during inspiration with flail chest.

c. Prepare a chart comparing the cause and effects of spontaneous pneumothorax, tension pneumothorax, and flail chest on ventilation and cardiovascular activity.

Infant Respiratory Distress Syndrome

Infant respiratory distress syndrome (IRDS), also called hyaline membrane disease, is a common cause of neonatal deaths, particularly in premature infants. With improved methods of testing for lung maturity and supportive treatment to maintain the infant's life, the mortality rate has decreased in recent years.

PATHOPHYSIOLOGY

During the third trimester of fetal development, the alveolar surface area and lung vascularity greatly increase in preparation for independent lung function immediately after birth. Surfactant, which reduces surface tension in the alveoli and promotes expansion, is first produced between 28 and 36 weeks of gestation depending on the maturity of the individual lung. It has been shown that in utero stress hastens the maturation of lung tissue. Infant lung maturity can be assessed by measuring the surfactant level of the fetus with a test such as the lecithin-sphingomyelin (L/S) ratio in amniotic fluid, which is obtained by amniocentesis. Initially sphingomyelin is high, then it decreases and lecithin increases until the ratio represents adequate surfactant function at around 35 weeks of gestation. Normally, the first few inspirations after birth are difficult as the lungs are inflated; then breathing becomes easier. Without adequate surfactant, each inspiration is very difficult because the lung totally collapses during each expiration, thereby requiring use of the accessory muscles and much energy. The poorly developed alveoli are difficult to inflate, and an inadequate blood supply further deters the production of surfactant by alveolar cells (see Fig. 17–4). Diffuse atelectasis results, which decreases pulmonary blood flow and leads to reflex pulmonary vasoconstriction and severe hypoxia (Fig. 17–20). Poor lung perfusion and lack of surfactant lead to increased alveolar capillary permeability, with fluid and protein (fibrin) leaking into the interstitial area and alveoli, forming the "hyaline membrane" and further decreasing oxygen diffusion. Some of the surviving neonates experience brain damage due to severe hypoxia.

A vicious cycle develops as acidosis develops from respiratory impairment and metabolic factors. The strenuous muscle activity required to breathe requires more oxygen than is available, and this leads to anaerobic metabolism and increased lactic acid. In turn, acidosis causes pulmonary vasoconstriction and impairs cell metabolism, reducing the synthesis and secretion of surfactant.

ETIOLOGY

Infant respiratory distress syndrome is usually related to premature birth, but other factors are involved. It occurs more commonly in male children and following cesarean delivery. Infants born to diabetic mothers are predisposed to this syndrome.

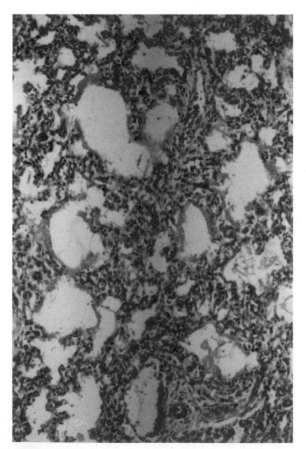

FIGURE 17–20. Infant respiratory distress syndrome. Photomicrograph of lung tissue with infant respiratory distress syndrome and atelectasis. (Courtesy of R.W. Shaw, M.D., North York General Hospital, Toronto, Ontario.)

SIGNS AND SYMPTOMS

There may be respiratory difficulty at birth or shortly after birth. Signs include a persistent respiratory rate of more than 60 breaths per minute, nasal flaring, subcostal and intercostal retractions, rales, and low body temperature. Chest retractions are quite marked in a neonate because of the soft chest wall. As infant respiratory distress syndrome continues, respirations become more rapid and shallow, frothy sputum and expiratory grunt develop, blood pressure falls, and cyanosis and peripheral edema become evident. Signs of severe hypoxemia are decreased responsiveness, irregular respirations with periods of **apnea**, and decreased breath sounds.

DIAGNOSTIC TESTS

Arterial blood gas analysis is helpful in monitoring both oxygen and acid-base balance. Initially, hypoxemia (low Pao_2) and metabolic acidosis (low serum HCO_3^-) are present. Respiratory acidosis (high Pco_2) develops as ventilation becomes more difficult. Chest radiographs indicate areas of congestion and atelectasis.

TREATMENT

Supportive measures such as oxygen therapy, fluid and electrolyte replacement, appropriate nutrition, and medications (e.g., synthetic lung surfactant, colfosceril) to increase lung compliance can be used for a time until the lungs mature. Mechanical ventilation is helpful for a short time, but long-term ventilator use has led to pneumothorax, permanent lung damage, and infections.

Adult Respiratory Distress Syndrome

Adult respiratory distress syndrome (ARDS) is also known as shock lung, wet lung, postperfusion lung, and a variety of other names related to specific causes. A multitude of agents, such as severe pulmonary infection or systemic sepsis, prolonged shock, burns, aspiration, and smoke inhalation may cause ARDS. The onset of respiratory distress usually occurs 1 to 2 days after an injury or other precipitating event. In many cases, it is associated with multiple organ dysfunction or failure secondary to a severe insult to the body.

PATHOPHYSIOLOGY

The basic changes in the lungs result from injury to the alveolar wall and capillary membrane, leading to release of chemical mediators, increased permeability of alveolar capillary membranes, increased fluid in the interstitial area and alveoli, and damage to the surfactant-producing cells. These events result in decreased diffusion of oxygen, difficulty in expanding the lungs, and diffuse atelectasis. Reductions in tidal volume and vital capacity occur. Damage to lung tissue progresses as increased numbers of neutrophils migrate to the lungs, releasing proteases and other mediators. Hyaline membranes form in the alveoli, platelet aggregation and microthrombi develop in the pulmonary circulation, and ultimately diffuse necrosis and fibrosis occur throughout the lungs.

ETIOLOGY

Severe or prolonged shock may cause ARDS because of ischemic damage to the lung tissue. Inflammation in the lungs arises directly from such events as inhalation of toxic chemicals or smoke; excessive oxygen concentration in inspired air; toxins from systemic infection, particularly by gram-negative organisms; fat emboli; explosions; aspiration of highly acidic gastric contents; or lung trauma. Other causes include DIC, cancer, acute pancreatitis, and uremia.

SIGNS AND SYMPTOMS

Early signs may be masked by the effects of the primary problem. Onset is usually marked by dyspnea, restlessness, rapid shallow respirations, and increased heart rate. Arterial blood gas measurements indicate a significant decrease in Po_2. As lung congestion increases, the accessory muscles are used, rales can be heard, productive cough with frothy sputum may be evident, and lethargy and confusion develop. A combination of respiratory and metabolic acidosis evolves as diffusion is impaired and anaerobic metabolism is required.

TREATMENT

The underlying cause must be successfully treated, and supportive respiratory therapy must be maintained until the causative factors are removed and healing occurs. Administration of fluid may be limited to minimize alveolar edema, although this may be difficult in patients with multisystem failure.

Acute Respiratory Failure

PATHOPHYSIOLOGY

Acute respiratory failure (ARF) can be the end result of many pulmonary disorders. It occurs when Pao_2 is less than 50 mm Hg (severe hypoxemia) or $Paco_2$ is greater than 50 mm Hg (hypercapnia) and serum pH is decreasing (less than 7.3). Normal values are approximately 80 to 100 mm Hg for oxygen and 35 to 45 mm Hg for carbon dioxide. The abnormal values mentioned are considered inadequate for the body's metabolic needs at rest. The precise figures used for these criteria may vary somewhat with the cause of the problem, but the significant factor is the trend or progressive changes in the values that occur over time. Respiratory arrest refers to cessation of respiratory activity.

ARF can be related to ventilation and perfusion that are abnormal for any reason. It may be complicated by reflex pulmonary vasoconstriction due to hypoxia or acidosis, further impairing lung perfusion and increasing cardiac work load. The heart may be limited in its ability to compensate for reduced oxygen levels. Acidosis may be of respiratory origin, or it may be metabolic, related to the low oxygen levels. The ability of the kidneys to compensate for acidosis depends on the time available for this process to take place and the ability of the cardiovascular system to provide adequate circulation in the body. Both hypoxia and hypercapnia impair central nervous system function and lead to cardiac arrhythmias or arrest.

ETIOLOGY

ARF may result from acute or chronic disorders. Chronic conditions such as emphysema may lead to respiratory failure if the degenerative tissue changes progress to the point where ventilation and gas exchange are minimal. ARF may also develop in an earlier stage of emphysema or other chronic lung disease if it is complicated by pneumonia or pneumothorax or central nervous system depression caused by narcotics or other depressant drugs. Acute respiratory failure may occur with many acute respiratory disorders such as chest trauma (flail chest or tension pneumothorax), pulmonary embolus, or acute asthma. ARF is a serious threat in patients with many neuromuscular diseases such as myasthenia gravis, amyotrophic lateral sclerosis, or muscular dystrophy (see Chapter 20).

SIGNS AND SYMPTOMS

The signs may be masked or altered by the primary problem. Manifestations include rapid, shallow, often labored respirations. General signs of hypoxia and hypercapnia include headache, tachycardia, lethargy, and confusion.

TREATMENT

As in many other situations, the primary problem must be resolved and supportive treatment must be given to maintain respiratory function.

Thinkabout 17-16

a. Compare the factors contributing to infant respiratory distress syndrome and ARDS.

b. Describe the basic pathophysiology of respiratory distress syndrome and its initial effect on arterial blood gases.

c. Using an example, explain how respiratory failure may develop and explain why this is life threatening.

d. Explain how severe hypoxia and hypercapnia affect the central nervous system and the level of response.

CASE STUDIES

CASE STUDY A
Influenza and Pneumonia

Mrs. AH has had an acute episode of influenza A, complicated by pneumococcal pneumonia. She lives in a seniors' apartment building, where a number of residents have had influenza in the past month.

a. State the cause of influenza and describe briefly how it affects the lungs.

b. Describe the normal mechanisms that defend against infection in the respiratory tract.

c. Explain why it can be expected that a number of residents in such a building would be affected by influenza.

d. What precautions could be taken by the residents to avoid the infection?

e. What precautions could you take in your particular profession to reduce the risk of respiratory infection for yourself, your colleagues, and your patients?

f. Explain why antibacterial drugs are not directly effective in cases of influenza. Why may they be prescribed?

g. Explain why Mrs. AH is predisposed to develop pneumonia.

Mrs. AH was admitted to the hospital after she developed severe chest pain and appeared confused to friends. Pneumococcal pneumonia was suspected.

h. Describe the appropriate diagnostic tests that would be used for Mrs. AH and give the rationale for each.

i. Mrs. AH indicates that the chest pain increases on inspiration or coughing. Explain the probable cause of this chest pain and of her confusion.

j. Describe how other signs and symptoms would probably change as pneumonia develops and give the rationale for each (include the relevant respiratory and systemic signs).

k. Predict the values of arterial blood gases in Mrs. AH in the early stage of pneumococcal pneumonia and in the advanced stage if two lobes are involved (use general descriptions such as increased slightly or greatly, not specific figures).

l. Explain how Mrs. AH can compensate to maintain a normal serum pH.

m. List several reasons why Mrs. AH may become dehydrated.

n. Explain several ways in which dehydration could complicate Mrs. AH's status.

o. Describe several treatment measures that would be helpful in this case.

CASE STUDY B
Acute Asthma

Eight-year-old BJ has had asthma for 2 years since he had acute bronchitis. He was tested for allergies and demonstrated marked responses to a number of animals, pollens, and molds. BJ also has a history of asthma related to exposure to very cold weather.

a. Describe the pathophysiology of an acute asthma attack in BJ following exposure to cats.

b. Describe the early signs of an acute asthma attack and relate each of these to the changes taking place in the lungs.

c. If you were updating a medical and drug history for BJ, list several significant questions that should be asked.

d. Describe what precautions you would take if you were treating or dealing with BJ and include your reasons. Describe your actions if BJ had an attack while he was with you.

e. State and explain the effects of a prolonged asthma attack.

f. Explain the factors contributing to severe hypoxia and acidosis in a prolonged attack.

g. Define status asthmaticus.

h. Explain why BJ is likely to have frequent respiratory infections.

i. Suggest several measures that BJ can take to reduce anxiety and perhaps the risk of an asthma attack.

j. Explain how a beta$_2$-adrenergic agent is helpful in treating asthma and how it is usually administered.

CASE STUDY C
Emphysema

Mr. KY, age 71, has had significant emphysema for 6 years. He has reduced his cigarette smoking since mild congestive heart failure was diagnosed (right-sided heart failure—refer to Chapter 16). He has been admitted to the hospital with a suspected closed pneumothorax and respiratory failure.

a. Describe the pathophysiologic changes in the lungs with emphysema, and explain how these affect oxygen and carbon dioxide levels in the blood.

b. Explain the possible role of smoking in Mr. KY's case and its general effects on respiratory function (consider effects on cardiovascular function also).

c. What significant characteristics related to emphysema and heart failure would you expect to observe in Mr. KY?

d. Explain how a pneumothorax has probably occurred in the presence of emphysema.

e. Explain how a pneumothorax has precipitated respiratory failure, using the effects on lung function and gas exchange in your answer. Include the criteria for respiratory failure.

f. Explain why caution must be exercised in administering oxygen to Mr. KY.

g. Mr. KY is resting quietly. Suggest three complications of immobility that could develop in Mr. KY and one preventive measure that could be taken for each.

h. Explain how congestive heart failure develops from emphysema.

i. Describe respiratory therapy that might be helpful to Mr. KY.

With aggressive treatment, Mr. KY recovered and returned home.

j. Suggest some reasons why Mr. KY may not receive adequate nutrition and hydration at home.

k. Suggest other support measures that would be useful in this case.

CASE STUDY D
Cystic Fibrosis

MT, age 5 years, has cystic fibrosis, which was diagnosed following an intestinal obstruction after birth (meconium ileus). MT has frequent lung infections despite daily respiratory therapy. She is given pancrelipase with her meals and snacks to facilitate digestion and absorption. At a recent check-up, MT was found to be shorter and under the weight range for her age.

a. MT's parents would like to have another child. What is the probability that a future child would have cystic fibrosis? (Hint: What is the genetic status of each parent?)

b. Describe the basic pathophysiology of cystic fibrosis and briefly describe the various effects in the body.

c. Explain the possible effects on air flow of mucus obstructions in the lungs.

d. Explain why MT has frequent infections.

e. MT's parents are arranging a dental appointment for her. Describe any possible limitations in arranging the appointment and list what precautions should be taken when she arrives for the appointment.

f. State several criteria that would be helpful in maintaining adequate nutrition for MT.

g. If MT does not take pancrelipase regularly, she has steatorrhea (frequent loose, fatty stools). Explain why this occurs and how it might affect her respiratory function if prolonged.

h. Using your basic knowledge of physiology, describe the possible effects on MT if she fails to digest and absorb adequate amounts of protein, calcium, vitamin D, vitamin K, and iron.

i. Explain why MT is likely to develop bronchiectasis at a later time, and describe the significant signs of its development.

j. Explain why MT may have a fluid-electrolyte imbalance if she has a high fever with a lung infection.

STUDY QUESTIONS

1. Explain the purpose of the specialized cells in the respiratory mucosa.

2. (a) Describe the function of the external intercostal muscles. (b) Describe the mechanism of and the energy required for quiet expiration and for forced expiration.

3. (a) Describe the location of the chemoreceptors that respond to elevated carbon dioxide levels and those that respond to low oxygen levels. (b) Which gas creates the primary respiratory drive under normal circumstances?

4. State and explain the effect of increased carbon dioxide levels on serum pH.

5. (a) Describe how carbon dioxide is transported in the blood. (b) Name a gas that can displace oxygen from hemoglobin.

6. What physiologic compensations are available for chronic hypoxia due to respiratory impairment and for chronic hypercapnia?

7. Explain how respiratory infection can cause serious respiratory obstruction in a young child and include examples.

8. (a) Name the organisms that commonly cause primary atypical pneumonia. (b) Compare the pathophysiologic changes in viral and pneumococcal pneumonia.

9. (a) Explain the significance and limitations of a positive tuberculin test. (b) Explain the conditions under which tuberculosis may be contagious. (c) What measures can be taken by health professionals to minimize the spread of infection?

10. (a) Explain how obstruction develops with chronic bronchitis. (b) Explain how acute asthma causes air trapping or atelectasis. (c) How does hypoxia and respiratory alkalosis develop in the early stages of an asthma attack? (d) Explain why serum pH is lowered when an asthma attack persists.

11. (a) Explain why the anteroposterior diameter of the chest is increased in a patient with emphysema. (b) Explain why hypercapnia may be a major problem in patients with emphysema. (c) Explain how each of the following develops in patients with emphysema: (1) cor pulmonale, (2) secondary polycythemia.

12. (a) Define meconium ileus. (b) Describe the effects of cystic fibrosis on the lungs and on the liver. (c) Explain several ways whereby permanent damage can occur in the lungs and in the pancreas.

13. (a) Explain why the lung is a common site for secondary cancer. (b) State two systemic signs or symptoms of cancer, two local respiratory signs, and two signs related to paraneoplastic syndrome. (c) Explain why the prognosis for lung cancer is poor (include three factors).

14. (a) List three factors predisposing to aspiration. (b) Describe the potential effects of aspirating vomitus.

15. (a) Describe the factors predisposing to atelectasis following abdominal surgery. (b) Describe the signs of atelectasis.

16. (a) Explain why pulmonary edema causes severe hypoxia. (b) Trace the path of a pulmonary embolus resulting from thrombophlebitis. (c) Compare the effects on respiration of a very small embolus and of a very large one.

17. (a) Describe the effects of a large open pneumothorax on respiratory function and on cardiovascular function. (b) Explain how covering an open pneumothorax improves oxygen levels. (c) Explain a possible cause of increased respiratory distress following the covering of an open pneumothorax.

18. (a) Explain how paradoxical motion develops with a flail chest injury and how it causes hypoxemia. (b) Explain why atelectasis does not occur directly with a flail chest injury.

19. (a) Compare the causes of infant and adult respiratory distress syndromes. (b) Describe the signs of infant respiratory distress. (c) Describe the criteria for a diagnosis of respiratory failure.

KEY TERMS

• •

abscesses	emulsification	ileostomy	pruritus
active transport	epigastric	impaction	retroperitoneal
adhesions	erythema	leukocytosis	rugae
aspiration	exocrine	mastication	serous
autodigestion	fecalith	mediastinal	sinusoids
bolus	gangrenous	melena	splenomegaly
calculi	gastrectomy	mesentery	steatorrhea
carcinogenic	gluconeogenesis	metastatic	stenosis
carrier	glycogen	multiparity	stricture
cholestasis	hematemesis	necrosis	tenesmus
chyme	hepatocytes	occult	ulcerogenic
colostomy	hepatotoxin	osmosis	vesicle
defecation	histamine	parietal	
diffusion	hyperbilirubinemia	peristalsis	
dysplasia	icterus	phagocytose	

REVIEW OF THE DIGESTIVE SYSTEM

Structures and Their Functions

The digestive system, sometimes called the gastrointestinal tract, alimentary tract, or gut, consists of a very long hollow tube extending through the trunk of the body and its accessory structures, the salivary glands, the liver and gallbladder, and the pancreas (Fig. 18–1). Inside this tube, ingested food and fluid, along with secretions from various glands are efficiently processed. First they are broken down into their separate constituents, then the desired nutrients, water, and electrolytes are absorbed into the blood for use by the cells and waste elements are eliminated from the body. Within this system the liver can reassemble the component pieces into new materials as needed by the body. For example, the proteins in milk are digested by enzymes in the digestive tract, producing the component amino acids, which are then absorbed into the blood. The individual amino acids are then used by the liver cells to produce new proteins, such as albumin or prothrombin, or they may circulate as they are in the amino acid pool in the blood to be taken up by individual cells as necessary.

The digestive tract is divided into two sections, the *upper* tract consisting of the mouth, esophagus, and stomach, and the *lower* tract consisting of the intestines. Although variations occur along the tube, the wall basically has five continuous layers. The inner layer is the mucosa, which includes the important mucus-producing cells. *Mucus* protects the tissues and facilitates the passage of the contents along the tube. The

epithelial cells of the mucosa have a rapid turnover rate because of the "wear-and-tear" associated with the food and secretions passing along the tract. The *submucosal* layer is composed of connective tissue, including blood vessels, nerves, lymphatics, and secretory glands. Two *muscle* layers, consisting of circular and longitudinal smooth muscle fibers, are responsible for motility in the tract. The outer layer of the wall comprises the visceral peritoneum or *serosa*.

The *peritoneum* is a very large **serous** membrane in the abdominal cavity. The **parietal** peritoneum covers the abdominal wall and the superior surface of the urinary bladder and uterus, whereas the *visceral* peritoneum encases the organs such as the stomach and intestines. Pain receptors connected to spinal nerves are located in the parietal peritoneum. The *peritoneal cavity* refers to the *potential* space between the parietal and visceral peritoneum. A small amount of serous fluid is present in the cavity to facilitate the necessary movement of structures such as the stomach. Numerous lymphatic channels drain excessive fluid from the cavity. The **mesentery** is a double layer of peritoneum that supports the intestines and conveys blood vessels and nerves to supply the wall of the intestine. The mesentery attaches the jejunum and ileum to the posterior (dorsal) abdominal wall. This arrangement provides a balance between the need for support of the intestines and the need for considerable flexibility to accommodate **peristaltic** movements and varying amounts of content. Serous membranes are normally thin, somewhat permeable, and highly vascular. For this reason, the peritoneal membranes are very useful as an exchange site for blood during peritoneal dialysis in patients with kidney

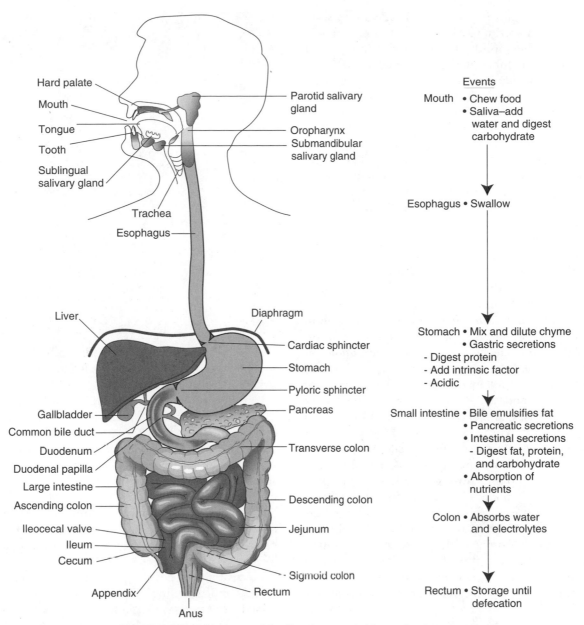

FIGURE 18-1. Anatomy of the digestive system with associated events.

failure (see Chapter 19). However, such an extensive membrane may also facilitate the spread of infection or malignant tumor cells through the abdominal cavity. The greater *omentum* is a layer of fatty peritoneum that hangs from the stomach like an apron over the anterior surface of the transverse colon and the small intestine. The lesser omentum is peritoneum that suspends the stomach and duodenum from the liver. When inflammation develops in the intestinal wall, the greater omentum with its many lymph nodes tends to adhere to the site, walling off the inflammation and temporarily localizing the source of the problem. Inflammation of the omentum and peritoneum may lead to scar tissue and the formation of **adhesions** between structures in the abdominal cavity such as loops of intestine, restricting motility and perhaps leading to obstruction. The

kidneys and pancreas are located posterior to the stomach against the abdominal wall and behind the parietal peritoneum. They are covered with peritoneum only on the anterior surface and are therefore referred to as **retroperitoneal.**

UPPER GASTROINTESTINAL TRACT

Food and fluid are taken into the body through the mouth, where the initial phase of mechanical breakdown and digestion takes place, and are then stored in the stomach where processing continues. The mouth is separated from the nasal cavity by the hard and soft palates. A large variety of microorganisms make up the resident flora of the mouth. In the mouth, or oral cavity (Fig. 18–2), **mastication** takes place as the teeth break down solid food and mix it with saliva. Salivary secretions from the parotid, sublingual, and submandibular glands enter the mouth through the salivary ducts, moisturizing and lubricating (with mucins) the food particles and facilitating the passage of solid material down the esophagus to the stomach. Saliva also contains the enzyme amylase, which begins the digestion of carbohydrate in the mouth (Table 18–1). Perhaps you have noted how chewing crackers can bring a sweet taste in the mouth as the starch is digested. The tongue and cheeks facilitate the movement and mixing of the food in the mouth. Chewing is usually considered a *voluntary* action, but reflex chewing can occur if voluntary control is lost. When food is ready to be swallowed, the tongue pushes the **bolus** of food back through the fauces (the passageway) to the pharyngeal wall, where receptors of the trigeminal and glossopharyngeal nerves relay the information to the swallowing center in the medulla. As the reflex is activated, *swallowing (or deglutition)* becomes an *involuntary* activity. The swallowing center coordinates the actions required to move food or fluid into the stomach, without **aspiration** into the lungs, by means of cranial nerves V, IX, X, and XII. The soft palate is pulled upward, the vocal cords are approximated, and the epiglottis covers the larynx. Respiration ceases, and the bolus is seized by the constricted pharynx. As the bolus of food moves into the esophagus, distending the wall, peristalsis is initiated, pushing the food down the esophagus. The distal part of the esophagus passes through the hiatus (opening) in the diaphragm to join the stomach in the abdominal cavity. The lower esophageal (gastroesophageal or cardiac) sphincter relaxes in advance of the bolus, allowing it to drop into the stomach. The pressure in this sphincter normally prevents reflux of gastric contents back up the esophagus. The esophagus is composed of skeletal muscle at the superior end that is gradually replaced by

TABLE 18–1 Major Digestive Enzymes and Their Actions

Enzyme	Source	Action
Salivary amylase	Parotid gland	Splits starch and glycogen into disaccharides
Pepsin	Gastric chief cells	Initiates splitting of proteins
Pancreatic amylase	Pancreas	Splits starch and glycogen into disaccharides
Pancreatic lipase	Pancreas	Splits triglycerides into fatty acids and mono-glycerides
Trypsin, chymo-trypsin carboxy-peptidase	Pancreas	Splits proteins into peptides
Pancreatic nucleases	Pancreas	Splits nucleic acids into nucleotides
Intestinal pepti-dase	Intestinal mucosa	Converts peptides into amino acids
Intestinal lipase	Intestinal mucosa	Converts fats into fatty acids and glycerol
Intestinal su-crase, maltase, lactase	Intestinal mucosa	Converts disaccharides into monosaccharides

smooth muscle fibers. The entire tube is lined with mucous membrane and is usually closed except when swallowing is in progress.

The stomach is an expansible muscular sac that acts as a reservoir for food and fluid. The outer surface is covered by visceral peritoneum. The stomach can hold 1.0 to 1.5 liters of food and fluid. When empty, the stomach wall falls into folds or **rugae.** The wall of the stomach consists of three smooth muscle layers—longitudinal, circular, and an additional oblique muscle layer—plus the mucosa and submucosa. The epithelial cells are tightly packed together to prevent penetration of acid or pepsin into the wall. Numerous glands are located in the mucosa, and there is a layer of thick protective mucus covering the inner surface. Constant mixing and churning of food occurs as secretions are added from the gastric glands. These secretions dilute the gastric contents, or **chyme,** and initiate the digestion of protein. The gastric glands located in the fundus of the stomach contain parietal cells that secrete *hydrochloric acid* and chief cells that secrete *pepsinogen,* which is converted to the active form, pepsin, by the action of hydrochloric acid. *Intrinsic factor,* required for the absorption of vitamin B_{12} in the ileum, is also produced by the parietal cells (see Chapter 16). The gastric secretions act as a defensive mechanism because of the highly acidic pH (around 2), which destroys many microorganisms that enter the stomach from the resident flora in the mouth or from food or utensils. Protective mucus is secreted by glands in the cardiac and pyloric areas. Also, enteroendocrine cells in the glands secrete a variety of chemicals, the most important of which is the hormone *gastrin,* which is released when food enters the stomach and then stimulates the parietal and chief cells. Depending to some extent on the type of food ingested,

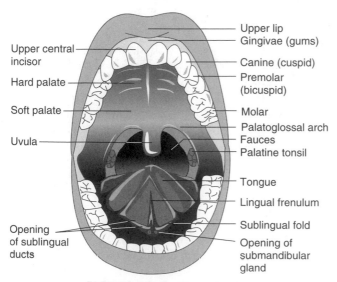

Upper lip
Gingivae (gums)
Canine (cuspid)
Premolar (bicuspid)
Molar
Palatoglossal arch
Fauces
Palatine tonsil
Tongue
Lingual frenulum
Sublingual fold
Opening of submandibular gland

Upper central incisor
Hard palate
Soft palate
Uvula
Opening of sublingual ducts

FIGURE 18–2. The oral cavity.

gastric emptying proceeds slowly, with small amounts of chyme (1 to 3 mL) passing intermittently through the pyloric sphincter into the duodenum.

LIVER

Secretions from the liver and the **exocrine** pancreas are added to the chyme in the duodenum through the ampulla of Vater and duodenal papilla (see Fig. 18–9). The **hepatocytes** of the liver constantly produce bile, a mixture of water, bile salts, bile pigment (conjugated bilirubin), cholesterol, and electrolytes including bicarbonate ions. The bile salts, formed from cholesterol, are essential for the **emulsification** of fats and fat-soluble vitamins (vitamins A, D, E, and K) before they are absorbed from the intestine. The majority of the bile salts are reabsorbed from the distal ileum and recycled to the liver through the enterohepatic circulation. Bicarbonate ions in bile assist in neutralizing gastric acid, increasing the pH of the small intestine so that intestinal and pancreatic enzymes can function. Bile produced by the hepatocytes flows through small canaliculi, draining into larger ducts until it reaches the right or left hepatic duct and then the common bile duct. The sphincter of Boyden usually directs the flow of bile into the gallbladder for storage but may allow it to flow onward into the duodenum. Following removal of the gallbladder, the storage facility is lost, but bile is secreted by the liver and small amounts continuously enter the duodenum.

The liver is a large organ covered by a fibrous capsule, distention of which causes a dull aching pain. The hepatocytes are arranged in lobules, and each lobule has plates of cells radiating from central veins, which eventually drain blood into the hepatic veins and inferior vena cava (see Fig. 18–11). The hepatocytes are supplied by blood from branches of the hepatic artery, carrying oxygen to the liver cells, and blood from the portal vein, which transports nutrients absorbed from the stomach and intestines (hepatic portal circulation) as well as venous blood from the pancreas and spleen. The blood from these two sources mixes in the **sinusoids,** channels passing between the plates of hepatocytes. The sinusoids are lined with endothelial cells and Kupffer's cells, which remove and **phagocytose** any foreign material and bacteria from the digestive tract before the blood enters the general circulation. The liver cells can regenerate, but if the organizational structure of the lobule with its unique arrangement of blood vessels and bile ducts is altered by necrosis and scar tissue, the regenerated areas may not be functional.

The liver is located in the upper right quadrant under the diaphragm and serves as the "metabolic factory" of the body. As blood flows through the sinusoids, absorbed nutrients may be taken up by the hepatocytes to be stored (e.g., the minerals iron and copper or vitamins A, B_6, B_{12}, folic acid, D, and K) or to be used in synthesizing other materials such as plasma proteins, blood-clotting factors, or lipoproteins. At the same time, the hepatocytes monitor many blood components such as glucose, iron, or amino acids, replacing those that have been depleted as the blood circulates through the body. An important function of the liver involves maintenance of blood glucose levels, glucose being essential for brain function. In conjunction with the hormone insulin, the liver responds to high blood glucose levels by converting glucose to **glycogen** (glycogenesis), which is stored in the liver. Alternatively, the hepatocytes break down liver glycogen to glucose (glycogenolysis) when blood glucose levels drop, stimulating glucagon secretion. **Gluconeogenesis**, the conversion of protein and fat into glucose, may take place when blood glucose levels drop, under the influence of hormones such as cortisol or epinephrine. The liver is also responsible for other metabolic activities such as the conversion of one amino acid into another, for use by various cells.

Other functions of the liver include inactivation of hormones, such as aldosterone and estrogen, and detoxification of drugs and alcohol before excretion. The detoxification process makes such substances less harmful and increases the solubility of many substances, facilitating their excretion. For example, ammonia, a nitrogen waste resulting from protein metabolism in the liver or in the intestine (from the normal bacterial action on amino acids) is converted into urea in the liver and is then excreted by the kidneys. Cholesterol is synthesized in the liver and is used in the production of steroid hormones such as cortisol or the sex hormones and bile salts. The liver is one of the sites where damaged or old erythrocytes are removed from the blood to facilitate the recycling of iron and protein from the hemoglobin (see Figs. 16–8 and 18–12). In addition, the hepatocytes secrete bile, which is vital for digestion and serves as a vehicle for the removal of bilirubin and excess cholesterol. The liver also serves as a blood reservoir because it is capable of releasing a large quantity of blood into the general circulation when blood volume is depleted.

PANCREAS

The pancreas lies posterior to the stomach with its head adjacent to the duodenum. The cells of the exocrine pancreas are arranged in lobules throughout the organ; they secrete digestive enzymes, electrolytes, and water into tiny ducts, which eventually drain into the main pancreatic duct that traverses the length of the pancreas. The pancreatic duct, carrying secretions from the exocrine pancreas, joins the common bile duct and then enters the duodenum. The major proteolytic enzymes in pancreatic secretions are trypsin and chymo-trypsin, carboxypeptidase, and ribonuclease (see Table 18–1). Also, pancreatic amylase aids in the digestion of carbohydrate, and lipase helps to digest fats. The enzymes are secreted in inactive form and are activated after they enter the duodenum. A trypsin inhibitor is produced by the pancreatic cells to reduce the risk of enzyme activation within the pancreas. Pancreatic secretions also contain bicarbonate ion, which assists in the neutralization of hydrochloric acid in the duodenum.

LOWER GASTROINTESTINAL TRACT

The small intestine has three sections, the duodenum, the jejunum, and the ileum, moving in a proximal to distal direction. The contents move slowly along the tube, influenced by both mixing and propulsive movements of the wall. Digestion continues in the duodenum as many enzymes are added to the chyme, and an alkaline pH is attained. The ileum is the major site of absorption of nutrients. The significant feature of the small intestine is the presence of plicae circulares, transverse folds of the mucosa covered with *villi* and *microvilli*. These numerous tiny projections greatly increase the absorptive surface area of the small intestine. Each villus is supplied with a capillary network, nerves, and a lacteal, a terminal lymphatic vessel that is essential for the absorption of lipids. At the base of the villi are the intestinal crypts, deep pockets from which new epithelial (simple columnar absorptive cells) cells arise. Cells in the crypts produce fluid with a pH of around 7, enzymes such as enterokinase, which activate pancreatic proenzymes, and hormones such as cholecystokinin. Other enzymes produced by the cells of the intestinal mucosa include peptidases, nucleosidases, lipase, sucrase, maltase, and lactase. Many goblet cells in the mucosa secrete large quantities of mucus into the intestine to protect the intestinal wall and to buffer the acid chyme.

The ileocecal valve marks the entry point from the ileum into the large intestine or colon. Hanging down at this point is a pouch, the cecum, from which the blind-ending appendix (vermiform appendix) extends. Moving superiorly from the cecum is the ascending colon, which becomes the transverse colon and then passes down the left side as the descending colon. This structure terminates as the sigmoid colon, rectum, and anal canal. The anus is the opening to the exterior. Absorption of large amounts of water and electrolytes takes place in the colon. This "recycling" process is of critical importance in maintaining the fluid and acid-base balances in the body because large volumes of fluids and ions such as bicarbonate and sodium are recovered from the added secretions as well as from ingested fluids. Large pouches or haustra in the colon wall allow for expansion as more solid material collects. General digestion and absorption of nutrients ceases in the colon. Resident bacteria assist in further breakdown of certain food materials (which is one cause of intestinal gas) and convert bilirubin to urobilinogen, which gives the feces the typical brown color. In the ileum, large masses of lymphoid tissue, called Peyer's patches, limit the spread of these bacteria into the small intestine. Some of these bacteria are beneficial to the human host, synthesizing vitamin K, for example, which is required for the production of clotting factors such as prothrombin and fibrinogen in the liver.

Colonic movements are slow to allow absorption of fluid and formation of the solid feces. The transverse and descending colon are marked by *mass movements*, strong peristaltic contractions that occur several times daily. Feces consists primarily of fiber and other indigestible material as well as sloughed mucosal cells and bacteria. Increased bulk or fiber in the intestine increases intestinal motility and the rate of passage, leading to a larger fecal mass and thus, more frequent **defecation,** or bowel movements. The rectum stores the solid feces until sufficient distention of the rectal wall stimulates the *defecation reflex*. Sensory nerve impulses from the stretch receptors are transmitted to the sacral spinal cord. The sacral parasympathetic nerves transmit motor impulses, which stimulate peristalsis and relax the internal anal sphincter. Pelvic muscles contract and voluntary relaxation of the external anal sphincter allows defecation to occur. If, under voluntary control, the external anal sphincter remains closed, the defecation reflex subsides temporarily. Elimination of feces can be assisted by increasing intra-abdominal pressure through voluntary contraction of the abdominal muscles and the diaphragm.

Thinkabout 18–1

a. Describe the purpose of mastication.

b. Where are carbohydrates digested? Name the enzymes responsible.

c. Explain why the liver receives blood from two sources.

d. State the likely times of glycogenolysis or glycogenesis relative to food intake or lack of intake.

e. Explain why the contents of the small intestine are relatively liquid and the contents of the descending colon are solid.

f. Describe one unique feature and the purpose of each of the following structures: mouth, stomach, small intestine, pancreas, and rectum.

g. Describe the benefits of mucus in the digestive tract.

Neural and Hormonal Controls

Stimulation of the *parasympathetic nervous system* (PNS), primarily through the vagus nerve (cranial nerve X), results in *increased motility* or peristalsis and *increased secretions* in the digestive system (Table 18–2; see also Chapter 20). During the initial cephalic phase before eating, pleasant smells, thoughts, or the sight of food can effect PNS stimulation. Conversely, emotions such as fear or anger stimulate the sympathetic nervous system (SNS), which inhibits gastrointestinal activity. SNS activity also causes vasoconstriction, leading to reduced secretions and regeneration of epithelial cells. The PNS through the facial (cranial nerve VII) and glossopharyngeal (cranial nerve IX) nerves maintains a continuous flow of saliva in the mouth, which is essential to keep the tissues moist and facilitates speech. A dry mouth for any reason leads to a sensation of thirst, a protection against dehydration. The sight, thought, or presence of food in the mouth stimulates increased salivary secretions, and these secretions usually continue for a time after swallowing, which is helpful in cleansing the mouth and teeth.

When food reaches the stomach, distention or stretching of the stomach and the increased pH associated with food intake activate the PNS, increasing peristalsis and gastric secretions. PNS stimulation also increases bile and pancreatic secretions. As digestion in the stomach progresses, peristaltic movements force very small amounts of chyme, 2 to 3 mL at a time, into the duodenum. Depending on the amount and type food involved, the stomach empties within 2 to 6 hours after a meal. Fluids pass through rapidly, whereas fats progress very slowly. The presence of food in the intestine stimulates intestinal activity but inhibits gastric activity through the *enterogastric reflex* to prevent overloading of the duodenum and to allow sufficient time for intestinal digestion and absorption. Food passes through the small intestine at a fairly constant rate. After eating there is a reflex increase in peristalsis around the ileocecal valve, which moves the ileal contents into the cecum and colon. Peristaltic movements in the colon are usually slow. The gastrocolic reflex stimulates a mass movement of the contents from the colon into the rectum when food enters the stomach.

Hormones play a major role in the process of digestion and absorption (see Table 18–2). *Gastrin* is secreted by mucosal cells in the pyloric antrum of the stomach in response to distention of the stomach or the presence of substances such as partially digested protein, alcohol, or caffeine in the stomach. Gastrin enters the blood and circulates, returning to stimulate the gastric cells to increase secretions, increase gastric motility, and relax the pyloric and ileocecal sphincters, thus promoting stomach emptying. In the presence of the chemical **histamine,** which is released from local mast cells, stimulation of the parietal cells by the PNS or gastrin leads to increased secretion of hydrochloric acid. Note that the histamine receptors on parietal cells are H_2 receptors, which differ from the H_1 receptors on cells involved in allergic responses. When chyme enters the duodenum, mucosal cells release hormones, two important ones being secretin and cholecystokinin (CCK). *Secretin* decreases gastric secretions and increases the bicarbonate ion content of pancreatic secretions and bile when the chyme is highly acidic. *CCK* inhibits gastric emptying, stimulates pancreatic secretions with increased digestive enzymes, and stimulates contraction of the gallbladder to increase bile flow into the duodenum. Variations in the digestive secretions and the rate of flow of chyme through the tract depend on the amount and type of food entering the digestive tract. For example, gastric emptying is delayed when the duodenum is full or when a meal high in fat content is ingested.

TABLE 18–2 Major Controls in the Digestive Tract and Their Effects

Hormone	Source	Stimulus	Effects
Gastrin	Gastric cells	Food in the stomach Protein, caffeine, or high pH of chyme	Increases gastric secretions and motility Promotes gastric emptying
Cholecystokinin	Intestinal mucosal cells	Protein and fat in the duodenum	Inhibits gastric secretions and motility, stimulates pancreatic enzyme secretion, stimulates gallbladder contractions and release of bile
Secretin	Intestinal mucosal cells	Acidic chyme in the duodenum	Stimulates bile and pancreatic secretions with high bicarbonate content
Neural controls			
Parasympathetic nervous system			Increases secretions and peristalsis
Sympathetic nervous system			Decreases secretions and peristalsis Stimulates vasoconstriction in the mucosa

Digestion and Absorption

Nutrients are broken down chemically into simple molecules that are absorbed along with electrolytes and water into the blood and transported to the liver through the hepatic portal system. Complex *carbohydrates* such as starches are digested first in the mouth and then in the intestine. They are broken down by enzymes into simple sugars (monosaccharides) such as glucose or fructose that are absorbed by **active transport** or facilitated **diffusion** in the intestine, primarily in the jejunum and ileum. The process of active transport requires cellular energy (adenosine triphosphate [ATP]) and a carrier molecule and therefore healthy cells with a good blood supply. On occasion, when a highly concentrated solution of glucose enters an empty stomach, glucose may diffuse quickly from the stomach into the blood. This rapid action can be effective in reversing hypoglycemia in a person with diabetes mellitus.

Proteins are first split into peptides or short chains of amino acids in the stomach and intestine and then further broken down by peptidases into amino acids, which are absorbed by active transport. *Lipids,* or *fats,* primarily triglycerides, must first be emulsified (dispersed into tiny droplets) by bile (the bile salt component) in the intestine; enzymes then act on them, forming monoglycerides and free fatty acids. These lipid-soluble molecules can diffuse across the cell membrane. Many recombine to form triglycerides again. Then, bound to protein, the lipids form chylomicrons, most of which diffuse into the lacteals or lymph capillaries in the microvilli. The lacteals join the lymphatic circulation, which eventually empties into the general circulation. Eventually the lipids reach the liver or adipose cells. Short-chain fatty acids may diffuse directly into the blood.

Fat-soluble vitamins (e.g., vitamins A, D, E, and K) or other lipid-soluble materials do not require digestion but are absorbed with the fats. If for any reason lipids are not absorbed, large molecules such as fat-soluble vitamins cannot be absorbed. Very small lipid-soluble molecules such as alcohol may be absorbed from the empty stomach into the blood by simple diffusion through the cell membranes. This may promote a high blood alcohol level within a short time following ingestion. The presence of food in the stomach delays such absorption. *Water-soluble vitamins* (e.g., vitamins B and C) and *minerals* (e.g., iron, copper, and zinc) diffuse into the blood. Vitamin B_{12} must be bound to intrinsic factor before absorption. *Electrolytes* (Na^+, K^+, Cl^-, HCO_3^-, and so on) may be absorbed by active transport or diffusion into the blood. *Water* is absorbed by osmosis. About 7000 mL of water is secreted into the digestive tract each day, and approximately 2300 mL is ingested in food and fluids. Of this amount, only 50 to 200 mL leaves the body in the feces. It is obvious that severe vomiting or diarrhea can quickly interrupt the recycling mechanism and affect fluid and electrolyte balance in the body. Drugs are primarily absorbed in the intestine, although some small acidic molecules such as aspirin may be absorbed in the stomach.

Thinkabout 18–2

a. Describe how the PNS affects the digestive tract, and name the major nerve responsible.

b. Give two reasons why it is important to control the rate of flow of chyme through the digestive tract.

c. State the source and purpose of gastrin.

d. State the final form in which carbohydrate and protein is absorbed into the blood.

e. Describe three general ways in which absorption of nutrients could be impaired.

COMMON MANIFESTATIONS OF DIGESTIVE SYSTEM DISORDERS

Anorexia, Nausea, and Vomiting

The manifestations of anorexia, nausea, and vomiting may be signs of digestive system disorders or of other conditions elsewhere in the body. For example, systemic infection, uremia (kidney failure), emotional responses such as fear, motion sickness, pressure in the brain, overindulgence in food, drugs, or pain may initiate these signs. However, nausea and vomiting are common indicators of gastrointestinal disorders, and the characteristics of the vomitus and the vomiting pattern can be helpful in diagnosis. Vomiting is also considered a body defense because it removes noxious substances from the body. Also, anorexia and vomiting can contribute to complications such as dehydration, alkalosis or acidosis, and malnutrition. Anorexia (loss of appetite) often precedes nausea and vomiting. Nausea is a generally unpleasant subjective feeling, which may be stimulated by distention, irritation, or inflammation in the digestive tract. Often, increased salivation, pallor, sweating, and tachycardia may occur with nausea and vomiting. Vomiting, or emesis, is the forceful expulsion of chyme from the stomach and sometimes from the intestine. The vomiting center in the medulla coordinates the activities involved in vomiting (Fig. 18–3). The vomiting center may be activated by distention or irritation in the digestive tract, by stimuli from various parts of the brain in response to unpleasant sights or smells, pain, or

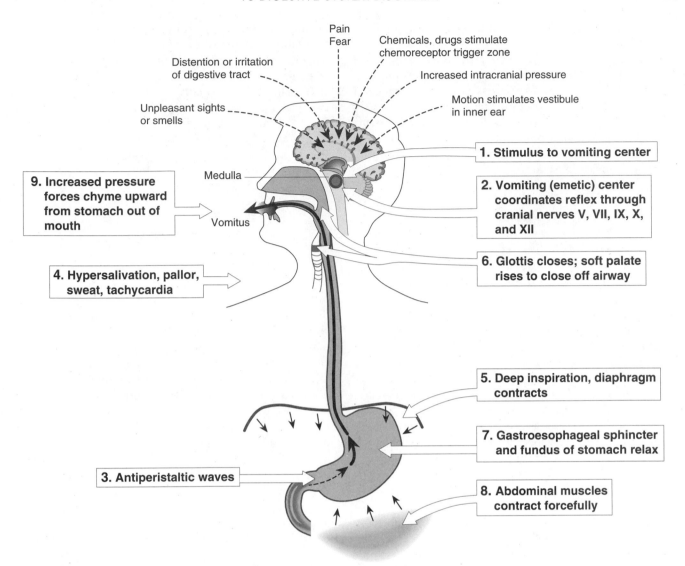

Pain
Fear

Chemicals, drugs stimulate
chemoreceptor trigger zone

Distention or irritation
of digestive tract

Increased intracranial pressure

Unpleasant sights
or smells

Motion stimulates vestibule
in inner ear

Medulla

1. Stimulus to vomiting center

**9. Increased pressure
forces chyme upward
from stomach out of
mouth**

Vomitus

**2. Vomiting (emetic) center
coordinates reflex through
cranial nerves V, VII, IX, X,
and XII**

**6. Glottis closes; soft palate
rises to close off airway**

**4. Hypersalivation, pallor,
sweat, tachycardia**

**5. Deep inspiration, diaphragm
contracts**

**7. Gastroesophageal sphincter
and fundus of stomach relax**

3. Antiperistaltic waves

**8. Abdominal muscles
contract forcefully**

FIGURE 18–3. The vomiting or emetic reflex.

ischemia, or by the vestibular apparatus of the inner ear (motion sickness). Sudden *projectile* vomiting without prior nausea or food intake may be associated with increased intracranial pressure (see Chapter 20). The chemoreceptor trigger zone in the medulla is stimulated by many drugs, toxins, and chemicals. Drugs may also cause vomiting by direct irritation of the digestive mucosa. Toxins may result from infecting microorganisms anywhere in the body. Toxic chemicals may be endogenous, as in kidney failure, or exogenous (from external sources).

The *vomiting reflex* includes taking a deep breath, closing the glottis and raising the soft palate, then ceasing respiration. This minimizes the risk of aspiration of vomitus into the lungs, where it may cause significant inflammation and obstruction of the airways. The gastroesophageal sphincter relaxes, and a strong contraction of the abdominal muscles squeezes the stomach against the diaphragm and forces the

gastric contents upward and out of the mouth. Reverse peristaltic waves in the proximal duodenum and antrum of the stomach promote expulsion of the contents. Retching may precede vomiting and involves the same reflex, but the chyme ascends in the esophagus and then falls back into the stomach. This process may take place several times before complete vomiting occurs. Recurrent vomiting can be exhausting and painful because the strong muscle contractions continue with each episode and the source of renewed energy—food—is not available. There is an increased risk of aspiration when the person is supine or unconscious or when the vomiting reflex is depressed by drugs because the vomitus may not be completely expelled. Also, the cough reflex may be suppressed. This is a common problem with postoperative vomiting or following heavy alcohol intake.

The characteristics of vomitus can be significant. The presence of blood leads to "coffee grounds" vomitus or

hematemesis, a brown, granular material resulting from the partial digestion in the stomach of protein in the blood. Blood, as a "foreign material," is irritating to the gastric mucosa. Yellow-stained vomitus often represents bile from the duodenum, whereas a deeper brown color may indicate content from the lower intestine, typical of recurrent vomiting in persons with intestinal obstruction. Recurrent vomiting of undigested food from previous meals indicates a problem with gastric emptying such as pyloric obstruction.

Diarrhea

Diarrhea is an excessive frequency of stools, usually of loose or watery consistency, and may be acute or chronic. The presence of blood, mucus, or pus in the stool may be helpful in diagnosing or monitoring a disease. Diarrhea is frequently associated with nausea and vomiting when infection or inflammation of the digestive tract develops, but in other cases it occurs alone. Often, diarrhea is accompanied by cramping pain. Large-volume diarrhea (secretory or osmotic) leads to a watery stool, resulting from increased secretions into the intestine. This type of diarrhea is often related to infections or to a rapid transit time, which limits reabsorption or increased osmotic pressure of the intestinal contents, causing them to retain water. A common cause of osmotic diarrhea is lactose intolerance, in which lactose remains undigested and unabsorbed inside the intestine, thereby increasing the osmotic pressure of the contents. Small-volume diarrhea often occurs in people with inflammatory bowel disease, and the stool may contain blood, mucus, or pus. The diarrhea may be accompanied by abdominal cramps and urgency. The differentiation between the two types of diarrhea is not always marked. Severe or prolonged diarrhea may lead to dehydration, electrolyte imbalance, and acidosis as well as malnutrition.

Steatorrhea is "fatty diarrhea," marked by frequent bulky, greasy, loose stools, often with a foul odor. These stools are associated with malabsorption syndromes such as celiac disease or cystic fibrosis, in which the food intake is not digested or absorbed. Fat is usually the first dietary component affected, and the presence of fat interferes with the digestion of other nutrients. The abdomen is often distended because of the bulk remaining in the intestines. Malnutrition is apparent in other tissues unless disguised by edema in these tissues due to hypoproteinemia.

Blood may occur in a normal stool or with diarrhea or constipation. *Frank* blood appears red because it has not been "digested" and usually results from lesions in the rectum or anal canal. **Melena** is a dark stool resulting from bleeding that has occurred higher in the digestive tract; the hemoglobin has been acted on by intestinal bacteria, providing the dark color. **Occult** blood refers to small, hidden amounts of blood that are not visible to the eye but are detectable on tests of a stool specimen (e.g., the guaiac test).

Gas develops normally in the digestive tract from swallowed air and digestive and bacterial action on food. Certain foods or alterations in motility also promote gas production. Excessive gas may become manifest as belching (expulsion through the mouth), abdominal distention and discomfort, or flatus (expulsion through the anus).

Constipation

Constipation refers to less frequent bowel movements with the passage of small hard stools. Bowel patterns differ with individuals, depending on factors such as diet and activity, and therefore abnormalities are related to the individual's normal pattern. Constipation may be an acute or chronic problem. In some individuals, periods of constipation may alternate with periods of diarrhea. In these cases, emptying of the bowel with diarrhea may lead to decreased peristalsis, which results in increased time available for reabsorption of fluid, leading to dry, hard feces. This dry mass then irritates the intestinal mucosa, leading to inflammation and increased secretions. Once the hard feces has been expelled, a period of diarrhea may follow.

Causes of constipation include inadequate dietary fiber, leading to inadequate bulk in the intestine and decreased peristalsis, inadequate fluid intake, failure to respond to the defecation reflex because of pain or timing, and muscle weakness and inactivity, which impede defecation. There are many other contributing factors. Neurologic disorders such as multiple sclerosis or spinal cord trauma predispose the individual to constipation. Drugs such as opiates (e.g., codeine) or anticholinergics (drugs that block the PNS) slow peristalsis. Obstruction due to tumors may delay passage and cause excessive reabsorption of fluid. Some antacids, iron medications, and bulk laxatives can predispose to constipation. Chronic constipation may lead to the development of hemorrhoids or diverticulitis. Severe constipation can lead to fecal impaction (retention of feces in the rectum and colon) and intestinal obstruction, usually indicated by pain and abdominal distention. In some cases, watery diarrhea masks a fecal impaction because fluid pushes past a well-lodged fecal plug.

Fluid and Electrolyte Imbalances

Dehydration and *hypovolemia* are common complications of digestive tract disorders. When vomiting and diarrhea occur, perhaps combined with insufficient fluid intake, fluid shifts from the blood into the digestive tract. If the loss persists, eventually intracellular fluid is decreased (see Chapter 6). Hypovolemia with impaired circulation and cellular dehydration may cause decreased function in all tissues and organs. Infants and the elderly are particularly vulnerable to losses incurred with vomiting and diarrhea because of the unique proportions and distribution of fluid in the body in these age groups and the decreased ability of the kidneys to compensate quickly for losses.

Electrolytes such as sodium are lost with both vomiting and diarrhea because both mucous and enzyme secretions contain large amounts of electrolytes. Gastric secretions are high in chloride ion. Diarrhea leads to significant losses of potassium ion. The effects of these imbalances may be reviewed in Chapter 6.

Acid-base imbalances are common with vomiting and diarrhea. Initially, vomiting leads to loss of hydrochloric acid, resulting in *metabolic alkalosis* due to loss of hydrogen ion and hypochloremia with increased serum bicarbonate levels (see Chapter 6). If vomiting is severe, there is a change to *metabolic acidosis*. Duodenal secretions containing large quantities of bicarbonate ion are lost, ketoacidosis develops owing to a glucose deficit, and lactic acid accumulates owing to hypovolemia and impaired tissue perfusion as well as increased muscle activity, all leading to acidosis. Metabolic acidosis also accompanies diarrhea because of heavy loss of bicarbonate ions in the stool and lack of absorption of fluid and glucose. The accompanying dehydration may limit the ability of the kidneys to respond to acidosis, leading to decompensation.

Thinkabout 18–3

a. List three specific causes of vomiting, including a variety of factors.

b. Describe the specific actions of the vomiting reflex that prevent aspiration.

c. Explain which arterial blood gases would be expected (1) in the early stage of vomiting, and (2) with diarrhea.

Pain

Many descriptors may be used for pain occurring with digestive tract disorders. A burning sensation frequently accompanies inflammation and ulceration in the upper digestive tract that is related to oral ulcerations when in the mouth or heartburn when substernal. Stretching of the liver capsule with swelling leads to a dull aching pain in the right upper quadrant. Cramping or diffuse pain is commonly associated with inflammation or distention or stretching of the intestines. Colicky and often severe pain results from recurrent smooth muscle spasm or contraction and occurs in response to severe inflammation or obstruction, for example, when the system attempts to propel an obstructing gallstone through the bile duct. These are all examples of visceral pain that arises from the organs in the digestive system and is often difficult to localize. Because these pain fibers are connected to the autonomic nervous system, autonomic responses such as pallor and sweating or nausea and vomiting frequently accompany this type of pain. Somatic pain is characterized by a steady, intense, often well-localized abdominal pain, which indicates involvement or inflammation of the parietal peritoneum. Somatic pain receptors are directly linked to spinal nerves and may cause a reflex spasm of the overlying abdominal muscles, which leads to a rigid abdomen or guarding. Referred pain is a common problem and may delay diagnosis because the source of the pain is perceived as a site distant from its origin. Referred pain results when visceral and somatic nerves converge at one spinal cord level, and the source of the visceral pain is then perceived as the same as that of the somatic nerve. Common sites of referred pain are seen in Figure 13–3.

Malnutrition

Nutritional deficits may be partial or general and have many causes related to gastrointestinal function. There may be a specific problem such as a vitamin B_{12} deficiency linked to a lack of intrinsic factor from the gastric mucosa. Iron deficiency may be caused by malabsorption, liver damage, or a bleeding ulcer. General malnutrition may result from chronic anorexia, vomiting, or diarrhea related to gastrointestinal malfunction or other systemic causes. For example, chronic inflammatory bowel disorders may cause anorexia, diarrhea, and malabsorption, or vomiting and diarrhea may be related to external factors such as cancer treatments (radiation and chemotherapy). "Wasting syndrome," or chronic diarrhea associated with acquired immune deficiency syndrome (AIDS), leads to malnutrition and dehydration. Interference with bile and pancreatic secretions by mucus plugs in persons with cystic fibrosis is another example of a systemic disease that may lead to malabsorption and malnutrition. In a child, growth and development may be delayed or impaired by malabsorption or malnutrition. At any stage, the outcomes include chronic fatigue, reduced resistance to infection, and impaired healing.

BASIC DIAGNOSTIC TESTS

Radiographs are useful diagnostic tools in digestive system disorders. X-ray films, often using a contrast medium such as barium (swallow or enema), are useful in outlining many gastrointestinal system structures and abnormalities, and ultrasound may demonstrate unusual masses. Computed tomography (CT) scans and magnetic resonance imaging (MRI) can be used to check liver and pancreatic abnormalities. Radioactive elements may be used to make tracer studies. Techniques such as fiberoptic endoscopy allow improved visualization or biopsy of various segments of the digestive tract, such as the esophagus.

Analysis of stool specimens or gastric washings can provide evidence of infection, bleeding, tumors, or malabsorption problems. Blood tests can be used to check liver function by evaluating serum protein levels, clotting times, serum liver enzymes, and bilirubin levels. Pancreatic problems may be detected by serum enzyme levels as well as stool analysis for enzymes and fat content. Blood tests can also be used to monitor tumor markers, for example, carcinoembryonic antigen (CEA) in patients with colon cancer, although these tests cannot stand alone as diagnostic tools or monitoring devices.

COMMON THERAPIES

Many digestive tract disorders require a team approach to assist with the many facets of the disease. *Dietary modifications* are helpful in the treatment of many gastrointestinal disorders. For example, a gluten-free diet is recommended for people with celiac disease, thus removing the source of the problem. Reduced intake of alcohol and coffee (caffeine) may promote the healing of ulcers, and increased fiber and fluid content may reduce constipation or minimize the risk of colon cancer. Limited fat content but increased caloric intake and vitamin supplements are recommended for patients with many malabsorption syndromes. When exacerbations have been shown to be stress-related, *stress reduction* techniques are useful in many patients with peptic ulcer or chronic inflammatory bowel disorders. These techniques are also very important in the treatment of adolescents or teenagers with digestive tract disorders because their social activities and body image may be affected by the disease. Severe or prolonged stress, whether resulting from a physical stressor such as infection or trauma or an emotional stressor such as fear or anger, does affect the digestive tract. These effects result from stimulation of the SNS, leading to vasoconstriction and possible ischemia of the mucosa, with subsequent inflammation and ulceration. Also, SNS stimulation decreases peristal-

sis, leading to prolonged contact of secretions and irritants with the mucosa. The stress response also promotes glucocorticoid secretion, which has catabolic effects if it is continued over a long term. High cortisol levels lead to reduced regeneration of the mucosa and delayed healing of any lesions. And a stressful environment predisposes the individual to poor nutritional habits, such as increased caffeine intake and indulgence in snack foods.

Drugs are used to treat many gastrointestinal disorders, and a great variety of medications are available, given the diversity of gastrointestinal problems. Many individuals treat themselves for minor digestive discomfort. It is always important to check specifically on self-prescribed medications when taking a patient history because many individuals do not think that over-the-counter drugs are of any importance. Such medications may mask signs of disease or may be the cause of a problem. If possible, it is better to identify and treat the cause of a problem rather than only the symptoms. Antacids are a common medication used for many purposes. The primary component of antacids is usually calcium carbonate, aluminum hydroxide, magnesium hydroxide, or a combination of these. Antiemetics, taken to relieve vomiting, include drugs such as dimenhydrinate (Gravol) or phenothiazines such as prochlorperazine (Compazine). Cannabinoids such as nabilone may be a successful antiemetic for cancer chemotherapy–induced vomiting. Acute constipation is treated with laxatives or enemas, of which there are many types. Bulk supplements (e.g., psyllium hydrophilic mucilloid [Metamucil]) or stool softeners (e.g., docusate sodium [Colace]) are most helpful particularly for recurrent constipation and are less likely to cause adverse effects than other laxatives. Chronic constipation is best treated by the addition of fiber and fluid to the diet, rather than persistent use of laxatives that may aggravate the problem. If diarrhea is not relieved by dietary changes, loperamide or narcotics such as codeine may reduce peristalsis and relieve cramps. Infections causing diarrhea are frequently self-limiting, but specific antimicrobial drugs may be required in some cases. Drugs such as sulfasalazine, an antibacterial and anti-inflammatory agent, may be used to treat acute episodes of inflammatory bowel disease. Anticholinergic drugs reduce PNS activity and may be used to reduce secretions and motility. Examples include pirenzepine, which inhibits gastric acid, and propantheline, which decreases gastrointestinal motility and spasm as well as gastric acid. Frequently used drugs whose purpose is to reduce gastric secretions include the histamine (H_2 receptor) antagonist group, which includes cimetidine. Trimebutine regulates abnormal intestinal motility and is useful for spastic colon (excessive activity) and paralytic ileus (insufficient activity).

Thinkabout 18-4

a. Describe and state the mechanism of (1) referred pain, and (2) colicky pain.

b. Describe the vomiting reflex, noting possible causes of aspiration during vomiting.

c. Explain why altered blood clotting times and serum protein levels may indicate the presence of liver disease.

d. Explain two ways in which severe or prolonged stress may contribute to ulcer formation in the digestive tract.

e. Explain how regular use of bulk laxatives can promote peristalsis and relieve constipation.

UPPER GASTROINTESTINAL TRACT DISORDERS

Disorders of the Oral Cavity

CONGENITAL DEFECTS

Cleft lip and cleft palate are common developmental abnormalities of the mouth and face and arise in the second or third month of gestation (Fig. 18–4). One or both defects may be present in various degrees of severity. Cleft lip, which may be unilateral or bilateral (on either side of the midline), results from failure of the maxillary processes to fuse with the nasal elevations or failure of the upper lip to fuse at some time between 4 and 8 weeks of fetal development. Cleft palate involves failure of the hard and soft palates to fuse between 7 and 12 weeks of gestation, creating an opening between the oral cavity and the nasal cavity. The infant has feeding problems because insufficient force can be developed in the mouth to suck, and the risk of aspirating fluid into the respiratory passages is high. Cleft lip and cleft palate appear to be multifactorial in origin and are related to a number of inherited as well as environmental factors. Surgical repair of the defect is necessary, followed by therapy as needed by a speech therapist or orthodontist. A multidisciplinary team is frequently required for a prolonged period when major clefts are present.

INFLAMMATORY LESIONS

Aphthous ulcers (aphthous stomatitis or canker sores) are a common problem. A member of the normal flora of the oral cavity, *Streptococcus sanguis*, may be involved.

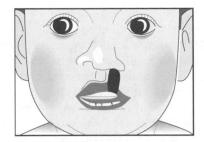

A Unilateral cleft lip
(complete)

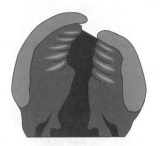

B Unilateral cleft palate and lip
(complete)

FIGURE 18–4. Cleft lip *(A)* and palate *(B)*.

These ulcers often accompany fevers, stress, or ingestion of certain foods. They are small, shallow painful lesions occurring on the movable mucosa, the buccal mucosa, the floor of the mouth, soft palate, and lateral borders of the tongue (see Fig. 18–2). The ulcers appear to be covered with a whitish exudate and have a red border. They heal spontaneously in a week or so.

INFECTIONS

Herpetic stomatitis may be associated with *herpes labialis* (cold sores or fever blisters). Herpes infection is usually caused by herpes simplex virus type 1 (HSV-1) and is transmitted by kissing or close contact, often in childhood. The initial infection is frequently asymptomatic, but the virus remains dormant in the body in a sensory ganglion, often the trigeminal nerve ganglion. When activated by stress, trauma, or another infection (such as a common cold), the virus migrates along the nerve to the skin or mucosa around the mouth, causing a burning or stinging sensation at the site followed by development of **vesicles** (blisters) as the virus reproduces and causes necrosis of the host cells. These vesicles rupture, leaving a shallow painful ulcer, which releases a clear fluid containing many organisms and then crusts over. The lesions heal spontaneously in a week or 10 days, when the virus again migrates along the trigeminal nerve to the sensory ganglion, where it enters a latent stage. Recurrences are common. In immunosuppressed patients, multiple lesions may develop in the oral cavity and pharynx (herpetic gingivostomatitis). The virus is often present in the saliva for some time after the vesicle has healed. Although no cure is available at present, the acute stage may be alleviated somewhat by prompt use of antiviral medications (e.g., topical acyclovir), thus decreasing the shedding of the virus and the risk of transmission as well as the discomfort. Herpes simplex virus may spread to the eyes, causing conjunctivitis and keratitis (see Chapter 20), either by contaminated fingers or through droplets sprayed from the mouth, for example, during dental treatment. Dental personnel are also vulnerable to *herpetic whitlow,* an acute and painful infection of the finger.

Oral candidiasis (thrush) is a common fungal infection that occurs particularly often in individuals who have taken broad-spectrum antibiotics or glucocorticoids and in those who have diabetes or are immunosuppressed. It is often an initial indication of infection in AIDS patients and may extend into the esophagus in such cases. The infection may also develop in young infants as they develop resident flora or from transmission from the mother. *Candida albicans* is often part of the normal resident flora of the mouth and is an opportunist under certain conditions. The infection appears as irregular patches of a white curdlike material on the mucosa, which can be wiped off to reveal **erythema** at the base. Nystatin, a topical antifungal agent, is the usual treatment.

Acute necrotizing ulcerative gingivitis (ANUG, trench mouth) is a common infection caused by anaerobic opportunistic bacteria in individuals in whom tissue resistance is decreased by stress, smoking, other pathologic conditions, or nutritional deficits. The gingivae around the mandibular anterior teeth (lower jaw) are affected, showing white pseudomembranous necrotic areas surrounded by red and swollen areas. The gingivae are painful and bleed easily. Debridement and antibiotics may be needed.

Syphilis may cause oral lesions that contain microorganisms and are highly contagious during the first and second stages (see Chapter 24). The primary stage is characterized by a chancre, a painless ulcer usually found on the tongue, lips, or palate. The lesion heals spontaneously (without treatment) in a week or two. The second stage may be manifested by red macules or papules on the palate similar to the typical skin rash occurring at this stage or by mucous patches, multiple, irregular loose white necrotic material on the mucosa, which is highly infectious. Again, this lesion heals spontaneously. Because these lesions may be missed, immediate treatment of the infection and control of transmission may be hampered. Both stages of syphilis are treated with penicillin, usually by injection, because the organism, *Treponema pallidum,* also exists in the general circulation of the individual.

DENTAL PROBLEMS

Dental caries (tooth decay or cavities) is considered an infection involving *Streptococcus mutans* (as the initiator), *Lactobacillus,* and other normal flora in the oral cavity. These bacteria act on sugars in ingested food to create large quantities of lactic acid that dissolves the minerals (calcium and phosphate) in tooth enamel, leading to erosion of the tooth surface. Fluoride as an anticaries treatment decreases the solubility of the minerals in enamel (fluorapatite replaces hydroxyapatite) and enhances the remineralization process. Excessive fluoride ingestion during tooth maturation can, however, cause hypocalcification of tooth enamel. If untreated, bacterial action and decay may continue to penetrate the tooth surface until the internal structures of the tooth are infected (pulpitis) or periapical abscesses form at the root of the tooth. *Gingivitis* or inflammation of the gingiva may result from increased plaque, which is a mass of bacteria and debris covering the tooth, or from poor oral hygiene or hormonal changes associated with pregnancy and the use of oral contraceptives. Periodontal disease may develop when there is an increase in activity of gram-negative anaerobic bacteria as they enter the plaque. There are different forms of *periodontitis* related to different causative organisms, patients of different ages, and different degrees of severity. A major destructive microbe in periodontal disease is *Porphyromonas gingivalis,* formerly identified as *Bacteroides oralis.* The subgingival areas are colonized by primarily gram-negative anaerobic bacteria, which ultimately destroy the periodontal attachment of the tooth and the surrounding alveolar bone. The mucosa is red and swollen and bleeds easily, and the teeth may feel loose. Major treatment is required to eradicate the infection and prevent loss of teeth.

HYPERKERATOSIS

An example of hyperkeratosis is *leukoplakia,* a whitish plaque or epidermal thickening of the mucosa that occurs frequently on the buccal mucosa, palate, or lower lip. The cause cannot always be identified but may be related to smoking or chronic irritation. These lesions require monitoring because in some cases epithelial dysplasia beneath the plaque develops into squamous cell carcinoma.

CANCER OF THE ORAL CAVITY

The common cancer of the oral cavity is *squamous cell carcinoma.* Lip cancer (usually on the lower lip) is obvious and accessible and has a good prognosis. Malignant tumors inside the oral cavity have a poor prognosis because they tend to be hidden and painless. They are more common in persons older than 40 years of age, particularly smokers, those with leukoplakia, or those with a history of alcohol abuse. Common sites in the oral cavity are the floor of the mouth and the lateral borders of the tongue. The carcinoma appears initially as a whitish thickening and then develops into either a nodular mass or an ulcerative lesion, which persists. Lip cancer usually spreads locally while intraoral cancer spreads first to the regional lymph nodes and nodes in the neck. *Kaposi's sarcoma* may occur in patients with AIDS. The typical lesion is a brownish or purple macular lesion, usually on the palate, which eventually becomes a nodular mass.

SALIVARY GLAND DISORDERS

The parotid gland is most frequently affected, both by infectious agents and tumors. Mumps is a viral infection leading to marked swelling of the gland, usually bilateral. It is less common now that a vaccine is available. Noninfectious parotitis may develop in debilitated or elderly patients who lack adequate fluid intake and mouth care. Tumors such as benign adenomas tend to affect the parotid glands of older individuals.

Thinkabout 18–5

Prepare a chart comparing the cause and characteristics of one inflammatory disorder, one infectious disorder, and one tumor of the oral cavity.

Dysphagia

There are many reasons for dysphagia or difficulty in swallowing (Fig. 18–5). Dysphagia may present as pain with swallowing, an inability to swallow larger pieces of solid material, or difficulty in swallowing liquids, depending on the cause of the problem. Dysphagia may result from a neurologic deficit, a muscular disorder, or a mechanical obstruction. *Achalasia* results from failure of the lower esophageal sphincter to relax owing to loss of innervation. This leads to accumulation of food and associated dilation of the lower esophagus as entry of food into the stomach is delayed. Often chronic inflammation develops in the esophagus, and reflux of this food may lead to aspiration when the person assumes a supine position. There is an increased risk of esophageal carcinoma following long-term achalasia.

Mechanical obstructions include *congenital atresia*, a developmental defect in which the upper and lower

esophageal segments are separated, the upper section ending in a blind pouch. Reflux of feedings occurs in the infant with congenital atresia, leading to aspiration. In many cases there is a connecting fistula from one of the segments to the trachea. Surgical correction is required as soon as possible to prevent aspiration and provide fluid and nutrients to the infant. **Stenosis** or narrowing of the esophagus may be a developmental or acquired defect; the acquired form is usually secondary to fibrosis associated with chronic inflammation or ulceration (esophagitis). Stenosis or **stricture** may also result from scar tissue following accidental ingestion of corrosive chemicals such as lye or other cleaning materials. Accidental ingestion of such damaging substances should not be treated by inducing vomiting to remove the chemical because this would cause additional tissue damage. Stenosis may require treatment with repeated mechanical dilation by bougies or surgery if food intake is severely limited by the obstruction. Esophageal *diverticula* are outpouchings of the esophageal wall that result either from congenital defects or from inflammation. The accumulated food in the pouch obstructs the flow of food down the esophagus, causes irritation, inflammation, and scar tissue in the wall, and often is regurgitated upward at a later time with possible aspiration into the respiratory tract. Signs of diverticula include dysphagia, foul breath, chronic cough, and hoarseness. Occasionally, ulcers may form in the esophageal wall and bleed. Other causes of dysphagia include *tumors*, which may be internal or external. Tumors in the esophagus either form circumferential strictures or grow out into the lumen of the esophagus. External tumors are located outside the esophagus, perhaps in a **mediastinal** lymph node, and compress the esophagus. Esophageal cancer is primarily *squamous cell carcinoma* and is most commonly found in the distal esophagus. Esophageal cancer is associated with chronic irritation due to, for example, chronic esophagitis, achalasia, hiatal hernia, alcohol abuse, and smoking. Unfortunately, the initial signs of dysphagia occur relatively late in the course of the disease, and the prognosis currently is poor.

Hiatal Hernia

In patients with hiatal hernia, part of the stomach is elevated and protrudes through the opening (hiatus) in the diaphragm into the thoracic cavity. Normally, the digestive tract is loosely attached to the diaphragm. Contributing factors to hiatal hernia include shortening of the esophagus, weakness of the diaphragm, or increased abdominal pressure (e.g., pregnancy). There are two types of hiatal hernia (Fig. 18–6). With a *sliding* hernia, the more common type, a portion of the stomach and the gastroesophageal junction move above the

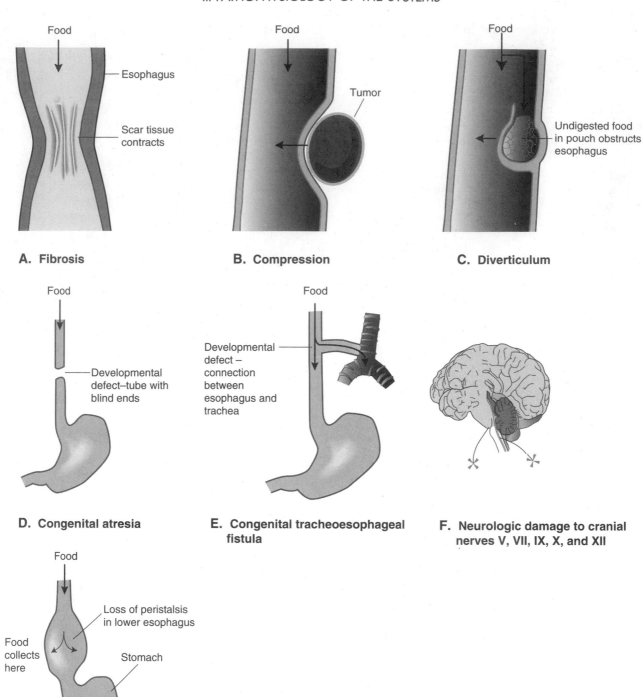

A. Fibrosis

Food

Esophagus

Scar tissue contracts

B. Compression

Food

Tumor

C. Diverticulum

Food

Undigested food in pouch obstructs esophagus

D. Congenital atresia

Food

Developmental defect–tube with blind ends

E. Congenital tracheoesophageal fistula

Food

Developmental defect – connection between esophagus and trachea

F. Neurologic damage to cranial nerves V, VII, IX, X, and XII

G. Achalasia

Food

Loss of peristalsis in lower esophagus

Food collects here

Stomach

FIGURE 18–5. Causes of dysphagia.

diaphragm, particularly when the person is in the supine position. In the standing position, the herniated portion slides back down into the abdominal cavity. With a *rolling* or *paraesophageal* hernia, part of the fundus of the stomach moves up through an enlarged or weak hiatus in the diaphragm. In this type of hernia, the blood vessels in the wall of the stomach may be compressed, leading to ulceration. Food often lodges in the pouch created by the herniated portion, leading to inflammation of the mucosa, reflux of food up the esophagus, and dysphagia as the mass of food enlarges and obstructs the passageway. Chronic esophagitis eventually may cause fibrosis and stricture. Often an incompetent gastroesophageal sphincter is associated with hiatal hernia, which increases the risk of reflux.

The signs of hiatal hernia include *heartburn* or *pyrosis,* a brief substernal burning sensation often accompanied by a sour taste in the mouth occurring after meals that results from reflux of the gastric contents up the esophagus. Frequent belching (gas) often accompanies this regurgitation. The discomfort is increased by lying down after eating, by bending over, or by coughing. Dysphagia is common either because of inflammation of the esophagus or because the mass of food collected in the pouch compresses the esophagus. Persistent mild substernal chest pain after meals is a frequent complaint because of inflammation or distention of the pouch. The manifestations can often be reduced by eating frequent small meals and avoiding a recumbent position after meals.

Gastroesophageal reflux (GER) is usually associated with hiatal hernia as well as with other conditions. GER depends on the competence of the lower esophageal sphincter (LES) or the relative pressures on either side of the LES. For example, either a decrease in LES pressure or an increase in intra-abdominal pressure allows more of the gastric contents to reflux back into the esophagus. Eliminating factors that reduce LES pressure such as caffeine, fatty foods, alcohol intake, cigarette smoking, and certain drugs may relieve the discomfort of hiatal hernia. Avoidance of spicy foods and ingestion of antacids may reduce the inflammation associated with reflux.

Gastritis

Gastritis is an inflammation of the stomach that may occur in many forms. It may be a mild transient irritation with only vague signs, or it may be an acute ulcerative or hemorrhagic episode. There are many causes of gastritis, among which are allergies, infections, excessive ingestion of alcohol, irritating foods, and drugs. Gastritis may be acute or chronic, and these terms represent two different entities.

ACUTE GASTRITIS

The gastric mucosa is inflamed and appears red and edematous. It may be ulcerated and bleeding if the mucosal barrier (the tightly packed epithelial cells and layer of thick mucus) is severely damaged or if the circulation is poor, reducing tissue resistance. Acute gastritis may result from infection by many types of microorganisms (e.g., bacteria and viruses), allergies to foods such as drugs or shellfish, ingestion of spicy or irritating foods such as hot peppers, particularly if the person is unaccustomed to these, heavy alcohol intake, ingestion of aspirin or other ulcerogenic drugs (especially on an empty stomach), ingestion of corrosives or toxic substances, or radiation or chemotherapy. The basic signs of gastrointestinal irritation are manifest. Anorexia, nausea, or vomiting develops, the severity of which varies with the particular situation. Hematemesis indicates ulceration and bleeding in the stomach. **Epigastric** pain, cramps, or general discomfort may be present. Depending on the cause, other signs may be present—for example, fever and headache usually accompany infection. In some cases, particularly with infections, diarrhea may develop (see next section on gastroenteritis). Acute gastritis is usually self-limiting, with complete regeneration of the gastric mucosa in a day or two. In persons with severe or prolonged vomiting, there is a danger of dehydration, electrolyte loss, and metabolic acidosis, which require supportive treatment. Certain infections may require treatment with antimicrobial drugs.

GASTROENTERITIS

Gastroenteritis refers to the involvement of the stomach and the intestines in the inflammatory process. It is

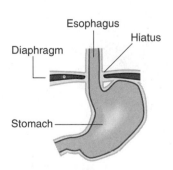
A. Normal stomach

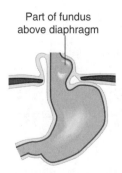
B. Sliding hiatal hernia

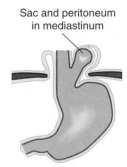
C. Paraesophageal hernia

FIGURE 18-6. Types of hiatal hernia.

usually due to infection but may also result from allergic reactions to foods or drugs. Many organisms in contaminated food and water are transmitted by the oral-fecal route. Common causes of food-borne infections are summarized in Table 18–3. Inflammation of the gastric mucosa stimulates vomiting, whereas diarrhea results when the inflammation causes increased motility, impaired absorption, and in some cases increased intestinal secretions. Nausea and abdominal cramps are usually present as well. Fever and malaise are common. The infection is usually self-limiting, although supportive treatment may be needed for fluid and electrolyte losses, particularly in young children and the elderly. A stool culture is helpful in identifying the causative organism in persistent cases.

CHRONIC GASTRITIS

Chronic gastritis is characterized by atrophy of the mucosa of the stomach with loss of the secretory glands. Infection with *Helicobacter pylori* is often present. Chronic gastritis is often associated with chronic peptic ulcers, alcohol abuse, and aging. Autoimmune disorders for example, pernicious anemia (see Chapter 16) are associated with a type of chronic gastric atrophy. The loss of the parietal cells leads to achlorhydria and

lack of secretion of intrinsic factor, which is required for the absorption of vitamin B_{12}. The signs of chronic gastritis are often vague and include mild epigastric discomfort, anorexia, or intolerance for certain foods, usually spicy or fatty foods. Persons with chronic gastritis have an increased risk of peptic ulcers and gastric carcinoma.

Thinkabout 18–6

a. Describe how each of the following entities causes dysphagia: achalasia, cancer of the esophagus, atresia.

b. Explain how chronic reflux of gastric contents into the esophagus may cause hiatal hernia.

c. Define pyrosis.

d. Explain how prolonged vomiting leads to acidosis and dehydration.

e. What is indicated by occult blood in the stool in a person with gastroenteritis?

TABLE 18–3 Common Infections Transmitted by Food and Water

Pathogen	Source	Incubation	Pathophysiology	Manifestations
Staphylococcus aureus	Food handlers Inadequate cooking or refrigeration of custards, salad dressing, cold meats	1–7 hours (2–4 average)	Enterotoxin (exotoxin), heat-stable	Sudden severe nausea, vomiting, and cramps, sometimes diarrhea. Subnormal body temperature and low blood pressure
Escherichia coli (Traveler's diarrhea)	Fecal contamination of food and water; EHEC type transmitted from undercooked ground beef	10–12 hours	Various strains may release enterotoxins (increase secretions) or invade the mucosa	Profuse watery diarrhea, sometimes with blood or mucus. Vomiting and abdominal cramps often present
Salmonella	Fecal contamination of food or undercooked or raw eggs, poultry, shellfish Contaminated work surfaces	6–72 hours	Organisms multiply in intestine, causing inflammation and ulceration	Sudden diarrhea, abdominal pain, and fever. Sometimes vomiting
Viral Rotavirus Norwalk	Oral-fecal Possibly fomites	24–72 hours	Inflammation and loss of villi	Vomiting and diarrhea, fever
Entamoeba histolytica (amoebic dysentery)	Fecal contamination of water and vegetables	2–4 weeks	Protozoan parasite with cyst stage and active trophozoite stage; may invade mucosa, causing abscesses	Diarrhea with blood and mucus, may alternate with constipation. Fever and chills
Clostridium botulinum	Spores in poorly canned food or prepared meat	12–36 hours	Neurotoxin (exotoxin) causes nerve paralysis	Visual problems, dysphagia, then flaccid paralysis and respiratory failure. Possibly early vomiting or diarrhea

Peptic Ulcer

GASTRIC AND DUODENAL ULCERS

Pathophysiology

Peptic ulcers occur most commonly in the proximal duodenum (duodenal ulcers) but are also found in the antrum of the stomach (gastric ulcers) or lower esophagus (Fig. 18–7). Peptic ulcers usually appear as single, small round cavities that penetrate the submucosa. Ulcers may eventually erode more deeply into the muscularis and eventually may perforate the wall. An area of inflammation surrounds the crater. When the erosion invades a blood vessel wall, bleeding takes place. Bleeding may involve persistent loss of small amounts of blood or massive hemorrhage, depending on the size of the blood vessel involved. Chronic blood loss may be detected by the presence of iron-deficiency anemia or occult blood in the stool. Healing of peptic ulcers is difficult because the lesion cannot be isolated from the irritants in the environment. During the healing process, granulation tissue forms deep in the cavity, and new epithelial tissue regenerates from the edges. This granulation tissue often breaks down because it is subject to damage by the chyme. Because a longer time is often required for healing, more fibrous scar tissue develops at the site. The ulcers tend to recur because predisposing factors remain or the scar tissue itself interferes with the blood supply to the area.

The development of peptic ulcers begins with a breakdown of the mucosa, which results from an imbalance between the mucosal defense system and forces that are potentially damaging to it. Also, the bacterium *H. pylori* is present in the majority of persons with peptic ulcer, although its precise role is not understood. Given the material that is ingested by the stomach and the fact that the powerful and highly acidic gastric secretions can digest protein in food, it is remarkable that the gastric defenses can maintain the integrity of the tissues as well as they do. Once acid or pepsin penetrates the mucosa, the tissues are exposed to continued damage because acid diffuses into the gastric wall. Many factors may contribute to the decreased resistance of the mucosa or to excessive hydrochloric acid or pepsin secretion. Impaired mucosal defenses seem to be a more common factor in gastric ulcer development, whereas increased acid secretion is a predominant factor in duodenal ulcers. The mucosal barrier may be damaged by an inadequate blood supply, which interferes with the rapid regeneration of the epithelium and the production of sufficient mucus as well as reducing the secretion of alkaline bicarbonate ions in the protective mucus and secretion of protective prostaglandins. Defenses also may be decreased by excessive glucocorticoid secretion with its catabolic effects, or by substances that break down the mucus layer such as refluxed bile, aspirin, nonsteroidal anti-inflammatory drugs (NSAIDs), or alcohol. Any break in the barrier allows acid to penetrate and damage the underlying cells.

The other main factor contributing to ulcer development, increased acid-pepsin secretions, is associated with increased gastrin secretion; increased vagal stimulation; increased number of acid-pepsin secretory cells in the stomach; increased stimulation of acid-pepsin secretion by alcohol, caffeine, or certain foods; and interference with the normal feedback mechanism that reduces acid-pepsin secretion when the stomach is empty. Severe or prolonged stress appears to affect both sides of the balance, reducing mucosal blood flow and motility, leading to stasis of chyme, and increasing glucocorticoid effects. Also, stress may promote behavioral factors that are often implicated in ulcer development such as increased caffeine and alcohol intake, cigarette smoking, and altered eating patterns, which often include both irregular hours for intake and ingestion of irritating foods.

Several complications are frequently associated with peptic ulcer. The ulcer may erode a blood vessel, causing *hemorrhage*, a very common complication (see Fig. 18–7B). Rupture of a small blood vessel causes continued loss of small amounts of blood usually apparent as occult blood in the stool, whereas erosion of a large blood vessel leads to massive hemorrhage, indicated by hematemesis and shock. Hemorrhage may be the first sign of a peptic ulcer. A second potential complication, *perforation* occurs when the ulcer erodes completely through the wall, allowing chyme to enter the peritoneal cavity (Fig. 18–7D). This process results in chemical *peritonitis*, inflammation of the peritoneal membranes and other structures in the abdominal cavity. Eventually this inflammation causes increased permeability of the intestinal wall, passage of bacteria and their toxins into the peritoneal cavity, and bacterial peritonitis. Hemorrhage is not necessarily present when perforation occurs. Thirdly, *obstruction* of the digestive tract may result later from stricture due to scar tissue around the pylorus or duodenum, particularly in people with protracted or recurrent ulceration.

Etiology

Peptic ulcers are common, particularly among males. A genetic factor seems to be involved in the development of duodenal ulcers; also, these are more common in persons with blood group O. Gastric ulcers are more common in older individuals, in those with scar tissue present, and in those who regularly take ulcerogenic anti-inflammatory medications (aspirin or NSAIDs). Multiple factors such as those listed are usually involved in the etiology.

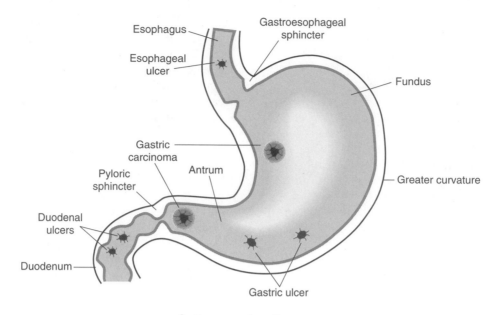

A   **Common locations**

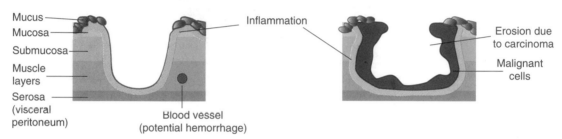

B   **Peptic ulcer**   **C**   **Gastric carcinoma**

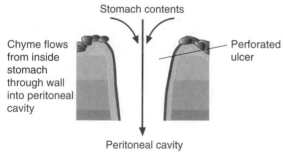

D   **Perforated ulcer**

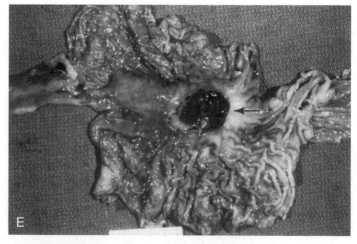

FIGURE 18–7. *A*, Typical locations of peptic ulcer and gastric carcinoma. *B–D*, Development of ulcers. *E*, Bleeding peptic ulcer. (Courtesy of R.W. Shaw, M.D., North York General Hospital, Toronto, Ontario.)

Signs and Symptoms

Epigastric burning or aching pain is common with ulcers, usually 2 to 3 hours after meals and at night. This cyclic pain is usually relieved by ingestion of food or antacids. Intake of spicy foods may initiate pain at mealtime. Heartburn, nausea, vomiting, and weight loss may occur. Vomiting is most likely to occur after intake of alcohol or particularly irritating food. In some patients, weight gain occurs because the person discovers that more frequent food intake relieves the discomfort between meals.

Treatment

Treatment usually consists of antimicrobial drugs (tetracycline or amoxicillin), metronidazole, and bismuth subsalicylate to eradicate *H. pylori.* An H$_2$ receptor antagonist such as cimetidine may be used to reduce acid secretion. In some individuals, a coating agent such as sucralfate or anticholinergic agents may be helpful. Reducing exacerbating factors such as excessive coffee intake is useful. Vagotomy may be performed to reduce acid secretions in refractory cases. Surgery (partial **gastrectomy** or pylorroplasty) may be required in patients with perforated or bleeding ulcers.

STRESS ULCERS

Stress ulcers result from severe trauma such as burns or head injury or with serious systemic problems such as hemorrhage or sepsis. Ulcers associated with burns are often called Curling's ulcers, those with head injury are termed Cushing's ulcers, and others may be referred to as ischemic ulcers. Multiple ulcers, usually gastric ulcers, form within hours of the precipitating event as the blood flow to the mucosa is greatly reduced, leading to reduced secretion of mucus and epithelial regeneration. The mucosal barrier is lost, and acid diffuses into the mucosa. In people with Cushing's ulcers, increased vagal stimulation of acid secretion often occurs. The first indicator of stress ulcers is usually hemorrhage because of their rapid onset and masking by the primary problem. Prophylactic medications are usually administered as soon as possible to minimize the risk of stress ulcer development in cases of trauma.

Gastric Cancer

PATHOPHYSIOLOGY

Gastric cancer arises primarily in the mucous glands, most tumors occurring in the antrum or pyloric area with some affecting the lesser curvature of the stomach or cardia (see Fig. 18–7). The lesion is most often an ulcerative type with an irregular crater and a raised margin. Other forms of gastric cancer may infiltrate the gastric wall causing thickening or may appear as a protruding mass or polyp. Early gastric carcinoma refers to a lesion confined to the mucosa and submucosa, whereas advanced gastric carcinoma involves the muscularis layer. Eventually the tumor extends into the serosa and spreads to the lymph nodes (regional and supraclavicular) and to the liver and ovaries. Gastric cancer is asymptomatic in the early stages and usually is not diagnosed until it is well advanced, at which point the prognosis is poor.

ETIOLOGY

Geographic differences are marked in the development of gastric carcinoma, which has a high incidence in Japan, Iceland, Chile, and Hungary, but a significant decline is evident in the United States. Diet appears to be a key factor because a move to a different location results in a change in risk level to that associated with the new area. Food preservatives such as nitrates or nitrites and smoked foods increase the risk. Genetic influences play a role in that the risk is increased in family members and individuals with blood group A. The presence of chronic atrophic gastritis in an individual also increases the likelihood of cancer developing.

SIGNS AND SYMPTOMS

Manifestations are usually vague and mild until the cancer is advanced. The initial signs include anorexia, feelings of indigestion or epigastric discomfort, weight loss, fatigue, or a feeling of fullness after eating. Incidental tests may reveal occult blood in the stool or iron-deficiency anemia and precipitate a search for the cause and earlier diagnosis.

TREATMENT

Surgery (gastric resection) combined with chemotherapy and radiation is the usual treatment and may relieve symptoms when used as a palliative measure.

Dumping Syndrome

Dumping syndrome may occur following gastric resection (e.g., partial gastrectomy), in which, because the pyloric sphincter is removed, control of gastric emptying is lost. Large quantities of ingested food are rapidly "dumped" into the intestine. The storage stage in the stomach, which includes appropriate dilution of chyme by gastric secretions, is missed. The hyperosmolar chyme draws more fluid from the vascular compartment into the intestine (Fig. 18–8), adding to the intestinal distention and increasing intestinal motility. These changes lead to signs occurring *during or shortly after meals,* including abdominal cramps, nausea, and diarrhea. The concurrent hypovolemia causes dizziness or weakness, rapid pulse, and sweating. In addition, individuals with dumping syndrome may experience *hypoglycemia 2 to 3 hours after meals.* The rapid gastric emptying and absorption leads to high blood glucose levels and increased insulin secretion, which results in a rapid drop in blood glucose level with no reserve nutrients advancing slowly from the stomach. Rebound hy-

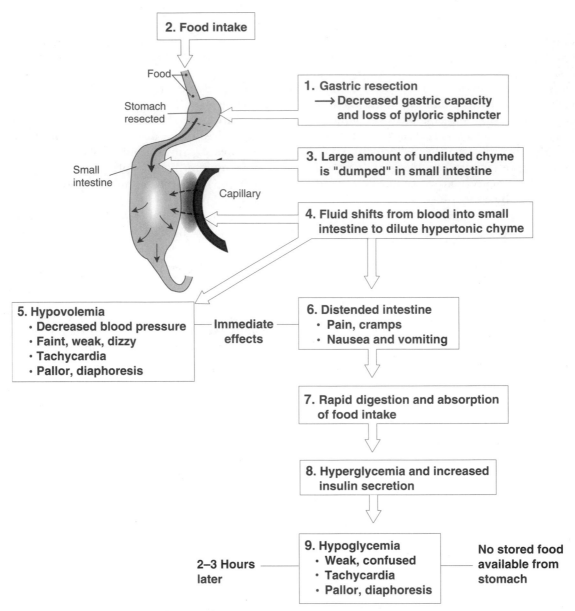

FIGURE 18–8. Dumping syndrome (postgastrectomy).

poglycemia then develops several hours after eating with tremors, sweating, and weakness. These problems can usually be resolved by dietary changes, including consumption of frequent small meals that are high in protein and low in simple carbohydrates. Also, fluids should be taken between meals rather than with meals. These measures reduce the hypertonicity of the chyme and the fluctuations in blood glucose. In some cases, medications may be used to decrease intestinal motility.

Pyloric Stenosis

Narrowing and obstruction of the pyloric sphincter may be a developmental defect in infants, or it may be acquired later in life, usually because of the presence of fibrous scar tissue. In the congenital form, the pyloric muscle is hypertrophied and can be palpated as a hard mass in the abdomen. Signs of stenosis usually appear within several weeks after birth, first as episodes of regurgitation of some food and then as projectile vomiting occurring immediately after feeding and failure to gain weight. Vomitus may be ejected some distance from the infant and does not contain bile. Stools become small and infrequent. The infant is often irritable because of persistent hunger and may become dehydrated. Surgery is required to remove the obstruction. In persons with acquired pyloric obstruction, interference with gastric emptying leads to a persistent feeling of fullness and then to an increased incidence of vomiting with or after meals, the vomitus typically containing food from prior meals.

Thinkabout 18–7

a. List and explain three factors that predispose to peptic ulcer formation.

b. Suggest reasons why the prognosis for gastric cancer is poor.

c. Explain why dizziness, weakness, and tachycardia may occur (1) immediately after a meal in a postgastrectomy patient, and (2) 2 to 3 hours after eating.

DISORDERS OF THE LIVER AND PANCREAS

Gallbladder Disorders

The gallbladder and biliary tract are frequently affected by one or more interrelated problems involving the formation of gallstones (Fig. 18–9). *Cholelithiasis* refers to gallstone formation, masses of solid material or **calculi** that form in the bile. *Cholecystitis* refers to inflammation of the gallbladder and cystic duct, and *cholangitis* is inflammation usually related to infection of the bile ducts. *Choledocholithiasis* pertains to obstruction by gallstones of the biliary tract.

PATHOPHYSIOLOGY

Gallstones may consist primarily of cholesterol or bile pigment (bilirubin) or may be of mixed content, including calcium salts (Fig. 18–10). The content of the stone depends on the primary factor predisposing to calculus formation. Cholesterol stones appear white or crystalline, whereas bilirubin stones are black. Calculi vary in size and shape and may form initially in the bile ducts, gallbladder, or cystic duct. Once a focus or nucleus forms, the stone tends to grow as additional solutes are deposited on it, particularly if bile flow is sluggish. Small stones may be silent and may be excreted in the bile, whereas larger stones are likely to obstruct the flow of bile in the cystic or common bile ducts. Gallstones tend to form when the bile contains a very high concentration of a component such as cholesterol or a deficit of bile salts. Inflammation or infection in the biliary structures may provide a focus for stone formation or may alter the solubility of the constituents,

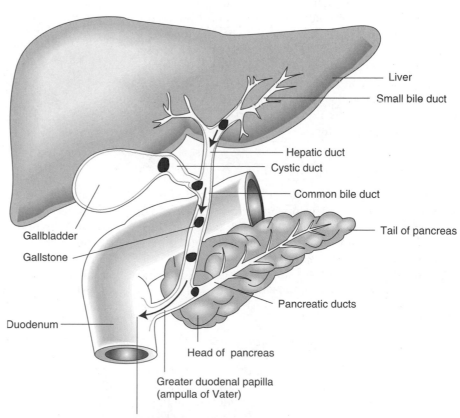

FIGURE 18–9. The biliary ducts and pancreas with possible locations of gallstones.

Labels: Liver · Small bile duct · Hepatic duct · Cystic duct · Common bile duct · Tail of pancreas · Pancreatic ducts · Head of pancreas · Greater duodenal papilla (ampulla of Vater) · Major duodenal papilla (sphincter of Oddi) · Duodenum · Gallstone · Gallbladder

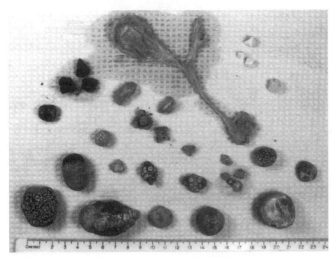

FIGURE 18–10. Examples of gallstones. (Courtesy of Paul Emmerson and Seneca College of Applied Arts and Technology, Toronto, Ontario.)

fostering the development of a calculus. Whether inflammation or infection is primary or secondary to stone formation is not always clear. The presence of gallstones may cause irritation and inflammation in the gallbladder wall, and this susceptible tissue may then be infected. Infecting organisms are usually *Escherichia coli* or enterococci, which usually gain access to the gallbladder from the portal veins or adjacent lymph nodes. Gallstones are frequently asymptomatic, or they may cause acute or chronic cholecystitis. When a stone obstructs bile flow in the cystic or common bile duct, biliary colic develops, consisting of severe spasms of pain associated with strong muscle contractions attempting to move the stone along. Obstruction of the biliary system at the sphincter of Oddi may also cause pancreatitis because the pancreatic secretions are backed up or bile refluxes into the pancreatic ducts.

ETIOLOGY

Cholesterol gallstones occur more commonly in women and tend to develop in individuals with high cholesterol levels in the bile. High-risk factors include obesity, high cholesterol intake, **multiparity**, and the use of oral contraceptives or estrogen supplements. Bile pigment stones are more common in individuals with hemolytic anemia, alcoholic cirrhosis, or biliary tract infection.

SIGNS AND SYMPTOMS

Gallstones are frequently asymptomatic. However, larger calculi may obstruct a duct at any time, causing sudden severe waves of pain (biliary colic) in the upper right quadrant or epigastric area, often radiating to the back and right shoulder. Nausea and vomiting are usu-

ally present. The pain usually increases for some time and then may decrease if the stone moves on. If the pain continues, and jaundice develops as the bile backs up into the liver and blood, surgical intervention may be necessary. There is also a risk of a ruptured gallbladder if obstruction persists.

Acute cholecystitis is usually associated with some degree of obstruction and inflammation. Severe pain is often precipitated by eating a fatty meal; fever, **leukocytosis**, and vomiting accompany the pain. Chronic cholecystitis is manifested by milder signs, although the course may be punctuated by acute episodes. Signs often include intolerance to fatty foods, excessive belching, bloating, and mild epigastric discomfort.

TREATMENT

The gallbladder and gallstones may be removed surgically. In many cases the stones are fragmented by such methods as extracorporeal shock wave lithotripsy (using high-energy sound waves), sometimes assisted by administration of bile acids.

Thinkabout 18–8

a. Define cholelithiasis and choledocholithiasis.
b. List three factors predisposing to cholesterol gallstones.
c. Describe how a cholesterol stone forms.
d. Describe the pain typical of an acute episode of gallstone obstruction and give the rationale for it.

Jaundice

Jaundice (**icterus**) is the yellowish color of the skin and other tissues that results from high levels of bilirubin in the blood. The color is usually apparent first in the sclera or white area of the eye. Bilirubin is a product of the hemolysis of red blood cells (RBCs) and the breakdown of hemoglobin (see Fig. 16–8). Jaundice or **hyperbilirubinemia** can be a sign of many different types of primary disorders. These disorders are classified in three groups (see Fig. 18–12). *Prehepatic* jaundice results from excessive destruction of red blood cells and is associated with hemolytic anemias or transfusion reactions. Liver function is normal but is unable to handle the additional bilirubin. *Physiologic jaundice of the newborn* is common 2 to 3 days after birth. Increased hemolysis of red blood cells combined with the immature infant liver leads to a transient mild hyperbilirubinemia. *Intrahepatic* jaundice occurs with liver disease such as hepatitis or cirrhosis. It is related to impaired uptake of bilirubin from the blood and decreased conjugation of bilirubin by the hepatocytes (Fig. 18–11). *Posthepatic* jaundice is caused by obstruction of bile flow into the gallbladder or duodenum and subsequent backup of bile into the blood. Congenital atresia of the bile ducts, obstruction due to cholelithiasis, inflammation of the liver, or tumors all lead to posthepatic jaundice. The type of jaundice present may be indicated by increases in the serum bilirubin level and changes in the stools. These are summarized in Figure 18–12. For example, serum levels of unconjugated bilirubin (indirect-reacting) are elevated in prehepatic jaundice, whereas posthepatic jaundice results from increased amounts of conjugated bilirubin (direct) in the blood. In patients with liver disease both intrahepatic and posthepatic jaundice may be present because inflammation or infection both impairs hepatocyte function and ob-

structs the bile canaliculi, leading to elevations in the blood of both unconjugated and conjugated bilirubin. In persons with posthepatic jaundice, the obstruction prevents bile from entering the intestine, interfering with digestion and resulting in a light-colored stool. Also, the bile salts that enter the blood and tissues as bile backs up cause irritation and **pruritus** (itching) of the skin. Treatment depends on removing the cause. Phototherapy is effective in mild forms, whereby exposure to ultraviolet light promotes the conjugation of bilirubin.

Hepatitis

Hepatitis refers to inflammation of the liver. It may result from a local infection (viral hepatitis), from an infection elsewhere in the body (e.g., infectious mononucleosis or amebiasis), or from chemical or drug toxic-

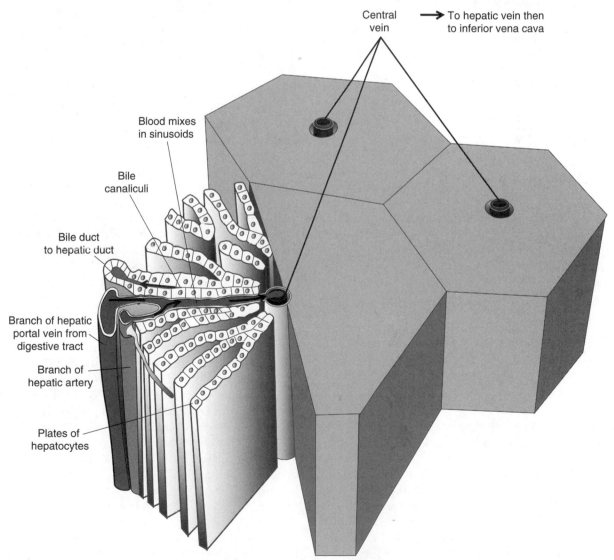

FIGURE 18–11. Structure of liver lobule.

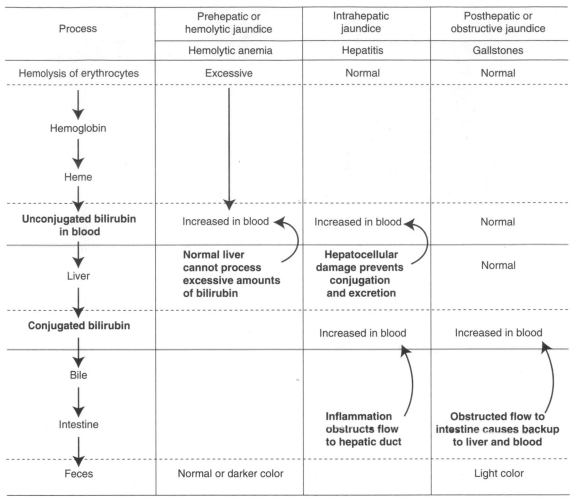

Process	Prehepatic or hemolytic jaundice	Intrahepatic jaundice	Posthepatic or obstructive jaundice
	Hemolytic anemia	Hepatitis	Gallstones
Hemolysis of erythrocytes	Excessive	Normal	Normal
Hemoglobin			
Heme			
Unconjugated bilirubin in blood	Increased in blood	Increased in blood	Normal
Liver	**Normal liver cannot process excessive amounts of bilirubin**	**Hepatocellular damage prevents conjugation and excretion**	Normal
Conjugated bilirubin		Increased in blood	Increased in blood
Bile			
Intestine		**Inflammation obstructs flow to hepatic duct**	**Obstructed flow to intestine causes backup to liver and blood**
Feces	Normal or darker color		Light color

FIGURE 18–12. Types of jaundice.

ity. Mild inflammation impairs hepatocyte function, whereas more severe inflammation and **necrosis** may lead to obstruction of blood and bile flow in the liver as well as impaired liver cell function. Given the many functions of the liver, damage to the liver cells has extensive effects in the body. Fortunately the liver has a good functional reserve and excellent regenerative powers.

VIRAL HEPATITIS

Pathophysiology

Although a number of viruses may affect the liver cells, hepatitis is considered to result from infection by a group of viruses that specifically target the hepatocytes. These include hepatitis A virus, hepatitis B virus, hepatitis C virus, hepatitis D virus, and hepatitis E virus. The liver cells are damaged in two ways—by direct action of the virus (e.g., hepatitis C) or by cell-mediated immune responses to the virus (e.g., hepatitis B). Cell injury results in inflammation and necrosis in the liver. Both the hepatocytes and the liver appear swollen, and dif-

fuse necrosis may be present. With severe inflammation, biliary stasis may develop, leading to backup of bile into the blood. The degree of inflammation and damage varies. Some mild cases show few manifestations, but in other cases fulminant hepatitis develops with massive necrosis and liver failure. Depending on the severity of the inflammation, the hepatic cells may regenerate, or fibrous scar tissue may form in the liver. Scar tissue often obstructs the channels used for blood and bile flow, interfering with the unique organization of the liver lobule, and leading to further damage from ischemia. *Chronic* inflammation occurs with hepatitis types B, C, and D and is defined as persistent inflammation and necrosis of the liver for more than 6 months. This type of disease eventually causes permanent liver damage and cirrhosis. There is also an increased incidence of hepatocellular cancer associated with chronic hepatitis. Hepatitis types B, C, and D may exist in a **carrier** state, in which asymptomatic individuals carry the virus in their hepatocytes but can transmit the infection via their blood to others. Carriers may be individuals who have never had active disease or have a chronic low-grade infection.

Etiology

The viruses causing hepatitis vary in their characteristics, mode of transmission, incubation time, and effects. These are summarized in Table 18–4. There may be other viruses causing hepatitis that have not yet been identified.

Hepatitis A

Also called *infectious hepatitis*, hepatitis A is caused by a small RNA virus called the hepatitis A virus or HAV. It is transmitted primarily by the oral-fecal route, often from contaminated water or shellfish. Outbreaks may occur in day care centers. Sexual transmission has occurred in the homosexual population. HAV has a relatively short incubation period of 2 to 6 weeks. HAV causes an acute but self-limiting infection and does not have a carrier or chronic state. Fecal shedding of the virus (the contagious period) begins several weeks before the onset of signs (Fig. 18–13). At this time, the first antibodies, IgM-HAV, appear, followed shortly by the second group of antibodies, IgG-HAV, which remain in the serum for years providing immunity against further infection. A vaccine is available for those who are traveling to an endemic area. Gamma globulin provides temporary protection and may be administered to those just exposed to HAV.

Hepatitis B

Formerly called serum hepatitis, this form of hepatitis is caused by the hepatitis B virus (HBV), a partially double-stranded DNA virus. The whole virion is often called a Dane particle. This virus is more complex and consists of three antigens—two core antigens (HBcAg and HBeAg) and one surface antigen (HBsAg). Each antigen stimulates antibody production in the body (see Fig. 18–13). These serum antigens and antibodies are useful in diagnosing and monitoring the course of hepatitis, including the development of chronic hepatitis. For example, large amounts of HBsAg are produced by infected liver cells early in the course of the infection. When this antigen persists in the serum it poses a high risk of continued active infection and damage to the liver (chronic disease). Also, a carrier state is common for HBV, in which the individual is asymptomatic but is contagious for the disease. Hepatitis B has a relatively long incubation period, averaging about 2 months. Long incubation periods make it more difficult to track sources and contacts for infections. Also a window or prolonged lag time occurs before the serum markers or symptoms become present, during which time the virus cannot be detected but can be transmitted to others. HBV is transmitted primarily by infected blood but is found in many body secretions. Intravenous drug abusers have a high incidence of HBV. Hemodialysis increases the risk, as does exposure to blood or body fluids by health care workers if suitable precautions are not taken. Sexual transmission has been noted, and HBV can be passed to the fetus during pregnancy. A HBV vaccine is available for long-term protection for those in higher risk groups, including health professionals, and is now routinely administered to children. HBV immune globulin is available as a temporary measure.

Hepatitis C

Formerly called non A–non B or NANB hepatitis, hepatitis C is the most common type of hepatitis transmitted by blood transfusions. The virus is a single-

TABLE 18-4 Types of Hepatitis

Disease	Agent	Transmission	Incubation Period	Serum Markers	Carrier/Chronic
Viral Hepatitis					
Hepatitis A (infectious)	HAV (RNA virus)	Oral-fecal	2–6 weeks	anti-HAV IgM anti-HAV IgG	None
Hepatitis B (serum)	HBV (DNA double-strand virus)	Blood and body fluids	1–6 months (average 60–90 days)	HBsAg, anti-HBs HBcAb IgM HBcAb IgG HBeAg, HBeAb	Carrier and chronic
Hepatitis C (non A–non B)	HCV (RNA virus)	Blood and body fluids	2 weeks to 6 months (average 6–9 weeks)	anti-HCV	Carrier and chronic
Hepatitis D chronic (delta)	HDV (defective RNA virus requires presence of HBV)	Blood and body fluids	? 2–10 weeks	anti-HDV IgM anti-HDV IgG	Chronic
Hepatitis E	HEV (RNA virus)	Oral-fecal	2–9 weeks	HE Ag	
Toxic Hepatitis	Hepatotoxins; chemicals or drugs	Direct exposure	Days to months		Acute or chronic
Chronic Noninfectious Hepatitis	Autoimmune, metabolic, idiopathic			Various autoantibodies	Chronic

A. Hepatitis A

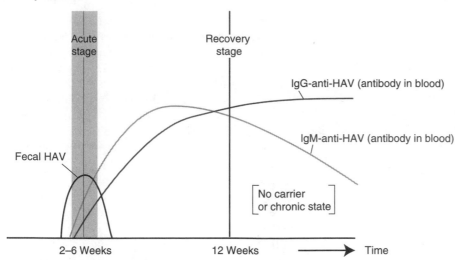

B. Hepatitis B — Acute

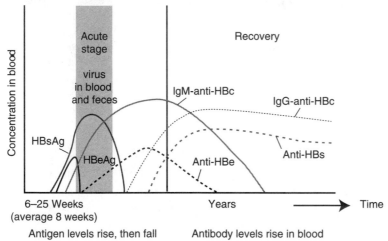

C. Hepatitis B — Chronic Infection

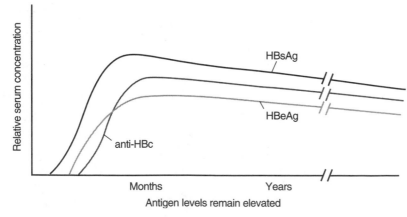

FIGURE 18-13. Serologic changes seen with hepatitis.

stranded RNA virus. It also causes chronic disease and may exist in a carrier state. HCV infection increases the risk of hepatocellular carcinoma.

Hepatitis D

The agent for hepatitis D is also called delta virus. This incomplete RNA virus requires the presence of hepatitis B virus (HBsAg) to replicate and produce active infection. HDV usually increases the severity of HBV infection. HDV is also transmitted by blood and has a high incidence in intravenous drug abusers.

Hepatitis E

Hepatitis E is caused by HEV, a single-stranded RNA virus, and is spread by the oral-fecal route. It is similar to HAV and lacks a chronic or carrier state. It is more common in developing countries, where it causes a fulminant hepatitis that has a high mortality rate in pregnant women.

Signs and Symptoms

The manifestations of acute hepatitis vary from mild or asymptomatic to severe disease that is often rapidly fatal in fulminant cases. The course of hepatitis has three stages: first, the preicteric or prodromal stage, next, the icteric or jaundice stage, and last, the posticteric or recovery stage. Onset of the *preicteric* stage may be insidious, with fatigue and malaise, anorexia and nausea, and general muscle aching. Sometimes fever, headache, a distaste for cigarettes, and mild upper right quadrant discomfort are present. Serum levels of liver enzymes (e.g., aspartate aminotransferase [AST] or alanine aminotransferase [ALT]) are elevated. The *icteric* stage marks the onset of jaundice as serum bilirubin levels rise. As biliary obstruction increases, the stools become light in color, the urine becomes darker, and skin becomes pruritic. The liver is tender and enlarged (hepatomegaly), causing a mild aching pain. In severe cases, blood clotting times may be prolonged because the synthesis of blood clotting factors is impaired. This stage tends to last longer in patients with hepatitis B. The posticteric or recovery stage is marked by a reduction in signs, although this period may extend over some weeks. On average, the acute stage of hepatitis A lasts 8 to 10 weeks, whereas hepatitis B is prolonged over 16 weeks.

Treatment

There is no method of destroying viruses in the body at this time. Gamma globulin, if available, may be helpful when given early in the course. Supportive measures such as rest and a diet high in protein, carbohydrate,

and vitamins are most useful. Chronic hepatitis may be treated with glucocorticoids to suppress the immune reaction and decrease inflammation. Otherwise, gradual destruction of the liver occurs. Interferon may be of value in patients with chronic hepatitis B and C.

TOXIC OR NONVIRAL HEPATITIS

A variety of **hepatotoxins** such as chemicals or drugs may cause inflammation and necrosis in the liver. These reactions may be direct toxic effects of the substance or an immune response (hypersensitivity) to certain materials. Toxic effects may result from sudden exposure to large amounts of a substance or from long-term exposure, perhaps in the workplace. Hepatotoxic drugs include acetaminophen, halothane, phenothiazines, and tetracycline. Toxic chemicals include solvents such as carbon tetrachloride, toluene, or ethanol. Reye's syndrome, which occurs when aspirin is used in conjunction with viral infections, also causes toxic effects on the liver (see Chapter 20). Hepatocellular damage can result from either of two processes, inflammation and necrosis or **cholestasis**. The signs of toxicity are similar to those of infectious hepatitis. It is important to remove the toxic chemical from the body as quickly as possible to reduce the risk of permanent liver damage.

Thinkabout 18-9

a. Explain how prehepatic jaundice might develop and the expected change in serum bilirubin.
b. Describe two ways in which hepatitis A differs from hepatitis B.
c. Describe how serum markers may indicate the presence of chronic viral hepatitis.
d. Define a carrier of hepatitis and explain why a carrier is considered hazardous.

Cirrhosis

PATHOPHYSIOLOGY

Cirrhosis refers to a disorder in which the liver demonstrates extensive diffuse fibrosis and loss of lobular organization. Nodules of regenerated hepatocytes may be present but are not necessarily functional because the vascular network and biliary ducts are distorted. Cirrhosis is a progressive disorder and leads eventually to liver failure. Even if the primary cause is removed, further damage is likely because fibrosis interferes with the blood supply to liver tissues, or the bile may back up, leading to ongoing damage. Initially the liver is enlarged, but then it becomes small and shrunken as fibrosis proceeds. In many cases, degenerative changes are silent until the disease is well advanced.

Cirrhosis may be classified by the structural changes that take place (e.g., micronodular or macronodular) or by the cause of the disorder. In some cases, cirrhosis may be linked to specific underlying disorders, particularly congenital problems or inherited metabolic disorders. The three general categories of cirrhosis are first, alcoholic liver disease (the largest group, also called portal or Laennec's cirrhosis), secondly, biliary cirrhosis, associated with disorders causing obstruction of bile flow, and thirdly, postnecrotic cirrhosis, linked with chronic hepatitis or long-term exposure to toxic materials. Liver biopsy and serologic tests may determine the cause and extent of the damage.

The effects of cirrhosis evolve from two factors: (1) the loss of liver cell functions, and (2) interference with blood and bile flow in the liver. Major functional losses in persons with cirrhosis include decreased processing of bilirubin and production of bile, impaired digestion and absorption of nutrients, particularly fats and fat-soluble vitamins, decreased production of blood-clotting factors and plasma proteins, impaired glucose metabolism, inadequate storage of iron and vitamin B_{12}, decreased inactivation of hormones such as aldosterone and estrogen, and decreased removal of toxic substances such as ammonia and drugs. These changes are linked with clinical signs in Table 18–5. Altered blood chemistry, including abnormal levels of electrolytes or amino acids, and excessive ammonia or other toxic chemicals affect the central nervous system, leading to hepatic encephalopathy. Serum ammonia levels correlate well with the clinical signs of encephalopathy. Ammonia is an end-product of protein metabolism in the liver or intestine, and then is converted by liver cells into urea for excretion by the kidneys. The ingestion of a meal high in protein or an episode of bleeding in the digestive tract may cause a marked elevation in serum ammonia concentration and may lead to severe encephalopathy.

As bands of fibrous tissue develop in the liver, blood flow becomes obstructed, leading to high pressure in the portal veins or *portal hypertension*. The backup of blood progresses through the hepatic portal system of veins, causing congestion in the spleen (**splenomegaly**), intestinal walls, and stomach (Fig. 18–14). Because the esophageal veins have several points of anastomosis or collateral channels to join with the gastric veins, the increased pressure of blood extends into the esophageal veins, creating large distended and distorted veins or varices near the mucosal surface of the esophagus. These veins are easily torn by food passing down the esophagus. Hemorrhage of these *esophageal varices* is a

TABLE 18–5 Common Manifestations of Liver Disease

Signs or Symptoms	Pathophysiology
Fatigue, anorexia, indigestion, weight loss	Metabolic dysfunction in the liver, such as decreased gluconeogenesis
	Decreased bile for digestion and absorption
	Portal hypertension leading to edema of intestinal wall, interfering with digestion and absorption
Ascites	Portal hypertension, elevated aldosterone and ADH levels, decreased serum albumin, lymphatic obstruction in liver
General edema	Elevated aldosterone and ADH levels, decreased serum albumin
Esophageal varices, hemorrhoids	Portal hypertension and collateral circulation
Splenomegaly	Portal hypertension
Anemia	Decreased absorption and storage of iron and vitamin B_{12}, malabsorption, splenomegaly, bleeding
Leukopenia, thrombocytopenia	Splenomegaly, possible bone marrow depression
Increased bleeding, purpura	Decreased absorption of vitamin K, decreased production of clotting factors by liver, thrombocytopenia
Hepatic encephalopathy tremors, confusion, coma	Metabolic dysfunction with inability to remove ammonia from protein metabolism and other toxic substances
Gynecomastia, impotence, irregular menses	Impaired inactivation of sex hormones (e.g., estrogen) leads to imbalance
Jaundice	Impaired extraction and conjugation of bilirubin
	Decreased production of bile and obstruction of bile flow
Pruritus	Bile salts in the tissues due to biliary obstruction

common complication of cirrhosis. The high pressure in the portal veins in conjunction with other factors also affects fluid shifts in the hepatic portal system, leading to *ascites* (Fig. 18–15). Ascites is an accumulation of fluid in the peritoneal cavity that causes abdominal distention. Portal hypertension increases the hydrostatic pressure in the veins, the increased serum aldosterone levels result in increased sodium ion and water in the extracellular compartment, and the decreased serum levels of albumin lower the plasma osmotic pressure. All these factors contribute to a shift of fluid out of the blood and into the peritoneal cavity. The fibrous tissue in the liver also interferes with bile flow out of the liver, leading to obstructive jaundice with elevated conjugated as well as unconjugated bilirubin levels in the blood.

The progressive changes that occur in biliary and postnecrotic cirrhosis are directly linked to inflammation, necrosis, and fibrosis associated with the primary condition. In patients with *alcoholic liver disease*, or portal cirrhosis, there are several stages in the development of hepatocellular damage related to the effects of alcohol. Alcohol and its metabolites, such as acetaldehyde, are

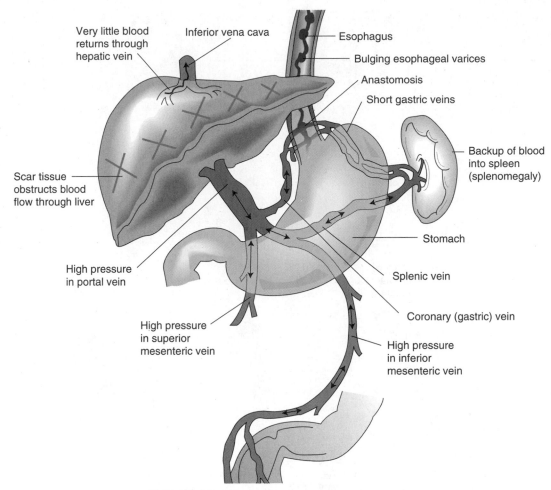

Very little blood returns through hepatic vein

Inferior vena cava

Esophagus

Bulging esophageal varices

Anastomosis

Short gastric veins

Backup of blood into spleen (splenomegaly)

Scar tissue obstructs blood flow through liver

High pressure in portal vein

Stomach

Splenic vein

High pressure in superior mesenteric vein

Coronary (gastric) vein

High pressure in inferior mesenteric vein

FIGURE 18–14. Development of esophageal varices.

toxic to the liver cells and alter many metabolic processes in the liver. Secondary malnutrition may aggravate the damaging effects on liver cells. The initial change in alcoholic liver disease is the accumulation of fat in liver cells, causing *fatty liver.* Other than enlargement of the liver or hepatomegaly, this stage is asymptomatic and is reversible if alcohol intake is reduced. In the second stage, *alcoholic hepatitis,* inflammation and cell necrosis occur. Fibrous tissue forms, an irreversible change. Acute inflammation may develop when alcohol intake generally increases to a higher level or "binge drinking" becomes more excessive. This second stage may also be asymptomatic, or it may become manifest with mild symptoms such as anorexia, nausea, and liver tenderness. In some patients with an episode of excessive alcohol intake, there may be sufficient damage to precipitate liver failure, encephalopathy, and death. The third stage, or *end-stage cirrhosis,* is reached when fibrotic tissue replaces normal tissue, significantly altering the basic liver structure to the extent that little normal function remains. Signs of portal hypertension or impaired digestion and absorption are the usual early indicators of this stage.

SIGNS AND SYMPTOMS

Initial manifestations of cirrhosis are often mild and vague and include such signs as fatigue, anorexia, weight loss, anemia, and diarrhea. Dull aching pain may be present in the upper right quadrant. As cirrhosis advances, ascites and peripheral edema develop, increased bruising is evident, esophageal varices form, and eventually jaundice and encephalopathy occur (see Table 18–5). An imbalance in sex hormone levels secondary to impaired inactivation mechanisms leads to spider nevi on the skin, testicular atrophy, impotence, gynecomastia, and irregular menses. Complications involve ruptured esophageal varices leading to hemorrhage, circulatory shock and acute hepatic encephalopathy. Acute encephalopathy is manifest by asterixis, a "hand-flapping tremor," and by confusion, disorientation, convulsions, and coma. Chronic encephalopathy is characterized by personality changes, memory lapses, irritability, and disinterest in personal care. Another complication of cirrhosis is the presence of frequent infections, perhaps respiratory or skin infections. These infections are encouraged by excessive fluids in the

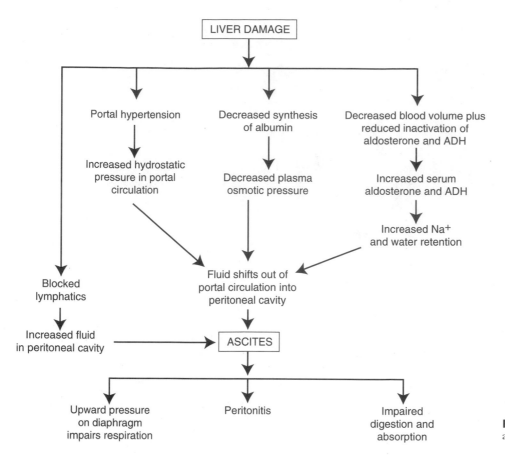

FIGURE 18-15. Development of ascites with cirrhosis.

tissues that interfere with the diffusion of nutrients and thus lead to delayed tissue regeneration and healing. Also, a decreased protein level and anemia impair tissue maintenance. Pruritus and associated scratching of the skin may damage the skin barrier, leading to infection.

TREATMENT

Supportive or symptomatic treatment such as avoiding fatigue and exposure to infection is necessary. Dietary restrictions may include restrictions on protein and sodium intake. High carbohydrate intake and vitamin supplements are necessary. Serum electrolytes may have to be balanced, possibly requiring the use of diuretics (e.g., furosemide) to reduce body fluids. Antibiotics such as neomycin are useful to reduce intestinal flora and control serum ammonia levels. Ruptured esophageal varices need emergency treatment. Portocaval shunts may be used to reduce portal hypertension. Liver transplants are becoming more common. Occasionally part of an adult's liver has been successfully transplanted into a child.

Cancer of the Liver

Primary malignant tumors are relatively rare in the liver. The most common tumor is hepatocellular carci-

noma secondary to hepatitis B or C. Tumors may also result from prolonged exposure to **carcinogenic** chemicals. Secondary or metastatic cancer is very common in the liver, particularly cancers that arise from areas served by the hepatic portal veins or that spread along the peritoneal membranes (see Fig. 5–6). The signs of liver cancer initially are mild and general and are similar to those of other liver diseases; they include anorexia and vomiting, fatigue, weight loss, and hepatomegaly. Because of the minimal early indications, the cancer is usually advanced by time of diagnosis. Chemotherapy is the usual treatment.

Thinkabout   18–10

a. Describe the structure of the liver as it is altered by cirrhosis.

b. At which stage(s) is alcoholic liver disease reversible and why?

c. State the rationale for each of the following manifestations of cirrhosis: excessive bleeding, ascites, jaundice, weight loss.

Acute Pancreatitis

PATHOPHYSIOLOGY

Pancreatitis is an inflammation of the pancreas resulting from **autodigestion** of the tissues. It may occur in acute or chronic form. The autodigestion follows activation of the pancreatic enzymes within the pancreas itself. It appears that activation of the proenzyme trypsinogen into trypsin is the trigger; in turn, trypsin converts other proenzymes and chemicals into active forms. The activated enzymes, trypsin, and the proteases amylase and lipase digest the pancreatic tissue, leading to massive inflammation and necrosis. The pancreas is composed of delicate tissue and lacks a fibrous capsule that might contain the effects of autodigestion for a time. In some cases, pseudocysts or pancreatic **abscesses** may develop if the local inflammatory response is successful in localizing the injury. However, in many cases, enzymatic destruction of tissue progresses around the pancreas. Fat necrosis occurs (lipase), binding calcium ions, and blood vessels are eroded by elastase (a protease), leading to hemorrhage. In addition to this enzyme activity, the damaging products released by tissue necrosis lead to widespread inflammation of the peritoneal membranes. The inflammatory response, including vasodilation and increased capillary permeability, leads to hypovolemia and circulatory collapse. The severe pain associated with the autodigestion of nerves and the inflammation contributes to shock (neurogenic shock). Chemical peritonitis develops as the inflammation spreads, eventually resulting in bacterial peritonitis as intestinal bacteria escape through the more permeable membranes (see Fig. 18–20). If the inflammatory process is not controlled quickly, sepsis may result from the escape of bacteria and toxins from the intestines into the general circulation. Other complications which may cause death are adult respiratory distress syndrome and acute renal failure.

ETIOLOGY

Although many factors may precipitate acute pancreatitis, the two major causes are gallstones and alcohol abuse. Gallstones may obstruct the flow of bile and pancreatic secretions into the duodenum or cause reflux of bile into the pancreatic duct, thus activating trypsinogen. Alcohol appears to stimulate an increased secretion of pancreatic enzymes and contract the sphincter of Oddi, blocking flow, but there may be other mechanisms. Alcoholics do have chronic pancreatitis, and the acute episode may be an exacerbation of the chronic form rather than a separate entity.

SIGNS AND SYMPTOMS

Sudden onset of acute pancreatitis may follow intake of a large meal or a large amount of alcohol. Severe epigastric or abdominal pain radiating to the back is the primary symptom. Pain increases when the individual assumes a supine position. Signs of shock—low blood pressure, pallor and sweating, rapid but weak pulse—develop as inflammation and hemorrhage cause hypovolemia. Low-grade fever is common until infection develops, when body temperature may rise significantly. Abdominal distention and decreased bowel sounds occur as peritonitis leads to decreased peristalsis and paralytic ileus.

DIAGNOSTIC TESTS

Serum amylase level rises within the first 12 to 24 hours and falls after 48 hours. Serum lipase is also elevated and remains so for approximately a week. Hypocalcemia is common as calcium ions bind to fatty acids in areas of fat necrosis. Leukocytosis is an indicator of inflammation and infection.

TREATMENT

All oral intake is stopped, and bowel distention is relieved to reduce pancreatic stimulation. Shock as well as electrolyte imbalances are treated. Analgesics such as meperidine may be given for pain relief (not morphine, which causes spasm of the sphincter of Oddi).

Carcinoma of the Pancreas

Pancreatic (exocrine) cancer is increasing in incidence in North America. The major risk factor appears to be cigarette smoking. The common form of the neoplasm is adenocarcinoma, which arises from the epithelial cells in the ducts. A tumor at the head of the pancreas usually causes obstruction of biliary flow as well as pancreatic flow, leading to weight loss and jaundice as early manifestations. Cancer of the body and tail of the pancreas frequently remains asymptomatic until it is well advanced and involves the nearby structures, such as the liver, stomach, lymph nodes, or posterior abdominal wall and nerves. Liver failure resulting from hepatobiliary obstruction is frequently the cause of death.

Thinkabout 18–11

a. Explain why the liver is a common site of secondary cancer.

b. Explain the concept of autodigestion and describe two specific effects of this process in the pancreas.

LOWER GASTROINTESTINAL TRACT DISORDERS

Celiac Disease

Celiac disease, also called celiac sprue or gluten enteropathy, is a malabsorption syndrome that is considered primarily a childhood disorder. However, it may also occur in adults, usually at middle-age. There is a related disorder, tropical sprue, that is probably bacterial in origin and frequently occurs in epidemics in tropical areas. Celiac disease appears to be linked to genetic factors and consists of a defect in the intestinal enzymes that prevents further digestion of gliadin, a breakdown product of *gluten*. Gluten is a constituent of certain grains, wheat, barley, rye, and oats. Combining the digestive block with an immunologic response in the person results in a toxic effect on the intestinal villi. The villi atrophy, resulting in decreased enzyme production and less surface area available for absorption of nutrients. Thus, the end result of celiac disease is malabsorption and malnutrition. In an infant, the first signs of the disorder usually appear as cereals are added to the diet around 4 to 6 months of age. Malabsorption syndromes are manifested by steatorrhea, muscle wasting, and failure to gain weight. Irritability and malaise are common. Fortunately, celiac disease can usually be treated by maintaining a gluten-free diet, using corn and rice for grains. The intestinal mucosa returns to normal after a few weeks without gluten intake.

Chronic Inflammatory Diseases or Inflammatory Bowel Disease

Crohn's disease and ulcerative colitis are chronic inflammatory diseases, the causes of which are unknown. A genetic factor appears to be involved because there is a higher familial incidence and inflammatory bowel disease (IBD) is much more common among certain groups, namely, whites, particularly Ashkenazic Jews (from Eastern Europe). Investigative studies on an immunologic abnormality continue because many individuals have factors such as anticolon antibodies or HLA and a cytokine, interleukin (IL) in the blood as well as T-lymphocytes that are cytotoxic to the mucosa. In many patients, particularly those with ulcerative colitis, there are manifestations of immune abnormalities elsewhere in the body, including iritis, ankylosing spondylitis, and nephrolithiasis. There are many similarities between Crohn's disease and ulcerative colitis, and there may be an overlap in their clinical presentation. Both diseases occur in both males and females. Crohn's disease often develops in childhood or adolescence, whereas ulcerative colitis more frequently appears in the second or third decade. These diseases are characterized by remissions and exacerbations as well as considerable diversity in the severity of clinical effects.

CROHN'S DISEASE (REGIONAL ILEITIS OR REGIONAL ENTERITIS)

Pathophysiology

Crohn's disease may affect any area of the digestive tract but occurs most frequently in the small intestine, particularly the terminal ileum and sometimes the colon. Inflammation occurs in a characteristic distribution called "skip lesions" with affected segments clearly separated by areas of normal tissue (Fig. 18–16). Initially, inflammation occurs in the mucosal layer with the development of shallow ulcers. The ulcers tend to coalesce to form fissures separated by thickened elevations or nodules, giving the wall a typical "cobblestone" appearance. The progressive inflammation and fibrosis may affect all layers of the wall (transmural), leading eventually to a thick, rigid "rubber hose" wall. This change leaves a narrow lumen ("string sign"), which may become totally obstructed. Granulomas indicative of chronic inflammation may be found in the wall and in the regional lymph nodes. The damaged wall impairs the ability of the small intestine to process and absorb food. Also, the inflammation stimulates intestinal motility, decreasing the time available for digestion and absorption.

Other complications are common. Adhesions between two loops of intestine may develop when the subserosa is inflamed. The ulcers may penetrate the intestinal wall, causing abscesses to form. Fistulas, a connecting passage between two structures, may form as the ulcer erodes through the intestinal wall. Fistulas may be found between two loops of intestine (see Fig. 18–16), between the intestine and the bladder, or between the intestine and the skin.

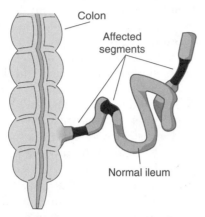

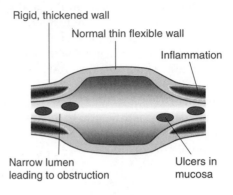

A. "Skip lesions" — distribution of affected segments alternating with normal segments of bowel

B. Changes in the intestinal wall

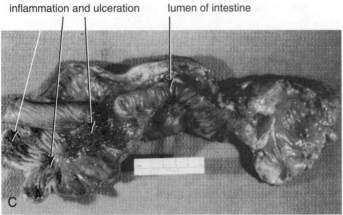

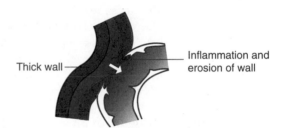

D. Fistula–abnormal opening between two structures

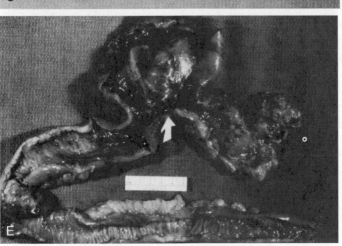

FIGURE 18–16. Regional ileitis (Crohn's disease). *A*, "Skip lesions." *B*, Narrowing and obstruction. *C*, Photograph showing narrowing ("garden-hose") and inflammation-ulceration of bowel. *D*, Diagram of fistula. *E*, Photograph of fistula. (*C* and *E* courtesy of R.W. Shaw, M.D., North York General Hospital, Toronto, Ontario.)

Signs and Symptoms

The course of Crohn's disease is variable. Exacerbations are marked by diarrhea with cramping abdominal pain. The stool is typically soft or semi-formed. Melena may occur if the ulcers erode blood vessels. Anorexia, weight loss, and fatigue are associated with malabsorption and malnutrition. Children have delayed growth and sexual maturation due to lack of adequate protein and vitamins, particularly fat-soluble vitamins A and D. Also, treatment with glucocorticoids hampers growth. In addition, many psychological implications are associated with this type of chronic illness.

ULCERATIVE COLITIS

Pathophysiology

The inflammation commences in the rectum and progresses in a continuous fashion proximally through the colon. The small intestine is rarely involved. The mucosa and submucosa are inflamed, commencing at the base of the crypts of Lieberkuhn (mucus-secreting goblet cells). The tissue becomes edematous and friable, and ulcerations develop. In an attempt to heal, granulation tissue forms, but it is vascular and fragile and bleeds easily. When the ulcers coalesce, large areas of the mucosa become denuded, but there are residual "bridges" of intact mucosa over the ulcers. This tissue destruction interferes with the absorption of fluid and electrolytes in the colon. In severe acute episodes, a serious complication, *toxic megacolon,* may develop, as inflammation impairs peristalsis, leading to obstruction and dilation of the colon. A concern with long-term ulcerative colitis is the increased risk of colorectal carcinoma, which may be predicted by preceding metaplasia and **dysplasia** in the mucosa.

Signs and Symptoms

Diarrhea is present, consisting of frequent watery stools marked by the presence of blood and mucus and accompanied by cramping pain. During severe exacerbations, blood and mucus alone may be passed frequently, day or night, accompanied by **tenesmus**. Fever and weight loss may be present. Rectal bleeding may be considerable and contributes to severe iron deficiency anemia.

Treatment

Exacerbations are often precipitated by physical or emotional stressors. It is helpful to identify and remove, if possible, the specific factors that apply in each individual. It is beneficial to use a team approach to the treatment of IBD because it involves multiple aspects of care. Specific measures usually include anti-inflammatory medications such as sulfasalazine (sulfapyridine with 5-aminosalicylic acid) or glucocorticoids. These may be administered systemically, both orally and parenterally, or topically as an enema or suppository. In some refractive cases, other immunosuppressive agents may be used. Antimotility agents are used in some patients with mild disease or following bowel resection. Nutritional supplements are frequently required, particularly during acute episodes. Total parenteral nutrition (intravenous) may be required during severe exacerbations. The recommended diet is usually high in protein, vitamins, and calories but low in fat. Low-bulk diets reduce intestinal stimulation during exacerbations. Antibiotics are required for secondary infection. Surgery (resection or **ileostomy**, a procedure to create an artificial opening on the surface of the abdomen) is necessary for complications such as obstruction or fistulas or severe exacerbations that do not respond to medication. In some cases surgical intervention may provide a temporary rest for the intestine and can be reversed to normal at a later time.

Thinkabout 18–12

a. Describe the characteristics of steatorrhea.

b. Explain how the pathologic changes seen in celiac disease lead to malabsorption.

c. Prepare a chart comparing Crohn's disease and ulcerative colitis by location and characteristics of the lesions, manifestations, and potential complications.

d. Explain several ways in which an adolescent's growth and development could be impaired by the presence of Crohn's disease.

Appendicitis

A common acute problem in young adults, appendicitis is an inflammation of the vermiform appendix (see Fig. 18–1). It may be secondary to obstruction of the appendiceal lumen by a **fecalith** or foreign material, or it may be due to twisting or spasm, and sometimes it develops for unknown reasons. Initially, the appendiceal wall is inflamed, and purulent exudate forms. The increasing congestion and pressure within the appendix leads to ischemia and necrosis of the wall, resulting in increased permeability that allows bacteria and toxins to escape through the wall into the surrounding area. This breakout of bacteria leads to abscess formation or bacterial peritonitis. An abscess may develop when the adjacent omentum temporarily walls off the inflamed area by adhering to the appendiceal surface. In some cases, the inflammation and pain subside temporarily but then recur. Peritonitis, usually localized, develops as the bacteria leak through the inflamed wall of the appendix and spread along the peritoneal membranes. The wall appears blackish in color as gangrene develops (infection in necrotic tissue). Eventually, the appendix ruptures or perforates, releasing its contents into the peritoneal cavity. This leads to generalized peritonitis, which may be life-threatening (see Fig. 18–20).

In classic cases, general periumbilical pain related to the inflammation and stretching of the appendiceal wall occurs initially. Nausea and vomiting are common, and then the pain becomes more severe and localized in the lower right quadrant (LRQ), accompanied by LRQ tenderness (at McBurney's point midway between the umbilicus and the iliac crest). Localized pain results from involvement of the parietal peritoneum over the appendix. The location of the appendix does vary among individuals, and this can be diagnostically misleading. Sometimes appendicitis develops "silently." Following rupture, the pain usually subsides temporarily as the pressure is relieved but then recurs as a steady, severe abdominal pain as peritonitis develops. Low-grade fever and leukocytosis occur as inflammation develops. Other signs indicating the onset of peritonitis include a rigid "boardlike" abdomen, tachycardia, and hypotension. Treatment requires surgical removal of the appendix and administration of antibiotics.

Diverticular Disease

Diverticular disease refers to various problems related to the development of diverticula. A *diverticulum* is a herniation or outpouching of the mucosa through the muscle layer of the colon wall, frequently in the sigmoid. Usually multiple diverticula are present. *Diverticulitis* refers to inflammation of the diverticula, and *diverticulosis* is asymptomatic diverticular disease. It is a common problem in the Western world, affecting primarily older individuals. Diverticula form at gaps between bands of longitudinal muscle that coincide with openings in the circular muscle bands that permit passage of blood vessels through the wall. Congenital weakness of the wall may also be a contributing factor. These weaker areas bulge outward when pressure is increased frequently inside the lumen of the intestine, for example, in the presence of strong muscle contractions. Consistent low-residue diets, irregular bowel habits, and aging lead to chronic constipation and then to muscle

hypertrophy in the colon with elevated intraluminal pressures and finally to the gradual development of diverticula.

In many cases, diverticular disease remains asymptomatic. Sometimes there is mild discomfort, diarrhea, or constipation and flatulence, which can be excused for other reasons. With diverticulitis, inflammation, related to stasis of feces in the pouches, develops in the diverticula. Lower left quadrant cramping or steady pain and tenderness with nausea and vomiting indicate inflammatory disease. A slight fever and elevated white blood cell count accompany the discomfort. During acute episodes of diverticulitis, food intake is reduced, and antibiotics are taken as required. Diverticular disease is treated by increasing the bulk in the diet and encouraging regular bowel movements without constipation. Potential complications include intestinal obstruction, perforation with peritonitis, and abscess formation.

Colorectal Cancer

In the United States, colorectal cancer ranks high as a cancer killer in individuals older than 50 years. Most malignant neoplasms develop from adenomatous polyps, of which there are a diversity of types. A polyp is a mass that protrudes into the lumen, and many polyps represent genetic abnormalities. As polyps increase in size, they carry an increased risk of dysplasia and malignant changes. The presence of familial multiple polyposis (Fig. 18–17) or long-term ulcerative colitis in a patient or occurrence of colorectal cancer among close relatives increase the risk of cancer developing. Environmental factors such as diet also appear to play a major role in carcinogenesis. High fat and sugar intake are thought to produce carcinogenic substances, whereas low-fiber diets increase risk because they prolong the contact time of the mucosa with carcinogens.

Carcinomas are distributed about equally in the right or ascending colon, the left or descending colon, and the distal sigmoid and rectum. In recent years an increasing number of tumors have been found in the right colon because lesions in this location are more difficult to diagnose easily at an early stage by routine rectal digital examination or proctosigmoidoscopy. Tumors in the sigmoid and rectum are more easily accessible. Carcinomas may manifest differently, for example, as circumferential or annular constrictive "napkin-ring" growths (see Fig. 18–17), which are common in the left colon, or as projecting polypoid masses, common in the right colon. Flat ulcerating lesions occur less frequently. All types of carcinomas invade the wall, the mesentery, and the lymph nodes and metastasize to the liver.

Although most carcinomas remain asymptomatic until they are well advanced, the initial signs of colorectal cancer depend largely on the location of the growth as related to the characteristics of the feces at that point. For example, an annular lesion in the rectosigmoid area, where the fecal mass is relatively solid, causes partial obstruction with dilation of the proximal colon (see Fig. 18–17). Vague cramping pain, small flat pellets or "ribbon" stool, and a feeling of incomplete emptying are common signs of cancer in this location. Cancer in the right colon, where the fecal material is liquid, does not cause obstruction but often becomes manifest by systemic signs such as fatigue, weight loss, or iron deficiency anemia. An unexplained change in bowel habits, such as alternating diarrhea and constipation, may be a sign of malignancy. Bleeding may be indicated by occult blood or melena if it arises from the proximal colon. Regular testing of stool specimens for occult blood has been suggested as a useful screening tool. Frank (red) blood and mucus on or near the surface of the stool usually are related to bleeding from a lesion in the rectum. Staging of colorectal cancer is based on Dukes' classification, which assesses the extent of invasiveness of the neoplasm into the intestinal wall, involvement of lymph nodes, and the presence of distant metastases (see Chapter 5). Category A tumors are localized in the mucosa and submucosa, whereas category D tumors have widespread metastases. Colorectal cancer is treated by surgical removal of the involved area, usually requiring a **colostomy**, an artificial opening into the abdominal wall where feces may be continually collected in a bag. Both curative and palliative surgery may be accompanied by radiation and chemotherapy.

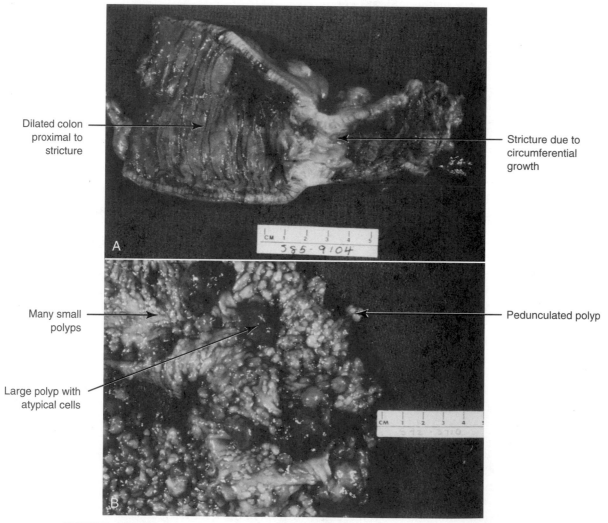

Dilated colon proximal to stricture

Stricture due to circumferential growth

Many small polyps

Pedunculated polyp

Large polyp with atypical cells

FIGURE 18–17. Colorectal cancer. *A,* Photograph showing circumferential malignant growth (cancer) obstructing flow of feces and causing proximal dilation of the colon. *B,* Photograph showing polyposis and malignant changes. (Courtesy of R.W. Shaw, M.D., North York General Hospital, Toronto, Ontario.)

Thinkabout 18–13

a. Describe, in the order in which they develop, each stage of the pain seen with acute appendicitis, including the location and type of pain and the reason for it.

b. Define the term diverticulitis and explain how diverticula develop and become inflamed.

c. State two factors that predispose a patient to colorectal cancer.

d. Explain why the signs of colorectal cancer vary with the location of the tumor.

Intestinal Obstruction

Intestinal obstruction refers to a lack of movement of the intestinal contents through the intestine. This impairment develops more frequently in the small intestine but can occur in the large intestine as well. Depending on the cause and location, obstruction may manifest as an acute problem or a gradually developing situation. For example, twisting of the intestine could cause sudden total obstruction, whereas a tumor leads to progressive obstruction. Because of its smaller lumen, obstructions are more common and occur more rapidly in the small intestine. There are two kinds of causes. *Mechanical* obstructions are those resulting from tumor, adhesions, hernias, or other tangible obstructions (Fig. 18–18). *Functional* or adynamic obstructions result from neurologic impairment such as spinal cord injury or lack of propulsion in the intestine and are frequently referred to as *paralytic ileus.*

PATHOPHYSIOLOGY

When mechanical obstruction of the flow of intestinal contents occurs, gases and fluids accumulate in the area proximal to the blockage, distending the intestine (Fig. 18–19). Gases arise primarily from swallowed air but also from bacterial activity in the intestine. Increasing strong contractions of the proximal intestine develop in an effort to move the contents onward. The increasing pressure in the lumen leads to more secretions entering the intestine and also compresses the veins in the wall, preventing absorption as the intestinal wall becomes edematous. The intestinal distention leads to persistent vomiting with additional loss of fluid and electrolytes. With small intestinal obstructions, there is no opportunity to reabsorb fluid and electrolytes, and hypovolemia quickly results.

If the obstruction is not removed, the intestinal wall becomes ischemic and necrotic as the arterial blood supply to the tissue is reduced by the pressure. If twisting of the intestine (e.g., volvulus) occurs, or if immediate compression of arteries (e.g., intussusception or strangulated hernia) results from the primary cause of obstruction, the intestinal wall becomes necrotic and gangrenous very rapidly. Gangrene refers to bacterial invasion and colonization of necrotic tissue. The obstruction promotes rapid reproduction of intestinal bacteria, some of which produce endotoxins. As the wall becomes necrotic and more permeable, intestinal bacteria or toxins can leak into the peritoneal cavity (peritonitis) or into the blood supply (bacteremia and septicemia). In time, perforation of the necrotic segment may occur. Also, ischemia and necrosis of the intestinal wall eventually lead to decreased innervation and cessation of peristalsis. A decrease in bowel sounds indicates this change.

Functional obstruction or paralytic ileus usually results from neurologic impairment. Peristalsis ceases and distention of the intestine occurs as fluids and electrolytes accumulate in the intestine. In this type of obstruction, reflex spasms of the intestinal muscle do not occur, but the remainder of the process is similar to that of mechanical obstruction.

ETIOLOGY

Functional obstruction or paralytic ileus is common following abdominal surgery, in which the effects of the anesthetic combined with inflammation or ischemia in the operative area interfere with conduction of nerve impulses. It may also occur in the initial stage of spinal cord injuries or with hypokalemia, mesenteric thrombosis, toxemia, or inflammation related to ischemia, pancreatitis, peritonitis, or infection in the abdominal cavity.

Mechanical obstruction may result from adhesions (from prior surgery, infection, or radiation) that twist or constrict the intestine, from hernias (protrusion of a section of intestine through an opening in the muscle wall), or from strictures due to scar tissue. Tumors, foreign bodies, intussusception (telescoping of a section of bowel inside an adjacent section), or volvulus (twisting of a section of intestine on itself) are other common causes of obstruction. In many cases, the cause of intussusception or volvulus is unknown. Intussusception may occur secondary to polyps or tumors that pull a section of bowel forward with them. Volvulus may be linked to adhesions. Hirschsprung's disease or congenital megacolon is a condition in which parasympathetic innervation is missing from a section of the colon,

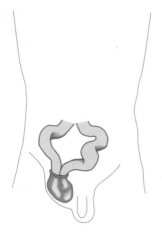

A. Inguinal hernia

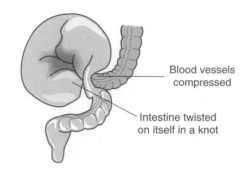

Blood vessels compressed

Intestine twisted on itself in a knot

B. Volvulus

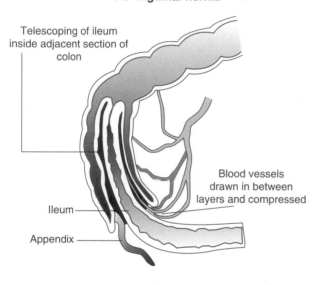

Telescoping of ileum inside adjacent section of colon

Blood vessels drawn in between layers and compressed

Ileum

Appendix

C. Intussusception

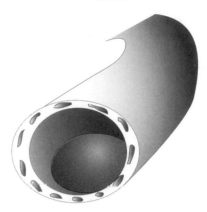

D. Tumor

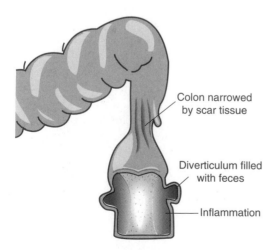

Colon narrowed by scar tissue

Diverticulum filled with feces

Inflammation

E. Diverticulitis

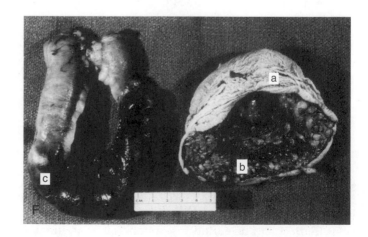

FIGURE 18–18. *A–E,* Causes of intestinal obstruction. *F,* Photograph of hernia with infarcted intestine. The sac consists of the abdominal wall covered by skin (a) at a site weakened by scar tissue, forming a protrusion into which a loop of intestine is compressed (b). This protrusion obstructs the blood flow to the intestinal wall (c) (infarcted area) as well as the flow of feces inside the intestine. (Courtesy of R.W. Shaw, M.D., North York General Hospital, Toronto, Ontario.)

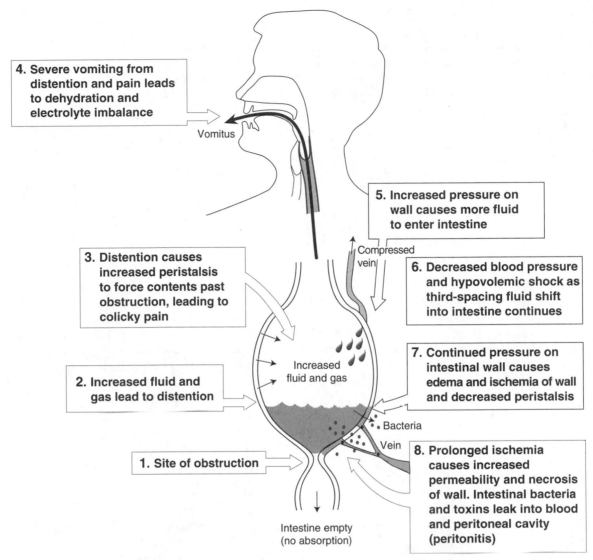

FIGURE 18-19. Effects of intestinal obstruction.

impairing motility and leading to constipation and eventually obstruction. This condition often occurs in conjunction with other anomalies. Gradual obstruction may develop from chronic inflammatory conditions such as Crohn's disease or diverticulitis.

SIGNS AND SYMPTOMS

With mechanical obstruction of the small intestine, severe colicky abdominal pain develops as peristalsis increases initially. Borborygmi (audible rumbling sounds due to movement of gas in the intestine) and intestinal rushes can be heard as the intestinal muscle forcefully contracts in an attempt to propel the contents forward. The signs of paralytic ileus differ significantly in that bowel sounds decrease or are absent, and pain is steady. Vomiting and abdominal distention occur quickly with obstruction of the small intestine. Vomiting is recurrent and consists first of gastric contents and then bile-stained duodenal contents. Restlessness and diaphoresis with tachycardia are typically present initially. As hypovolemia and electrolyte imbalances progress, signs of dehydration, weakness, and confusion are apparent, as well as signs of shock. Obstruction of the large intestine develops slowly and signs are mild. Constipation and mild lower abdominal pain are common, followed by abdominal distention, anorexia, and eventually vomiting and more severe pain.

TREATMENT

The underlying cause is treated, and fluids and electrolytes are replaced. Surgery and antimicrobial therapy are required as soon as possible for any strangulation, whereas paralytic ileus may need decompression by suction.

Peritonitis

Peritonitis is an inflammation of the peritoneal membranes. It may result from chemical irritation or directly from bacterial invasion of the sterile peritoneal cavity. Chemical irritation, unless resolved quickly, ultimately leads to bacterial peritonitis. It is usually an acute condition and requires treatment of the primary cause as well as the effects. The incidence of peritonitis and septicemia has decreased with the prophylactic use of antibiotics, but peritonitis remains a threat in many situations.

PATHOPHYSIOLOGY

Inflammation of the peritoneal membranes may commence with the presence of chemical irritants such as bile, chyme, or foreign objects in the peritoneal cavity. This inflammation then increases the permeability of the intestinal wall, permitting bacteria to enter the peritoneal cavity (Fig. 18–20). Necrosis or perforation of the intestinal wall also allows infection directly by enteric organisms. Initially, when local inflammation develops, the peritoneum and omentum tend to produce a thick, sticky exudate, which helps the adjacent tissues to stick together and temporarily seal the area, localizing the source of the problem. In some cases, the inflammation subsides and an abscess forms that may flare up at a later time. This local inflammation may also reduce peristalsis in the area, decreasing the risk of spreading toxins or bacteria at the time. However, unless the original cause of the problem is removed, it is likely that the inflammation or infection will spread.

The peritoneum consists of a large unlimited expanse of highly vascular tissue covering the viscera and lining the abdominal cavity. This structure provides a means of rapid dissemination of irritants or bacteria throughout the abdominal cavity. Also, the many blood vessels in the membranes can leak large volumes of fluid into the peritoneal cavity when inflammation leads to vasodilation and increased permeability of the blood vessels in the membrane. Hypovolemic shock results as this process of "third-spacing" occurs (see Chapter 16). The fluid, protein, and electrolytes sequestered in the peritoneal cavity are not recycled into the circulating blood and therefore are of no value to body fluid balance. Nausea and vomiting, resulting from the intestinal irritation and pain, add to the fluid loss. Abdominal distention is evident, and the typical, rigid boardlike abdomen develops as reflex abdominal muscle spasm occurs in response to involvement of the parietal peritoneum. Also, the inflamed membranes permit intestinal bacteria and toxic materials to migrate into the blood and then into the general circulation. When inflammation persists, nerve conduction is impaired, and peristalsis decreases, leading to obstruction of the intestines (paralytic ileus).

ETIOLOGY

Chemical peritonitis may result from the enzymes released with pancreatitis, urine leaking from a ruptured bladder, chyme spilled into the peritoneal cavity from a perforated ulcer, bile escaping from a perforated gallbladder, or from blood or any other foreign material in the cavity. Bacterial peritonitis may be caused by direct trauma affecting the intestines, a ruptured appendix, or intestinal obstruction, particularly when blood vessels are compressed and the wall becomes gangrenous. Any abdominal surgery may lead to the potential complication of peritonitis. Pelvic inflammatory disease in women, in which infection ascends through the uterus and into the fallopian tubes, which provide direct access to the peritoneal cavity, is another common cause (see Chapter 24). By no means are the causes limited to this list.

SIGNS AND SYMPTOMS

Sudden, severe, generalized abdominal pain occurs with localized tenderness at the site of the underlying problem. The pain tends to increase with any movement, and breathing is often restricted by the individual. Vomiting is common. Signs of dehydration and hypovolemia, including decreased skin turgor, dry buccal mucosa, pallor, low blood pressure, agitation, and tachycardia are present. Fever and leukocytosis occur as the inflammation and infection develop. Abdominal distention is common, and a rigid abdomen signals involvement of the parietal peritoneum. Decreased bowel sounds indicate the onset of paralytic ileus and secondary obstruction.

TREATMENT

Depending on the primary cause of the peritonitis, surgery may be required. Massive doses of antibiotics specific to the major causative organism are needed as well as replacement of fluids and electrolytes. Nasogastric suction to relieve abdominal distention is often required, as is treatment to combat paralytic ileus when appropriate.

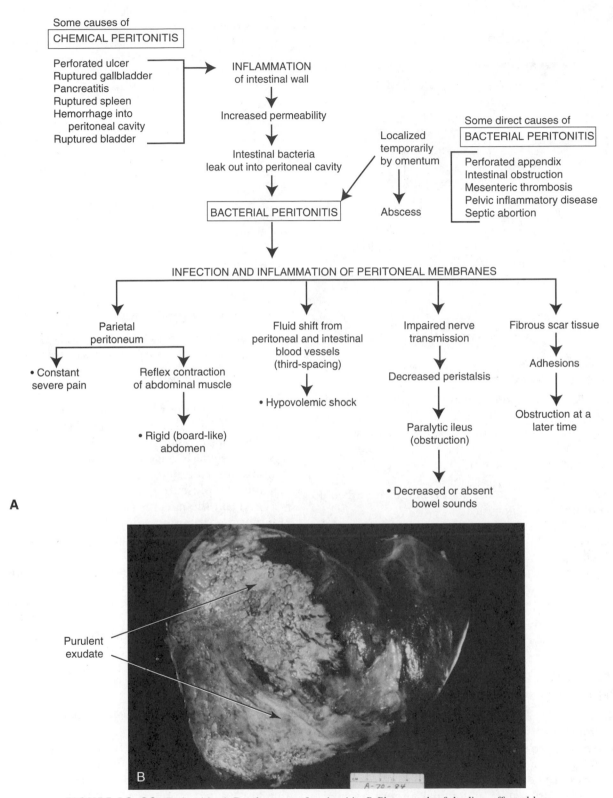

FIGURE 18–20. Peritonitis. *A,* Development of peritonitis. *B,* Photograph of the liver affected by acute peritonitis resulting from a ruptured appendix; liver is covered by a purulent exudate. (Courtesy of R.W. Shaw, M.D., North York General Hospital, Toronto, Ontario.)

Thinkabout 18–14

a. Explain why the characteristics of the pain differ with mechanical and functional obstruction.

b. Explain how each of the following conditions causes an intestinal obstruction: (1) intussusception, (2) adhesion, (3) inguinal hernia.

c. Explain (1) how an obstruction can lead to bacterial peritonitis, and (2) how peritonitis can lead to obstruction.

d. Explain the cause of hypovolemic shock with peritonitis.

e. What factors lead to metabolic acidosis with bacterial peritonitis?

CASE STUDIES

CASE STUDY A
Gastroenteritis

Baby K, age 14 months, has vomiting and diarrhea and is crying continuously because of what appears to be severe abdominal pain. The suspected cause is gastroenteritis due to *Staphylococcus aureus* from a milk custard that had not been properly stored.

a. Briefly describe how *S. aureus* in the custard could cause vomiting and diarrhea.

b. Describe the fluid and electrolyte imbalances that can be expected in Baby K.

c. What arterial blood gases would you expect to find in this case of gastroenteritis?

d. Describe the signs of dehydration that can be expected in a child.

e. Explain why a young child can quickly develop vascular collapse if vomiting and diarrhea are severe.

CASE STUDY B
Peptic Ulcer and Peritonitis

Ms. X, age 76, has been admitted to the emergency department with severe generalized abdominal pain and vomiting. No significant findings were immediately evident to indicate a cause. Six hours later, Ms. X 's blood pressure began to drop, and her pulse was rapid but thready. Exploratory abdominal surgery revealed a perforated gastric ulcer and peritonitis.

a. Describe the process by which an ulcer develops.

b. Suggest several possible factors contributing to ulcer formation.

c. Explain why peptic ulcer may not be diagnosed in an early stage of development.

d. Describe the process of perforation of an ulcer and the development of bacterial peritonitis.

e. Explain why Ms. X showed signs of shock.

Following surgery, Ms. X had no bowel sounds, and her abdomen was distended.

f. Describe how paralytic ileus could have developed.

g. Ms. X was given antibiotics, intravenous fluids, and intravenous alimentation (total parenteral nutrition). Explain the reason for each of these treatments.

h. Explain why older individuals may have difficulty in compensating for fluid and electrolyte imbalances.

i. List other potential complications of immobility for which Ms. X is at risk during a prolonged recovery.

CASE STUDY C
Hepatitis B and Cirrhosis

JB, age 35, has had chronic hepatitis B for 9 years. The origin of his acute infection was never ascertained.

a. Describe the pathophysiology of acute hepatitis B infection.

b. If JB had known about his exposure, could any treatment measures have been undertaken at the time?

c. Describe two signs of the preicteric stage and three signs of the icteric stage of acute hepatitis B infection.

d. What serum markers remain high when chronic hepatitis B is present?

e. Explain the circumstances under which JB could transmit the virus (including the various stages of the disease [preicteric, icteric, and so on] as well as the mode of transmission).

f. Explain how cirrhosis develops from chronic hepatitis B.

g. Explain why the early stage of cirrhosis is relatively asymptomatic.

JB's cirrhosis is now well advanced. He has developed ascites, edema in the legs and feet, and esophageal varices. His appetite is poor, he is fatigued, and he has frequent respiratory and skin infections. Jaundice is noticeable.

h. What factors predispose JB to each of the manifestations listed above?

i. If a cure for hepatitis B were discovered at this point, how would this affect JB's prognosis?

j. JB has been admitted with hematemesis and shock due to ruptured esophageal varices. Explain why each of the following events occur: (1) excessive bleeding from trauma, (2) increased serum ammonia levels, (3) flapping tremors and confusion.

CASE STUDY D
Crohn's Disease

Mr. PT, age 19, has had Crohn's disease affecting the ileum and part of the jejunum for 5 years and has had numerous exacerbations.

a. Describe the pathophysiology of Crohn's disease.

b. Suggest several possible exacerbating factors associated with Crohn's disease.

c. Describe the common signs of an exacerbation.

d. Explain how nutritional deficits may occur with Crohn's disease.

e. PT has delayed growth (he is much shorter than his classmates). Suggest several specific contributing factors to retarded growth in a young person.

f. PT has developed a fistula between the ileum and the bladder. Describe the effect of a fistula.

g. There is considerable risk of intestinal obstruction developing in PT at some point in the near future. Explain how this obstruction could gradually form.

h. Suggest several manifestations, with the reason for each, of an acute obstruction in the ileum.

i. Describe the potential complications that might occur if an intestinal obstruction is not treated promptly.

STUDY QUESTIONS

1. (a) List the defense mechanisms that reduce the risk of infection in the oral cavity. (b) State the locations of resident (normal) flora in the digestive tract. (c) State the approximate pH of gastric secretions and two purposes served by this pH.

2. (a) Explain how the liver responds to high blood glucose levels. (b) Describe six functions of the liver (include a variety of functions).

3. (a) What is the major site of absorption and form of the major groups of nutrients? (b) What is the major site of absorption of water and electrolytes? (c) Which substances are absorbed primarily by active transport and which are absorbed by osmosis? (d) Explain why tissue damage hinders active transport.

4. Describe the location and role of the parasympathetic nervous system in defecation.

5. (a) Explain the purpose of the enterogastric reflex. (b) Describe two results of excessively rapid flow of chyme through the digestive tract.

6. (a) Name the common electrolytes lost because of diarrhea. (b) State the major effect on the body of sodium loss and of potassium loss. (c) State and explain what arterial blood gases may be expected in the presence of severe vomiting.

7. Define steatorrhea and explain several possible causes of this manifestation.

8. Explain several ways in which severe stress can affect the digestive tract.

9. Explain how an H_2-antagonist (drug) affects gastric function.

10. Explain how dysphagia may result from (a) stricture, (b) diverticulitis.

11. Explain why hiatal hernia is aggravated by (a) intake of a large meal, and (b) lying down after a meal.

12. (a) Explain several mechanisms by which intestinal infection can cause diarrhea. (b) Explain how fluid balance and acid-base balance are altered by diarrhea.

13. (a) Explain why peptic ulcers often do not heal quickly but tend to persist or recur. (b) Describe the common differences between gastric ulcer and gastric cancer. (c) Explain why abdominal cramps occur with the dumping syndrome.

14. (a) Define cholecystitis. (b) List factors that predispose to cholelithiasis. (c) Trace a gallstone on its path from a bile canaliculus to the duodenum and note the different possible effects caused by obstruction at various locations.

15. (a) State a common cause of posthepatic jaundice and the significant change in serum bilirubin that occurs with it. (b) Describe the common manifestations of acute hepatitis. (c) Describe how chronic hepatitis may affect liver tissue. (d) Define fulminant hepatitis and its possible outcomes.

16. (a) Describe the three common types of cirrhosis and give one cause of each. (b) State the rationale for each of the following signs of cirrhosis: nausea, abdominal pain (upper right quadrant), esophageal varices, hepatic encephalopathy.

17. Describe possible obstructive effects of liver cancer.

18. Explain two causes of shock resulting from acute pancreatitis.

19. (a) Explain why malnutrition may develop from Crohn's disease. (b) Explain the process by which chronic bleeding may cause anemia. (c) Explain, using an example, how a fistula develops in patients with Crohn's disease. (d) Compare the characteristics of diarrhea typical of Crohn's disease and ulcerative colitis.

20. Describe the pathophysiology involved in the various stages of acute appendicitis.

21. Explain how a long-term low-residue diet contributes to the development of diverticula.

22. (a) List the common early signs of colorectal cancer, relating each to a particular site. (b) Explain why the prognosis for colorectal cancer is relatively poor.

23. (a) Explain how intestinal obstruction results from (i) volvulus, (ii) paralytic ileus, (iii) tumor. (b) Explain how hypovolemia develops with intestinal obstruction.

24. (a) Explain how the peritoneal membranes may provide a defense in the early stage of acute appendicitis. (b) Explain how the structure of the peritoneal membrane may be a disadvantage after the appendix ruptures. (c) Explain how shock develops with acute peritonitis.

CHAPTER

19

Urinary System Disorders

KEY TERMS

active transport	embolus	nocturia	pyuria
anastomosis	frequency	oliguria	renal colic
anuria	glucosuria	orthostatic hypotension	retroperitoneal
autoregulation	hematuria	osmosis	semipermeable
azotemia	hyperkalemia	osteodystrophy	membrane
calculi	hypertension	osteoporosis	tetany
dialysate	immunosuppression	polyuria	ultrafiltration
diffusion	infarction	proteinuria	urgency
dysuria	necrosis		

REVIEW OF THE URINARY SYSTEM

The purpose of the urinary system is to remove metabolic wastes, hormones, drugs, and other foreign material and to regulate water, electrolytes, and acid-base balance in the body. Other functions include the secretion of erythropoietin, the activation of vitamin D, and the regulation of blood pressure through the renin-angiotensin-aldosterone system.

Thinkabout 19–1

What is the purpose of erythropoietin? of vitamin D?

The two kidneys are bean-shaped structures, each the size of a fist, located behind the peritoneum (that is, **retroperitoneally**) on the posterior abdominal wall. The kidneys are covered by a fibrous *capsule* and are embedded in fat, with the superior portion also protected by the lower ribs (Fig. 19–1).

Inside each kidney is the *cortex* or outer layer, in which the majority of the glomeruli are located, and the *medulla* or inner section of tissue, which consists primarily of the tubules and collecting ducts. Inside the medulla lies the *renal pelvis* and calyces, through which urine flows into the ureter (Fig. 19–2).

Each kidney consists of over a million *nephrons*, the functional units of the kidney (Fig. 19–3). The *glomeru-*

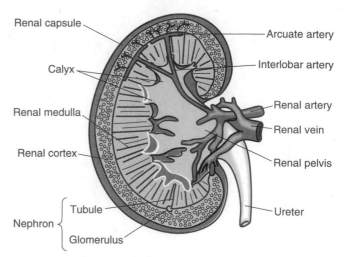

FIGURE 19–2. Anatomy of the kidney.

lus consists of Bowman's capsule surrounding a network of capillaries. These form the filtration unit for the blood. During *filtration* a large volume of fluid including wastes, nutrients, electrolytes, and other dissolved substances passes from the blood into the tubule. Cells and protein remain in the blood (Table 19–1). When the filtration pressure increases, more filtrate forms, and more urine is probably produced. The filtrate flows into the *tubules*. The tubule consists of three parts, the proximal convoluted tubule, the loop of Henle, and the distal convoluted tubule. Here *reabsorption* of essential nutrients, water, and electrolytes takes place and *secretion* of certain wastes and electrolytes occurs. The collecting ducts transport the urine to the renal pelvis.

Reabsorption is one process that takes place in the tubules. In the proximal convoluted tubule, most of the water is reabsorbed into the blood in the peritubular capillaries along with glucose and other nutrients and some electrolytes. Reabsorption of nutrients and electrolytes involves primarily the use of **active transport**, or cotransport, which requires carrier molecules and an energy source. If a substance such as glucose is present in excessive amounts in the filtrate, it is not all reabsorbed into the blood through the peritubular capillaries and therefore is present in the urine. This limit on reabsorption is called the *transport* or *tubular* maximum (e.g., approximately 310 mg/min for glucose). Thus, persistent **glucosuria** is an indication of diabetes mellitus. Water is reabsorbed by **osmosis.** As the filtrate progresses through the loop of Henle and the distal convoluted tubule, electrolytes and water are adjusted to the body's current needs. Concurrently, the acid-base balance of the blood is maintained with removal of excess acids and replacement of buffers such as bicarbonates (see Chapter 6). Active secretion of some wastes and drugs from the blood into the filtrate also occurs in the distal tubule (Fig. 19–4).

Hormones control the reabsorption of fluid and elec-

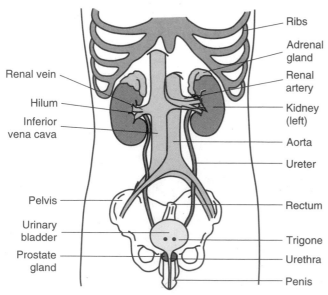

FIGURE 19–1. Gross anatomy of the urinary system (male).

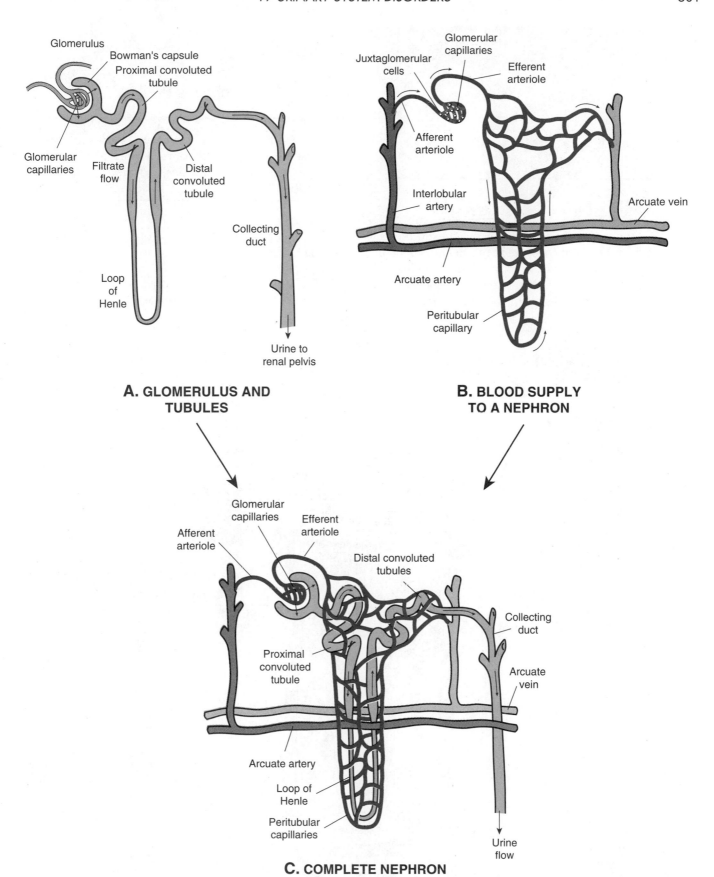

A. GLOMERULUS AND TUBULES

B. BLOOD SUPPLY TO A NEPHRON

C. COMPLETE NEPHRON

FIGURE 19-3. The nephron: *A,* Glomerulus and tubules; *B,* blood supply to the nephron; *C,* complete nephron.

TABLE 19–1	Composition of Blood, Filtrate, and Urine		
Substance	**Plasma**	**Filtrate**	**Urine**
Water (L)	180	180	1.4
Glucose (mg/L)	1000	1000	0
Protein (mg/L)	40,000	0–trace	0–trace
Urea (mg/L)	260	260	18,000
Na^+ (mEq/L)	142	142	128
K^+ (mEq/L)	5	5	60
HCO_3^- (mEq/L)	28	28	14

Thinkabout 19–2

Which of the following substances does the body normally retain? Which does it normally excrete? (1) glucose, (2) sodium ions, (3) bicarbonate ions, (4) acids?

trolytes (see Chapter 6). Antidiuretic hormone (ADH) controls the reabsorption of water by altering the permeability of the distal convoluted tubule and collecting duct. Aldosterone controls sodium reabsorption and water by exchanging sodium ions for potassium or hydrogen ions in the distal convoluted tubule.

The organization of the nephrons within a kidney is complex. The blood vessels and the collecting tubules and ducts for the filtrate must be functionally integrated to fulfill the purpose of the system. Scar tissue can interfere with blood or filtrate flow and thus can

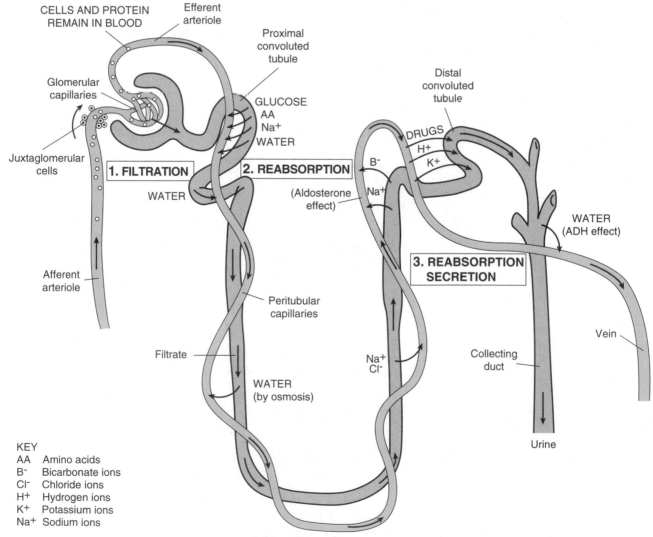

FIGURE 19–4. Formation of urine.

lead to secondary damage and progressive destruction of the kidney.

Blood enters and leaves the kidney at the hilum through the renal artery and vein. About 25 percent of the cardiac output enters the renal arteries from the aorta; thus the kidneys are processing a large volume of blood at any given time. Each renal artery passes through the pelvis, dividing several times during its passage (see Fig. 19–2). No **anastomoses** or junctions exist between the interlobar and arcuate arteries, meaning that no alternative blood supply is available to a lobe of the kidney that is deprived of its blood supply, perhaps by an **embolus** (e.g., a blood clot). Any obstruction to blood flow would therefore cause that particular lobe to undergo **necrosis** and **infarction.**

The interlobar arteries divide several times, eventually forming the *afferent arterioles,* which supply the *glomerular capillaries* (see Fig. 19–3). The arrangement of blood vessels in the kidney is unique because the blood from the glomerular capillaries then flows into another arteriole, the *efferent arteriole,* and then into a second capillary network, the *peritubular capillaries.* The blood then flows into small veins and finally into the *renal vein.* This blood supply also provides nourishment for the renal tissues.

Thinkabout 19–3

a. Trace the movement of a glucose molecule in the renal artery through the kidney, naming each structure and process in sequence.

b. Trace the progress of an acid waste from the distal convoluted tubule to the point of excretion.

The purpose of the dual arterioles is to control the pressure in the glomerular capillaries and consequently the glomerular filtration pressure. This pressure determines the glomerular filtration rate (GFR). By constricting or dilating the arterioles, the amount of blood in the capillaries is adjusted, and filtration is normally maintained regardless of fluctuations in the systemic blood pressure. For instance, if the afferent arteriole is dilated and the efferent arteriole is constricted, pressure in the glomerular capillaries will increase, and GFR will increase (Fig. 19–5). The degree of constriction in the arterioles is controlled by three factors, local **autoregulation**, the sympathetic nervous system, and the renin-angiotensin mechanism. Autoregulation refers to the small local reflex adjustments

in the diameter of the arterioles that are made in response to minor changes in blood flow in the kidneys. This adjustment maintains the normal filtration rate. The second factor, the sympathetic nervous system (SNS), increases vasoconstriction in both arterioles when stimulated. Third, renin is secreted by the juxtaglomerular cells in the kidney when blood flow in the afferent arteriole is reduced (see Fig. 19–5). Through a series of enzyme reactions, renin acts on the plasma protein angiotensinogen to produce angiotensin II, which is a powerful systemic vasoconstrictor. If blood flow in the kidney is seriously impaired as it is when blood pressure drops, both the SNS and the renin-angiotensin mechanism are activated to restore blood pressure and blood flow.

Thinkabout 19–4

a. Describe the effect on blood pressure within the glomerular capillaries and on filtration if the afferent arteriole is severely constricted.

b. Describe the effect of prolonged severe vasoconstriction on the renal tissue.

Blood pressure is closely related to kidney function, and frequently it is elevated with renal disease. Whenever the blood flow or blood pressure in the afferent arteriole decreases, the *renin-angiotensin-aldosterone* triad is stimulated. Angiotensin not only causes systemic vasoconstriction, it also stimulates the secretion of aldosterone. This hormone increases the reabsorption of sodium and water to increase blood volume, thus increasing blood pressure. Serum renin levels can determine whether this mechanism is a factor in hypertension (high blood pressure), in which case renin-blocking drugs (beta-adrenergic blocking drugs) can be prescribed (see Chapter 16).

Thinkabout 19–5

Explain the effect on blood volume and urine volume of increased secretion of renin over a long period of time.

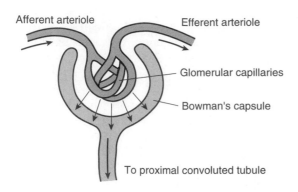

A. NORMAL FILTRATION

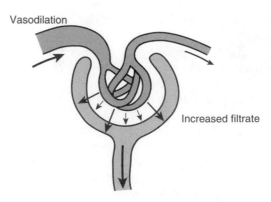

B. AFFERENT ARTERIOLE: DILATION

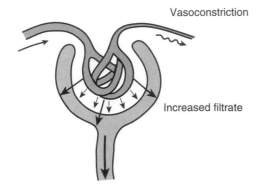

C. EFFERENT ARTERIOLE: CONSTRICTION

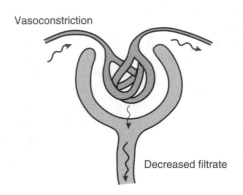

D. AFFERENT ARTERIOLE: CONSTRICTION

FIGURE 19–5. Control of glomerular filtration rate (GFR). *A,* Normal filtration; *B,* afferent arteriole: dilation; *C,* efferent arteriole: constriction; *D,* afferent arteriole: constriction.

When the filtrate has been processed in the tubules and collecting ducts, it is considered to be urine. Urine is transported through the collecting ducts to the renal calyces and pelvis and then into the ureters, where peristaltic movements assist its flow to the urinary bladder. The *bladder* is composed of smooth muscle lined with epithelium with rugae, or folds, that form an expandable sac. It is located retroperitoneally in the pelvic cavity. The bladder has openings for the two ureters to bring urine in and an outlet for the urethra through which urine flows out of the body. The triangular section outlined by these three openings is called the *trigone*.

Thinkabout 19–6

Locate the urinary bladder relative to the uterus and rectum in a female.

The female *urethra* is 3 to 4 cm long. It is relatively short and wide and opens into the perineum in front of the vagina and anus. The proximity of the urethra to these two sources encourages infection of the bladder. The male urethra is about 20 cm long and passes through the penis. At the base of the male bladder is the prostate gland, which plays a role in semen production and frequently is hypertrophied in older men, obstructing urine flow (see Chapter 24). The male urethra transports semen during sexual intercourse. The mucosa lining the urinary tract is continuous through the urethra, bladder, and ureter to the pelvis of the kidney. Organisms can enter the system through the urethra, and this continuous mucosa facilitates the spread of infection through the urinary tract.

Micturition (urination, voiding) occurs when a reflex is stimulated by increased pressure as the bladder distends. The reflex is transmitted by parasympathetic nerves extending to the sacral spinal cord. If the time is appropriate, the external and internal sphincters of the bladder and the pelvic diaphragm relax while the bladder muscle contracts, emptying the bladder.

INCONTINENCE AND RETENTION

Incontinence, or the loss of voluntary control of the bladder, has many causes. Young children have to learn voluntary control as the nervous system matures. Stress incontinence occurs when increased intra-abdominal pressure forces urine through the sphincter. This can occur with coughing or laughing but is most frequent in women after the urogenital diaphragm has become weakened by pregnancy or age. Spinal cord injuries or brain damage frequently interfere with voluntary neurologic control of the bladder.

Retention is an inability to empty the bladder. It may be accompanied by overflow incontinence. Note that a spinal cord injury at the sacral level blocks the micturition reflex, resulting in retention of urine or failure to void. Retention also may occur following anesthesia, either general or spinal.

Inability to control urine flow may be managed by wearing pads or briefs that contain the urine. A *catheter* is a tube in the urethra that drains urine from the bladder to a collecting bag outside the body. Catheters are common sources of infection in the urinary tract because they are irritating to the tissue and, when inserted, may be a means of introducing bacteria directly into the bladder.

DIAGNOSTIC TESTS

Urinalysis

The constituents and characteristics of urine may vary with dietary intake, drugs, and the care with which a specimen is handled. Urine normally is clear and straw-colored and has a mild odor. Urine pH is in the range of 4.5 to 8.0. The following lists offer general guidelines to abnormalities noted in freshly voided specimens. An "old" specimen will not provide accurate information. See the inside cover for normal values.

Appearance:

Cloudy—may indicate the presence of large amounts of protein, blood cells, or bacteria and pus.

Dark color—may indicate hematuria (blood), excessive bilirubin content, or highly concentrated urine.

Unpleasant or unusual odor—may indicate infection.

Abnormal constituents (present in significant quantities):

Blood (**hematuria**)—small (microscopic) amounts of blood are often associated with infection, inflammation, or tumors in the urinary tract.

Large numbers of red blood cells (gross hematuria) indicate increased glomerular permeability or hemorrhage in the tract.

Protein (**proteinuria**, albuminuria)—indicates the leakage of albumin or mixed plasma proteins into the filtrate owing to inflammation and increased glomerular permeability.

Bacteria (bacteriuria) and pus (**pyuria**)—indicate infection in the urinary tract.

Urinary casts (microscopic molds of the tubules, consisting of one or more cells, bacteria, protein, and so on)—indicate inflammation of the tubule.

Specific gravity indicates the ability of the tubules to concentrate the urine; a very low specific gravity (dilute urine) usually is related to renal failure (assuming normal hydration).

Thinkabout 19–7

a. List the normal constituents of urine.

b. Explain why hematuria and proteinuria reflect a glomerular problem rather than a tubular problem in the kidney.

Blood Tests

Like most other diseases, urinary tract disorders produce abnormalities that can be detected by various blood tests. Some of the more commonly used tests are described here.

Elevated serum urea (blood urea nitrogen [BUN]) and serum creatinine—indicate failure to excrete nitrogen wastes (resulting from protein metabolism) due to decreased GFR.

Metabolic acidosis (decreased serum pH and decreased serum bicarbonate)—indicates decreased GFR and failure of the tubules to control acid-base balance (see Chapter 6).

Anemia (low hemoglobin level)—indicates decreased erythropoietin secretion or bone marrow depression.

Electrolytes—depend on the related fluid balance: that is, retention of fluid if GFR is decreased may result in a dilution effect, and laboratory values are therefore not a true reflection of renal status.

Antibody level—Antistreptolysin O (ASO) or anti-

streptokinase (ASK) titer are used for diagnosis of poststreptococcal glomerulonephritis.
Renin levels—indicate a cause of hypertension.

Other Tests

Culture and sensitivity studies on urine specimens are used to identify the causative organism and select drug treatment when infection is suspected.

Clearance tests, such as creatinine or inulin clearance or radioisotope studies are used to assess GFR.

Radiologic tests, such as intravenous pyelography (IVP), angiography, ultrasound, computed tomography (CT), magnetic resonance imaging (MRI), and radionuclide imaging, may be used to visualize the structures and any abnormalities in the urinary system (see Ready Reference 4).

Cystoscopy visualizes the lower urinary tract and may be used in performing a biopsy or to remove kidney stones.

Biopsy may be used to acquire tissue specimens to allow microscopic examination of suspicious lesions in the bladder or kidney.

Thinkabout 19–8

What is the normal pH range for the blood and urine? What serum and urine pH would indicate that acidosis had developed?

DIURETIC DRUGS

Diuretics, or "water pills," are used to remove excess sodium ions and water from the body. They are prescribed for many disorders other than renal disease including hypertension, edema, congestive heart failure, and pulmonary edema. Diuretics increase the excretion of water through the kidneys, thereby increasing urinary volume. The most commonly used drug group inhibits sodium chloride reabsorption in the tubules. Examples of this group include hydrochlorothiazide, a mild diuretic, and furosemide, which is more potent. Because these drugs may cause excessive loss of potassium, patients may need dietary supplements such as bananas or potassium chloride tablets.

The major side effect of these drugs is excessive loss of electrolytes, which may cause muscle weakness or cardiac arrhythmias. Patients taking diuretics should be observed for **orthostatic hypotension** when moving from a supine to an upright position. Another group of diuretics, the potassium-sparing type (e.g., spironolactone), may be given in combination with thiazides to minimize the risk of **hyperkalemia** (high serum potassium levels). These drugs are usually administered in the morning because they cause urinary **frequency** for a period of time. This may limit other morning activities and appointments.

DIALYSIS

Dialysis provides an "artificial kidney," which can be used to sustain life after the kidneys fail. It is used to treat someone who has acute renal failure until the primary problem has been reversed, or it can be used for patients in end-stage renal failure, perhaps until a transplant becomes available. In people with renal transplants, it may be required if rejection occurs or between transplants (see Chapter 3). Dialysis is a demanding procedure for both the patient and the family. Diet, particularly protein, and fluid intake are severely restricted.

There are two forms of dialysis, peritoneal dialysis and hemodialysis (Fig. 19–6). Hemodialysis is usually provided in a hospital or a dialysis center. During the procedure the patient's blood moves from an implanted shunt or catheter in an artery, often in the arm, through a tube to a machine where the exchange of wastes, fluid, and electrolytes takes place. A **semipermeable membrane** separates the patient's blood from the dialysis fluid, and the constituents move between the two compartments. For example, wastes move from blood to the **dialysate** while bicarbonate ion moves into the blood from the dialysate. Blood cells and protein remain in the blood, unable to pass through the semipermeable membrane. Movement occurs by **ultrafiltration**, **diffusion** (by a concentration gradient), and osmosis. After the exchange has been completed, the blood is returned to the patient's vein. Heparin is administered to prevent clotting, requiring monitoring of blood clotting times. There are potential complications. The shunt may become infected, or blood clots may form. Eventually the blood vessels involved at the shunt become sclerosed or damaged, and a new site must be selected. Patients on dialysis have an increased risk of infection by hepatitis virus or human immunodeficiency virus (HIV). Hemodialysis is usually required three times a week, each session lasting about 3 to 4 hours. The patient may feel uncomfortable during the session because fluid and electrolyte balances change quickly, but usually he feels much better after the treatment.

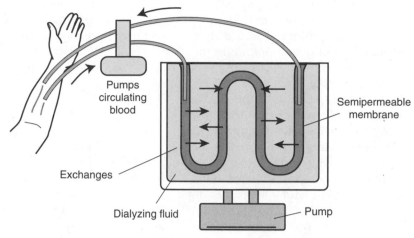

A. HEMODIALYSIS

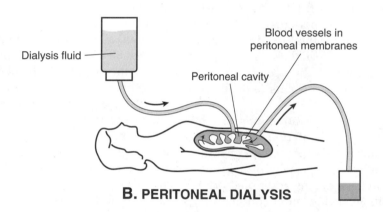

B. PERITONEAL DIALYSIS

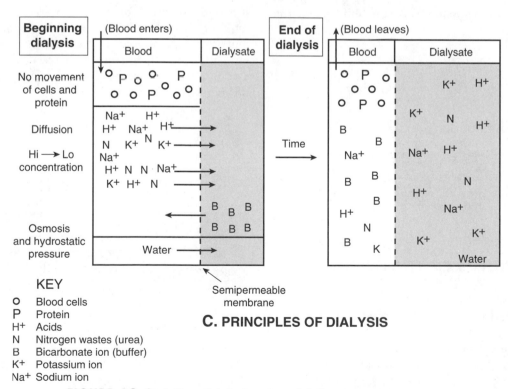

C. PRINCIPLES OF DIALYSIS

KEY

O Blood cells
P Protein
H+ Acids
N Nitrogen wastes (urea)
B Bicarbonate ion (buffer)
K+ Potassium ion
Na+ Sodium ion

FIGURE 19-6. *A,* Hemodialysis; *B,* peritoneal dialysis; *C,* principles of dialysis.

The feeling of well-being then dissipates gradually as wastes accumulate prior to the subsequent treatment.

Peritoneal dialysis can be administered in a dialysis unit or at home. It may be done at night while the patient sleeps or continuously while the patient is ambulatory (this is called continuous ambulatory peritoneal dialysis, or CAPD). In this procedure, the peritoneal membrane, which is very large, thin, and highly vascular, serves as the semipermeable membrane. A catheter with entry and exit points is implanted in the peritoneal cavity. The dialyzing fluid is instilled through the catheter into the cavity and remains there, allowing the exchange of wastes and electrolytes to occur by diffusion and osmosis. Then the dialysate is drained from the cavity by gravity into a container. This process requires more time than hemodialysis. However, the more continuous exchange process prevents excessive and sudden changes in fluid and electrolyte levels in the body, and the components of a dialysis solution can be adapted to individual needs. The major complication of peritoneal dialysis is infection resulting in peritonitis. Newer methods under investigation make use of charcoal absorbents and ultrafiltration techniques.

Prophylactic antibiotics are given with either form of dialysis whenever there is a risk of transient bacteremia, for example with any invasive procedure or tissue trauma. Fluid intake and diet, especially protein and electrolytes, must be monitored. Any additional problem occuring in the patient such as infection may also alter dialysis requirements. Caution is required with many drugs because toxic levels can build up in the blood.

Thinkabout 19–9

Explain why a dialysis solution would be low in urea but high in bicarbonate content.

DISORDERS OF THE URINARY SYSTEM

Urinary Tract Infections

Urinary tract infections (UTIs) are extremely common. Cystitis and urethritis are considered infections of the lower urinary tract, whereas pyelonephritis is an upper tract infection (Fig. 19–7). Most infections are *ascending*, arising from organisms in the perineal area and traveling along the continuous mucosa. Occasionally, pyelonephritis results from a blood-borne infection. The common causative organism is *Escherichia coli*, which is one of the normal flora of the intestine.

ETIOLOGY

Females are anatomically more vulnerable to infection than males because of the shortness and width of the urethra, its proximity to the anus, and the frequent irritation to the tissues caused by tampons, bubble bath, deodorants, and sexual activity. Older males with prostatic hypertrophy and retention of urine frequently develop infection. Because the male reproductive tract shares some of the structures of the urinary tract, any infection of the prostate or testes is likely to extend to the urinary structures.

Common causative factors in UTIs in both males and females include incontinence (incomplete emptying of the bladder), bladder retention of urine, and any obstruction to urine flow, which tends to result in growth of organisms because bacteria are not flushed out of the bladder by voiding. Urine provides an excellent medium for growth of organisms. Pregnancy, scar tissue, congenital defects, renal **calculi**, and vesicoureteral reflux all contribute to infection because the urine and any contaminants do not flow freely through and out of the system. Infection may result from decreased host resistance such as **immunosuppression,** impaired blood supply to the bladder (aging), or diabetes mellitus (vascular impairment and glucosuria). As mentioned earlier, instruments or catheters may directly introduce bacteria into the bladder and frequently traumatize the bladder wall, breaking the barrier to infection.

Thinkabout 19–10

a. List several factors that would predispose a pregnant woman with diabetes to cystitis.
b. Is the bladder normally sterile?

CYSTITIS

Pathophysiology

With cystitis, the bladder wall and urethra are inflamed, red, and swollen, and, in some cases, ulcerated. Bladder capacity is usually reduced.

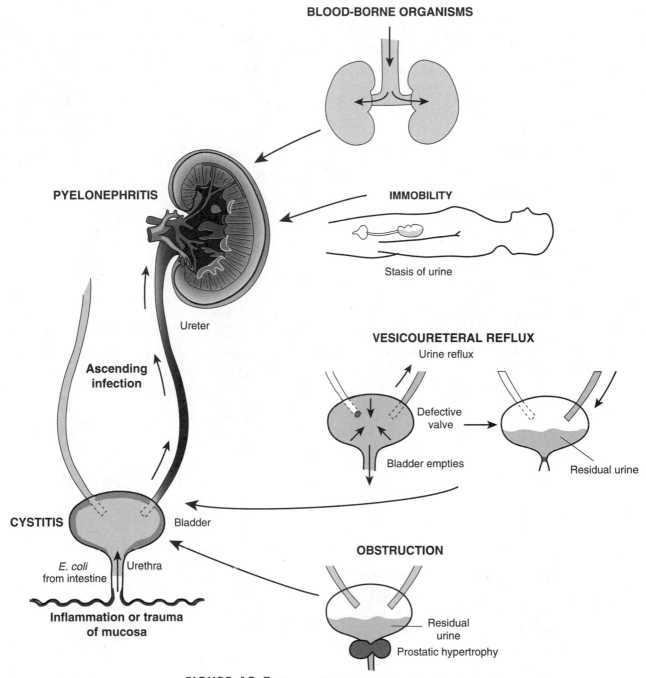

BLOOD-BORNE ORGANISMS

PYELONEPHRITIS

Ureter

IMMOBILITY

Stasis of urine

Ascending infection

VESICOURETERAL REFLUX

Urine reflux

Defective valve

Bladder empties

Residual urine

CYSTITIS

Bladder

E. coli from intestine

Urethra

Inflammation or trauma of mucosa

OBSTRUCTION

Residual urine

Prostatic hypertrophy

FIGURE 19–7. Causes of infection in the urinary tract.

Signs and Symptoms

Pain is common in the lower abdomen. **Dysuria, frequency,** and **urgency** are common as the inflamed bladder wall is irritated by urine. Systemic signs of infection may be present (fever, malaise, nausea, and leukocytosis). In some cases, the manifestations are very mild and may be unnoticed. Urinalysis indicates bacteriuria (more than 100,000 organisms per milliliter of urine), pyuria, and microscopic hematuria. The urine often appears cloudy and has an unusual odor.

PYELONEPHRITIS

Pathophysiology

One or both kidneys may be involved. The infection extends from the ureter and involves the renal pelvis and medullary tissue. Purulent exudate fills the kidney pelvis, and the medulla (tubules and collecting ducts) is inflamed and shows some evidence of necrosis. If the infection is severe, the exudate can compress the renal artery and vein and obstruct urine flow to the ureter. Bilateral obstruction is likely to result in acute renal failure (see Fig. 19–12).

Signs and Symptoms

Urinalysis results are similar to those for cystitis except that *urinary casts* consisting of leukocytes or renal epithelial cells are present, reflecting the involvement of the renal *tubule*. Pain associated with renal disease is usually a dull aching pain in the lower back or *flank* area resulting from inflammation that stretches the renal capsule. Systemic signs are usually more marked in pyelonephritis. The signs of cystitis such as dysuria are also present.

TREATMENT

UTIs are treated promptly with antibiotics such as trimethoprim-sulfamethoxazole (e.g., Bactrim). The patient is encouraged to increase fluid intake. The infection tends to recur unless the predisposing factors are removed. In some cases pockets of infection persist in the bladder. Therefore, it is essential to follow the course of antibiotics with *urinalysis* to ensure that the infection has been totally eradicated. Chronic cystitis tends to be asymptomatic and therefore can persist and spread to the kidneys, where it causes more damage.

To prevent permanent kidney damage, it is important to start treatment quickly and to follow up with urinalysis. Chronic pyelonephritis often causes insidious damage with areas of obstructive scar tissue that promote continued infection and eventually cause chronic renal failure.

Thinkabout 19–11

List the signs and symptoms of pyelonephritis that indicate that *infection* is present and those indicating that *kidney involvement* (local or systemic) exists.

Inflammatory Disorders

GLOMERULONEPHRITIS (ACUTE POSTSTREPTOCOCCAL GLOMERULONEPHRITIS)

There are many forms of glomerulonephritis. A representative form of glomerular or nephritic disease is acute poststreptococcal glomerulonephritis (APSGN), which follows streptococcal infection with certain types of group A beta-hemolytic *Streptococcus*. Organisms such as *Staphylococcus* may also cause the antecedent infection. Glomerulonephritis develops about 2 weeks after the infection. APSGN affects primarily children between the ages of 3 and 7 years, especially boys.

Pathophysiology

The antibodies formed from the earlier streptococcal infection form an antigen-antibody complex (type III hypersensitivity reaction), that lodges in the glomerular capillaries, activates complement, and causes an inflammatory response in both kidneys (Fig. 19–8). (See Chapter 3 for a review of the immune response.) This leads to increased capillary permeability and cell proliferation (Fig. 19–9) and results in leakage of protein and erythrocytes into the filtrate. When the inflammatory response is severe, the congestion and proliferation interfere with filtration in the kidney, causing decreased GFR and retention of fluid and wastes. The decreased blood flow in the kidney may also trigger renin secretion, which leads to elevated blood pressure and edema (see Fig. 19–11). Severe prolonged inflammation will causes scarring of the kidneys.

Signs and Symptoms

Flank or back pain develops as the kidney tissue swells and stretches the capsule. The urine becomes dark and cloudy ("smoky" or "coffee-colored") because of the protein and red blood cells retained in it. Urine output decreases (**oliguria**) as GFR declines. Facial and periorbital edema occurs initially followed by generalized edema as the colloid osmotic pressure of the blood drops and sodium and water are retained. General signs of inflammation are present, including malaise, fatigue, headache, anorexia, and nausea. Blood pressure is elevated owing to increased renin secretion and decreased GFR.

Diagnostic Tests

Blood tests show elevated serum urea and creatinine, decreased complement, and elevation of streptococcal exoenzymes antistreptolysin O (ASO) and antistreptokinase (ASK). Complement is probably a causative factor in the inflammatory damage that occurs in the kidney. Metabolic acidosis, with decreased serum bicarbonate and low serum pH, is present. *Urinalysis* confirms the presence of proteinuria, gross hematuria, and erythrocyte casts.

Treatment

Sodium restrictions may apply, and in severe cases, protein and fluid intake is decreased. In most cases, recovery takes place with minimum residual damage, although it is important to prevent future exposure to streptococcal infection and recurrent inflammation due to another hypersensitivity reaction. Prophylactic antibiotics may be needed. Some cases, particularly in adults, are not easily resolved. Acute renal failure or

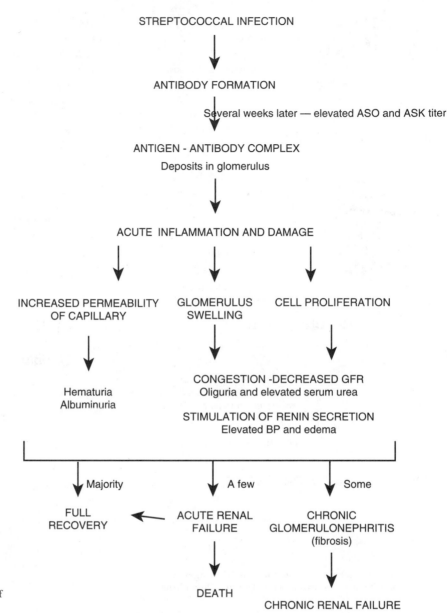

FIGURE 19-8. Development and course of poststreptococcal glomerulonephritis.

chronic glomerulonephritis may develop, which will gradually destroy the kidneys (through end-stage renal disease or uremia).

Thinkabout 19–12

a. Explain the development of inflammation in the kidney with APSGN.

b. Describe the signs of APSGN related to: (1) increased glomerular permeability, (2) decreased glomerular filtration rate.

NEPHROTIC SYNDROME (NEPHROSIS)

The nephrotic syndrome is secondary to a number of renal diseases as well as a variety of systemic disorders (e.g., systemic lupus erythematosus [SLE], exposure to toxins or drugs). However, lipoid nephrosis is a primary disease in young children.

Pathophysiology

The pathology is not well established. There is an abnormality in the glomerular capillaries and increased permeability that allows large amounts of plasma protein to escape into the filtrate. This results in marked hypoalbuminemia with decreased plasma osmotic pressure and subsequent generalized edema. Blood pressure remains low or normal in most cases because of

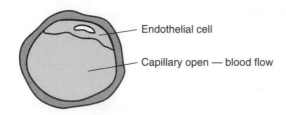

NORMAL GLOMERULUS

- Endothelial cell
- Capillary open — blood flow

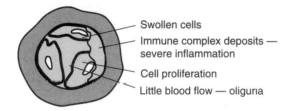

MILD GLOMERULONEPHRITIS

- Swollen endothelial cell and membrane
- Narrow capillary lumen — GFR decreases
- Immune complex deposits — inflammation
- RBC and protein leaks into filtrate — hematuria and proteinuria

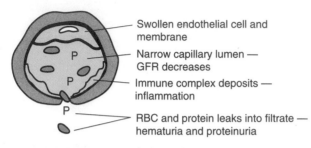

SEVERE GLOMERULONEPHRITIS

- Swollen cells
- Immune complex deposits — severe inflammation
- Cell proliferation
- Little blood flow — oliguria

= RBC

P = PROTEIN

FIGURE 19–9. Schematic representation of changes occurring in the nephron with acute poststreptococcal glomerulonephritis.

hypovolemia. The decreased blood volume also increases aldosterone secretion, leading to more severe edema. The other significant components of nephrotic syndrome are the high levels of cholesterol in the blood and lipoprotein in the urine. The cause of the hyperlipidemia and lipiduria is not totally clear.

Signs and Symptoms

The significant sign of nephrosis is the massive edema (anasarca) associated with weight gain and pallor. This excessive fluid throughout all tissues impairs appetite, breathing, and activity. Skin breakdown and infection may develop because arterial flow and capillary exchange are impaired.

Treatment

Glucocorticoids such as prednisone are prescribed to reduce the inflammation in the kidney. Nephrotic syn-

drome tends to recur and requires frequent monitoring and continued treatment. When administered long-term, glucocorticoids have significant negative effects on a child's growth (see Chapter 2 for long-term effects of therapy). Sodium intake may be restricted, but protein intake is usually increased.

Thinkabout 19–13

Compare the characteristics of the urine in a child with pyelonephritis, APSGN, and nephrotic syndrome.

URINARY TRACT OBSTRUCTIONS

Urolithiasis (Calculi or Kidney Stones)

Kidney stones are a common problem and frequently recur if the underlying disorder is not treated.

PATHOPHYSIOLOGY

Calculi can develop anywhere in the urinary tract. Most are composed of calcium salts, although a few are primarily uric acid or magnesium salts depending on the predisposing factor. Stones can be small or very large (e.g., *staghorn* calculus, which forms in the renal pelvis). Once any solid material or debris forms, deposits continue to build up on this nidus or focus and eventually form a large mass.

Calculi tend to form when there are excessive amounts of relatively insoluble salts in the filtrate. The solubility of calcium salts and uric acid varies with the pH of the urine. Calcium stones (phosphate or carbonate) form when calcium levels in the urine are high owing to hypercalcemia, especially if the patient's fluid intake is low or the urine is highly alkaline. Infection may cause stones consisting of mixed inorganic salts because in such cases the urine pH is alkaline and debris from the infection may act as a focus for the deposition of crystals. Uric acid stones develop with hyperuricemia (due to gout, high purine diets, or cancer chemotherapy), especially when the urine is acidic. Calcium oxalate stones may develop in people ingesting certain vegetarian diets that lead to increased levels of oxalate in the urine.

Stones usually cause manifestations only when they obstruct the flow of urine, (e.g., in the ureter). Calculi may lead to infection because they cause stasis of urine in the area and may also irritate the tissues. In the kidney, calculi may cause the development of hydronephrosis with dilation of calyces and atrophy of renal tissue related to the back pressure of urine behind the obstructing stone (Fig. 19–10).

Thinkabout 19–14

Explain how decreased fluid intake predisposes to calculi in the urinary tract.

SIGNS AND SYMPTOMS

Obstruction of the ureter causes an attack of "renal colic," consisting of intense spasms of pain in the flank area radiating into the groin that last until the stone passes or is removed. Pain may be accompanied by nausea and vomiting, cool moist skin, and rapid pulse. Radiologic examination confirms the location of the calculi.

TREATMENT

Small stones can be passed eventually. Newer methods of fragmentation of larger stones such as shockwave lithotripsy and laser lithotripsy have been quite successful and have decreased the need for invasive

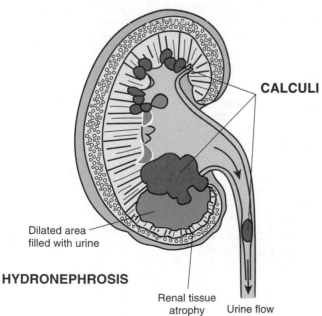

HYDRONEPHROSIS

Dilated area filled with urine

Renal tissue atrophy

Urine flow

CALCULI

FIGURE 19–10. Renal calculi and hydronephrosis.

surgery. Prevention of recurrence is of primary importance. Treatment of the underlying condition, adjustment of urine pH by ingestion of additional acidic or alkaline substances, and increased fluid intake all minimize the risk of recurrence.

Tumors

Benign tumors are rare in the urinary tract.

RENAL CELL CARCINOMA

Renal cell carcinoma is a primary tumor arising from the tubule epithelium. It tends to be asymptomatic in the early stage and often has metastasized to liver, lungs, bone, or central nervous system at the time of diagnosis. This cancer commonly occurs after age 50, more frequently in males and smokers.

The initial sign is usually hematuria, either gross or microscopic. Other manifestations include dull, aching flank pain, a palpable mass, anemia or erythrocytosis (depending on the tumor's effects on erythropoietin secretion), or paraneoplastic syndromes such as hypercalcemia (increased parathyroid hormone) or Cushing's syndrome (increased adrenocorticotropic hormone).

BLADDER CANCER

Malignant tumors of the bladder commonly arise from the transitional epithelium lining the bladder in the trigone area. This cancer tends to recur. The tumor is invasive through the wall to adjacent structures, and it metastasizes through the blood to liver and bone.

Bladder cancer has a high incidence in individuals working with chemicals in laboratories or industry, as well as in smokers and those with recurrent infections. The early sign is hematuria, gross or microscopic. Dysuria or frequency may develop. Treatment includes resection of the tumor, chemotherapy, and radiation. Instillation of BCG into the bladder following resection has reduced recurrences of superficial tumors (see Chapter 5).

VASCULAR DISORDERS

Nephrosclerosis

PATHOPHYSIOLOGY

Nephrosclerosis involves vascular changes in the kidney. Some vascular changes occur normally with aging.

These changes cause thickening and hardening of the walls of the arterioles and small arteries, and narrowing or occlusion of the lumina of the blood vessels. Such changes reduce the blood supply to the kidney, causing ischemia and atrophy, and also stimulate the secretion of renin, ultimately increasing the blood pressure (Fig. 19–11). It is often difficult to determine whether the primary lesion has developed in the kidney or whether it is secondary to hypertension (see Chapter 16) or diabetes (see Chapter 21) or other condition. In any case, a vicious cycle can develop with the kidneys and hypertension, and this must be broken to prevent renal failure or other complications of hypertension such as congestive heart failure.

TREATMENT

Drugs such as antihypertensive agents, diuretics, angiotensin-converting enzyme inhibitors (ACE inhibi-

tors), and beta blockers (which block renin release) all can assist in maintaining renal blood flow and reducing blood pressure. These drugs are discussed in Chapter 16. Sodium intake should be reduced as well. It is essential that the client understand that this is necessary long-term treatment because the damage to the kidneys is usually asymptomatic until complications develop in the late stage.

Thinkabout 19–15

List factors that may contribute to elevated blood pressure.

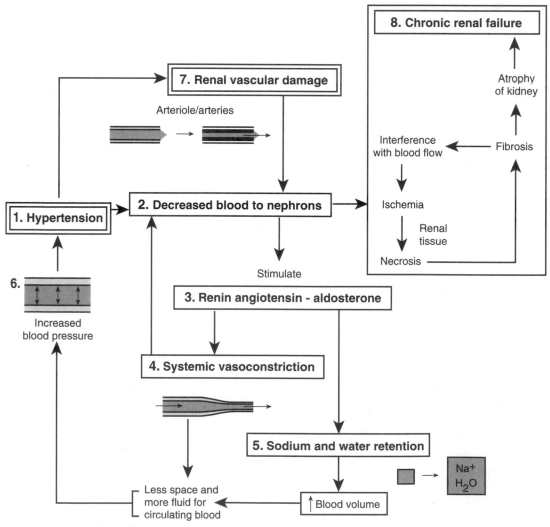

FIGURE 19–11. The relationship between hypertension and the kidney.

RENAL FAILURE

Acute Renal Failure

PATHOPHYSIOLOGY

The kidneys may fail suddenly for many different reasons. The failure is usually reversible if the primary problem is treated successfully. Dialysis may be used to replace the kidney function during this period. In some cases, the kidneys do sustain a degree of permanent damage. Acute renal failure usually develops rapidly. Either directly reduced blood flow into the kidney or inflammation and necrosis of the tubules cause obstruction and back pressure, leading to greatly reduced GFR and oliguria. Blood tests show elevated serum urea (BUN) and creatinine as well as metabolic acidosis, confirming the failure of the kidneys to remove wastes.

ETIOLOGY

There are numerous causes of acute renal failure (Fig. 19–12). They include acute bilateral kidney disease, such as glomerulonephritis, which reduces GFR, and severe and prolonged circulatory shock or heart failure, which results in tubule necrosis. The other major cause is nephrotoxins such as drugs, chemicals, or toxins, which cause tubule necrosis and obstruction of blood flow. Occasionally, mechanical obstructions such as calculi, blood clots, or tumors block urine flow beyond the kidneys and cause acute renal failure.

TREATMENT

It is important to reverse the primary problem as quickly as possible to minimize the risk of necrosis and permanent kidney damage. Recovery from acute renal failure is evidenced by increased urine output (diuretic stage). It may take a few months before the renal tubules recover totally, so fluid and electrolyte balance may not return to normal for some time.

Thinkabout 19–16

Focusing on the circulation through the nephron, explain why severely decreased blood flow in the afferent arteriole could cause tubule necrosis and obstruction.

Chronic Renal Failure

PATHOPHYSIOLOGY

Chronic renal failure is the gradual irreversible destruction of the kidneys over a long period of time. It may result from chronic kidney disease, such as pyelonephritis or congenital polycystic kidney disease, or from systemic disorders such as hypertension or diabetes. The gradual loss of nephrons is asymptomatic until it is well advanced because the kidneys normally have considerable reserve function. Once advanced, the progress of chronic renal failure may be slowed but cannot be stopped because the scar tissue and loss of functional organization tend to cause further degenerative changes.

There are several stages in chronic renal failure (Fig. 19–13) progressing from decreased renal reserve to insufficiency to end-stage renal failure or uremia. In the early stages of decreased reserve (around 60% nephron loss) there is a decrease in GFR, serum creatinine levels that are consistently higher than average but within normal range, serum urea levels that are normal, and no apparent clinical signs. The remaining nephrons appear to adapt, increasing their capacity for filtration.

The middle stage (around 75% nephron loss) or that of renal insufficiency is indicated by a change in blood chemistry and manifestations. At this point, GFR is decreased to approximately 20 percent of normal, and there is significant retention of nitrogen wastes (urea and creatinine) in the blood. Tubule function is decreased, resulting in failure to concentrate the urine and control the secretion and exchange of acids and electrolytes. Osmotic diuresis occurs as the remaining functional nephrons filter an increased solute load. This stage is marked by excretion of large volumes of dilute urine. Erythropoiesis is decreased, and the patient's blood pressure is elevated.

Uremia, or end-stage renal failure (more than 90% nephron loss), occurs when GFR is negligible. Fluid, electrolytes, and wastes are retained in the body, and all body systems are affected. In this stage, marked oliguria or **anuria** develops. Dialysis or a kidney transplant is required to maintain the patient's life.

SIGNS AND SYMPTOMS

The early signs of chronic renal failure include increased urinary output (**polyuria**), manifested as frequency and **nocturia**. General signs such as anorexia, nausea, anemia, fatigue, and exercise intolerance develop. Bone marrow is depressed and blood cell function impaired. High blood pressure is usually present. As the kidneys fail completely, oliguria develops, and the skin becomes dry, pruritic, and hyperpig-

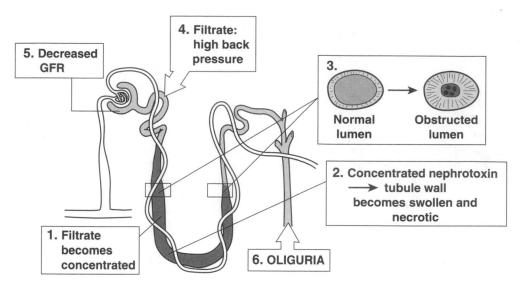

A. NEPHROTOXINS

5. Decreased GFR

4. Filtrate: high back pressure

3. Normal lumen → Obstructed lumen

2. Concentrated nephrotoxin ⟶ tubule wall becomes swollen and necrotic

1. Filtrate becomes concentrated

6. OLIGURIA

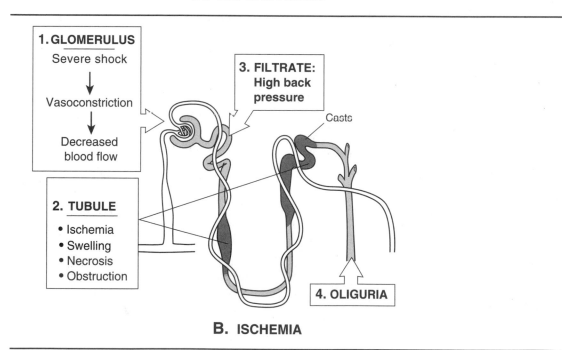

B. ISCHEMIA

1. GLOMERULUS
Severe shock
↓
Vasoconstriction
↓
Decreased blood flow

3. FILTRATE: High back pressure

Casts

2. TUBULE
• Ischemia
• Swelling
• Necrosis
• Obstruction

4. OLIGURIA

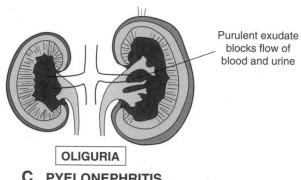

Purulent exudate blocks flow of blood and urine

OLIGURIA

C. PYELONEPHRITIS

FIGURE 19–12. Causes of acute renal failure. *A*, Nephrotoxins; *B*, ischemia; *C*, pyelonephritis.

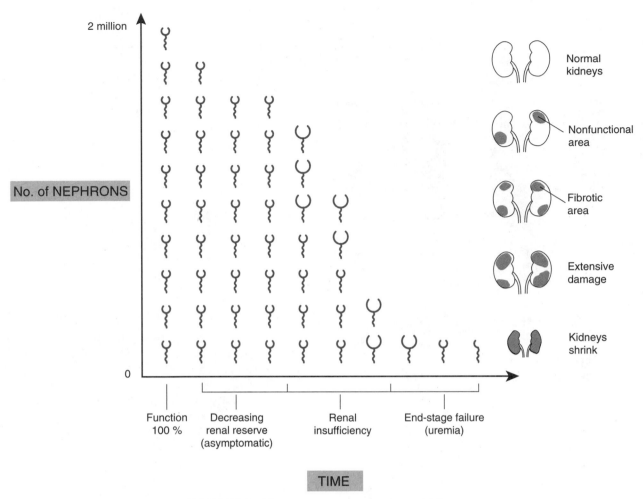

FIGURE 19-13. Development of chronic renal failure.

mented. Other signs in the uremic stage include peripheral neuropathy—abnormal sensations in the lower limbs, impotence and decreased libido in males, menstrual irregularities in females. Serious effects of uremia include encephalopathy (lethargy, memory lapses, seizures, tremors) and congestive heart failure. The failure of the kidney to activate vitamin D for calcium absorption and metabolism combined with urinary retention of phosphate ion leads to hypocalcemia and hyperphosphatemia with **osteodystrophy**, **osteoporosis**, and **tetany** (see Chapters 21 and 22). Uremic frost on the skin and a urinelike breath odor may develop in the terminal stage or if infection is present. Drug dosages usually need to be reduced in patients with uremia because of the kidney's decreased ability to excrete them. Systemic infections such as pneumonia are common owing to poor tissue resistance related to anemia, fluid retention, and low protein levels.

DIAGNOSTIC TESTS

Anemia, acidosis, and **azotemia** are the indicators of chronic renal failure. Metabolic acidosis be-

comes decompensated (serum pH below 7.35) in the late stage as GFR declines and tubule function is lost (see Chapter 6). Azotemia refers to the presence of nitrogen wastes in the blood, as indicated by elevated serum creatinine and urea levels. Serum electrolyte levels may vary depending on the amount of water retained in the body. Usually hyponatremia and hyperkalemia occur as well as hypocalcemia and hyperphosphatemia.

TREATMENT

Chronic renal failure affects all body systems. It is difficult to maintain control of the blood chemistry. Clients are subject to many complications, which in turn affect the uremia. For instance, a simple infection increases the wastes in the body, compromising all body systems. Intake of fluid, electrolytes, and protein must be restricted because the kidneys are limited in their ability to excrete excess wastes and fluid. Children with kidney failure have retarded growth. In the uremic stage dialysis or a transplant is required. Organ transplants are discussed in Chapter 3.

Thinkabout 19–17

a. Compare acute and chronic renal failure with respect to cause, reversibility, and urinary output at onset.

b. If uremia is untreated or if complications occur, metabolic acidosis can become decompensated. What change occurs in serum pH at this point, and what is the effect on overall cell metabolism in the body?

c. Why is there an increased risk of drug toxicity in the later stages of renal failure?

CASE STUDIES

CASE STUDY A
Nephrosclerosis and Chronic Renal Failure

Mr. H, age 68, has a long history of hypertension. He has had more headaches recently, his legs and feet are swollen, and he has noticed that more frequent voiding, both during the day and at night, is necessary. He constantly feels tired and does not feel hungry. Mr. H's blood pressure is 170/110, his pulse is 94, and he has gained 12 pounds in the last 2 months. Diagnostic test findings related to the blood and urine include elevated serum creatinine and urea levels, low serum bicarbonate, low hemoglobin, and hematocrit, and low serum sodium. The urine contains protein and has a very low specific gravity. The diagnosis is renal insufficiency or chronic renal failure due to nephrosclerosis.

1. Describe how nephrosclerosis leads to chronic renal failure.

2. Explain the cause of the edema and the weight gain.

3. State three factors contributing to fatigue.

4. Explain why Mr. H
    a. is voiding frequently.
    b. has a very dilute urine.

5. Explain why Mr. H has
    a. high blood pressure
    b. anemia
    c. metabolic acidosis

6. List the signs indicating that Mr. H has progressed into uremia or end-stage renal failure.

7. List three reasons why development of pneumonia is a high risk in Mr. H.

CASE STUDY B
Acute Poststreptococcal Glomerulonephritis

APSGN has been diagnosed in DK, age 4, a month after he was ill with tonsillitis. His face, abdomen, and legs are swollen, and he is not interested in his toys. He is short of breath when he moves about. His urine is dark and cloudy and is scant in volume.

1. Explain how DK's tonsillitis is probably related to the development of APSGN.

2. Explain why his urine is dark.

3. State two other significant characteristics you would expect to find in the urine.

4. State three abnormalities likely to be found on examination of DK's blood and explain the reason for each.

5. Explain why DK is producing very small amounts of urine.

6. Explain why acute renal failure could develop.

STUDY QUESTIONS

1. Trace the blood flow through the kidney, naming the blood vessels in order.

2. Trace the filtrate and the major changes in it, from Bowman's capsule to the urethra.

3. If the sympathetic nervous system causes vasoconstriction in the kidney, how does this increase blood pressure? How does it affect urine output?

4. Compare the signs of cystitis and pyelonephritis.

5. Compare the causes and pathophysiology of acute pyelonephritis, APSGN, and nephrotic syndrome.

6. How might urinary tract infections lead to calculus formation?

7. Compare the pathophysiology of acute and chronic renal failure.

8. Describe all the factors contributing to the lethargy of someone with chronic renal failure.

9. A client with chronic renal failure on hemodialysis is having extensive dental work performed. What precautions need to be taken for this client?

10. List the substances that should pass from the blood into the dialyzing fluid.

11. Why is protein intake restricted in patients with kidney disease?

12. Why would a respiratory infection such as pneumonia aggravate the effects of uremia?

13. Why would a child's growth and development be affected by chronic nephrosis and renal failure?

14. Differentiate the causes of frequent voiding associated with cystitis and with renal insufficiency.

15. Differentiate the causes of urinary retention and anuria.

CHAPTER
20
Neurologic Disorders

KEY TERMS

•••

afferent
amnesia
amniocentesis
anastomoses
anencephaly
anomalies
aphasia
asymptomatic
athetoid
atresia
autoregulation
baroreceptor
bifurcation
bilirubin
carrier
chemoreceptor

choreiform
clonic
cognitive
coma
contralateral
depolarizing
diplopia
disorientation
efferent
embolus
fissure
flaccid
foramina
fulminant
ganglion
gyrus

hyperreflexia
infarction
infratentorial
ipsilateral
ischemia
labile
neonates
neurotransmitter
nuchal rigidity
paralysis
paresis
paresthesia
permeability
petechia
photophobia
precursor

pressoreceptor
ptosis
repolarization
retina
scotoma
spastic
stenosis
stupor
sulcus
supratentorial
sutures
thrombus
tonic
transillumination
vesicle

REVIEW OF THE NERVOUS SYSTEM

The Brain

The brain is the communication and control center of the body. It receives many kinds of input, processes and evaluates it, decides on the response or action to be taken, and then initiates the response. Responses include both involuntary activity required to maintain homeostasis in the body (regulated by the autonomic nervous system) and voluntary actions (controlled by the somatic nervous system). With both reflex and voluntary activities, the individual is often not aware of the amount and diversity of input received or the integration or assessment of that input, but only of the response.

COVERINGS OF THE BRAIN

The brain is protected by the rigid bone of the skull, the three membranes or meninges, and the cerebrospinal fluid (CSF). The cranial and facial bones are connected by **sutures**, relatively immovable joints consisting of fibrous tissue. If pressure increases inside the skull in infants before the sutures fuse or ossify, the cranial bones may separate, causing the head to enlarge. There are a number of cavities or fossae in the skull as well as **foramina** and canals through which nerves and blood vessels pass. The largest opening, the foramen magnum, is located in the occipital bone at the base of the skull where the spinal cord emerges.

Meninges

The meninges are continuous connective tissue membranes covering the brain and spinal cord. They invaginate at four points, forming a supportive partition between portions of the brain. For example, the *falx cerebri* extends downward into the longitudinal **fissure** between the cerebral hemispheres, and the *tentorium cerebelli* separates the cerebral hemispheres from the cerebellum. The outer layer, the *dura mater*, is a tough, fibrous double-layered membrane that separates at specific points to form the dural sinuses, which collect venous blood and CSF for return to the general circulation (see Fig. 20–8). Beneath the dura is the *subdural space*, a potential space. The middle layer is the *arachnoid*, a loose weblike covering, and below this is the *subarachnoid space*, which contains the CSF as well as the cerebral arteries and veins. The arachnoid projects into the dural sinuses at several places around the brain as *arachnoid villi*, through which CSF can be absorbed into the venous blood. The *pia mater* is the inner layer. It is a very delicate connective tissue that adheres closely to the surface of the brain. Many small blood vessels are found in the pia.

Cerebrospinal Fluid

The CSF provides a cushion for the brain and spinal cord. Like plasma, it is a clear, almost colorless liquid, but it contains different concentrations of electrolytes and protein (Table 20–1). A change in the characteristics of the CSF is a useful diagnostic tool. For example, the presence of significant numbers of erythrocytes indicates bleeding. CSF is formed constantly in the choroid plexuses in the ventricles and then flows into the subarachnoid space, where it circulates around the brain and spinal cord and eventually passes through the arachnoid villi into the venous blood. To maintain a relatively constant pressure within the skull, it is important for equal amounts of CSF to be produced and reabsorbed at the same rate.

Blood-Brain Barrier

The blood-brain barrier is a protective mechanism provided primarily by relatively impermeable capillaries in the brain. It limits the passage of potentially damaging materials into the brain and controls the delicate but essential balance of electrolytes and proteins in the brain. This barrier is poorly developed in **neonates**, and therefore substances such as **bilirubin** (see the section on Rh factor incompatibility in Chapter 9) or other toxic materials can pass easily into the infant's brain, causing damage. When fully developed, the blood-brain barrier can be a disadvantage because it does not allow the passage of many essential drugs such as antibiotics into the brain.

Thinkabout 20–1

a. List in order the brain coverings and spaces, with their contents, from the brain tissue outward.

b. What is the effect of the production of more CSF than can be reabsorbed?

FUNCTIONAL AREAS OF THE BRAIN

Cerebral Hemispheres

The cerebral hemispheres make up the largest and most obvious portions of the brain. The outer surface is covered by elevations or **gyri** separated by grooves or **sulci**. The longitudinal fissure separates the two hemispheres. The surface or *cortex* consists of "gray matter," or nerve cell bodies. Beneath the gray matter is the white matter, composed of myelinated nerve fibers

TABLE 20–1 Characteristics of Normal Cerebrospinal Fluid

Appearance	Clear and colorless
Pressure	9–14 mm Hg or 150 mm H$_2$O
Red blood cells	None
White blood cells	Occasional
Protein	15–45 mg/dL
Glucose	45–75 mg/dL
Sodium	140 mEq/liter
Potassium	3 mEq/liter
Specific gravity	1.007
pH	7.32–7.35
Volume in the system at one time	125–150 mL
Volume formed in 24 hours	500–800 mL

bundled into tracts, which connect the hemispheres (corpus callosum) or occur as projection fibers, connecting the cortex to the spinal cord, or association fibers, connecting different gray areas in the brain.

Each hemisphere is divided into four major lobes, each of which has some specific functions (Fig. 20–1). Some complex functions such as language and memory involve many areas of the brain. Each hemisphere is concerned with voluntary movement and sensory function in the opposite (**contralateral**) side of the body, and these areas of the cortex have been well mapped. In Figure 20–1, note the large number of nerve cells required to innervate the face compared to the amount of cortex allocated to the trunk. The cells of the motor cortex of the frontal lobe initiate specific voluntary movements, and these cells are often referred to as upper motor neurons (UMNs). Their axons form the corticospinal tracts in the spinal cord. Because the crossover of most of these tracts occurs in the medulla, damage to the motor cortex in the left frontal lobe adjacent to the longitudinal fissure (on top of the head) results in **paralysis** or **paresis** of the muscles of the right leg. Similarly, the somatosensory cortex of the parietal lobe reflects specific areas of the body. Each sensory area of the cortex has an *association area* surrounding the primary cortex, in which the sensory input is interpreted. For example, the occipital lobe contains the primary visual cortex, which receives the stimuli from the eye, and the surrounding association cortex identifies the object seen. If the primary cortex is damaged, the person is blind, but if the association area is damaged, the person can see an object but cannot comprehend its significance.

The right and left hemispheres are generally similar in structure but not necessarily in function (Table 20–2). The term *dominant hemisphere* refers to the side of the brain that controls *language*, which in most people is the left hemisphere. There are two special areas involved in language skills. *Broca's area* is considered the motor or expressive speech area, in which the output of words, both verbal and written, is coordinated in an appropriate and understandable way. This area is located at the base of the premotor area of the frontal lobe. *Wernicke's area* is the integration center that comprehends language received, both spoken and written. This area is located in the posterior temporal lobe and

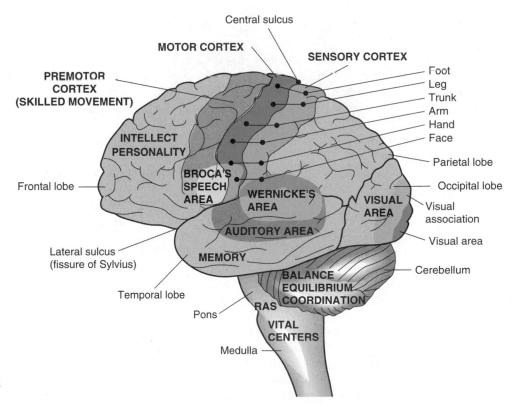

FIGURE 20–1. Functional areas of the brain.

TABLE 20–2 Major Functional Areas of the Brain	
Area	**Function**
Frontal Lobe	
Prefrontal area	Intellectual function and personality
Premotor cortex	Skilled movements
Motor cortex	Voluntary movements
Broca's area	Speech (expression)
Parietal Lobe	
Somatosensory area	Sensation (e.g., touch, pain)
Occipital Lobe	
Visual Cortex	Vision
Temporal Lobe	
Auditory cortex	Hearing
Olfactory cortex	Smell
Wernicke's area	Comprehension of speech
	Memory
Cerebellum	Body balance and position, coordinated movement
Medulla Oblongata	Control and coordination centers for respiration and cardiovascular activity
	Swallow reflex center, vomiting reflex, cough reflex
	Nuclei of five cranial nerves
Hypothalamus	Autonomic nervous system
	Link with endocrine system
	Control of body temperature, fluid balance
	Centers for thirst, hunger
Thalamus	Sensory sorting center
Basal Nuclei	Coordination and control of body movement
Reticular Activating System	Arousal or awareness
Limbic System	Emotional responses

has connecting fibers to the visual and auditory areas. The left hemisphere also appears to be responsible for mathematical ability and problem-solving and logical reasoning abilities. The right hemisphere has greater influence on artistic abilities, creativity, spatial relationships and emotional and behavioral characteristics.

The *basal nuclei* (sometimes called the basal ganglia) are clusters of cell bodies or gray matter located deep among the tracts of the cerebral hemispheres. These are part of the *extrapyramidal system* (EPS) of motor control, which controls and coordinates skeletal muscle activity, preventing excessive movements and initiating accessory and often involuntary actions such as arm-swinging when walking. Two additional nuclei located in the midbrain, the substantia nigra and the red nucleus, are also connected to the basal nuclei and the EPS.

The *limbic system* consists of many nuclei and connecting fibers in the cerebral hemispheres that encircle the superior part of the brain stem. The limbic system is responsible for emotional reactions or feelings, and for this purpose it has many connections to all areas of the brain. Part of the hypothalamus is involved with the limbic system. It provides the link for the autonomic responses such as altered blood pressure or nausea that

occur when one experiences fear, excitement, or an unpleasant sight or odor. Any **cognitive** decision arising from the higher cortical centers may be accompanied by an emotional aspect mediated through the limbic center.

Diencephalon

The diencephalon is the central portion of the brain. It is surrounded by the hemispheres and contains important structures such as the thalamus and the hypothalamus. The *thalamus* consists of many nerve cell bodies, the major function of which is to serve as a sorting and relay station for incoming sensory impulses. From the thalamus, connecting fibers transmit impulses to the cerebral cortex and other appropriate areas of the brain. The *hypothalamus* is responsible for the maintenance of homeostasis in the body, controlling the autonomic nervous system and much of the endocrine system through the hypophysis or pituitary gland. It is responsible for the regulation of body temperature, intake of food and fluid, and the regulation of sleep cycles. The hypothalamus is also the key to the stress response and plays major roles in emotional responses through the limbic system and in biologic behaviors such as the sex drive (libido).

Brainstem

The inferior portion of the brain, called the brainstem, is the connecting link to the spinal cord. The *pons* is composed of bundles of afferent and efferent fibers. Several nuclei of cranial nerves are also located in the pons. The *medulla oblongata* contains the vital control centers regulating respiration and cardiovascular function as well as the coordinating centers governing the cough reflex, swallowing, and vomiting. The medulla is the location of the nuclei of several cranial nerves and is the site of crossover of the majority of fibers of the corticospinal tracts (decussation of the pyramids), which results in the contralateral control of muscle function. The *reticular formation* is a network of nuclei and neurons scattered throughout the brainstem that has connections to many parts of the brain. The *reticular-activating system (RAS)* is part of this formation and determines the degree of arousal or awareness of the cerebral cortex. In other words, these neurons decide which sensory impulses the brain ignores and which it notices. Many drugs can affect the activity of the RAS, thus increasing or decreasing the input to the brain.

Cerebellum

The cerebellum is located dorsal to the pons and medulla, below the occipital lobe. It functions to coordinate movement and maintain posture and equilibrium by continuously assessing and adjusting to input from the pyramidal system, the proprioceptors in joints and muscles, the visual pathways, and the vestibular pathways from the inner ear.

Thinkabout 20-2

a. Describe the specific location and function of each of the following: the somatosensory area, the RAS, Wernicke's area, the basal nuclei, and the visual association area.

b. Describe white matter—what it is and what its function is—and give an example of it.

c. Predict the effects of brain damage occurring in the left frontal lobe, the cerebellum, and the hypothalamus.

BLOOD SUPPLY TO THE BRAIN

Blood is supplied to the brain by the internal carotid arteries and the vertebral arteries (see Fig. 16–27). Each *internal carotid* artery is a branch of a common carotid artery (right or left) and includes the carotid sinus, which is the location of the **pressoreceptors** or **baroreceptors** that monitor blood pressure and the **chemoreceptors** that check blood pH and oxygen levels. At the base of the brain, each internal carotid artery divides into an anterior and middle cerebral artery (see Fig. 20–7). The *anterior cerebral artery* supplies the frontal lobe, and the *middle cerebral artery* supplies the lateral part of the cerebral hemispheres, primarily the temporal and parietal lobes. The *vertebral arteries* join to form the *basilar artery,* which supplies branches to the brainstem and cerebellum as it ascends. At the base of the brain, the basilar artery divides into the right and left *posterior cerebral* arteries, which supply blood to the occipital lobes. **Anastomoses** between these major arteries at the base of the brain are provided by the *anterior communicating artery* between the anterior cerebral arteries, and the *posterior communicating arteries* between the middle cerebral and posterior cerebral arteries. This arrangement forms the *circle of Willis* and provides an alternative source of blood if the internal carotid or vertebral artery is obstructed. This circle of arteries surrounds the pituitary gland and optic chiasm. The anterior, middle, and posterior cerebral arteries follow a course over the surface of each hemisphere, with many branches penetrating into the brain substance.

Blood flow in the cerebral arteries is relatively constant because the brain cells constantly use oxygen and glucose (essential nutrients for neurons) and have little storage capacity. **Autoregulation,** through which vasodilation results from increased carbon dioxide levels or decreased blood pressure, is important in the brain. Also, the pressoreceptors (baroreceptors) and chemoreceptors protect the brain from damage related to abnormal blood pressure or pH. As mentioned earlier, venous blood collects in the dural sinuses and then drains into the right and left internal jugular veins.

CRANIAL NERVES

There are 12 pairs of cranial nerves. They originate primarily from the brainstem and pass through foramina in the skull to serve structures in the head and neck, including the eyes and ears. The vagus nerve (cranial nerve X) serves a more extensive area, branching to innervate many of the viscera. A cranial nerve may consist of motor fibers only (with associated sensory fibers from proprioceptors in the skeletal muscles) or of sensory fibers only, or it may be a mixed nerve containing both motor and sensory fibers (Table 20–3). Four cranial nerves (III, VII, IX, X) include parasympathetic fibers.

Thinkabout 20-3

a. Explain why the circle of Willis is important.

b. Describe the effect of an obstruction in the middle cerebral artery.

c. How will a lack of glucose or oxygen affect brain function, and why?

d. What are the different types of fibers and the functions of cranial nerves II, III, and IX? Describe the effects of damage to each.

The Spinal Cord and Peripheral Nerves

SPINAL CORD

The spinal cord is protected by the bony vertebral column, the meninges, and the CSF. The cord is continuous with the medulla oblongata and ends at the level of the first lumbar vertebra. Beyond this extends a bundle of nerve roots known as the cauda equina. This arrangement is significant because there is little risk of damag-

TABLE 20–3 Major Components of Cranial Nerves

Number	Name	Type of Fibers	Function
I	Olfactory	Sensory	Special sensory—smell
II	Optic	Sensory	Special sensory—vision
III	Oculomotor	Motor	Eye movements
			Four extrinsic eye muscles
			Upper eyelid—levator palpebrae muscle
		PNS	Iris—pupillary constrictor muscle
			Ciliary muscle—accommodation
IV	Trochlear	Motor	Eye movements—superior oblique eye muscle
V	Trigeminal	Sensory	General sensory—eye, nose, face and oral cavity, teeth
		Motor	Muscles of mastication with sensory proprioceptive fibers; speech
VI	Abducens	Motor	Eye movements—lateral rectus eye muscle
VII	Facial	Sensory	Special sensory—taste, anterior two-thirds of tongue
		Motor	Muscles of facial expression
			Scalp muscles
		PNS	Lacrimal gland, nasal mucosa, salivary glands (sublingual and submandibular)
VIII	Vestibulocochlear	Sensory	Special sensory—hearing and balance (inner ear)
IX	Glossopharyngeal	Sensory	Special sensory—Taste, posterior one-third of tongue
			General sensory—pharynx and soft palate (gag reflex)
			Sensory—carotid sinus for baroreceptors and chemoreceptors
		Motor	Pharyngeal muscles—swallowing
		PNS	Salivary gland (parotid)
X	Vagus	Sensory	Special Sensory—Taste, pharynx, posterior tongue
			General sensory—external ear and diaphragm
			Visceral sensory—Viscera in thoracic and abdominal cavities
		Motor	Pharynx and soft palate—swallowing and speech
		PNS	Heart and lungs; smooth muscle and glands of digestive system
XI	Spinal accessory	Motor	Voluntary muscles of palate, pharynx, and larynx
			Head movements—sternocleidomastoid and trapezius muscles
XII	Hypoglossal	Motor	Muscles of tongue

constitute the white matter surrounding an internal butterfly-shaped core of gray matter or nerve cell bodies. In the gray matter, the anterior horns consist of cell bodies of motor neurons, whose axons leave the spinal cord through the ventral root of the spinal nerves to innervate the skeletal muscles. The posterior horns contain association neurons. The white matter is composed of **afferent** and **efferent** fibers organized into tracts as well as communicating fibers running between the two sides of the cord. Each tract is assigned a unique position in the white matter (a cross-section of the cord would illustrate the "map" of tracts; see Fig. 20–16*B*). The name of the tract is based on its source and destination, and the fibers in it transmit one type of impulse. For example, the lateral spinothalamic tract is made up of *ascending* fibers, which conduct pain or temperature *sensations* relayed from spinal nerves and receptors on the opposite side of the body, to the thalamus. The *descending* tracts are of two types. The *pyramidal* or corticospinal tracts conduct impulses concerned with voluntary movement from the motor cortex *(upper motor neurons)* to the *lower motor neurons* in the anterior horn at the appropriate level of the spinal cord. Most of these tracts cross in the medulla. The *extrapyramidal* tracts carry impulses that modify and coordinate voluntary movement and maintain posture. Lower motor neurons may receive both stimulatory and inhibitory input from upper motor neurons as well as from interneurons in the cord. The sum of the input determines what activity occurs in the spinal nerves and skeletal muscles.

SPINAL NERVES

Thirty-one pairs of spinal nerves emerge from the spinal cord, carrying motor and sensory fibers to and from the organs and tissues of the body. They are named by the location in the vertebral column where they emerge (see Fig. 20–16) and are numbered within each section. For example, there are eight pairs of cervical nerves, numbered C1 to C8. Each spinal nerve is connected to the spinal cord by two short roots. The ventral or anterior root is made up of efferent or motor fibers from the lower motor neurons in the anterior horn. The dorsal or posterior root consists of afferent or sensory fibers from the dorsal root **ganglion**, where sensory fibers from peripheral receptors have already synapsed. The area of sensory innervation of the skin by a specific spinal nerve is called a *dermatome*, and these can be drawn on a "map" of the body surface (see Fig. 20–17). Assessment of sensory awareness using the dermatome map can be a useful tool in determining the level of damage to the spinal cord.

There are four *plexuses* where fibers from several spinal nerves branch and then re-form in different

ing the cord when a needle is inserted into the subarachnoid space below the first lumbar level (L3–L4) to obtain a sample of CSF *(lumbar puncture).*

The cord consists of the nerve fibers or *tracts* that

combinations to become specific peripheral nerves. These are the cervical, brachial, lumbar, and sacral plexuses. This networking means that the phrenic nerve, for example, consists of fibers from C3 to C5 and the sciatic nerve contains fibers from L4 to L5 and S1 to S3. Also, the fibers in each spinal nerve can be distributed in several peripheral nerves. This dispersal pattern can minimize the effects of damage to one spinal segment.

REFLEXES

Reflexes are automatic rapid involuntary responses to a stimulus. A simple reflex involves a sensory stimulus from a receptor conducted along an afferent nerve fiber, a synapse in the spinal cord, and an efferent impulse conducted along a peripheral nerve to elicit the response. For example, touching a very hot object with the hand results in an immediate movement away from the object. At the same time, connecting neurons or interneurons transmit the sensory information up to the brain to initiate follow-up action. Many reflexes controlling visceral activities or posture take place continuously, *without* the individual's awareness. In addition, each individual has *acquired* or learned reflexes, such as those developed when one learns to ride a bicycle. Certain reflexes, such as the patellar or knee-jerk reflex, are useful in diagnosis. Absent, weak, or abnormal responses may indicate the presence of a neurologic problem and sometimes can show the location of spinal cord damage.

Thinkabout 20–4

a. At which level would a lumbar puncture occur and why?

b. Describe the general location of the cervical spinal nerves.

c. Describe a dermatome and its purpose.

d. Describe the components of a simple reflex, in sequence, relating it to a specific example.

The Neuron and Conduction of Impulses

NEURONS

Neurons or nerve cells are highly specialized, nonmitotic cells that conduct impulses throughout the CNS and the body. They require glucose and oxygen for metabolism. There are many variations in the specific structural characteristics of each neuron depending on its function. The cell body has a variable number of processes or extensions depending on the type of neuron involved. These processes make up nerves and tracts. The dendrite is the receptor site, which conducts impulses toward the cell body. The cell body contains the nucleus. The axon conducts impulses away from the cell body toward an effector site or connecting neuron, where it can release neurotransmitter chemicals at its terminal point.

Many nerve fibers are covered by a myelin sheath, which insulates the fiber and speeds up the rate of conduction. The myelin sheath, which wraps many layers of its plasma membrane around the axon, is formed by Schwann cells. The nucleus and cytoplasm of the Schwann cell form the neurilemma or sheath of Schwann around the myelin. Gaps between the Schwann cells comprise the nodes of Ranvier, where axon collateral branches may emerge and where stimuli may affect the axon.

Regeneration of Neurons

Neurons cannot undergo cell division. If the cell body is damaged, the neuron dies. In the peripheral nervous system, axons may be able to regenerate if the cell body is viable. After damage occurs to the axon, the section distal to the injury degenerates because it lacks nutrients and is removed by macrophages and Schwann cells. The Schwann cells then attempt to form a new tube at the end of the remaining axon. The cell body becomes larger and synthesizes additional proteins for the growth of the replacement axon. The new growth does not always occur appropriately or make its original connections because the surrounding tissue may interfere.

CONDUCTION OF IMPULSES

A stimulus increases the **permeability** of the neuronal membrane, allowing sodium ions to flow inside the cell, thus **depolarizing** it and generating an action potential. The change to a positive electrical charge inside the membrane leads to increased permeability of the adjacent area, and the impulse thus moves along the membrane. Recovery or **repolarization** occurs as potassium ions move outward; then the normal permeability of the membrane is restored, and the sodium-potassium pump returns the sodium and potassium ions to their normal locations (see Fig. 6–3 in Chapter 6). In myelinated fibers this action potential is generated only at the nodes of Ranvier, and therefore the impulse can "skip" along very rapidly (saltatory conduction). Generally, the larger axons conduct impulses more rapidly than smaller ones. The synapse provides the connection between two or more neurons or a neuron and an effector site. Very complex "electrical circuits" exist in the nervous system, with multiple synapses on any one neuron. The electrical activity of the brain can be monitored by attaching electrodes to the scalp and measuring the brain waves by means of an electroencephalogram or EEG (see Fig. 20–10).

SYNAPSES AND CHEMICAL NEUROTRANSMITTERS

The common synapse involves the release of chemical **neurotransmitters** from **vesicles** in the synaptic buds of the axons (Fig. 20–2). These transmitters may stimulate or inhibit the conduction of the impulse. A typical synapse consists of the terminal axon of the presynaptic neuron containing the vesicles and the receptor site on the membrane of the postsynaptic neuron. The axon and the receptor site are separated by the fluid-filled synaptic cleft. When the stimulus reaches the axon, the neurotransmitter is released from the vesicles and flows across the cleft to act on the receptor in the postsynaptic membrane, creating a stimulus. Receptors are quite specific for each transmitter. Neurotransmitters are either inactivated by enzymes or taken up by the axon to prevent continued stimulation. Because there are usually many impulses from a variety of neurons arriving at one postsynaptic neuron, that neuron can process the input and then transmit the net result of the information to the next receptor site.

There are many chemical neurotransmitters in the body. Acetylcholine is present at neuromuscular junctions and in the autonomic nervous system, the peripheral nervous system, and, less commonly, the central nervous system. The catecholamines include norepinephrine, epinephrine, and dopamine and are present in the brain. Norepinephrine is a neurotransmitter in the sympathetic nervous system (SNS), whereas both norepinephrine and epinephrine, when released from the adrenal medulla with SNS stimulation, circulate in the blood and interstitial fluid, ultimately diffusing into the synaptic cleft and stimulating the appropriate receptors in the SNS. Other neurotransmitters include serotonin, histamine, and gamma-aminobutyric acid (GABA). The roles of many neurotransmitters in mental illness as well as other pathologies are being studied intensively. For example, norepinephrine and dopamine are excitatory, and thus low levels may be linked to depression. The enkephalins and beta-endorphins are of great interest because they can block the conduction of pain impulses in the spinal cord and brain (see Chapter 13). Drugs have been developed that can mimic the effects of natural chemical neurotransmitters, stimulating specific receptors and promoting similar effects. Other drugs are designed to bind to certain receptors but not stimulate them. These drugs block the action of normal neurotransmitters, thus inhibiting the activity initiated by them. Drugs can also affect neurotransmission by either inhibiting the enzymes that normally inactivate transmitters or interfering with the uptake of neurotransmitters into the axons for recycling.

Thinkabout 20–5

a. If postsynaptic membrane permeability is increased, is the neuron more easily stimulated or less excitable?

b. Explain the effect of the myelin sheath and the nodes of Ranvier on the conduction of impulses.

c. Briefly describe, in the correct sequence, the events that occur in synaptic transmission.

d. Can any chemical neurotransmitter stimulate any receptor?

The Autonomic Nervous System

The autonomic system incorporates the sympathetic and parasympathetic systems. They generally have antagonistic effects, thereby providing a fine balance that aids in maintaining homeostasis in the body (see Table 20–4).

The autonomic system provides motor and sensory innervation to smooth muscle, cardiac muscle, and glands. Although the individual is largely unaware of this involuntary activity, it is integrated with somatic activity by the higher brain centers. The neural pathways in the motor fibers of the autonomic system are different because each involves two neurons and a ganglion. The *preganglionic* fiber is located in the brain or spinal cord. This axon then synapses with the second neuron in the *ganglion* outside the CNS, and this *postganglionic* fiber continues to the effector organ or tissue.

SYMPATHETIC NERVOUS SYSTEM

The SNS, or thoracolumbar nervous system, increases the general level of activity in the body, increasing cardiovascular, respiratory, and neurologic functions. It is basic to the fight-or-flight or stress response and is augmented by the increased secretions of the adrenal medulla in response to

Neurotransmitters

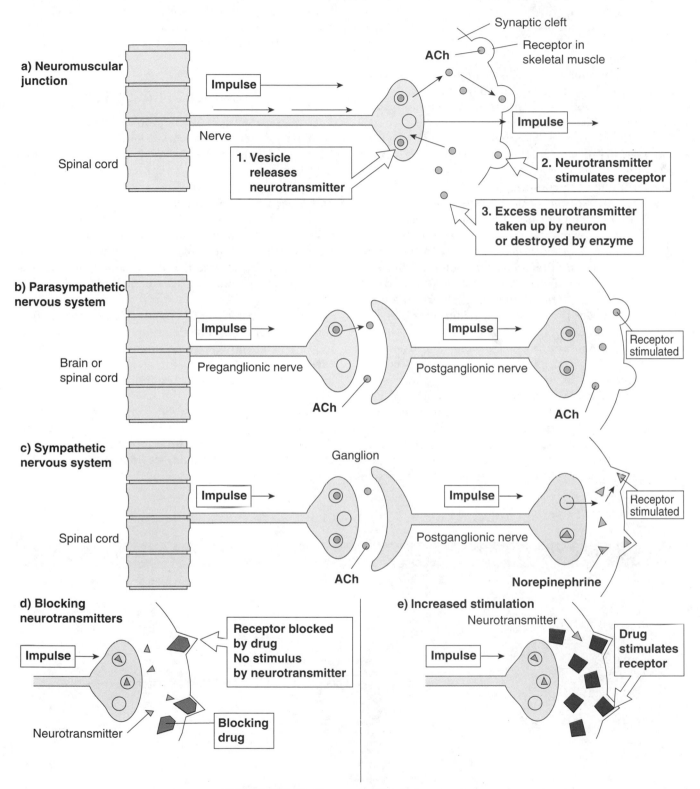

FIGURE 20-2. Neurotransmitters at the synapse.

SNS stimuli. The preganglionic fibers of the sympathetic nerves arise from the thoracic and the first two lumbar segments of the spinal cord. The *ganglia* are located in two *chains* or trunks, one on either side of the spinal cord. Here there are synapses to postganglionic fibers or connecting fibers to other ganglia in the chain.

The neurotransmitters and receptors are important in the autonomic nervous system because they are closely linked to drug actions. The neurotransmitter released by preganglionic fibers at the ganglion is acetylcholine (ACh), hence these fibers are termed *cholinergic* fibers. Most SNS postganglionic fibers release *norepinephrine* or *adrenaline (adrenergic* fibers). The postganglionic fibers to sweat glands and blood vessels in skeletal muscle are cholinergic.

Several types of *adrenergic receptors* in the tissues respond to norepinephrine and epinephrine. Norepinephrine acts primarily on *alpha* (α) receptors, and epinephrine acts on both *alpha* and *beta* (β) receptors. The major sites of the receptors and the effects of stimulation are summarized in Table 20–4. An organ or tissue may have more than one type of receptor, but one type usually is present in greater numbers and exerts the dominant effect. Drugs may be used to stimulate these receptors or to prevent stimulation (see Fig. 20–2). For example, beta$_1$-adrenergic receptors (beta$_1$-type sympathetic receptors) are located in cardiac muscle. With SNS stimulation, epinephrine stimulates these receptors, resulting in an increased heart rate and force of contractions. In a patient with a damaged heart, drugs such as beta$_1$-adrenergic blocking agents (beta blockers) may be used to block these receptors, thus preventing the stimulation and exces-

sive heart activity. Or a patient may require a drug that can stimulate the beta receptors to improve heart function (a beta-adrenergic drug). The best drugs are specific for one type of receptor in one organ or tissue because they do not alter function in other areas of the body. In other words, the more specific the drug action, the more mild the adverse or side effects of the drug.

PARASYMPATHETIC NERVOUS SYSTEM

The parasympathetic nervous system (PNS or craniosacral nervous system) dominates the digestive system and aids in the recovery of the body following sympathetic activity. There are two locations of PNS preganglionic fibers—cranial nerves III, VII, IX, and X at the brainstem level, and the sacral spinal nerves. The vagus nerve (cranial nerve X) provides extensive innervation to the heart and digestive tract. In the PNS the ganglia are scattered and located close to the target organ, and the neurotransmitter at both preganglionic and postganglionic synapses is ACh.

There are two types of cholinergic receptors. Nicotinic receptors are always stimulated by ACh and are located in all postganglionic cholinergic neurons in the PNS and SNS. Muscarinic receptors are located in all effector cells and may be stimulated or inhibited by ACh depending on the organ. Like the pharmacologic effects initiated in the SNS, cholinergic blocking agents reduce PNS activity, whereas cholinergic or anticholinesterase agents (which prevent the enzyme cholinesterase from breaking down ACh) increase PNS activity.

TABLE 20–4	Effect of Stimulation of the Autonomic Nervous System			
Area	**SNS Receptor**	**Sympathetic**	**Parasympathetic**
Cardiovascular			
Heart	β-1 (beta-1)	Increases rate and force of contractions	Decreases rate and contractility
Blood vessels	α-1 (alpha-1)		
Skin, mucosa, viscera		Vasoconstriction	No innervation
Skeletal muscle	β2	Vasodilation	No innervation
Adrenal Medulla		Secretion of epinephrine and norepinephrine	No innervation
Respiratory System	β-2	Bronchodilation (smooth muscle)	Bronchoconstriction
Eye	α-1	Pupil dilation (radial muscle)	Pupil constriction (sphincter or circular muscle)
Sweat Glands	α-1	Increased secretion	
Digestive System	α-2		
Secretions		Decreased	Increased
Peristalsis		Decreased	Increased
Sphincters	α-1	Constricts	Relaxes
Urinary System			
Sphincters of bladder	α-1	Constricts	Relaxes
Renin	β-1	Increased secretion	
Male Genitalia	α-1	Ejaculation	Erection

Thinkabout 20–6

a. Compare the location of the ganglia and the junction of PNS and SNS peripheral nerve fibers with those in the CNS.

b. Explain how the PNS and SNS affect cardiovascular activity and blood pressure.

c. List the synapses in which ACh is the neurotransmitter.

d. Which part of the autonomic nervous system promotes digestion and absorption? How does this occur?

e. Briefly describe the action and effect of a drug classified as an alpha$_1$-adrenergic blocking agent.

f. Briefly describe where a cholinergic drug acts and how it affects the postsynaptic receptors. Give two examples of its possible effects on function.

GENERAL EFFECTS OF NEUROLOGIC DYSFUNCTION

The effects of neurologic damage due to different causes have many similarities because specific areas of the brain and spinal cord have established functions. Therefore, damage to a certain area from a tumor or head injury, for example, can result in the same neurologic loss and signs. Also, the effects of increased pressure within the CNS are basically similar regardless of the cause. To facilitate study and prevent repetition, these common effects are discussed in this section and are then referred to in the subsequent sections on specific disorders. Some unique variations in effects of damage to the nervous system do occur, given the diversity of pathologic conditions and the possible combinations of effects.

Local (Focal) Effects

Local effects are signs related to the specific area of the brain or spinal cord where the lesion is located (see Fig. 20–1). Examples are paresis or paralysis of the right arm resulting from damage to a section of the left frontal lobe, or loss of vision resulting from damage to the occipital lobe. With an expanding lesion such as a growing tumor or hemorrhage, additional impairment is noted as the adjacent areas become involved.

Supratentorial and Infratentorial Lesions

Supratentorial lesions occur in the cerebral hemispheres above the tentorium cerebelli. A lesion in this location leads to a specific dysfunction in a discrete area, perhaps numbness in a hand. The lesion must become very large before it affects consciousness. An **infratentorial** lesion is located in the brainstem or below the tentorium. A relatively small lesion in this location can affect many motor and sensory fibers because they are bundled together when passing through the brainstem, resulting in widespread impairment. Also, respiratory and circulatory function as well as the level of consciousness can be impaired by a small lesion in this area.

Left and Right Hemispheres

Certain effects of brain damage are unique to the left or right hemisphere. These occur in addition to focal effects. In most individuals, damage to the left hemisphere leads to loss of logical thinking ability, analytical skills, other intellectual abilities, and communication skills. Right-sided brain damage impairs appreciation of music and art and causes behavioral problems. Spatial orientation and recognition of relationships may be deficient, leading to interference with mobility and "neglect" of the contralateral side of the body (which is not recognized as "self").

Level of Consciousness

Normally, a person is totally aware of surrounding activities and incoming stimuli and is oriented to time, place, and people; the person can respond quickly and appropriately to questions, commands, or events. One of the early changes noted in those with acute brain disorders is a decreasing level of consciousness or responsiveness. The cerebral cortex and the RAS in the brainstem determine consciousness. Usually extensive supratentorial lesions must be present in the cerebral hemispheres to cause loss of consciousness, whereas relatively small lesions in the brainstem (infratentorial lesions) can affect the RAS. Space-occupying masses in the cerebellum can also compress the brainstem and RAS. It is wise to remember that many systemic disorders, such as acidosis or hypoglycemia, can depress the CNS, reducing the level of consciousness. Various levels of reduced consciousness may present as lethargy, confusion, **disorientation**, memory loss, unresponsiveness to verbal stimuli, or difficulty of arousal. Standard categories using tools such as the *Glasgow Coma Scale* provide consistency in the medical assessment (Table 20–5).

TABLE 20–5 Glasgow Coma Scale

Criteria	Maximum	Example—0700 Hours	Example—0900 Hours	Example—1100 Hours
Eye Opening				
Spontaneous	4			
Response to speech	3	x	x	
Response to pain	2			
None	1			x
Motor Response				
Obeys commands	6	x		
Localizes pain	5		x	
Normal flexion (to pain)	4			
Abnormal flexion (decorticate)	3			
Abnormal extension (decerebrate)				
None (flaccid)	2			x
	1			
Verbal Response				
Oriented to time and place	5			
Confused	4	x		
Inappropriate words	3		x	
Incomprehensible	2			
None	1			x
Score	15	13	11	4
	(Good, normal)			

The lowest level is loss of consciousness or **coma,** in which the affected person does not respond to painful or verbal stimuli and the body is flaccid, although some reflexes are present. The terminal stage, deep coma, is marked by a loss of all reflexes, fixed and dilated pupils, and slow and irregular pulse and respirations. A diagnosis of *brain death* is often required because these individuals can be maintained artificially on cardiopulmonary support systems. The criteria for brain death include cessation of brain function including function of the cortex and the brainstem (e.g., a flat or inactive electroencephalogram [EEG]), absence of brainstem reflexes or responses, and absence of spontaneous respirations when ventilator assistance is withdrawn. The criteria also include establishment of the certainty of irreversible brain damage by confirming the cause of the dysfunction. Drug overdose or hypothermia can cause loss of brain activity temporarily; thus a longer time period and additional testing are required before brain death can be confirmed in these individuals.

Motor Dysfunction

Damage to the upper motor neurons in the cerebral cortex (frontal lobe) or to the corticospinal tracts in the brain interferes with voluntary movements, thus causing weakness or paralysis on the opposite (**contralateral**) side of the body. This contralateral effect is determined by the crossover of the corticospinal tracts in the medulla. The area affected, such as a leg or arm, depends on the specific site of damage. Muscle tone and reflexes may be increased (**hyperreflexia**) because the intact spinal cord continues to conduct impulses with no moderating or inhibiting influences sent from the brain (**spastic** paralysis). This frequently leads to contractures in the affected limbs.

Damage to the lower motor neurons in the anterior horns of the spinal cord results in weakness or paralysis on the same side of the body at and below the level of damage. In the area of damage the muscles are usually **flaccid** (lack tone), and reflexes are absent (flaccid paralysis). If the cord distal to the damage is intact, some reflexes in that area may be present and hyperactive (hyperreflexia).

Lower motor neurons are also located in the nuclei of *cranial nerves* in the brainstem, and similarly, **ipsilateral** weakness or flaccid paralysis may result from damage to any cranial nerves containing motor fibers (see Table 20–3).

Two involuntary motor responses that occur with severe brain trauma include *decorticate* and *decerebrate* posturing. Decorticate responses include rigid flexion in the upper limbs with adducted arms and internal rotation of the hands. The lower limbs are extended. This response may occur with severe damage in the cerebral hemispheres. Decerebrate responses occur with brainstem lesions and CNS depression due to systemic effects. Both the upper and lower limbs are extended, as is the head, and the body is arched.

Sensory Deficits

Sensory loss may involve touch, pain, temperature, and position as well as the special senses of vision, hearing, taste, and smell. The somatosensory cortex in the parietal lobe (see Fig. 20–1), which receives and localizes basic sensory input from the body, is mapped to correspond to receptors in the skin and skeletal muscles of various body regions. The specific site of damage determines the deficit. Mapping of the dermatomes (see Fig. 20–17) assists in the evaluation of spinal cord lesions. Damage to the cranial nerves or their nuclei or to the assigned area of the brain may interfere with vision or other special senses.

Visual Loss—Hemianopia

Because of the unique visual pathway, loss of the visual fields depends on the site of damage in the visual pathway (Fig. 20–3). At the optic chiasm, the fibers in each optic nerve come together and then divide. If the optic chiasm is totally destroyed, vision is lost in both eyes. Partial loss can result in a variety of effects depending on the particular fibers damaged. Fibers from the medial (inner) half of each **retina** cross over to the other hemisphere, whereas fibers from the lateral or outer half of the retina remain on the same side. Thus, the optic tract coursing from the optic chiasm to the occipital lobe on one side includes fibers from half of each eye. If the optic tract or occipital lobe is damaged, vision is lost from the medial half of one eye and the lateral half of the other eye; this is called *homonymous hemianopia*. The overall effect is loss of the visual field on the side opposite to that of the damage. In other words, damage to the left occipital lobe means loss of the right

visual field because the left half of both retinas receives light waves from the right side of the visual field. If you were caring for this patient, it would be best to stand on the patient's left side.

Language Disorders

Aphasia refers to an inability to comprehend or to express language. There are many types of aphasia, the main types being expressive, receptive, and global (Table 20–6). Many variations and combinations may occur in individual cases. Dysphasia refers to partial impairment, which is more common, but the term aphasia is frequently used to refer to both partial and total loss of communicating ability. *Expressive* or *motor aphasia* results in an impaired ability to speak or write fluently or appropriately. Such a person may be unable to find any intelligible words or construct a meaningful sentence. This type of aphasia occurs when Broca's area in the dominant frontal lobe (usually the left lobe) is damaged (see Fig. 20–1). *Receptive* or *sensory aphasia* is an inability to read or understand the spoken word. This category does not include hearing or visual impairment. The source of the problem is the inability to process information in the brain. The individual may be capable of fluent speech, but frequently it is meaningless. Damage to Wernicke's area in the left temporal lobe results in receptive aphasia. *Global aphasia* commonly describes a combination of expressive and recep-

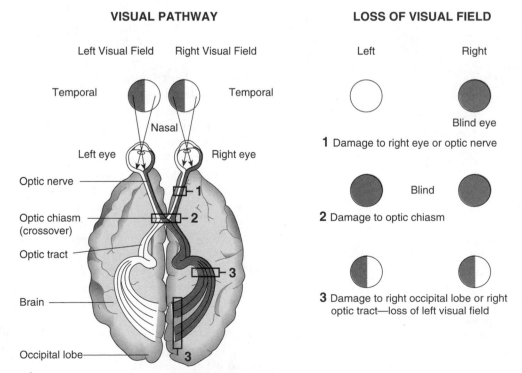

FIGURE 20–3. The visual pathway.

TABLE 20–6 Aphasia

Type	Site of Damage	Effect
Expressive (motor)	Broca's area Left frontal lobe	Cannot speak or write fluently or appropriately
Receptive (sensory)	Wernicke's area Left temporal lobe	Unable to understand written or spoken language
Global	Broca's and Wernicke's areas and communication fibers	Cannot express self or comprehend others' language

tive aphasia resulting from major damage to the brain, Broca's area, Wernicke's area, and many communicating fibers throughout the brain.

Other types of language disorders include *dysarthria*, in which words cannot be articulated clearly; this is a motor dysfunction that usually results from cranial nerve damage or muscle impairment. *Agraphia* refers to impaired writing ability, and *alexia* is impaired reading ability. *Agnosia* is the term used to refer to loss of recognition or association. For example, visual agnosia indicates an inability to recognize objects. Thorough testing is required before a specific diagnosis can be made of any of these disorders.

Thinkabout 20–7

a. Compare normal function and coma using two characteristics of these levels of consciousness.

b. Describe two possible areas of CNS damage that probably will lead to flaccid paralysis.

c. Describe the effects on motor function of damage to the lateral surface of the frontal lobe.

d. Describe the characteristics of receptive aphasia and state the usual location of the lesion.

Seizures

Seizures or convulsions are caused by spontaneous discharge of neurons in the brain. This state may be precipitated by inflammation, hypoxia, or bleeding in the brain. Often the seizure is focal or is related to the particular site of the irritation, but it may become generalized. Frequently it is manifested by involuntary repetitive movements or abnormal sensations. Seizures are described in more detail in a later section of this chapter.

Increased Intracranial Pressure

The skull contains brain tissue, blood, and CSF. The volume of each of these normally remains relatively constant, thus maintaining a normal pressure inside the cranial cavity. Temporary fluctuations in blood flow and blood pressure may occur with activities such as coughing or bending over. Because the brain is encased in the rigid, nonexpandable skull, any increase in fluid such as blood or inflammatory or purulent exudate or any additional mass such as a tumor leads to an increase in pressure in the brain. The result is that less blood can enter the "high pressure" area in the brain, and eventually the brain tissue itself is compressed. Both of these effects decrease the function of the neurons, both locally and generally. The pressure increases at the site of the problem initially but gradually is dispersed throughout the CNS by means of the continuous flow of fluid, leading to widespread loss of function. Changes in intracranial pressure (ICP) can be directly monitored by instruments placed in the ventricles (invasive procedures) or indirectly by methods such as radiologic examinations or assessment of the level of consciousness and vital signs.

Increased ICP is common in many neurologic problems, including brain hemorrhage, trauma, edema, infection, tumors, and excessive amounts of CSF (Fig. 20–4). All of these problems create the same general set of manifestations. A summary of these effects is provided in Table 20–7.

EARLY SIGNS

Initially, when ICP increases, the body attempts to compensate for it by shifting more CSF to the spinal cavity, for example, and increasing venous return from the brain. These compensation mechanisms are effective for only a short time. The resulting hypoxia triggers arterial vasodilation through local autoregulation reflexes in an attempt to improve the blood supply to the brain. However, this adds to the fluid volume inside the skull and is also effective for only a short time. Because of these compensatory mechanisms, ICP is often significantly elevated before signs become apparent. If the cause of the increased pressure has not been removed, the *first* indication of increased ICP is usually a *decreasing level of consciousness* or decreased responsiveness. Additional early indications of increased ICP include *severe headache* due to stretching of the dura and large blood vessels and *vomiting*—often projectile vomiting not associated with food intake—which is the result of pressure stimulating the emetic center in the medulla. *Papilledema* may be present, caused by increased pressure and swelling of the optic disc. This can be observed by looking through the pupil of the eye at

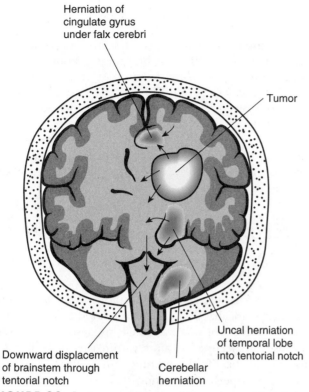

Herniation of cingulate gyrus under falx cerebri

Tumor

Downward displacement of brainstem through tentorial notch

Cerebellar herniation

Uncal herniation of temporal lobe into tentorial notch

FIGURE 20-4. Increased intracranial pressure and herniation.

VITAL SIGNS

If the pressure elevation continues, cerebral **ischemia** develops, which stimulates a powerful response (Cushing's reflex) from the vasomotor centers in an attempt to increase the blood supply to the brain. Systemic vasoconstriction occurs to increase systemic blood pressure and force more blood into the brain to relieve the ischemia. The baroreceptors respond to the increased blood pressure by slowing the heart rate, and the chemoreceptors respond to the low carbon dioxide levels that accompany the accelerated systemic circulation by reducing the respiratory rate. In other words, the brain responds to ischemia by one mechanism while feedback control for blood pressure uses other mechanisms to respond to conditions in the rest of the body. As ICP continues to rise, so does systemic blood pressure (Fig. 20–5). An increasing *pulse pressure* (the difference between systolic and diastolic pressures) is significant in people with ICP. The widening gap in pulse pressure results from the slow heart rate and the intermittent but rapid on-off cycle of Cushing's reflex controlling systemic vasoconstriction. Eventually, severe ischemia and neuronal death prevent any circulatory control, and the blood pressure will drop. Various abnormal respiratory patterns develop, such as Cheyne-Stokes respirations with alternating apnea and periods of increasing and decreasing respirations, depending on the site of the lesion.

the retina, where the optic disc provides a "window" into the brain (see Fig. 20–21). The optic nerve (cranial nerve II) is similar to a projection of brain tissue in that it is surrounded by CSF and meninges and enters the eye at the optic disc, where it reflects any increased ICP from the brain. These early manifestations continue to increase in severity as long as pressure continues to rise.

VISUAL SIGNS OF INTRACRANIAL PRESSURE

In addition to papilledema and specific reflex changes, several other significant indicators of in-

TABLE 20-7 Effects of Increased Intracranial Pressure	
General Signs	**Rationale**
Decreasing level of consciousness	Pressure on RAS (brainstem) or cerebral cortex
Headache	Stretching or distortion of meninges or walls of large blood vessels
Vomiting	Pressure on emetic center in medulla
Vital signs	
Increasing blood pressure with increasing pulse pressure	Cushing's reflex response to cerebral ischemia causes systemic vasoconstriction
Slow heart rate	Response to increasing blood pressure
Signs affecting vision	
Papilledema	Increased pressure of CSF causes swelling around the optic disc
Pupil, fixed and dilated	Pressure on cranial nerve III (oculomotor)

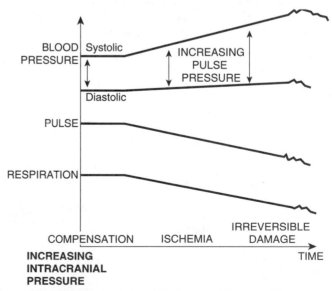

FIGURE 20-5. Vital signs with increased intracranial pressure.

creasing ICP are seen in the eyes. Pressure on cranial nerve III (oculomotor nerve) affects the size and response of the pupils. Usually one pupil ipsilateral to the lesion becomes fixed (unresponsive to light) and dilated as the PNS fibers in the affected cranial nerve III become nonfunctional. With additional pressure both pupils become fixed and dilated (or "blown"). Other signs include **ptosis** or "droopy eyelid," which is another effect of pressure on the third cranial nerve because innervation to the muscle of the upper eyelid is impaired; abnormal or excessive eye movements such as nystagmus may also result from increased pressure.

CHANGES IN CEREBROSPINAL FLUID

The pressure of CSF is elevated (above 20 mm Hg) in patients with increased ICP. The composition of the fluid may vary with the cause of the problem (see Table 20–1). It may be pinkish in color and contain erythrocytes, suggesting that hemorrhage is occurring. A cloudy, yellowish fluid may indicate infection, whereas abnormal protein levels may reflect the presence of a neoplasm.

HERNIATION

When a mass such as a blood clot or tumor becomes large enough, it may displace brain tissue, leading to herniation. There are several different types of herniation (see Fig. 20–4). In transtentorial or central herniation, the cerebral hemispheres, diencephalon, and midbrain are displaced downward. The resultant pressure affects the flow of blood and CSF, the RAS, and respiration. Uncal (uncinate) herniation occurs when the uncus of the temporal lobe is displaced downward past the tentorium cerebelli, creating pressure on the third cranial nerve, the posterior cerebral artery, and the RAS. Cerebellar or tonsillar (infratentorial) herniation develops when the cerebellar tonsils are pushed downward through the foramen magnum, compressing the brainstem and vital centers and causing death.

Thinkabout 20–8

a. List the early signs of increased ICP.
b. Explain why headache occurs with ICP.
c. Describe the usual changes in vital signs resulting from increased ICP.
d. Explain why a lesion in the brainstem is more critical than one in the cerebral hemisphere.

Diagnostic Tests

Computed tomographic (CT) scans, magnetic resonance imaging (MRI), cerebral angiography, Doppler ultrasound for assessing patency of the carotid and intracerebral vessels, and EEGs provide useful information. Lumbar puncture is useful to examine the CSF for raised ICP and altered components.

Clinical assessment routinely includes the use of tools such as the Glasgow coma scale to assess the level of consciousness and a checklist of normal reflexes.

ACUTE NEUROLOGIC PROBLEMS

Brain Tumors

Tumors are an example of a space-occupying lesion that causes localized dysfunction related to its location and the effects of increased ICP, as described earlier, because of space constraints within the skull. Benign tumors can be life-threatening unless they are in an accessible superficial location where they can be removed. Most primary malignant tumors arise from one of the neuroglial or glial cells (gliomas), the supportive or parenchymal cells in the CNS (see Fig. 5–10). These tumors are classified according to the cell of derivation (such as astrocytoma) and the location of the tumor. In addition, tumors may develop in the meninges or pituitary gland, causing similar neurologic effects resulting from pressure on the brain. Primary malignant tumors very rarely metastasize outside the CNS, but multiple tumors may be present within the CNS. Secondary brain tumors are quite common, usually metastasizing from breast or lung tumors, and they cause effects similar to those of primary tumors.

PATHOPHYSIOLOGY

Primary malignant tumors, particularly astrocytomas, do not usually have well-defined margins but are invasive and have irregular projections into adjacent tissue that are difficult to remove totally. There is usually an area of inflammation around the tumor. As the mass expands, it compresses and distorts the tissue around it, eventually resulting in herniation. A relatively small tumor in the brainstem or cerebellum can compress the medulla within a short time. However, tumors in the cerebral hemispheres, particularly in "silent" areas, may grow quite large before their effects are noticeable.

ETIOLOGY

Brainstem and cerebellar tumors are common in young children, and research into the etiology of these tumors continues, particularly with regard to prenatal parental exposure to carcinogens and to embryonic development. Adults are affected more frequently by tumors in the cerebral hemispheres; predisposing factors to these tumors have not been established.

SIGNS AND SYMPTOMS

The specific site of the tumor determines the focal signs. If the tumor grows rapidly, signs of ICP develop quickly, often beginning with morning headaches. Over time, these headaches increase in severity and frequency. Lethargy and irritability may develop as well as personality and behavioral changes. In some cases, seizures are the first sign, as the tumor irritates the surrounding tissue. Brainstem or cerebellar tumors may affect several cranial nerves, perhaps causing unilateral facial paralysis or visual problems. Unlike other forms of cancer, brain tumors do not cause the usual signs of malignancy because they do not metastasize outside the CNS, and they must be removed because they will cause death before they are large enough to cause general effects.

TREATMENT

Surgery is the treatment of choice, often accompanied by radiation and chemotherapy. The prognosis for many types of tumors is improving as new drugs are developed. In some cases, surgery and radiation may cause substantial damage to normal tissue in the CNS.

Thinkabout 20-9

a. List the specific signs of dysfunction that would be expected in a young child with a cerebellar tumor.

b. Choose a possible tumor site in one cerebral hemisphere and list the signs (focal and general) that would be expected as the tumor grows.

c. Explain why a tumor in the cerebral hemisphere may grow quite large before any signs appear, but a brainstem tumor causes signs in the early stages.

d. Explain why the general signs of cancer, such as weight loss and anemia, do not develop with brain tumors.

e. Explain why the brain is a common site of metastatic cancer from the lung.

Vascular Disorders

TRANSIENT ISCHEMIC ATTACKS
Pathophysiology

A transient ischemic attack (TIA) results from a temporary localized reduction of blood flow in the brain. It may result from partial occlusion of an artery related to atherosclerosis or from a small **embolus**, a vascular spasm, or local loss of autoregulation. The brain must have a constant source of glucose and oxygen. TIAs may be useful if they serve as a warning and lead to diagnosis and treatment of a problem prior to the occurrence of a cerebrovascular accident (CVA, stroke).

Signs and Symptoms

The manifestations are directly related to the location of the ischemia. The patient remains conscious. Intermittent short episodes of impaired function such as muscle weakness in an arm or leg, visual disturbances, or numbness and **paresthesia** in the face may occur. Transient aphasia or confusion may develop. The attack may last a few minutes or longer but rarely lasts more than 1 to 2 hours, and then the signs disappear. Repeated attacks are frequently a warning of the development of atherosclerosis.

CEREBROVASCULAR ACCIDENTS
Pathophysiology

A CVA is an **infarction** of brain tissue that results from lack of blood. The tissue necrosis may be an outcome of total occlusion of a cerebral blood vessel by atheroma or embolus, or it may be the consequence of a ruptured cerebral vessel (Fig. 20–6A). Five minutes or less of ischemia causes irreversible cell damage. A central area of necrosis develops surrounded by an area of inflammation, and function in this area is lost immediately.

The development and effects of a stroke vary with the cause. There are three common categories (Table 20–8). Occlusion of an artery by an atheroma is the most common cause. (*Atherosclerosis* may be reviewed in Chapter 16.) Atheromas frequently develop in the large arteries such as the carotids. This condition causes gradual narrowing of the arterial lumen by plaque and **thrombus**, leading to possible TIAs and eventually infarction. The second type of stroke is a sudden obstruction due to an *embolus* lodging in a cerebral artery. Thrombus may break off an atheroma, or mural thrombus may form inside the heart following a myocardial infarction and then break away. Emboli can also result from other materials, such as tumors, air, or infection (endocarditis). The third class

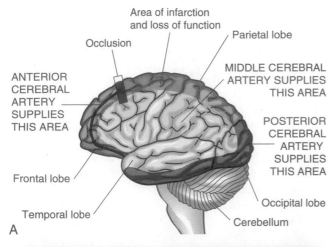

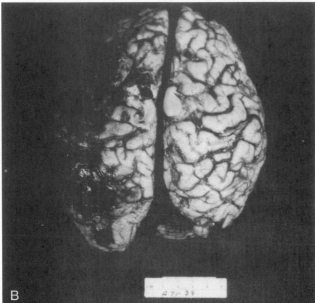

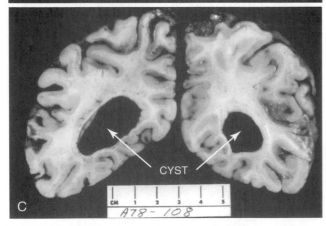

FIGURE 20–6. *A,* Effects of cerebrovascular accident (CVA). *B,* External superior surface of the brain showing acute hemorrhagic infarction. Note blood vessels on surface of brain. *C,* Cut surface of brain showing cyst from healed infarction. (Courtesy of R.W. Shaw, M.D., North York General Hospital, Toronto, Ontario.)

of stroke involves intracerebral *hemorrhage,* usually caused by rupture of a cerebral artery in a patient with severe hypertension (see Chapter 16). Hemorrhagic strokes are frequently more severe and destructive than others, affecting large portions of the brain (see Fig. 20–6*B*). Because of the increased ICP, the effects are evident in both hemispheres and are complicated by the secondary effects of bleeding in addition to the disrupted blood supply. The presence of free blood in interstitial areas affects the cell membranes and can lead to significant secondary damage as vasospasm, electrolyte imbalances, acidosis, and cellular edema develop.

It is important to minimize the inflammation and pressure in the brain and to institute therapy to maintain adequate perfusion to limit the area of permanent damage. Collateral circulation may have developed in areas gradually affected by atherosclerosis (see Chapter 16). Because neurons do not regenerate, an area of residual scar tissue and often cysts remain, with a permanent loss of neurons in that area (see Fig. 20–6*C*). In many cases, because specific functions result from integrated output from many areas, it is possible with intensive therapy for a person with a stroke to develop new neural pathways in the brain or to relearn a task, thus recovering some lost function.

Etiology

The risk factors for atherosclerosis are discussed in Chapter 16 and apply similarly to CVA. Emboli may arise from atheromas in the large arteries such as the carotids or from cardiac disorders associated with the left ventricle such as acute myocardial infarction, atrial fibrillation, endocarditis, or an implant such as a prosthetic valve. Severe or long-term hypertension or arteriosclerosis in the elderly increase the risk of intracerebral hemorrhage.

Signs and Symptoms

Signs and symptoms depend on the location of the obstruction, the size of the artery involved, and the functional area affected (see Fig. 20–6*A*). The presence of collateral circulation may diminish the size of the affected area. There are "silent" areas of the brain, in which dysfunction resulting from small infarctions is not obvious. Obstruction of small arteries may not lead to obvious signs until several small infarctions have occurred. Occlusion of large arteries such as the internal carotid artery or the middle cerebral artery or a hemorrhage may cause severe widespread effects, including coma, loss of consciousness, or death. In some cases, the effects of a stroke develop slowly over a

TABLE 20–8 Types of Cerebrovascular Accidents

	Thrombus	Embolus	Hemorrhage
Predisposing condition	Atherosclerosis in cerebral artery	Atherosclerosis or systemic source (e.g., heart)	Hypertension Arteriosclerosis
Onset	Gradual—may be preceded by transient ischemic attacks Occurs often at rest	Sudden	Sudden Occurs often with activity
Increased ICP	Minimal	Minimal	Present
Effects	Localized—may be less permanent damage if collateral circulation has been established	Localized unless multiple emboli are present	Widespread and severe—often fatal

period of hours. Initially, flaccid paralysis is present; spastic paralysis develops several weeks later as the nervous system recovers from the initial insult. Generally, the functional deficits increase during the first 48 hours as inflammation develops at the site and then subside as some neurons around the infarcted area recover.

Specific local signs depend on the area affected (see Figs. 20–1 and 20–6). Occlusion of an anterior cerebral artery affects the frontal lobe. Common signs include contralateral muscle weakness or paralysis and sensory loss in the leg, confusion, and loss of problem-solving skills with personality changes. The middle cerebral artery supplies a large portion of the cerebral hemisphere, and therefore lack of blood supply leads to contralateral paralysis and sensory loss, primarily of the upper body and arm. Because the posterior cerebral artery supplies the occipital lobe, visual loss is likely. Aphasia develops if the left or dominant lobe is affected, whereas spatial relationships may be more severely impaired if the right side is damaged.

Treatment

Supportive treatment to maximize cerebral circulation and oxygen supply is usually initiated. A team approach to care is important to encourage recovery and minimize complications in patients in whom many basic functions are impaired. Speech, mobility, swallowing, and other functions may be affected in one individual. Correct positioning, frequent changes of position, and passive exercises to prevent muscle atrophy and contractures as well as skin breakdown are required (see Chapter 11). As soon as the vital signs are stable, a return to the sitting or standing position, with assistance, helps to maintain muscle tone and minimize perceptual deficits. Surgical intervention may be possible to relieve carotid artery obstruction. Also, the underlying problem (hypertension, atherosclerosis, or thrombus) can be treated. The prognosis varies considerably depending on the underlying causative factors, the artery affected, and the general health status of the individual.

CEREBRAL ANEURYSMS
Pathophysiology

An aneurysm is a localized dilation in an artery. Cerebral aneurysms are frequently multiple and occur at the points of **bifurcation** on the circle of Willis (Fig. 20–7). These "berry" aneurysms develop where there is

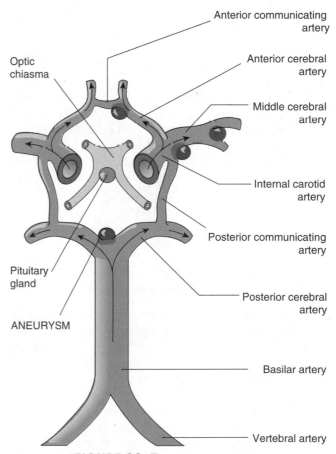

FIGURE 20–7. Cerebral aneurysm.

a weakness in the arterial wall at the bifurcation. The force of blood at this point leads to bulging in the wall, which is often aggravated by hypertension. Initially, the aneurysms are small and **asymptomatic**, but they tend to enlarge over the years until compression of the nearby structures, e.g., a cranial nerve, causes clinical signs or until rupture occurs. Rupture often results from a sudden increase in blood pressure associated with exertion, and bleeding occurs into the subarachnoid space (the location of the circle of Willis) and the CSF. This rupture may be a small leak or a massive tear. Blood is very irritating to the meninges and leads to an inflammatory response as well as irritation of the nerve roots passing through the meninges. Also, this free blood causes vasospasm in the cerebral arteries, further reducing perfusion and leading to additional ischemia. Hemorrhage from the ruptured vessel leads to increased ICP with its associated signs. No focal signs are present because the additional blood is dispersed through the system. Subarachnoid hemorrhages may be classified according to the clinical effects.

Thinkabout 20–10

a. Differentiate a TIA from a CVA with regard to the cause of each and the effects of each on function.

b. Describe the three causes of CVAs and the characteristic onset of signs with each.

c. Describe several factors that influence the degree of functional recovery that is attained following a CVA.

d. List common signs of an expanding aneurysm and of a bleeding aneurysm.

e. Why does a headache occur with a subarachnoid hemorrhage?

f. Explain why skin breakdown or ulcers may occur in a person who has had a stroke and list the common sites of these problems.

Signs and Symptoms

The enlarging aneurysm may cause pressure on the surrounding structures such as the optic chiasm or the cranial nerves, leading to loss of the visual fields (see Figs. 20–3 and 20–7) or other visual disturbances. The mass may also result in headache as tension increases on the blood vessel wall and meninges. A small leak is likely to cause headache, **photophobia** (increased sensitivity to light), and intermittent periods of dysfunction such as confusion, slurred speech, or weakness. **Nuchal rigidity,** or a stiff, extended neck, may develop because the escaped blood irritates the spinal nerve roots and causes muscle contractions in the neck. A massive rupture is manifested by an immediate severe "blinding" headache, vomiting, photophobia, and perhaps seizures or loss of consciousness. Death may occur shortly after rupture.

Treatment

An aneurysm that is diagnosed *before* rupture can be treated surgically as soon as possible by clipping or tying it off. In the interim, while the patient is waiting for surgery, it is important to prevent sudden increases in blood pressure. Surgical clipping of the aneurysm may also be done after rupture. Unfortunately, there is a substantial risk of rebleeding at the site of repair or from other aneurysms. Additional therapeutic measures focus on reducing the effects of increased ICP and cerebral vasospasm.

Infections

MENINGITIS

Pathophysiology

Meningitis is an infection of the meninges of the CNS. Because the membranes are continuous around the CNS and CSF flows in the subarachnoid space, infection spreads rapidly through the coverings of the brain (Fig. 20–8). Focal signs are absent because there is no localized infection. The inflammatory response to the infection leads to increased ICP, and the pia and arachnoid layers become edematous. The common bacterial infections lead to a purulent exudate that covers the surface of the brain and fills the sulci, causing the surface to appear flat. The exudate is present in the CSF, and the blood vessels on the surface of the brain appear dilated.

Etiology

Different age groups are susceptible to different organisms causing meningitis. In neonates, *Escherichia coli* is the most common causative organism; it is usually associated with a neural tube defect, premature rupture of the amniotic membranes, or a difficult delivery. In young children, meningitis results most frequently from bacterial infections due to *Haemophilus influenzae*, more often in the autumn or winter. *Neisseria meningitidis,* or *meningococcus,* the classic meningitis pathogen, is frequently carried in the nasopharynx of asymptomatic

TYPES OF HEMATOMAS AND THE MENINGES

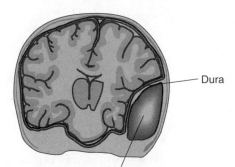

A. EXTRADURAL HEMATOMA
Blood fills space between dura and bone

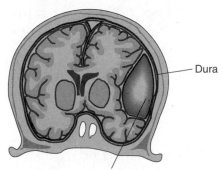

B. SUBDURAL HEMATOMA
Blood fills space beneath dura

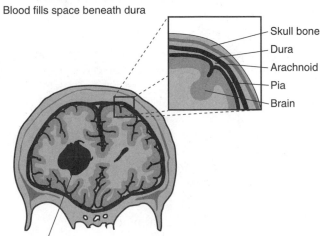

C. INTRACEREBRAL HEMATOMA

FIGURE 20–8. Types of hematomas.

carriers. Epidemics are common in schools or institutions where close contact between the children is likely to spread the organism. This type of meningitis occurs in children and young adults, more frequently in late winter and early spring. *Streptococcus pneumoniae* can cause meningitis in the elderly and in very young children. Meningitis may be secondary to other infections such as sinusitis or otitis, or it may result from an abscess located where the infection can spread through the bone to the meninges, for example, an abscessed tooth. Occasionally a virus such as mumps may lead to menin-

gitis. Any form of head trauma or surgery can result in meningitis from a variety of microorganisms.

Signs and Symptoms

Sudden onset of meningitis is common, with severe headache, back pain, photophobia, and nuchal rigidity (hyperextended stiff neck). These signs result from meningeal irritation. Two other clinical signs of meningeal irritation include *Kernig's sign* (resistance to leg extension when lying with the hip flexed) and *Brudzinski's sign* (neck flexion causes flexion of hip and knee). Vomiting, irritability, and lethargy progressing to **stupor** or seizures are common early indicators of increased ICP. Fever and chills with leukocytosis indicate infection. Meningococcal infections result in a **petechial** rash or extensive ecchymoses over the body. Different signs, including feeding problems, irritability, lethargy, a typical high-pitched cry, and bulging fontanelles, occur in the newborn.

Potential complications include hydrocephalus, if CSF flow is blocked by pus or adhesions, and cranial nerve damage. In some cases, damage to the cerebral cortex may occur, resulting in mental retardation, seizures, or motor impairment. In **fulminant** cases due to highly virulent organisms, disseminated intravascular coagulation develops with associated adrenal hemorrhage. These cases often result in vascular collapse or shock and death.

Diagnostic Tests

Examination of CSF, obtained by lumbar puncture, confirms the diagnosis. If meningitis is present, the CSF pressure will be elevated; it will appear cloudy and usually contains increased leukocytes. The causative organism in the CSF or blood must be identified to ensure adequate and effective treatment.

Treatment

Aggressive antimicrobial therapy is required as well as specific treatment measures for ICP and seizures as needed. With prompt diagnosis and treatment, the majority of patients survive. The mortality rate in neonatal meningitis is high, and there is some risk of permanent brain damage in very young children. Vaccines are available as a preventive measure for some types of meningococcal and *H. influenzae* meningitis, especially when outbreaks occur.

BRAIN ABSCESS

An abscess is a localized infection, frequently occurring in the frontal or temporal lobes. Onset tends to be insidious, with local and general signs of increased pressure developing in a manner similar to that seen in other disorders. A medical history may be helpful in making the diagnosis. Abscesses usually result from spread of organisms from the ear, throat, lung, or sinus infections, or directly from a site of injury or surgery. Common organisms are staphylococci, streptococci, and pneumococci. Often both surgical drainage and antimicrobial therapy are required.

ENCEPHALITIS

Encephalitis is considered an infection of the parenchymal or connective tissue in the brain and cord, particularly the basal ganglia. Occasionally chemicals may cause inflammation of the tissue. Necrosis and inflammation develop in the brain tissue, often resulting in some permanent damage. The signs are similar to those of meningitis. Encephalitis is usually of viral origin but may be related to other organisms. Western equine encephalitis is an arboviral infection spread by mosquitoes that occurs more frequently in the summer months. Early signs of infection include severe headache, lethargy, vomiting, and fever. Herpes simplex encephalitis occurs occasionally and is more dangerous, arising from spread of herpes simplex virus type 1 (HSV-1) from the trigeminal nerve ganglion. This virus causes extensive necrosis and hemorrhage in the brain, often involving the frontal and temporal lobes. Early treatment with an antiviral drug such as acyclovir may control the infection. Otherwise, treatment is supportive.

Thinkabout 20–11

a. List the significant signs of developing meningitis.

b. Describe the changes that occur in the CSF with meningitis.

c. Why does an abscess cause focal signs but meningitis does not?

Many other specific infections affect the nervous system, including rabies, poliomyelitis, tetanus, neurosyphilis, and herpes zoster (shingles).

INFECTION-RELATED SYNDROMES

Reye's Syndrome

Pathophysiology

The cause of Reye's syndrome has not yet been fully determined, but it appears to be linked to a viral infection in children such as influenza that is treated with aspirin (ASA). The number of cases has decreased since awareness of this potential danger has been heightened, and drugs such as acetaminophen have replaced aspirin in the treatment of fever associated with viral infections. The major pathologic changes occur in the brain and the liver. A noninflammatory cerebral edema develops, leading to increased ICP. The liver enlarges and shows fatty changes in the tissue and then progresses to acute liver failure. Jaundice is not present, but serum levels of liver enzymes are elevated. The resultant metabolic abnormalities include hypoglycemia, increased lactic acid, and elevated serum ammonia, which causes acute encephalopathy. Brain function is severely impaired by cerebral edema and the effects of high ammonia levels. In some cases, the kidneys are also affected by fatty degenerative changes, leading to increases in serum urea and creatinine.

Signs and Symptoms

Encephalopathy initially causes lethargy, headache, and vomiting, which are quickly followed by disorientation and hyperreflexia, hyperventilation, seizures, stupor, or coma.

Treatment

Treatment is supportive. The mortality rate is high if diagnosis and treatment are not initiated quickly.

Guillain-Barré Syndrome

Pathophysiology

Guillain-Barré syndrome is also known as postinfectious polyneuritis, acute idiopathic polyneuropathy, and acute infectious polyradiculoneuritis. The precise cause is unknown, but evidence indicates that an abnormal immune response, perhaps an autoimmune response, precipitated by a preceding viral infection or immunization, may be responsible. It is an inflammatory condition of the peripheral nervous system. Local inflammation with accumulated lymphocytes, demyelination, and axon destruction occur. These changes lead to impaired nerve conduction, particularly in the efferent (motor) fibers, although afferent (sensory) and autonomic fibers may also be involved. If the cell body remains alive through the acute period, the axon can regenerate. Initially, the inflammatory and degenerative process affects the peripheral nerves in the legs; then it ascends to involve the spinal nerves to the trunk and neck and frequently includes the cranial nerves as well. The critical period develops when the ascending paralysis involves the diaphragm and respiratory muscles. Recovery is usually spontaneous, with the manifestations diminishing in reverse descending order. That is, motor function is regained first in the upper body and then gradually improves in the trunk and the lower extremities.

Signs and Symptoms

Progressive muscle weakness and areflexia beginning in the legs leads to an ascending flaccid paralysis. This may be accompanied by paresthesia or pain and general muscle aching. As paralysis advances upward, vision and speech may be impaired. This process may occur rapidly over a few hours or several days. If swallowing and respiration are affected, a life-threatening situation develops. Many patients sustain autonomic system impairment, manifested as cardiac arrhythmias, **labile** blood pressure, or loss of sweating capability.

Treatment

Treatment is primarily supportive, and a ventilator is required in many cases. The use of immunoglobulin therapy or plasmapheresis, in which IgG immunoglobulin is separated and removed from the patient's blood, in the early stage may shorten the acute period of the disease in some patients and hasten recovery. Physiotherapy throughout the recovery period is essential to maximize functional restoration.

Head Injuries

Head injuries may involve skull fractures, hemorrhage, and edema or direct injury to brain tissue. An injury may be very mild, causing only bruising of the tissue, or it can be severe and life-threatening, causing destruction of brain tissue and massive swelling of the brain. The skull protects the brain but can also destroy it by means of bone fragments that penetrate or compress the brain tissue and by its inability to expand to relieve pressure.

TYPES OF HEAD INJURY

In *closed* head injuries the skull is not fractured in the injury, but trauma still occurs to the brain tissue, and blood vessels may be ruptured by the force exerted against the skull (Fig. 20–9). *Open* head injuries are those involving fractures or penetration of the brain by missiles or sharp objects. *Linear* fractures are simple cracks in the bone. *Comminuted* fractures result from several fracture lines and often are not complicated. *Compound* fractures involve trauma in which the brain tissue is exposed to the environment and is likely to be more severely damaged because bone fragments may penetrate the tissue and infection is more probable. *Depressed* skull fractures involve displacement of a piece of bone below the level of the skull, thereby compressing the brain tissue. With this type of fracture, the blood supply to the area is frequently impaired, and considerable pressure is exerted on the brain. *Basilar* fractures occur at the base of the skull.

Concussion is a reversible interference with brain function, usually resulting from a mild blow to the head. This causes sudden excessive movement of the brain, disrupting neurologic function and leading to loss of consciousness. **Amnesia** or memory loss and headaches may follow a concussion, but usually recovery occurs within 24 hours, and no permanent damage occurs. A *contusion* is a bruising of brain tissue with rupture of small blood vessels and edema. It usually results from a blunt blow to the head. There may or may not be residual damage, depending on the force of the blow and the degree of tissue injury.

PATHOPHYSIOLOGY

Primary brain injuries are direct injuries such as lacerations or crushing of the neurons, glial cells, and blood vessels of the brain. Secondary injuries result from the effects of cerebral edema, hemorrhage or hematoma, cerebral vasospasm, infection, and ischemia related to systemic factors. Primary injuries may involve a laceration or compression of brain tissue by a piece of bone or foreign object or perhaps rupture or compression of the cerebral blood vessels. Because the brain is not tightly held in place, the application of unusual force may rotate or shift it inside the skull. The brain tissue may be damaged by the rough inner surface of the skull or by the movement of the lobes of the brain against each other (shearing injury). In some cases, an area of the brain opposite the side of direct damage is injured as the brain bounces off the skull. This is a *contrecoup* injury, which may occur in acceleration or deceleration injuries in which the skull and brain hit a solid object. Such action causes the brain to rebound against the opposite side of the skull usually, causing minor damage. Any trauma to the brain tissue causes loss of function related to that specific area. Cell damage and bleeding then lead to inflammation and vasospasm around the site of the injury, creating increased pressure, further general ischemia, and further dysfunction.

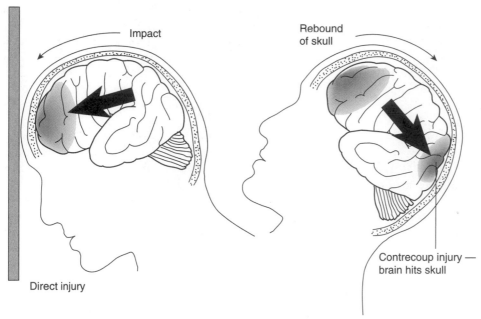

A. Closed Injury — Direct and Contrecoup Injury

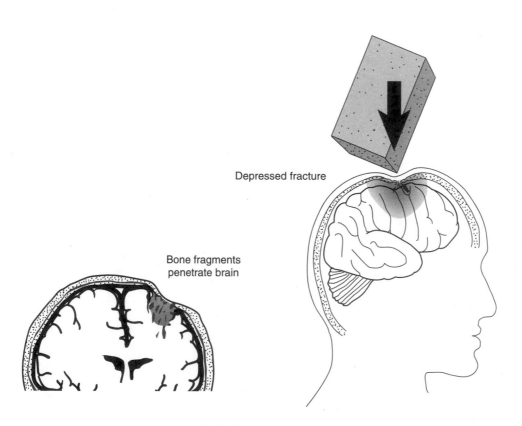

B. Open Injury

FIGURE 20–9. Types of head injury—closed and open.

A *hematoma* is a collection of blood in the tissue that develops from ruptured blood vessels either immediately after the injury or after some delay (see Fig. 20–8). It may also develop after surgery. *Epidural* (extradural) *hematoma* results from bleeding between the dura and the skull, usually from tearing of the middle meningeal artery in the temporal region. Signs of trouble usually arise within a few hours of injury when the person loses consciousness following a brief period of responsiveness. A *subdural hematoma* develops between the dura and the arachnoid. Frequently, there is a small tear in a vein, which causes blood to accumulate slowly. A hematoma may be acute (signs present in about 24 hours) or subacute (pressure develops over a week or so). A chronic subdural hematoma may occur in an elderly person, in whom brain atrophy allows more space for a hematoma to develop. Also, a tear in the arachnoid can allow leakage of CSF into the subdural space (hygroma), creating additional pressure. An _intracerebral hematoma_ resulting from contusions or shearing injuries may develop several days following injury. In all types of hematomas, the bleeding leads to local pressure on adjacent tissue and general increased ICP. When the blood accumulates slowly, the blood cells undergo hemolysis. The contents of this cell breakdown exert osmotic pressure, drawing more and more water into the area, increasing the size and pressure of the mass, and raising the ICP. Herniation may result from an untreated mass. Any bleeding in the brain may precipitate cerebral vasoconstriction (vasospasm), leading to further ischemia and more damage to the neurons.

Other factors that may cause secondary brain damage include infection, which is usually a high risk with open head injuries, and hypoxia related to systemic injury or shock. Respiratory or cardiovascular impairment may cause additional ischemia in the brain.

After the bleeding and inflammation subside, there may be some recovery of the neurons in the area surrounding the direct damage. The central area of damage undergoes necrosis and is replaced by scar tissue or a cyst.

ETIOLOGY

The majority of head injuries occur in young adults as a result of sports injuries and accidents involving cars or motorcycles. Many of these incidents are associated with excessive alcohol intake. A high blood alcohol level can impede neurologic assessment by masking the signs of injury. The effects of other systemic injuries such as a chest injury or shock can do the same thing. Alcohol, because of its dehydrating effects, tends to delay the onset of cerebral edema and ICP, but there may be a greater increase in ICP at a later time.

SIGNS AND SYMPTOMS

The person with a head injury manifests the appropriate focal signs and the general signs of increased ICP. Seizures frequently occur. Cranial nerve damage may be evident, particularly in those with basilar fractures. Other signs may include otorrhea and rhinorrhea (leakage of CSF from the ear and nose, respectively). This leakage occurs with fractures and with tearing of the meninges, allowing fluid to pass out of the subarachnoid space. Similarly, blood may leak through torn vessels and meninges (e.g., otorrhagia). This sign indicates the presence of a fracture

and a meningeal tear, which potentially allow microorganisms to enter the brain, causing meningitis or an abscess.

Individuals with head injuries may be examined and released from the hospital if no brain damage is apparent. It is usually suggested that the person's family or friends continue to perform a simplified head injury routine for the next day or so in case delayed hematoma formation occurs. This routine involves wakening the person periodically to check the level of consciousness, checking for reactive pupils, and watching for vomiting or any change in movement, sensation, or behavior. Headache, irritability, and fatigue are often present for a few days in persons with minor injuries.

If the individual is unconscious for a prolonged period of time other problems may develop. Immobility may cause complications such as pneumonia or decubitus ulcers (see Chapter 11). Fever may be a sign of hypothalamic impairment or of cranial or systemic infection. Stress ulcers may develop from increased gastric secretions.

TREATMENT

CT scans are useful in determining the extent of brain injury. Agents such as glucocorticoids, which decrease edema, and antibiotics, which reduce the risk of infection, are helpful. Surgery may be necessary to reduce ICP. Blood and oxygen may be administered to protect the remaining brain tissue. Treatment of any other injuries is important, particularly if those injuries interfere with respiration or circulation.

The prognosis for recovery from a head injury is more positive now with the use of improved surgical techniques, monitoring devices, and drug therapies. There may be residual damage in specific areas of the brain, resulting in motor or sensory deficits. Seizures, focal or generalized, are a common sequelae because of the increased irritability of tissue around the scar. Often, general fatigue, frequent headaches, and memory loss are present for some time following recovery.

Thinkabout 20–12

a. Differentiate an open head injury from a closed head injury.

b. Describe the location, common source, and time of development of a subdural hematoma.

c. Describe three significant signs of an injury to the right occipital lobe, including one specific focal sign and two general signs.

TABLE 20–9 Classification of Seizures

I. Partial seizures (focal)
   a. Simple
      1. Motor (includes Jacksonian)
      2. Sensory (visual, auditory, etc.)
      3. Autonomic
      4. Psychic
   b. Complex (impaired consciousness)
      1. Temporal lobe or psychomotor
   c. Partial leading to generalized seizures
II. Generalized (both hemispheres affected with loss of consciousness)
   a. Tonic-clonic (grand mal)
   b. Absence (petit mal)
   c. Myoclonic
   d. Infantile spasms
   e. Atonic (akinetic)
   f. Lennox-Gestaut syndrome (febrile seizures)
III. Unclassified

Seizure Disorders

Seizures result from uncontrolled, excessive discharge of neurons in the brain. The activity may be localized or generalized. Seizure disorders are characterized by recurrent seizures, sometimes called convulsions. Epilepsy is the old term for recurrent seizures. Seizure disorders are classified by their location in the brain and their clinical features, including EEG patterns during and between seizures. The international classification of seizures is summarized in Table 20–9. This is a commonly accepted classification incorporating newer terminology and dividing seizures into two basic categories, generalized and partial.

Generalized seizures have foci or origins in the deep structures of both cerebral hemispheres and the brainstem and cause loss of consciousness, whereas *partial* seizures have a single or focal origin, often in the cerebral cortex, and may or may not involve altered consciousness. However, partial seizures may progress into generalized seizures. Seizures may be primary (idiopathic) or secondary (acquired) with an identified cause, such as post-traumatic syndrome. Seizures can be categorized on other grounds because they may result from an abnormality in the brain or from systemic causes such as hypoglycemia or withdrawal from certain drugs. They may be a temporary problem, as with febrile seizures in an infant, or they may be chronic and occur frequently. An individual can have more than one type of seizure. For example, absence seizures, which are common in children, may decrease or be replaced by tonic-clonic or psychomotor seizures. Common types of seizures are described later under Signs and Symptoms.

PATHOPHYSIOLOGY

A seizure results from a sudden uncontrolled discharge of neurons, which causes abnormal motor or sensory activity and possibly loss of consciousness. The neurons in the epileptogenic focus are hyperexcitable and have a lowered threshold for stimulation. Any physiologic change such as alkalosis or other sensory stimulus such as flashing lights can easily activate the "irritable" neurons, and in turn these focal cells stimulate the surrounding normal cells, spreading the activity. Each seizure lasts for a few seconds or minutes, and the excessive activity of the neurons then ceases spontaneously. The altered pattern of electrical activity or brain waves during a seizure can be demonstrated on an EEG, indicating the type of seizure and its focus (Fig. 20–10). Also, observation of the seizure by bystanders, particularly its initial effects, is useful in identifying the origin or focus of the seizure.

A. FOCAL SEIZURE, LEFT FRONTAL LOBE

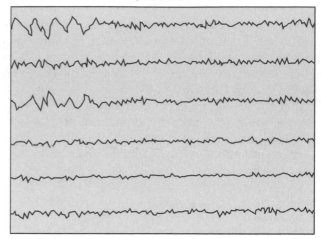

B. GENERALIZED TONIC-CLONIC SEIZURE

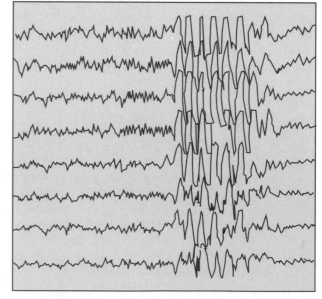

FIGURE 20–10. Electroencephalogram and seizures.

Complications may arise from generalized (grand mal) tonic-clonic seizures if they are severe and frequent. Injuries may occur during a seizure. Recurrent or continuous seizures without recovery of consciousness are termed *status epilepticus*. This condition may lead to serious consequences if it is not treated promptly. Respiration is impaired during a generalized tonic-clonic seizure, and skeletal muscle activity is intense, and the combination of these events in status epilepticus can lead to severe hypoxia, hypoglycemia, and acidosis, possibly resulting in brain damage.

ETIOLOGY

Many seizure disorders are idiopathic and are commonly referred to as epilepsy when they are recurrent. Children often have absence seizures starting around the age of 5. Children with congenital disorders such as cerebral palsy may have seizures as part of the disability. Acquired seizures following head injury or infection are more common now because improved treatment of these primary conditions has led to a higher survival rate. A seizure may be initiated by a tumor or hemorrhage in the brain or by a high fever in an infant or young child. Some systemic disorders such as renal failure or hypoglycemia may precipitate a seizure in an individual who has no prior history of seizures. Drugs such as cocaine or the effects of withdrawal from alcohol can precipitate seizures.

Precipitating factors or triggers of an individual seizure may include physical stimuli such as loud noises or bright lights or biochemical stimuli such as stress, excessive fluid retention (premenstrual), hypoglycemia, or hyperventilation (alkalosis). Awareness and avoidance of the potential precipitating factors in an individual can reduce the frequency of seizures.

SIGNS AND SYMPTOMS
Absence (Petit Mal) Seizures

Absence seizures are generalized seizures that are more common in children beginning about the age of 5 years. The seizure lasts for 5 to 10 seconds and may occur many times during the day. There is a brief loss of consciousness and sometimes transient facial movements, such as twitches of the eyelids or lip smacking. Usually the child simply stares into space for a moment and then resumes the activity previously pursued. No memory of the episode is retained.

Tonic-Clonic (Grand Mal) Seizures

Tonic-clonic seizures are generalized seizures that may occur spontaneously or following simple seizures. Some individuals have prodromal signs such as nausea or muscle twitching prior to the seizure. Frequently an aura, such as a peculiar visual or auditory sensation, precedes the loss of consciousness. With loss of consciousness, the individual falls to the floor, and the body is affected by a strong **tonic** muscle contraction, resulting in a rigid body with extended limbs. A cry escapes as the abdominal and thoracic muscles contract, forcing air out of the lungs. The jaws are clenched tightly, and respiration ceases during this period. The tonic stage is followed by the **clonic** stage, in which the muscles alternately contract and relax, resulting in a series of forceful jerky movements involving the entire body. Also, there may be increased salivation (foaming at the mouth) and frequently bowel and bladder incontinence. The contractions gradually subside, and consciousness returns. Usually the person is confused and fatigued; the muscles ache, and he falls into a deep sleep in this postictal period. The aura may be remembered but not the entire seizure (amnesia). Hypoxia is common at this time because of interference with respiration during the seizure and because some airway obstruction may be present owing to excess saliva or tongue position. Also, the contracting muscles have presented an increased demand for oxygen during the seizure. The increased levels of lactic acid and carbon dioxide contribute to acidosis. Recurrent tonic-clonic seizures without full return to consciousness are termed status epilepticus, as mentioned earlier and carry an increased risk of complications.

Simple Partial or Focal Seizures

Focal seizures arise from an epileptogenic focus, often related to an area of damage in the cortex. They are manifested by repeated motor activity such as turning the head or eye away from the focus, or by a sensation such as tingling that begins in one area and may spread. Auditory or visual experiences such as ringing in the ears or a sensation of light may occur if the focus is in the appropriate area. Memory and consciousness remain. A *jacksonian seizure* is a focal motor seizure in which the clonic contractions begin in a specific area and spread progressively, that is, "march" up the arm and then to the face.

Complex Partial, Temporal Lobe, or Psychomotor Seizures

Children and adults may have complex partial seizures. They usually arise from the temporal lobe but may involve the limbic system or frontal lobe. Sometimes an aura is present, such as the perception of an odd odor. The seizure itself consists of bizarre behavior, perhaps repetitive and purposeful but inappropriate—for example, waving or clapping the hands. Frequently, visual or auditory hallucinations or feelings of déjà vu (perceiving strange surroundings as familiar) occur. The person is unresponsive to people or activities during the seizure, and afterward he or she is amnesic and drowsy.

TREATMENT

Any primary cause should be treated, and factors that precipitate seizures in an individual should be determined and avoided. Anticonvulsant drugs such as phenytoin (Dilantin) are prescribed to raise the threshold for neuronal stimulation and prevent seizures. In many cases, anticonvulsant drugs are combined with sedatives such as phenobarbital to allow a reduction in the dosage and side effects of the drugs while simultaneously decreasing the occurrence of seizures. Phenytoin may cause gingival hyperplasia, which can create difficulty in maintaining good oral hygiene as well as creating a cosmetic problem for the patient. Many anticonvulsant drugs reduce leukocyte counts, thus predisposing the patient to infection. Different types of seizures require different medications, and it may be necessary to try several drugs to find the one that offers optimum control. It is essential to continue medication as prescribed at set intervals and without omissions because sudden withdrawal can cause more severe seizures or status epilepticus with its risk of brain damage.

Once a seizure begins, it cannot be stopped. When tonic-clonic seizures occur, it is important to prevent injury to the person without forcibly restraining him or her. Force can lead to injury because the muscle contractions and movements are strong. Similarly, one should not attempt to place an object between the lips. If possible, the person should be placed on the floor on his or her side to prevent falls and to prevent the tongue from falling back, obstructing the airway. Single episodes require no additional medical treatment. Prolonged or recurrent seizures are life-threatening and require hospital treatment with medications such as intravenous diazepam, oxygen, and fluids.

Thinkabout 20–13

a. Describe how a seizure develops in the brain tissue.
b. Differentiate a partial seizure from a general seizure and give an example of each.
c. Describe factors that should be avoided if you have a patient with a history of seizures.
d. List the sequence of events in a generalized tonic-clonic seizure.

CONGENITAL AND GENETIC NEUROLOGIC DISORDERS

Hydrocephalus

PATHOPHYSIOLOGY

Hydrocephalus is a condition in which excess CSF accumulates, compressing the brain tissue and blood vessels. The condition is sometimes called "water on the brain." The infant's head enlarges beyond the normal size as the amount of fluid increases. Excess CSF occurs because more is produced than is absorbed. There are two types of hydrocephalus. The first, *noncommunicating* or *obstructive hydrocephalus,* occurs in babies when the flow of CSF through the ventricular system is blocked, usually at the aqueduct of Sylvius or the foramen magnum (Fig. 20–11). This condition usually results from a fetal developmental abnormality such as **stenosis** or a neural tube defect. In many neonates an associated myelomeningocele or Arnold-Chiari malformation is present. Most cases are apparent shortly after birth, but some may not be diagnosed until later in childhood. The obstruction leads to increased back pressure of fluid in the ventricles of the brain, which gradually dilates or enlarges the ventricles and compresses the blood vessels and brain tissue. In the second type, *communicating hydrocephalus,* the absorption of CSF through the subarachnoid villi is impaired, resulting in increased pressure of CSF in the system. In neonates, the skull can expand to some degree in the early stages of hydrocephalus to relieve the pressure, but if it is not treated quickly, the brain tissue will be permanently damaged. In older children and adults, ICP can increase more rapidly than in neonates when CSF flow is blocked because the sutures of the skull are fused. The amount of brain damage that results depends on the rate at which pressure increases and the time that elapses before relief occurs. Other factors may also be present in a particular patient that increase the risk of damage. Brain damage may result in major physical disability as well as intellectual impairment because all areas of the brain are affected.

ETIOLOGY

As mentioned earlier, congenital abnormalities are the most frequent cause of hydrocephalus, due to stenosis or **atresia** at the connecting channels between the ventricles or a thickened arachnoid membrane. Obstruction may also develop at any age from tumors, infection, or scar tissue. Meningitis can also cause obstructive hydrocephalus during the acute infection or lead to fibrosis in the meninges, impairing absorption.

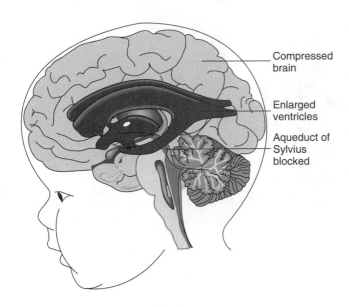

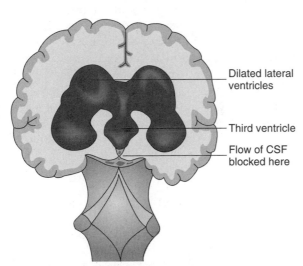

FIGURE 20–11. Hydrocephalus.

SIGNS AND SYMPTOMS

The signs of increasing CSF depend on the age of the patient. In the *neonate* or very young *infants,* in whom the sutures have not yet closed, the head can enlarge and the fontanels bulge in the early stages of hydrocephalus. Recording head size is a standard procedure following birth. With current brief hospitalization periods, this measurement may not be followed up, but it can provide a basic reference point if a problem is suspected. Scalp veins appear dilated, and the eyes show the "sunset sign," in which the white sclera is visible above the colored pupil. Pupil response to light is sluggish. The infant is lethargic but irritable and difficult to feed. A high-pitched or shrill cry often occurs when the infant is moved or picked up. It is important to diagnose and treat such a child as soon as possible to minimize brain damage.

In older children and adults the head cannot enlarge, and the signs of increased ICP develop as the volume of CSF expands. Depending on the underlying cause, other manifestations may be present.

TREATMENT

Surgery is usually performed to remove an obstruction or provide a shunt for CSF from the ventricle into the peritoneum or other extracranial site. Shunts are subject to blockage or infection and thus require continued close monitoring to prevent further brain damage.

Thinkabout 20–14

a. Differentiate between communicating and non-communicating hydrocephalus.
b. Explain the effects of ventricular dilation.
c. Explain why there are no focal signs of hydrocephalus in neonates.

Spina Bifida

PATHOPHYSIOLOGY

Spina bifida refers to a group of neural tube defects, which are congenital anomalies of varying severity. The neural tube develops during the fourth week of gestation, beginning in the cervical area and progressing toward the lumbar area. The basic problem is failure of the posterior spinous processes on the vertebrae to fuse, which may permit the meninges and spinal cord to herniate, resulting in neurologic impairment. Any number of vertebrae can be involved, and the lumbar area is the most common location. There are three common types (Fig. 20–12). The first, *spina bifida occulta*, develops when the spinous processes do not fuse, but herniation of the spinal cord and meninges does not occur. The defect may not be visible, although often a dimple or a tuft of hair is present on the skin over the site. The defect may be diagnosed on routine x-ray examination or when mild neurologic signs become manifest during tension on the cord during a growth period. The second type, *meningocele*, refers to the same bony defect, but herniation of the meninges occurs out through the defect, and the meninges and CSF form a sac on the surface. **Transillumination** confirms the absence of nerve tissue in the sac. Neurologic impairment is usually not present, although infection or rupture of

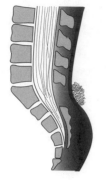

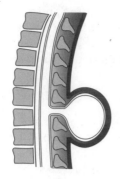

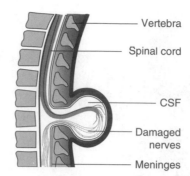

A. Spina bifida occulta   **B.** Meningocele   **C.** Myelomeningocele

FIGURE 20-12. Spina bifida.

the sac may lead to further neurologic damage. *Myelomeningocele* is the most serious form of spina bifida. With this defect, herniation of the spinal cord and nerves along with the meninges and CSF occurs, resulting in considerable neurologic impairment. The location and extent of the herniation determine how much function is lost. This defect is often associated with hydrocephalus.

DIAGNOSTIC TESTS

The presence of spina bifida can be diagnosed prenatally by ultrasound. **Amniocentesis**, in which the presence of alpha-fetoprotein (AFP) that has leaked into the amniotic fluid surrounding the fetus can be demonstrated, may indicate spina bifida. AFP may also be found in the maternal blood.

ETIOLOGY

Spina bifida appears to have a multifactorial basis, with a combination of genetic and environmental factors contributing to its development. There is a high familial incidence of spina bifida as well as associated defects such as **anencephaly** (absence of the cerebral hemispheres). Environmental factors include exposure to radiation, gestational diabetes, and deficits of vitamin A or folic acid. At present, it is recommended that folic acid supplements be taken before conception and for the first 6 weeks of pregnancy as a preventive measure.

SIGNS AND SYMPTOMS

Meningocele and myelomeningocele are visible as a protruding sac over the spine. In myelomeningocele, the extent of the neurologic deficit depends on the level of the defect (see Fig. 20–16); sensory and motor function at and below the level of the herniation are impaired. Some degree of muscle weakness or paralysis is present. Bladder and bowel control are usually impaired. Depending on the level of damage and the

availability of reflex and sphincter control, there may be fecal and urinary incontinence.

TREATMENT

Controversy continues about the timing of the surgical repair of the sac—whether it should take place immediately or be delayed. Rupture and infection are potential complications. The decision also depends on the presence of other **anomalies** that may be present in the infant. Following repair, ongoing assistance and therapy are required to manage the neurologic deficits. Community services as well as the Spina Bifida Association, which has many local chapters, provide continuing support for the parents and the child.

Cerebral Palsy

PATHOPHYSIOLOGY

Cerebral palsy (CP) is a group of disorders marked by some degree of motor impairment resulting from brain damage in the perinatal period. The clinical presentation is highly variable and depends on the specific areas in the brain where trauma has occurred. The damage may occur before, during, or shortly after birth and is nonprogressive. Although all children have altered mobility, which provides the basis for classifying cerebral palsy, an assortment of other problems is often present in any individual. Pathologically, the brain tissue is affected by malformation, mechanical trauma, hypoxia, hemorrhage, hypoglycemia, hyperbilirubinemia, or some other factor, resulting in necrosis of brain tissue. In some cases, generalized necrosis and atrophy of brain tissue have occurred, whereas in other cases only one or two localized areas of the brain are affected.

ETIOLOGY

Single or multiple factors may be implicated in the development of cerebral palsy. Hypoxia or ischemia is the major cause of brain damage; it may occur prenatally, perinatally, or postnatally. It may be associated with placental complications or a difficult delivery or with vascular occlusion, hemorrhage, aspiration, or respiratory impairment in the premature infant. High bilirubin levels due to problems such as prematurity or Rh blood incompatibility may cause *kernicterus*, in which accumulated bilirubin crosses the blood-brain barrier and damages the neurons. Other causes of cerebral palsy include infection or metabolic abnormalities such as hypoglycemia in either the mother or the child.

SIGNS AND SYMPTOMS

Cerebral palsy is classified on the basis of the motor disability that results (Table 20–10). There are three major groups. The first and largest group includes those with *spastic paralysis*, which results from damage to the pyramidal tracts (diplegia) or the motor cortex (hemiparesis) or from general cortical damage (quadriparesis). The second group is *dyskinetic* disease, which results from damage to the extrapyramidal tract, basal nuclei, or cranial nerves. This form of cerebral palsy is manifest by **athetoid** or **choreiform** *type* movements and loss of coordination with fine movements. The third group, *ataxic* cerebral palsy, commonly develops from damage to the cerebellum. In some cases the effects are evident at birth, whereas in others the delay in motor development or abnormal muscle tone does not become apparent for several months. Persistence of early reflexes, such as the Moro reflex, may indicate cerebral palsy.

Spasticity is manifested by increased muscle tone or resistance to passive movement with excessive reflex responses. Unilateral use of the hands or feet and asymmetric body movements are indications of abnormality. Writhing movements or facial grimaces may indicate athetoid cerebral palsy. Feeding difficulties and constant tongue thrusting are signs of motor dysfunction and may interfere with nutrition and growth. The position of the child's limbs when resting or when held up is often unusual (e.g., scissors position of the legs).

Many associated problems in addition to the motor deficit may be present, which depend on the other areas of brain damage. Intellectual function may be impaired. Generally, one-third of those with cerebral palsy are considered to have normal intelligence, one-third are mildly impaired, and one-third are more severely disabled. Communication and speech development is very difficult because of motor disability, possible impaired mentation, and visual or hearing deficits. A number of children have learning disabilities and behavioral problems such as attention deficit, spatial disorientation, and hyperactivity. Seizures, primarily of the generalized tonic-clonic type, are common. Visual problems such as astigmatism and strabismus occur frequently.

TREATMENT

Early stimulation programs are helpful in encouraging motor skills, coordination, and intellectual development. Assessment and therapy by speech and language pathologists can help the parents deal with feeding and swallowing problems, positioning the child correctly, reducing the effects of tongue-thrusting, and encouraging communication. Specialists in early education for developmentally handicapped children can work with the child and the family to develop and maximize motor skills, eye-hand coordination, and reflex responses. As the child develops, simple exercises can be instituted to help him learn to recognize familiar objects or sounds, to associate cause with effect, and to identify likes and dislikes. Hearing and vision require monitoring in the early stages, and some form of communication must be developed as soon as possible. Many new devices and techniques are now available to promote communication. Family members can be trained to provide effective and efficient care for the child, and physiotherapy can reduce the incidence of complications. Exercise therapy and devices such as braces can improve mobility and reduce deformities. Appropriate medication to control seizures prevents complications. Technologic advances including computers provide aids for many different problems and enable many individuals to live more independently as well as to develop individual interests and skills. In many areas, children with cerebral palsy are being integrated into mainstream classes in schools and into other activities as well.

TABLE 20–10 Cerebral Palsy			
Type	**Percent Cases**	**Area of Damage**	**Effects**
Spastic	65%–75%	Motor cortex or pyramidal tracts	Paralysis Hyperreflexia and increased muscle tone
Dyskinetic	20%–25%	Basal nuclei or extrapyramidal tracts	Loss of motor control and coordination Athetoid or choreiform movements
Ataxic	5%	Cerebellum	Gait disturbance Loss of balance
Mixed	13%	All of above	Some of each of above

Thinkabout 20–15

a. Compare Down's syndrome (see Chapter 7) and cerebral palsy with regard to cause and effects on motor and cognitive abilities.

b. Describe the factors that could interfere with communication in a child with cerebral palsy.

CHRONIC DEGENERATIVE DISORDERS

Multiple Sclerosis

PATHOPHYSIOLOGY

Multiple sclerosis (MS) involves a progressive demyelination of the neurons of the brain, spinal cord, and cranial nerves. It affects all types of nerve fibers—motor, sensory, and autonomic—and occurs in diffuse patches throughout the system (Fig. 20–13). Intellectual functions are not usually affected. Multiple sclerosis is

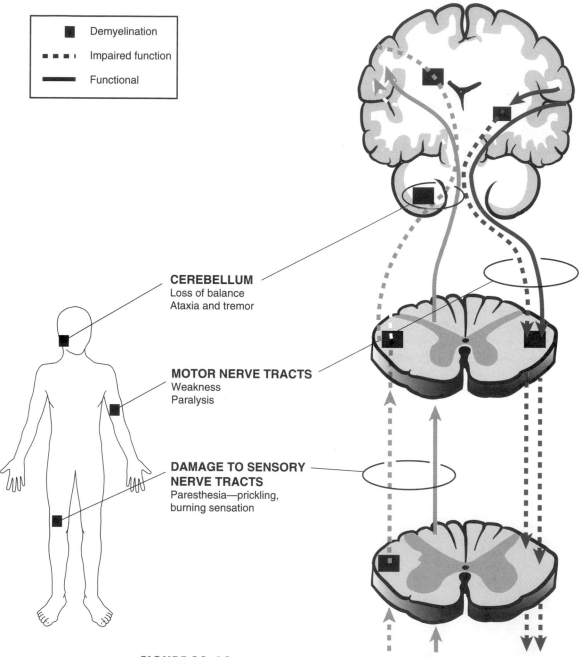

- ◼ Demyelination
- ▪▪▪▪ Impaired function
- ——— Functional

CEREBELLUM
Loss of balance
Ataxia and tremor

MOTOR NERVE TRACTS
Weakness
Paralysis

DAMAGE TO SENSORY NERVE TRACTS
Paresthesia—prickling, burning sensation

FIGURE 20–13. Multiple sclerosis—distribution of lesions.

characterized by remissions and exacerbations. The earliest lesion occurs as an inflammatory response and loss of myelin around the venules in the white matter of the brain or spinal cord. Later, larger areas of inflammation and demyelination, termed plaques, become visible, primarily in the white matter. Loss of myelin interferes with the conduction of impulses in the affected fibers. Initially, the area of plaque appears pinkish and edematous, but then it becomes gray and scarred. Each plaque varies in size, and several may coalesce into a single patch. The initial inflammation may subside, and neural function may return to normal for a short time until another exacerbation occurs. In time, neural degeneration becomes irreversible, and function is lost permanently. With each recurrence, additional areas of the CNS are involved. Multiple sclerosis varies in severity, occurring in mild and slowly progressive patterns in some individuals and in rapidly progressive forms in others.

ETIOLOGY

The onset of symptoms usually occurs in individuals between 20 and 40 years of age, and the disease is more common in females. The cause is unknown. Multiple sclerosis appears to have both genetic and environmental components and is perhaps an immunologic disorder with a familial tendency. It occurs more frequently in people of European descent, and there is an increased risk for close relatives of affected individuals. The environmental factors have not yet been determined, although it is thought that climate may play a role in that the disease is more common in temperate zones and in individuals who grow up in temperate climates. Viral infection and an abnormal immune response have also been suspected.

SIGNS AND SYMPTOMS

The manifestations are determined by the areas of demyelination that occur in each individual. Initially, weakness in the legs often occurs, related to plaques on the corticospinal tract. If the cranial nerves are affected, **diplopia** (double vision), **scotoma** (a spot in the visual field), or dysarthria (poor articulation) may occur. Areas of numbness, burning, or tingling develop if the sensory nerve fibers are damaged. As the number of plaques increases with each exacerbation, progressive weakness and paralysis extending to the upper limbs, loss of coordination, and bladder and bowel dysfunction occur. Sensory deficits include paresthesias as well as loss of position sense involving the upper body and face as well as the legs. The clinical picture and mode of progression vary greatly among individuals. Later in the course of the disease, depression or euphoria may develop. Complications related to immobility such as respiratory infection, decubitus ulcers, and contractures are common as the disease progresses.

DIAGNOSTIC TESTS

There is no definitive test for multiple sclerosis, and a long delay may precede the diagnosis. The multiplicity of effects based on the history and examination point to the correct diagnosis. MRI studies may detect CNS lesions. Many patients have elevated IgG levels in the CSF.

TREATMENT

No specific treatment is available at this time, although new measures are being investigated. Interferon-beta appears to reduce the frequency and severity of exacerbations in some patients through its effects on the immune system. The number of exacerbations can be reduced by avoiding excessive fatigue and stress, injury, or infection. Glucocorticoids may help to control acute signs during exacerbation. Therapy and exercise to maintain mobility are considered important. Achieving a balance between rest and activity is important. Special problems such as constipation or incontinence require individual attention. It is important to maintain communication and interest by addressing issues such as visual impairment or speech disorders early in the course of the disease. Intervention by a speech and language pathologist early in the course of the disease can maximize communication and assist with some feeding problems.

Thinkabout 20–16

a. Relate the following early signs of multiple sclerosis to the location of plaques: diplopia, tremors in the legs, facial weakness.

b. Relate the frequency of exacerbations to the progress of the disease.

Parkinson's Disease (Paralysis Agitans)

PATHOPHYSIOLOGY

In Parkinson's disease dysfunction of the extrapyramidal motor system occurs because of progressive degenerative changes in the basal nuclei, principally in the substantia nigra. In this condition a decreased number of neurons in the substantia nigra secrete dopamine, an inhibitory neurotransmitter, leading to an imbalance between excitation and inhibition in the basal nuclei. The excess stimulation affects movement and posture by increasing muscle tone and activity, leading to resting tremors, muscular rigidity, difficulty in initiating movement, and postural instability. Also, many patients with Parkinson's disease have a reduced number of cortical neurons, which is associated with dementia. Diagnosis depends on the physical manifestations because no specific diagnostic test is available at this time.

ETIOLOGY

Primary or idiopathic Parkinson's disease usually develops after age 60 and occurs in both males and females. Inheritance is not a factor in its development, and the current focus of investigation is on the possible damaging effects of viruses or toxins on cells. Secondary parkinsonism may follow encephalitis, trauma, or vascular disease. Drug-induced Parkinson's disease is linked particularly to use of the phenothiazine class of drugs (e.g., chlorpromazine). In these cases, the effects may be reversible or diminished when the drug is discontinued.

SIGNS AND SYMPTOMS

Early signs include fatigue, weakness and muscle aching, decreased flexibility, and less spontaneous change in facial expression. A more obvious sign is tremors in the hands at rest. As the disease advances, further motor impairment, increased muscle rigidity, difficulty in initiating movement (bradykinesia), and a lack of associated movements occur. Associated movements might include loss of arm-swinging when walking or spontaneous postural adjustments when sitting. The face of the patient resembles a mask, and blinking of the eyelids is reduced, resulting in a blank staring face. The characteristic standing posture is stooped, leaning forward with the head and neck flexed (Fig. 20–14). Festination, or a propulsive gait (short, shuffling steps with increasing acceleration) occurs as the person's postural reflexes are impaired, leading to falls. As orthostatic hypotension develops, the threat of falls increases.

Other functions are affected as the voice becomes low and devoid of inflection (the person speaks in a monotone), and dysarthria develops. Chewing and swallowing become difficult, prolonging eating times and causing recurrent drooling. Autonomic dysfunction is manifested in the later stages by urinary retention, constipation, and orthostatic hypotension. Uri-

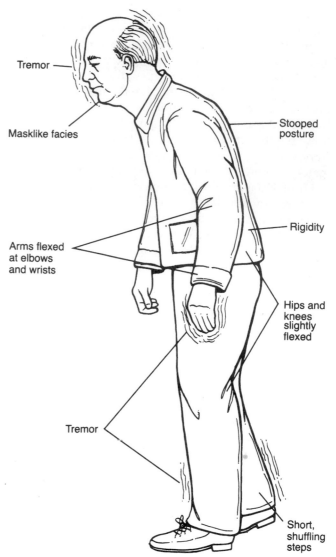

FIGURE 20–14. Parkinson's disease. (From Monahan FD, Drake T, Neighbors M: Nursing Care of Adults. Philadelphia, W.B. Saunders, 1994.)

nary tract and respiratory infections are common complications.

TREATMENT

Dopamine replacement therapy has been used to reduce the motor impairment. Levodopa (L-Dopa), a **precursor**, is administered because dopamine itself does not cross the blood-brain barrier. Several drugs under investigation now show promise. The swallowing and speech impairments need early attention from a speech and language pathologist to maintain function as long as possible. Physiotherapy is helpful in maintaining general mobility. Constant monitoring and immediate treatment of respiratory and urinary tract infections can reduce the risk of damage to the organs involved.

Thinkabout 20–17

a. Describe the pathophysiology of Parkinson's disease.

b. Describe three common manifestations that can be observed in a person with Parkinson's disease.

c. List several reasons why adequate nutrition and hydration may be difficult to maintain in a person with Parkinson's disease.

d. If adequate nutrition and hydration are not maintained, what potential complications may ensue?

Amyotrophic Lateral Sclerosis (Lou Gehrig's Disease)

The name of the disease is indicative of the pathology, amyotrophic meaning muscle wasting and sclerosis referring to the degenerative "hardening" of the lateral corticospinal tracts. The cause has not been identified, although a gene related to the familial form of the disease (which occurs in about 10 percent of cases) has been located. The disease affects primarily individuals between 40 and 60 years of age, particularly males. Although the disease is not a common one, it has attracted public attention because there is no means of preventing the continuous and rapid decline of motor function while cognitive function remains intact. Also, amyotrophic lateral sclerosis (ALS) has been the focus of consideration by the public and legislative and medical groups of ethical issues related to euthanasia for patients with such diseases.

PATHOPHYSIOLOGY

Amyotrophic lateral sclerosis is a progressive degenerative disease affecting both upper motor neurons in the cerebral cortex and lower motor neurons in the brainstem and spinal cord. The loss of upper motor neurons leads to spastic paralysis and hyperreflexia, whereas damage to lower motor neurons results in flaccid paralysis, with decreased muscle tone and reflexes. Sensory neurons, cognitive function, and cranial nerves III, IV, and VI to the eye muscles are not affected. There is no indication of inflammation around the nerves. The loss of neurons occurs in a diffuse and asymmetrical pattern but proceeds without remission. Although no specific test is available to confirm the presence of the disease, many tests are required to eliminate other possible diagnoses.

SIGNS AND SYMPTOMS

Initially, in most cases the upper extremities manifest weakness and muscle atrophy, with loss of fine motor coordination commencing with the distal fibers. Stumbling and falls are common. Muscle cramps or twitching may result from an imbalance of antagonistic muscles. The weakness and paralysis progress throughout the body. Dysarthria develops as the cranial nerves controlling speech are lost. Eventually, swallowing and respiration are impaired, and a ventilator is required.

TREATMENT

At this time, no specific treatment is available to slow the degenerative process. A well-balanced program of moderate exercise and rest is helpful. It is advisable to use electronic communication devices relatively early in the course of the disease. A team approach to care can minimize the complications of immobility and sustain function as long as possible and can also support the family. The team may include a respiratory therapist, nutritionist, speech pathologist, physiotherapist, psychologist, social worker, and others.

Myasthenia Gravis

PATHOPHYSIOLOGY

Myasthenia gravis is an autoimmune disorder that impairs the receptors for acetylcholine (ACh) at the myoneural (neuromuscular) junction. The specific cause is not known, although many patients have thymus disorders such as benign tumors. Women are more frequently affected than men, and the age of onset is between 20 and 30 years. In myasthenia gravis, IgG autoantibodies to ACh receptors form, blocking and ultimately destroying the receptor site, thus preventing any further stimulation of the muscle. This change leads to skeletal muscle weakness and rapid fatigue of the affected muscles. The facial and ocular muscles are usually affected initially, followed by the arm and trunk muscles.

DIAGNOSTIC TESTS

Several tests are available, including electromyography and an assay of serum antibodies. The Tensilon test uses edrophonium chloride, a short-acting anticholinesterase inhibitor, to prolong the action of ACh at the myoneural junction, resulting in a short period of increased skeletal muscle function.

SIGNS AND SYMPTOMS

Muscle weakness is noticeable in the face and eyes, and fatigue develops quickly when the muscles are being used. Diplopia and ptosis impair vision, and speech becomes a monotone with a nasal tone. Spontaneous facial expressions are lost, and the face appears to droop sadly. Attempts to smile may appear more like a snarl. Chewing and swallowing become difficult as the weakness progresses and the risk of aspiration increases. The head droops as the neck muscles become involved. As the arms become weaker, it is difficult for the person to comb hair, brush the teeth, or prepare and eat food. Muscle fatigue becomes more marked as the day progresses.

Upper respiratory infections occur more frequently and tend to be prolonged because it becomes more difficult to remove secretions. *Myasthenic crisis* may occur in the presence of additional stress such as infection, trauma, or alcohol intake. This state involves an increase in weakness and fatigue, and respiratory impairment may develop.

TREATMENT

Anticholinesterase agents such as pyridostigmine or neostigmine may be used to temporarily improve neuromuscular transmission. These agents prolong the action of ACh at the neuromuscular junction and facilitate activities such as eating. Glucocorticoids such as prednisone are effective in suppressing the immune system.

Thinkabout 20–18

a. Explain why a person with myasthenia gravis might prefer a soft diet. List several potential complications of a continued soft diet.

b. Describe how oral hygiene might be affected by myasthenia gravis.

c. Compare the pathophysiology, significant early signs or symptoms, and course of amyotrophic lateral sclerosis, myasthenia gravis, multiple sclerosis, and Guillain-Barré syndrome.

Huntington's Disease

PATHOPHYSIOLOGY

Huntington's disease or chorea is an inherited disorder that does not become manifest until midlife. Maternal inheritance delays onset later than inheritance from fathers. Progressive atrophy of the brain occurs, with degeneration of neurons, particularly in the basal ganglia and the frontal cortex. There is depletion of GABA, an inhibitory neurotransmitter in the basal nuclei and substantia nigra. Levels of ACh in the brain also appear to be reduced.

ETIOLOGY

This condition is inherited as an autosomal dominant trait (there is an approximately 50% probability of having an affected child) and is carried on chromosome 4. Until recently, there were no diagnostic tests available to identify affected individuals prior to onset of symptoms, and therefore children with a high risk of inheritance were born to affected individuals before the disease was diagnosed. This combination of factors has increased the incidence of the disorder through the years.

SIGNS AND SYMPTOMS

At the onset, restlessness and choreiform (rapid, jerky) movements in the arms and face are common. There may also be early indications of intellectual impairment such as loss of problem-solving skills, poor judgment, inability to concentrate, and memory lapses. With progressive degeneration, rigidity and akinesia develop, making any movement difficult. Personality changes, moodiness, and behavioral disturbances become more marked as dementia progresses.

DIAGNOSTIC TESTS

The presence of the defective gene can be detected by DNA analysis.

TREATMENT

No therapy is available to slow the progress of the disease. Symptomatic therapy such as physiotherapy or drugs may reduce the choreiform movements and maintain mobility for a longer time.

Alzheimer's Disease

Alzheimer's disease is a common form of *dementia*, which can be defined as a progressive loss of intellectual function to the point where it interferes with work, relationships, and personal hygiene. Dementias can result from many conditions including vascular disease, infections, toxins, and genetic disorders. Dementia involves loss of memory, especially short-term or recent memory, and confusion about the events in long-term memory. Personality changes, lack of initiative, repetitive behavior, and impairments in judgment, abstract thinking, and problem-solving abilities are characteristics.

PATHOPHYSIOLOGY

Typical changes in Alzheimer's disease include cortical atrophy and widening of the sulci, particularly in the frontal and temporal lobes. Atrophy leads to dilated ventricles. Neurofibrillary tangles in the neurons and senile plaques are found in very large numbers in the affected parts of the brain. The plaques, which disrupt neural conduction, contain fragments from beta-amyloid precursor protein (βAPP), and the role of this protein is a focus of current research. Some neurofibrils and plaques have been found in the brains of elderly people whose cognitive function is not impaired, and therefore it appears that the numbers and distribution of the plaques are the significant factors. There is also a deficit of the neurotransmitter ACh in the brain. No definitive diagnostic tests are available, and the diagnosis is based on observations as well as the ruling out of other possible causes.

ETIOLOGY

Early-onset or presenile Alzheimer's disease develops between the ages of 30 and 60 and is known to be inherited. The defective gene has been located on chromosome 14 and can be detected with a blood test. Some other cases of familial Alzheimer's disease have been traced to genes on chromosomes 19 and 21. Other forms of Alzheimer's disease (senile dementia) affect people over 65 years old and appear to be multifactorial in origin, involving a combination of genetic (linked to chromosome 19) and environmental factors such as aluminum toxicity or slow viruses. Further studies are in progress.

SIGNS AND SYMPTOMS

Onset tends to be insidious with gradual loss of memory and lack of concentration. Cognitive function continues to decline, and behavioral changes such as irritability, hostility, and mood swings are common. In time, it becomes difficult to manage the activities of daily living, including preparing meals, dressing, and maintaining personal hygiene, and the person may

become confused and lost even in familiar territory. Degenerative changes may gradually interfere with motor function. In the late stage, the person does not recognize his or her family, lacks awareness or interest in the environment, and may be incontinent.

TREATMENT

No specific treatment is available. Symptomatic treatment of specific problems such as depression or anxiety may be given. A team approach to care is helpful in prolonging independence and supporting the family. Social workers, psychologists, and speech therapists can provide direction and assistance. A daily routine and secure surroundings facilitate care.

Thinkabout 20–19

List the early signs of Alzheimer's disease.

SPINAL CORD PROBLEMS

Herniated Intervertebral Disc

PATHOPHYSIOLOGY

Herniation involves protrusion of the nucleus pulposus, the inner gelatinous component of the intervertebral disc, through a tear in the annulus fibrosus, the tough outer covering of the disc (Fig. 20–15). Such

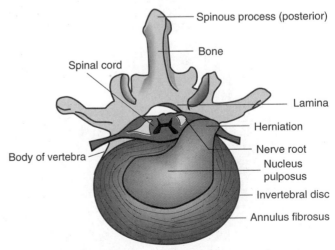

FIGURE 20–15. Herniated intervertebral disc.

protrusions exert pressure on the spinal nerve root or spinal cord at the site, interfering with nerve conduction. The tear in the capsule may occur suddenly or develop gradually. Depending on which site is involved, sensory, motor, or autonomic function can be impaired. The most common location is the lumbosacral discs at L4 to L5 or L5 to S1. Some herniations involve cervical discs between C5 and C7. If pressure on the nerve tissue or blood supply is prolonged and severe, permanent damage to the nerve tissue may result.

ETIOLOGY

A person may be predisposed to herniation because of degenerative changes in the intervertebral disc re-sulting from age or metabolic changes. The herniation usually is caused by trauma or poor body mechanics, leading to excessive stress on the muscles, for example, by improper lifting of heavy objects or during transfer of a patient.

SIGNS AND SYMPTOMS

Signs depend on the location and extent of the protrusion (Figs. 20–16 and 20–17). In most cases the effects are unilateral; however, large protrusions may cause bilateral effects. Because of pressure on the sensory nerve fibers in the dorsal root, lumbosacral herniations cause pain in the lower back, radiating down one or both legs (sciatic nerve pain). Actions such as cough-

A. THE SPINAL CORD

B. CROSS-SECTION OF THE SPINAL CORD SHOWING TRACTS

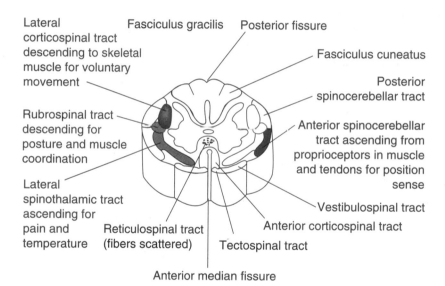

FIGURE 20–16. Functional areas of the spinal cord.

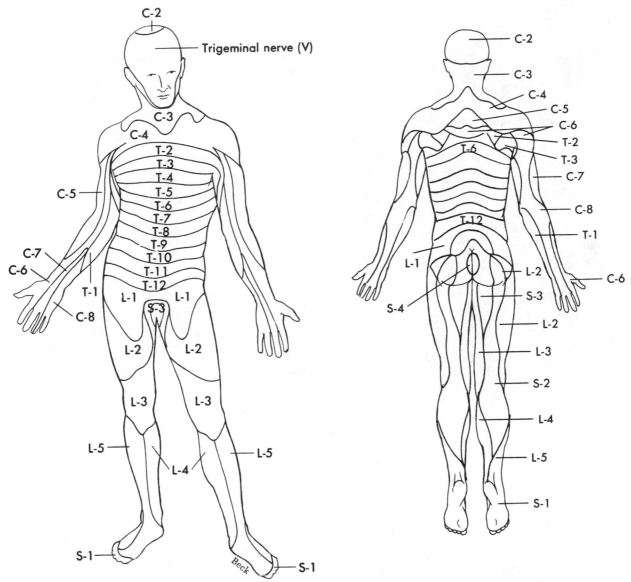

FIGURE 20–17. Dermatomes. (From Thibodeau GA: Anatomy and Physiology. St. Louis, Times Mirror/Mosby College Publishing, 1987.)

ing or straight leg raising usually aggravate the pain. Paresthesia or numbness and tingling may occur. If the nerve compression is extensive, muscle weakness develops. Also, interference with micturition (bladder emptying) may develop.

Similarly, a herniated disc in the cervical region causes pain in the neck and shoulder that radiates down the arm. Sensory impairment, reduced neck movement, and weakness may accompany the pain. The pressure may lead to skeletal muscle spasm in the neck or back, further increasing the pain.

DIAGNOSTIC TESTS

Myelography with contrast dye confirms the herniation, as do CT scans or MRI.

TREATMENT

Conservative treatment, including bed rest, application of heat, ice, or traction, or drugs such as analgesics, anti-inflammatory agents, and skeletal muscle relaxants usually comprise the initial approach. Surgery, including laminectomy or diskectomy, may be required if compression persists.

Spinal Cord Injury

Injury to the spinal cord usually results from fracture or dislocation of the vertebrae. This trauma then compresses, stretches, or tears the spinal cord (Fig. 20–18). The supporting ligaments and the intervertebral disc

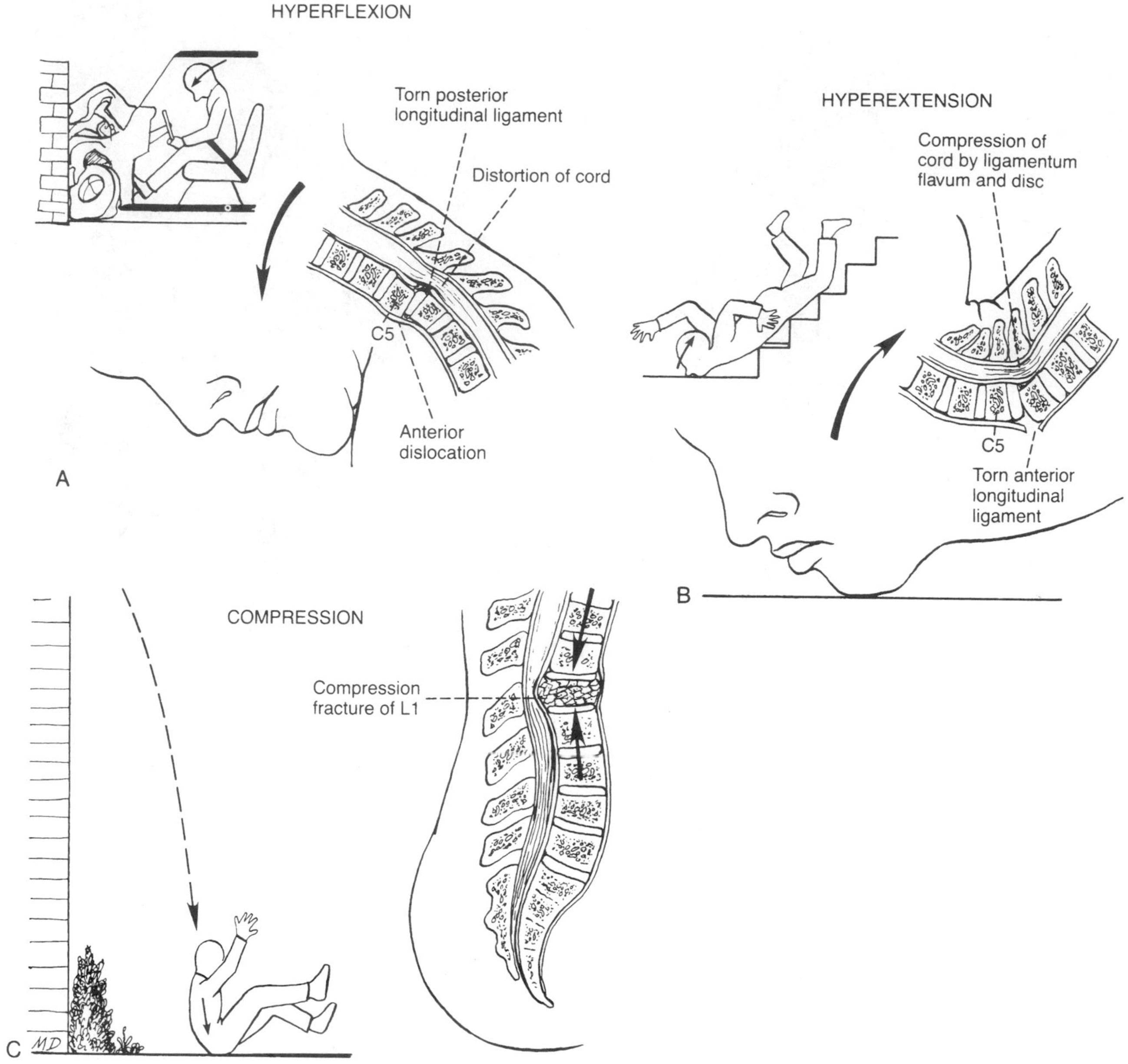

FIGURE 20-18. Types of spinal cord injuries. (From Copstead LC: Perspectives on Pathophysiology. Philadelphia, W.B. Saunders, 1995.)

may be damaged also. Most injuries occur in mobile areas of the spine, C1 to C7 and T12 to L2 (see Fig. 20–16). Cervical injuries may result from hyperextension or hyperflexion of the neck, with possible fracture. Usually damage to the disc and ligaments occurs, leading to dislocation, loss of alignment of the vertebrae, and compression or stretching of the spinal cord. Dislocation of any vertebra may crush or compress the spinal cord and compromise the blood supply. Compression fractures cause injury to the spinal cord when great force is applied to the top of the skull or to the feet and is then transmitted up or down the spine. This may happen when diving into an empty pool or jumping from a height and landing on one's feet, or when an

object falls on one's head when in an upright position. The shattered bone is compressed and protrudes to exert pressure horizontally against the cord. The sharp edges of bone fragments may lacerate or tear nerve fibers and blood vessels. Vertebral fractures may be classified as simple (single line break), compression (the bone is crushed or shattered in multiple fragments), wedge (an angular section of bone is displaced), or dislocation (the vertebra is forced out of its normal position). Spinal cord damage also may result directly from penetration injuries such as stab or bullet wounds. Because these injuries are often unstable, immediate appropriate immobilization is essential to prevent secondary damage.

A. DURING SPINAL SHOCK (PERIOD IMMEDIATELY FOLLOWING INJURY)

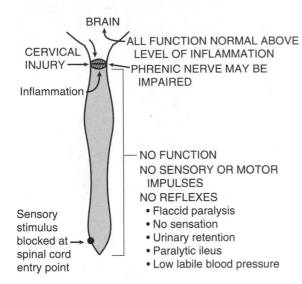

B. OVERVIEW OF PERMANENT EFFECTS – POSTSPINAL SHOCK

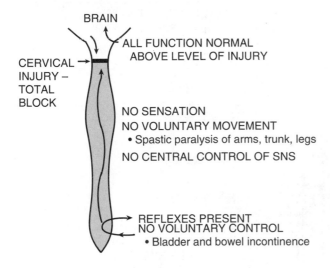

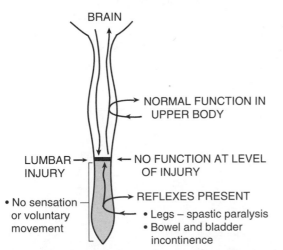

FIGURE 20–19. Effects of spinal cord damage.

PATHOPHYSIOLOGY

Damage to the spinal cord may be temporary or permanent. Nerves in the spinal cord do not regenerate. Reversible damage includes bruising when mild edema and minor bleeding temporarily impair conduction of nerve impulses. Compression of the cord must be relieved quickly to maintain adequate blood supply. Prolonged ischemia and necrosis lead to permanent damage. Laceration of nerve tissue by bone fragments usually results in permanent loss of conduction in the affected nerve tracts. Complete transection (severing) or crushing of the cord causes irreversible loss of all function at and below the level of injury. Partial transection or crushing injuries may allow for recovery of some function.

As with any trauma, bleeding and inflammation develop locally, creating additional pressure and further interfering with blood flow. Edema and hemorrhage extend for several segments above and below the level of injury. Initially, the loss of function may appear to be more extensive because of this additional compression, but as the edema subsides, there may be partial recovery of function. When injury occurs in the cervical region, this inflammation may extend upward to C3 to C5, interfering with phrenic nerve innervation to the diaphragm and therefore with respiration. In addition, tissue damage leads to increased secretion of norepinephrine in the area, which causes vasoconstriction, leading to additional local ischemia and necrosis. In the initial period following the injury, conduction of impulses ceases in the nerve tracts and in the gray matter, a period known as *spinal shock* (a form of neurogenic shock). Depending on the extent of the injury and the amount of resultant bleeding, the inflammation gradually subsides, damaged tissue is removed by phagocytes, and scar tissue forms. During this period, reflex activity resumes in the spinal cord below the level of injury, and any undamaged tracts continue to conduct impulses through the level of damage (Fig. 20–19).

ETIOLOGY

Most spinal cord injuries occur in young men and result from motorcycle or automobile accidents. The second most common cause is sports (e.g., diving, football). The other major cause of injury is falls, and the elderly are included in this group.

SIGNS AND SYMPTOMS

During the initial period of spinal shock all neurologic activity ceases at, below, and slightly above the level of injury (see Fig. 20–19). No reflexes are present, including skeletal muscle, sensory, and autonomic system (bladder and bowel function). This condition may persist for days or months. Recovery from spinal shock is indicated by the gradual return of reflex activity below the level of injury. In most cases, hyperreflexia develops because the normal inhibitory or "dampening" impulses cannot reach the levels below the injury. Gradually the extent of permanent damage is revealed. Voluntary motor activity and sensory impulses are blocked at the level of damage. The specific effects of permanent damage depend on the level at which the spinal cord trauma occurred (see Figs. 20–16 and 20–17). For example, cervical injuries affect motor and sensory function in the arms, trunk, and legs as well as respiratory function, SNS function (T1–L2) and sacral parasympathetic fibers. Paralysis of all four extremities is termed quadriplegia, whereas paraplegia refers to paralysis of the lower part of the trunk and legs. Trauma in the lumbar region interferes with function in the lower extremities and the sacral parasympathetic nerves. Many injuries are incomplete, and the permanent effects vary considerably among individuals.

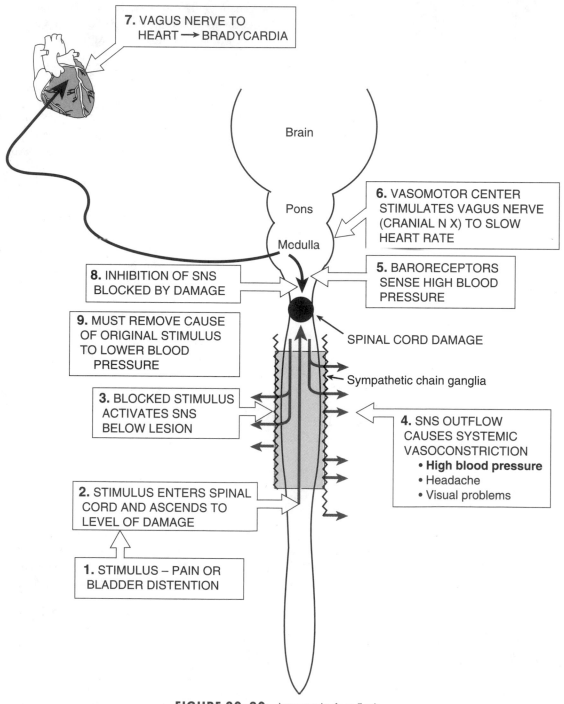

FIGURE 20–20. Autonomic dysreflexia.

During the period of spinal shock, the signs include flaccid paralysis and sensory loss at and below the injured area, an absence of all reflexes, and loss of central control of autonomic function. In patients with cervical injury, this includes loss of control of vasomotor tone, blood pressure, diaphoresis and body temperature, and bowel and bladder emptying. Blood pressure is low and labile. Urinary retention and paralytic ileus are present. Following recovery from spinal shock and return of reflexes, spastic paralysis and sensory deficit are present below the level of damage. Reflex or neurogenic bladder and bowel function are present as well (urinary incontinence and reflex defecation). Partial cord injuries can lead to different patterns of impairment, for example, ipsilateral paralysis and contralateral loss of pain and temperature sensation, depending on the point of decussation and the location of the specific tracts. In patients with cervical injuries, respiratory function may continue to be a matter of concern owing to phrenic nerve impairment and the loss of intercostal muscle innervation. Blood pressure and body temperature may be labile because central control of vasomotor tone and diaphoresis is lacking.

Stimulation of the sympathetic system may result in *autonomic dysreflexia* (Fig. 20–20). This potentially serious complication is caused by a sensory stimulus that triggers a massive sympathetic reflex response that cannot be controlled from the brain. The trigger may be any noxious stimulus in the body but most frequently is a distended bladder or decubitus ulcer. A sensory stimulus to the SNS below the level of injury can stimulate the entire chain of SNS ganglia, leading to excessive vasoconstriction with a sudden increase in blood pressure, severe headache, and visual impairment. However, bradycardia accompanies this syndrome as the baroreceptors sense the high blood pressure and respond through the vagus nerve by slowing the heart rate. Note that the excessive vasoconstriction cannot be reduced through the cardiovascular control center. Immediate resolution of this problem is needed to prevent a stroke or heart failure. This means finding and removing the cause of the stimulus and administering medication to lower the blood pressure.

Complications are common following spinal cord injury because of immobility and loss of function. Contractures may develop from muscle spasms, decubitus ulcers are common, and respiratory and urinary infections are frequent. Sexual function and reproductive capacity are likely to be affected. The sensory and psychological components of the sexual response are usually blocked by the injury. Many males have neurogenic reflex erections. Penetration depends on sustaining this reflex, which can be difficult. Many men, particularly those with high cord injuries, are infertile because sperm production in the testes is impaired. Women usually resume menstrual cycles once they have recovered from the acute trauma period, and they can bear children. Close monitoring of the pregnancy is necessary, and vaginal delivery may be difficult. With counseling and supportive mates, many individuals with spinal cord injury can develop or maintain sexual relationships.

TREATMENT

Surgery may be required to relieve pressure and repair tissues. Glucocorticoids may be needed to reduce edema and stabilize the vascular system. Other injuries require prompt treatment to minimize secondary damage due to decreased oxygen or circulation. Ongoing care is necessary to prevent the complications related to immobility. Early extensive rehabilitation is important to learn the best ways to use the remaining function, to prevent complications, and to assist in maximizing independence. A team approach can assist the patient in performing the activities of daily living as well as with ventilation and other body needs. Technology has provided myriad assistive devices, which can be tailored to the patient's individual needs.

 Thinkabout 20–20

a. Explain how a herniated intervertebral disc causes pain in the leg.

b. Compare the effects on motor function of a lumbar spinal cord injury immediately following the trauma and later (the permanent effect).

c. Explain why micturition may not occur immediately after an injury (urinary retention) but incontinence may develop later.

d. Explain several reasons why a cervical injury is much more serious than a lumbar injury.

MENTAL DISORDERS

Mental illness is classified using the Diagnostic and Statistical Manual of Mental Disorders (DSM) from the American Psychiatric Association. Mental health problems involve significant dysfunction in the areas of behavior or personality that interfere with the person's ability to function. Biochemical and structural abnormalities in the brain appear to contribute to these pathologies. Many disorders have a genetic component. Stressors may play a role in the development of the illness. Psychotic illness includes the more serious disorders such as schizophrenia, delusional disorders, and some affective or mood disorders. Many patients with psychotic disorders receive large doses of drugs with obvious side effects. Other common mental disorders include anxiety and panic disorders, which are less severe but nevertheless disruptive. This section provides a brief introduction to the pathophysiology of the common disorders.

Schizophrenia

PATHOPHYSIOLOGY

Schizophrenia includes a variety of syndromes, which present differently in different individuals. Although the etiology and pathogenesis have not been fully determined, some common changes do occur in the brains of schizophrenic patients. These include reduced gray matter in the temporal lobes, enlarged third and lateral ventricles, abnormal cells in the hippocampus (part of the limbic system), excessive dopamine secretion, and decreased blood flow to the frontal lobes. Some of these changes appear to be linked to the neurologic manifestations seen in schizophrenics, such as abnormal eye movements (staring or periodic jerky eye movements).

ETIOLOGY

Current theories focus on a genetic predisposition or brain damage in the fetus due to viral infection in the mother during pregnancy. Onset of schizophrenia usually occurs between the ages of 15 and 25 in men and between 25 and 35 in women.

SIGNS AND SYMPTOMS

Generally, disorganized thought processes are the basic problem. Communication is frequently impaired by poor language usage, including lack of appropriate association of thoughts, meaningless repetition of words or thoughts, or development of new words without accepted meanings (neologisms). Delusions or false beliefs and ideas are persistent. Delusions may include a belief in persecution by others or ideas of grandeur or power over others. Problem-solving ability is poor, and the attention span is brief. Hallucinations or abnormal sensory perceptions are frequent. The patient may withdraw socially from people and show little emotion, but he or she experiences mood swings and becomes anxious. Often personal care is minimal.

TREATMENT

Drugs are the major therapeutic modality, often in conjunction with psychotherapy and psychosocial reha-

bilitation. The antipsychotic drugs (major tranquilizers or neuroleptics) chlorpromazine (Thorazine), fluphenazine (Modequate), haloperidol (Haldol), and clozapine (Clozaril) act by decreasing dopamine activity in the brain. These drugs frequently cause side effects related to excessive extrapyramidal (EPS) activity (or Parkinson-like signs). Dystonia and tardive dyskinesia cause involuntary muscle spasms in the face, neck, arms, or legs. This may present as chewing or grimacing, repetitive jerky or writhing movements of the limbs, tremors, or a shuffling gait. With prolonged use and high doses of the drugs, tardive dyskinesia may be irreversible. Some of these side effects may be reduced by anti-Parkinson agents (anticholinergics), but these drugs also have adverse effects such as blurred vision and dry mouth.

Depression

Depression is classed as a mood disorder. Major depression or unipolar disorder is endogenous and is based on biologic factors or personal characteristics. Bipolar disorder involves alternating periods of depression and mania. Depression may also occur as an exogenous or reactive episode, a response to a life event. Depression also occurs secondarily to many systemic disorders, including cancer, diabetes, heart failure, and systemic lupus erythematosus. Depression is a very common disorder, and it is thought that many patients with milder forms do not receive treatment.

PATHOPHYSIOLOGY

Depression is classified as an affective or mood disorder based on disorganized emotions. It results from decreased activity by the excitatory neurotransmitters, norepinephrine and serotonin, in the brain. The exact mechanism has not yet been established.

SIGNS AND SYMPTOMS

Depression is indicated by a prolonged period of sadness marked by hopelessness and an inability to find pleasure in any activity. Lack of energy and loss of self-esteem and motivation interfere with daily activity. Some individuals may be irritable and agitated. The individual has difficulty in concentrating and solving problems. Sleep disorders such as insomnia usually accompany depression. Loss of appetite and libido (sex drive) are common.

TREATMENT

Antidepressant drugs that increase norepinephrine activity are effective in treating many cases of depression. Monamine oxidase (MAO) inhibitors such as tranylcypromine (Parnate) block the destruction of norepinephrine and serotonin by the enzyme MAO at the synapse. The tricyclic antidepressants (TCAs) such as amitriptyline (Elavil) block the reuptake of the neurotransmitters into the presynaptic neuron. A third group of drugs in common use, including fluoxetine (Prozac), blocks the reuptake of serotonin. These mechanisms allow the stimulation by excitatory neurotransmitters to continue in the brain. MAO inhibitors are associated with many interactions involving food and other drugs that may result in a hypertensive crisis (high blood pressure). Foods to be avoided include tyramine-containing substances such as chocolate, old cheese, beer, and red wine. Another method of treatment of depression involves electroconvulsive therapy (shock treatments), which increase norepinephrine activity.

Panic Disorder

PATHOPHYSIOLOGY

Panic disorder is an example of an anxiety disorder. A genetic factor has been implicated. There is evidence of an increased discharge of neurons in the temporal lobes. Biochemical abnormalities involving the neurotransmitters norepinephrine, serotonin, and GABA appear to be involved. Frequently, patients are fearful of having another panic attack, and this leads to increased irritability of the limbic system.

SIGNS AND SYMPTOMS

Repeated episodes of intense fear without provocation, which may last for minutes or hours, characterize this disorder. Palpitations or tachycardia, hyperventilation, sweating, sensations of choking or smothering, and nausea accompany the feeling of terror. Patients who anticipate attacks may develop a fear of open spaces or a fear of being in a place where no help is available (agoraphobia) and refuse to leave their homes.

TREATMENT

Psychotherapy combined with drug therapy consisting of antianxiety agents such as alprazolam (Xanax) or diazepam (Valium) is helpful. Antianxiety agents or minor tranquilizers such as the benzodiazepine drugs potentiate the activity of GABA, an inhibitory neurotransmitter. Large doses may be necessary, which can cause drowsiness and ataxia. These drugs have a wide safety margin when used appropriately. In some patients, tricyclic antidepressants may be prescribed.

Thinkabout 20-21

a. Compare three signs of schizophrenia with three signs of depression.
b. Explain how antipsychotic drugs act to reduce signs of mental illness.
c. Describe common signs of the extrapyramidal system side effects of antipsychotic drugs.
d. Describe a panic attack.

DISORDERS OF THE EYE AND EAR

The Eye

REVIEW OF NORMAL STRUCTURE AND FUNCTION

Visual information is received from light rays that pass through the transparent cornea and then through the lens, which focuses the image clearly on the light-sensitive nerve receptor cells of the retina. These visual stimuli are conducted by the optic nerves to the occipital lobe of the brain for interpretation and processing before they are sent to other areas of the brain.

The eye is well protected in the bony *orbit* of the skull. The eyelids *(palpebrae)* and eyelashes deflect foreign material in the air away from the eyes and protect the eye from excessive sunlight and drying. The levator palpebrae superior, the muscle of the upper eyelid, is controlled by the oculomotor nerve (cranial nerve III). The eyelids are lined with a thin mucous membrane, the *conjunctiva*, which continues over the sclera of the eye. The continual secretion of *tears* washes away particles and irritating substances. This watery secretion contains *lysozyme*, an antibacterial enzyme. The tears form in the *lacrimal gland* located on the superior lateral area of the orbit. They flow across the eye and drain into the lacrimal canals in the medial corner of the eye and then into the nasal cavity through the nasolacrimal duct. The tears keep the external tissues of the eye moist and healthy.

Six skeletal muscles *(extrinsic muscles)* control the movement of the eyeball in the bony orbit. They originate on the orbit and insert onto the sclerae on the outside of the eyeball. There are four straight (rectus) muscles and two angled (oblique) muscles, which are coordinated to move and rotate the eye and are under the control of cranial nerves III, IV, and VI.

The eyeball consists of a spherical three-layered wall

filled with fluid (Fig. 20–21). The anterior portion of the three layers differs from the posterior section because these tissues must permit the passage of light rays. The outer layer is a tough fibrous coat, the posterior portion of which is the sclera and the anterior portion the cornea. The *sclera* is visible as the "white" of the eye, and the *cornea* is a transparent bulging portion through which light rays pass (if you look at another person's eye from the side, you can observe the curve of the cornea). The cornea does not contain blood vessels but is nourished by the fluids around it and oxygen diffusing from the atmosphere. This source of oxygen is a concern for individuals wearing contact lenses. The middle layer of the eye, or *uvea,* is made up of the *choroid,* a dark, vascular layer adjacent to the sclera in the posterior portion of the eye. The dark color absorbs the light, preventing reflection of light within the orbit. The numerous blood vessels in the choroid supply nutrients to the outer layers of the retina. In the anterior part of the eye, the choroid develops into the ciliary body and iris. The *ciliary body* consists of the *ciliary muscle,* which controls the shape of the lens to focus the image of near and distant objects accurately and clearly on the retina, and the *ciliary processes,* which secrete aqueous humor, the fluid in the anterior cavity of the eye. The *iris* is a circular structure surrounding the *pupil,* an opening through which light rays pass into the interior of the eye. The iris is pigmented and gives the eye its distinctive brown or blue tone. The iris contains two muscles that control the size of the pupil. The circular or sphincter muscle contracts in response to parasympathetic stimuli or excessive light on the retina, resulting in a constricted or small pupil. PNS fibers reach the iris from cranial nerve III. Under SNS control, the radial muscles of the iris, when contracted, cause the pupil to dilate or open. This function is easier to remember if it is associated with the stress or fight-or-flight response, in which sympathetic stimulation leads to pupil dilation. The *suspensory ligament* connects the lens to the ciliary body. The *lens* is a transparent biconvex structure made up of an elastic capsule surrounding an orderly arrangement of fibers. The shape of the lens is altered as the contraction of the ciliary muscle alters tension on the suspensory ligament. This adjustment in lens curvature or *accommodation* bends the light rays *(refraction)* entering the eye sufficiently to focus a sharp image on the retina.

The inner coat of the wall of the eye is the *retina.* This multilayered coat is present only in the posterior two-thirds of the eye because light rays passing through the lens cannot bend to reach the retina if it is present in the anterior part of the eye. The retina

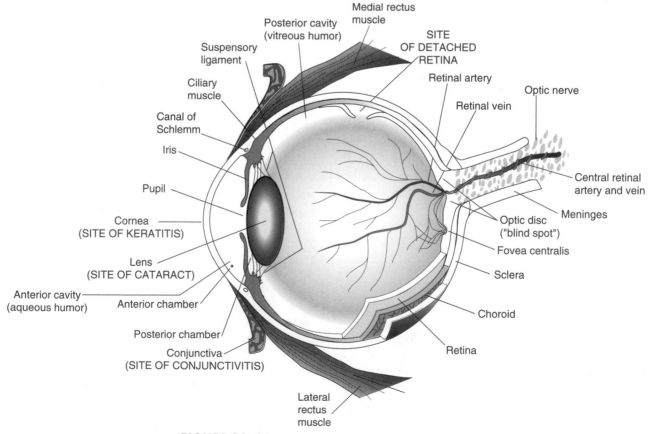

FIGURE 20–21. The structures of the eye and sites of eye problems.

consists of a pigmented layer and several layers of neurons. Innermost are the rods and cones, which are light-sensitive _photoreceptor_ cells. _Rods_ are specialized for dim light, and _cones_ are color sensitive. There are three types of cones, red, green, and blue, which determine color perception. _Color blindness_ is common in males and results from a deficit of one type of cone owing to an abnormal gene on the X chromosome (sex-linked recessive gene). The light energy is absorbed by the rods and cones and converted into electrical energy in the neurons. The nerve impulses eventually converge in the fibers of the _optic nerve_ (cranial nerve II), which carries visual information to the _occipital lobe_ of the brain (see Fig. 20–3). At the optic chiasm, half of the fibers from each optic nerve cross to pass to the occipital lobe in the opposite hemisphere. Therefore, the left occipital lobe receives images from the right visual field. The optic nerve leaves the eye at the _optic disc_ in the posterior portion of the eye. Because the optic nerve is essentially a projection of brain tissue surrounded by CSF and meninges, it reflects pressure in the brain (see earlier section, Increased Intracranial Pressure). The central retinal artery and vein, which supply the retina and other structures, also pass through the optic disc. There are no rods or cones at the optic disc, forming the "blind spot." In the center of the posterior retina is the macula lutea, a yellowish area containing a depression, the _fovea centralis_, which is an area containing many cones that provides the most acute vision.

The eye is divided into two cavities by the lens and ciliary body. The _posterior cavity_ is the space between the lens and the retina, and it contains the transparent jellylike _vitreous humor_. This material is formed during embryonic development and holds the retina approximated against the choroid to ensure diffusion of nutrients as well as to maintain the shape and size of the eyeball. The _anterior cavity_ between the cornea and the lens is further divided into the _anterior chamber_, extending from the cornea to the iris, and the _posterior chamber_, between the iris and the lens. The chambers are connected through the pupil. The anterior cavity is filled with _aqueous humor_, which is continuously secreted by the ciliary processes into the posterior chamber. It flows through the pupil into the anterior chamber and drains into the reticular network and canal of Schlemm (see Fig. 20–23). This canal encircles the eye at the junction of the cornea and iris and returns the fluid to the blood. To maintain normal intraocular pressure inside the eye, the amount of aqueous humor formed should equal the amount reabsorbed. Normal pressure maintains the shape of the eye. The aqueous humor supplies nutrients to the lens and cornea, which lack blood vessels.

To review the physiology of vision, light rays from an object pass through the cornea, where they are re-fracted, and then through the aqueous humor and pupil. The curvature of the lens is adjusted to refract the light rays so that they converge on the retina, providing a sharp image of the object. The light continues through the transparent aqueous humor to the retina, where the photoreceptor neurons, the rods and cones, are stimulated. The light energy is converted into an electrical stimulus, which is transmitted by the optic nerve to the occipital lobe of the brain, where the image is identified and integrated with other information. The double image projected from different angles by the two eyes provides a wider visual field, and the central overlap of visual fields provides depth perception.

Thinkabout 20–22

a. Explain why one may have a "runny nose" when crying.

b. Describe the outer layer of the eye, naming and locating the parts and describing the function of each.

c. List the parts of the eye that do not contain blood vessels and explain how they are nourished.

d. List the components of the eye that are transparent.

e. Explain the effect of sudden fear or anger on the size of the pupil.

f. List the functions of the oculomotor nerve.

g. Describe the location and function of the photoreceptor cells.

h. Describe the type of impulses carried by the optic nerve.

DIAGNOSTIC TESTS

The Snellen chart or similar eye charts, consisting of lines of progressively smaller letters and numbers, measure visual acuity. Visual field tests are used to check central and peripheral vision. Tonometry assesses intraocular pressure by checking the resistance of the cornea. An ophthalmoscope can be used to examine the interior structures, and gonioscopy measures the angle of the anterior chamber. Muscle function and coordination can also be tested.

Neurologic damage to the visual pathway is covered in the second section of this chapter, Acute Neurologic Problems. _Retinopathies_ are discussed in Chapter 16 under hypertension and in Chapter 21 under diabetes mellitus.

STRUCTURAL DEFECTS

Structural defects interfere with the focusing of a clear image on the retina. In *myopia*, nearsightedness, the image is focused in front of the lens, perhaps because the eyeball is too long (Fig. 20–22). *Hyperopia*, or farsightedness, develops if the eyeball is too short and the image is focused behind the retina. In cases of myopia and hyperopia the blurred image can be corrected with a lens that refocuses the image on the retina, such as a concave lens for myopia. *Presbyopia* refers to farsightedness associated with aging, when the loss of elasticity reduces accommodation. *Astigmatism* develops from an irregular curvature in the cornea or lens. *Strabismus* (squint or cross-eye) results from a deviation of one eye, resulting in double vision (*diplopia*). This may be caused by a weak or hypertonic muscle, a short muscle, or a neurologic defect. In young children, strabismus must be treated immediately to prevent the development of *amblyopia,* the suppression by the brain of the visual image from the affected eye. *Nystagmus* is an involuntary abnormal movement of one or both eyes. It may be a back and forth rhythmic motion or jerky movement or circular motion. This abnormality may result from neurologic causes, from inner ear or cerebellar disturbances, or from drug toxicity. Trauma to the cranial nerves can cause paralysis of the extraocular muscles, leading to diplopia or paralysis of the upper eyelid (*ptosis*).

INFECTIONS AND TRAUMA

Conjunctivitis is a superficial inflammation or infection involving the conjunctiva. Allergies or irritating chemicals may cause inflammation. Organisms such as *Staphylococcus aureus* may cause the highly contagious "pinkeye," which occurs frequently in children. The sclera of the eye appears red, and there is a discharge. Severe pain and photophobia (sensitivity to light) develop when the cornea is involved because it has numerous pain receptors (trigeminal nerve—cranial nerve V). *Chlamydia trachomatis* causes infection in the reproductive tract and may infect the eyes of newborns, who

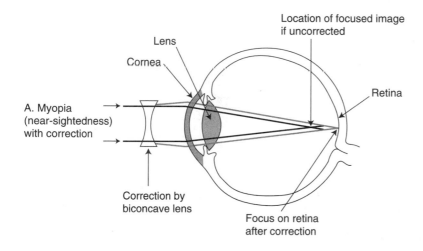

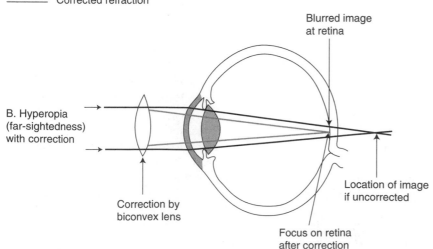

FIGURE 20-22. Refraction defects in the eye.

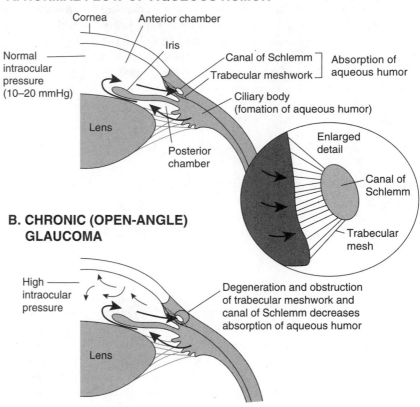

A. NORMAL FLOW OF AQUEOUS HUMOR

Cornea
Anterior chamber
Iris
Normal intraocular pressure (10–20 mmHg)
Canal of Schlemm
Trabecular meshwork
Absorption of aqueous humor
Ciliary body (fomation of aqueous humor)
Lens
Posterior chamber
Enlarged detail
Canal of Schlemm
Trabecular mesh

B. CHRONIC (OPEN-ANGLE) GLAUCOMA

High intraocular pressure
Degeneration and obstruction of trabecular meshwork and canal of Schlemm decreases absorption of aqueous humor
Lens

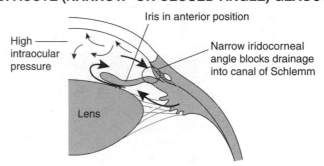

C. ACUTE (NARROW- OR CLOSED-ANGLE) GLAUCOMA

Iris in anterior position
High intraocular pressure
Narrow iridocorneal angle blocks drainage into canal of Schlemm
Lens

FIGURE 20–23. Glaucoma.

are routinely given medication after birth to prevent this. Herpes virus is dangerous because it may cause *keratitis* with corneal ulceration and eventual scarring and loss of vision.

Trauma to the cornea may also cause scarring. Penetration injuries may cause damage to the internal structures or loss of the vitreous humor.

GLAUCOMA

Pathophysiology

Glaucoma results from increased intraocular pressure caused by an excessive accumulation of aqueous humor. *Narrow-angle* glaucoma occurs when the angle between the cornea and the iris is decreased by factors such as an abnormal anterior insertion of the iris. With aging, the lens enlarges, pushing the iris more forward and to the side. This anatomic position may block the outflow of aqueous humor when the pupil is dilated and the thickened iris fills the narrow angle (Fig. 20–23). Pressure inside the eyeball can increase significantly within an hour of pupil dilation, blocking drainage of fluid. This leads to *acute* glaucoma, in which there is a sudden marked increase in intraocular pressure. *Chronic* glaucoma, sometimes referred to as wide-angle or open-angle glaucoma, is a common degenerative disorder. The trabecular network and canal of Schlemm become obstructed, and the outflow of aqueous humor gradually diminishes. Intraocular pressure increases slowly and usually asymptomatically. The increased pressure compresses the blood flow to the retinal cells, causing ischemia and damage to the retinal cells. The anterior portion of the retina is affected first, including the receptor cells for peripheral vision. If pressure inside the eyeball continues to increase, more of the retina and the optic nerve will be damaged. When observed through the pupil, the optic disc appears eroded or "cupped" as the optic nerve fibers are compressed. Damage to the retina and optic nerve is irreversible, and eventually blindness results.

Etiology

Chronic glaucoma develops frequently in older individuals, usually beginning after age 50. Narrow-angle glaucoma may be caused by a developmental abnormality, aging, or scar tissue in the eye from trauma or infection.

Signs and Symptoms

Chronic glaucoma has an insidious onset. Increased intraocular pressure is the initial indicator of chronic glaucoma. Routine screening tests are recommended as individuals age because this is often the only sign. Loss of peripheral vision may not be noticed initially except by a screening test because individuals automatically adjust the direction of the eyes to focus on an object. As pressure increases, corneal edema and altered light refraction lead to blurred vision and the appearance of "halos" around lights. Mild eye discomfort develops as the corneal pain receptors are stimulated by the increased pressure.

Acute episodes of glaucoma may be triggered by pupil dilation resulting from adrenergic drugs such as those used for colds or hay fever (vasoconstrictors or decongestants, which may cause pupil dilation), stress, or prolonged periods in darkened rooms. As intraocular pressure rises rapidly, eye pain, nausea, and headache develop, vision is blurred, and the cornea appears bulging and cloudy. The pupil is dilated and unresponsive to light.

Treatment

Chronic glaucoma is treated by administration of eyedrops to reduce secretion of aqueous humor (e.g., timolol or betaxolol, beta-adrenergic blocking agents) or eyedrops to constrict the pupil (e.g., pilocarpine, a miotic or cholinergic agent). It is essential to maintain treatment, administering the medication on a regular basis, to control intraocular pressure and minimize the risk of retinal damage. If the condition is unresponsive to drugs, laser trabeculoplasty or trabeculectomy to deepen the anterior chamber and increase the drainage of aqueous humor may be required.

Acute glaucoma, if severe, may require surgery such as removal of part of the iris to open a passageway for drainage into the canal of Schlemm (iridectomy). Laser iridotomy is a popular noninvasive procedure.

CATARACTS

Cataracts are a progressive opacity or clouding of the lens. The size, site, and density of the opacity varies among individuals and may differ in one individual's two eyes. The changes may be caused by degeneration related to aging or by metabolic abnormalities such as diabetes.

Blurred vision that progresses over the visual field and becomes darker with time is the only indicator. The rate at which impairment develops varies considerably, and a cataract in one eye may advance more quickly than one in the other eye. When advanced to the point of interfering with the person's ability to function or work, the damaged lens can be removed and replaced by an artificial intraocular lens. Prior to surgery tests are essential to assess retinal function, intraocular pressure, and the possible presence of other lesions such as tumors. Cataract surgery is usually day surgery, and the patient is quickly ambulatory. Extracapsular extraction is the most common procedure; it leaves the posterior capsule in place to receive the lens implant and stabilize the eye structures to reduce the risk of subsequent retinal detachment. Peripheral iridectomy may be included to prevent postoperative glaucoma.

DETACHED RETINA

A detached retina is an acute problem, which occurs when the retina tears because of marked myopia, degeneration with aging, or scar tissue that creates tension on the retina. The tear allows vitreous humor to flow behind the loose retinal portion (see Fig. 20–21). As increased vitreous humor continues to seep behind the retina, an increasing portion of the retina is lifted away from the choroid. The retinal cells cease to function as they are deprived of nutrients diffusing from the blood vessels of the choroid. This loss of function results in an area of blackness in the visual field. If separation continues, the retina is deprived of its source of nutrients in the choroid and dies. There is no pain related to the tear, but initially the patient may see light or dark floating spots in the visual field, resulting from blood or exudate leaking from the tear. Then a darkened or blind area develops, which increases in size with time. Typically, this event has been described as a "dark curtain" drawn across the visual field. Surgical intervention such as scleral buckling or laser therapy is required as soon as possible to close any holes and to reattach the retina in its proper position against the choroid to restore the source of nutrients to the retinal cells before irreversible damage occurs.

Thinkabout 20–23

a. Explain why infection or trauma involving the cornea is more serious than that involving the conjunctiva.

b. Describe the characteristic signs of cataract development and the rationale for it.

c. Compare wide-angle and narrow-angle glaucoma, including the pathophysiology and signs of each.

d. Explain the cause of blindness with cataract, acute glaucoma, detached retina, and damage to the optic chiasm.

The Ear

REVIEW OF NORMAL STRUCTURE AND FUNCTION

The ear is divided into three anatomic sections, the external ear, the middle ear, and the inner ear (Fig. 20–24). The *external* ear consists of the *pinna* or visible flap on the side of the head, and the *external auditory meatus* or canal. This canal passes through the temporal bone to the *tympanic membrane* or eardrum, which marks the separation between the external and middle ear. The middle ear consists of the *tympanic cavity*, a hollow area in the bone, which contains three tiny bones, the *ossicles*, comprising the *malleus, incus,* and *stapes*. The malleus is adjacent to the tympanic membrane, and the stapes fits against the oval window, a membrane connecting the middle ear and the inner ear. The middle ear cavity opens into the *auditory* or eustachian tube, which connects to the nasopharynx. This tube equalizes pressure in the middle ear with pressure in the external ear canal. This is important if atmospheric pressure changes suddenly, as when an airplane takes off. Chewing or swallowing helps to equalize the pressure on either side of the tympanic membrane. The middle ear cavity is also continuous with the *mastoid air cells* in the mastoid process of the temporal bone around the ear. A *continuous mucous membrane* lines the middle ear cavity, the mastoid cells, the auditory tube, and the respiratory tract. This is significant because it provides a path for direct spread of infection through these structures.

The inner ear is called the *labyrinth*. It is composed of two parts, the cochlea and the semicircular canals, joined by a vestibule. These structures consist of a bony labyrinth filled with a fluid, perilymph, inside of which is a membranous labyrinth filled with endolymph. The cochlea contains a complex arrangement of membranes surrounding the *organ of Corti,* where specialized hair cells provide stimuli to the sensory neurons for hearing. These neurons form the cochlear branch of the auditory nerve (cranial nerve VIII), which conducts impulses to the temporal lobe for reception and interpretation of sound. Some fibers from each ear cross to the auditory cortex in the opposite hemisphere, and some fibers remain on the same side, meaning that each auditory area receives some sound from each ear.

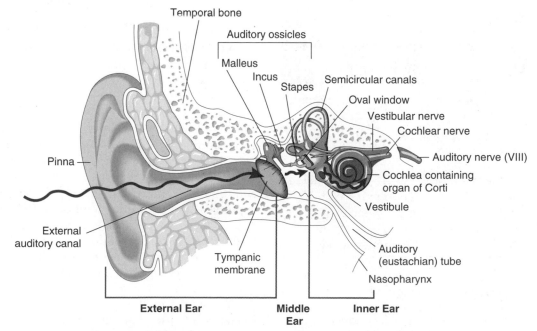

FIGURE 20–24. Structure of the ear and the hearing pathway.

The sound pathway begins with sound waves in the air. The height of a wave determines the loudness of the sound, and the number of sound waves per time period or frequency determines the pitch (high or low). Sound waves enter the external ear canal and strike the tympanic membrane, causing it to vibrate. Vibration of the tympanic membrane causes the malleus to vibrate, and then the incus and the stapes. The motion of the stapes against the oval window initiates movement of the perilymph and endolymph in the cochlea. These "water waves" stimulate movement of the membranes and hair cells in the organ of Corti, which converts the stimulus into a nerve impulse that is conducted to the auditory area of the brain, where the sound is received and interpreted. The semicircular canals in the inner ear include three structures, each at right angles to the other two; the sense of balance and equilibrium is focused in the crista ampullaris located in the ampulla of each semicircular canal and in the macula in the vestibule. These contain the receptor hair cells, which can be stimulated by motion of the fluid in response to head movements or position changes. Because of the arrangement of the canals, movement in any direction can be detected. Any stimulus is conducted by the vestibular branch of the auditory nerve to the medulla oblongata and other parts of the brain. Many additional connections to the cerebellum, to incoming proprioceptive impulses (joints, muscles, and tendons), and to visual stimuli are required for the coordination of righting reflexes to maintain body position.

Thinkabout 20–24

a. Describe the location of the middle ear, including its boundaries, and the openings from it. Describe the structures in the middle ear and their function.

b. Compare the advantages and disadvantages of the auditory tube and its relationship to the middle ear.

c. Describe the location of the auditory nerve receptors, and trace the connection to the brain.

d. Predict the effect on hearing capacity of damage to (1) the cochlea in the right ear, (2) the left auditory nerve, and (3) the left temporal lobe.

HEARING LOSS

There are two types of hearing loss, conduction deafness and nerve deafness. *Conduction* deafness occurs when sound is blocked in the external ear or middle ear. For example, an accumulation of wax or a foreign object in the external ear canal can block sound waves. Scar tissue or adhesions may impair the function of the tympanic membrane or ossicles. *Sensorineural* impairment develops with damage to the organ of Corti or the auditory nerve. Sensorineural loss may result from infection, particularly viral infection, including rubella, influenza, and herpes. Head trauma or neurologic disorders can affect the auditory nerve or temporal lobe. Ototoxic drugs such as the antibiotics streptomycin, neomycin, and vancomycin, the analgesics aspirin and ibuprofen, the diuretic furosemide, and some antineoplastic agents have caused temporary or permanent hearing loss. The early sign of toxicity is often tinnitus, a ringing or buzzing in the ears. Sudden very loud sounds or prolonged exposure to loud noise can damage the delicate hair cells because of the force exerted by excessive movement in response to the sound. This may be an occupational hazard, or it may be associated with loud music. Presbycusis is the sensorineural loss that occurs in the elderly owing to a reduced number of hair cells or receptor cells. *Congenital* deafness may be inherited or may result from infection or trauma during pregnancy or delivery. Hearing impairment in young children interferes with speech and social development. Tests comparing conduction by air through the external canal and conduction through the mastoid bone can assist in differentiating the type of deafness. Various types of hearing aids are available to improve hearing capacity. Cochlear implants are helpful in some cases of nerve damage.

EAR INFECTIONS

Otitis Media

PATHOPHYSIOLOGY

Otitis media is an inflammation or infection of the middle ear cavity. Exudate builds up in the cavity, causing pressure on the tympanic membrane and interfering with the movement of the membrane and the ossicles. Usually the auditory tube is obstructed by inflammation, preventing drainage of the fluid into the nasopharynx. Enlarged adenoids may compress the tube. The middle ear cavity is encased in rigid bone, and therefore increasing pressure eventually causes rupture of the tympanic membrane. Prolonged infection is likely to produce scar tissue and adhesions, leading to permanent conductive hearing loss. Chronic infection may lead to mastoiditis, infection involving the mastoid cells of the temporal bone.

ETIOLOGY

The mucosa of the middle ear cavity may become inflamed because of allergies or infection that spreads along the continuous mucosa from the nasopharynx and respiratory structures. This happens more easily in infants and young children because the auditory canal is shorter and wider and forms more of a right angle to the nasopharynx, thereby facilitating drainage of respiratory secretions into the auditory tube. Also, infants tend to spend more time in a recumbent position, and feeding in a supine position encourages reflux of fluid into the ear. As mucosal edema becomes more severe, the auditory tube becomes blocked, preventing drainage. Otitis media occurs more frequently in the winter months when there is an increase in respiratory infections. Common bacterial causes include *H. influenzae*, particularly in young children, pneumococci, beta-hemolytic streptococci, and staphylococci. Viral infection may also lead to otitis media, which is frequently complicated by a secondary bacterial infection.

SIGNS AND SYMPTOMS

Occasionally, otitis media is asymptomatic. More often, there is severe pain or earache (otalgia) related to the pressure on the tympanic membrane and on the nerve receptors in the cavity. The tympanic membrane appears red and bulging. An infant or young child tends to rub or pull at the ear to express distress. Mild hearing loss or a feeling of fullness is common. Signs of infection, such as fever and nausea, may be present. Rupture of the tympanic membrane results in a discharge from the external ear canal, accompanied by relief of pain.

TREATMENT

Antibacterials such as ampicillin are recommended, depending on the associated pathology. Decongestants may be useful in reducing the edema and obstruction in the auditory tube. Young children with recurrent otitis media may require insertion of drainage tubes through the tympanic membrane temporarily to relieve congestion. Surgery may be necessary to restore a functional tympanic membrane and ossicles (e.g., tympanoplasty) or to treat chronic mastoiditis (mastoidectomy). A person with an ear infection should use caution if he is planning to use air transportation because the pressures inside and outside the ear must be equalized to prevent additional damage (barotrauma). Chewing gum or swallowing during descent may help.

Otitis Externa

Otitis externa, sometimes called swimmer's ear, is an infection of the external auditory canal and pinna. It is usually of bacterial origin but occasionally is fungal. It may be associated with swimming, with irritation or the introduction of organisms when cleaning the ear, or with frequent use of earphones or earplugs. Pain, purulent discharge, and a hearing deficit are common signs of otitis externa. Otitis externa can be differentiated from otitis media because pain is usually increased with movement of the pinna.

OTOSCLEROSIS

Otosclerosis involves the resorption and subsequent development of additional bone in the middle ear cavity, which fixes the stapes to the oval window, blocking conduction of sound into the cochlea. It appears to develop from a genetic factor, primarily in young adult females. Surgical removal of the stapes (stapedectomy) and replacement by a prosthesis restores hearing.

MENIERE'S SYNDROME

Meniere's syndrome is an inner ear or labyrinth disorder common to adults. Excessive endolymph develops intermittently, interfering with the function of the hair cells in the cochlea and vestibule. The increased fluid appears to be of vascular origin. Each attack may last minutes or hours and causes severe vertigo, tinnitus, and unilateral hearing loss. Vertigo, a sensation of whirling and weakness, is often accompanied by loss of balance and falls, nausea and sweating, and nystagmus. Repeated occurrences lead to permanent damage to the hair cells, with permanent loss of hearing and vertigo (loss of balance and dizziness). Treatment consists of drugs such as diphenhydramine, diazepam, or antihistamines. Home exercise programs have assisted in reducing the individual's sensitivity to motion. In severe cases surgery may be helpful to provide a shunt, to remove excess endolymph, or to resect the vestibular nerve.

Thinkabout 20-25

a. Explain why infants and young children are predisposed to otitis media.

b. Explain why earache is often severe in persons with acute otitis media.

c. Explain two ways in which permanent hearing loss may develop with ear infections.

d. Differentiate conductive hearing loss from sensorineural loss and give an example of each.

e. Explain why Meniere's disease causes both hearing loss and vertigo.

CASE STUDIES

CASE STUDY A
Brain Tumor

Mr. AH, age 44, had a generalized tonic-clonic seizure unexpectedly at work. He had no history of seizures, trauma, infection, or other illness. Investigation revealed a tumor in the right parietal lobe. This was removed surgically, although the diffuse nature of the malignant mass prevented its complete elimination. Radiation treatment was recommended as follow-up.

a. Describe briefly several diagnostic tests that would be of value in this case.

b. Explain the basis of this seizure activity, and describe how it might be controlled.

c. Describe each stage in sequence of a generalized tonic-clonic seizure. Following surgery, Mr. AH demonstrated considerable weakness and sensory loss on his left side.

d. Relate the occurrence of each of these effects to the functional areas of the brain.

e. A few days after surgery, Mr. AH developed a bacterial infection at the operative site. Explain why this infection is likely to increase the motor and sensory deficits.

The infection was eradicated quickly with treatment, but the tumor did not respond to radiation and chemotherapy. As a result, several tumors in the brain grew relatively large during the next 2 months.

f. The cancer treatments caused severe anemia, nausea, and vomiting. Explain how these side effects could cause other complications (describe these clearly) for Mr. AH.

g. Suggest several types of therapy or assistance that would be helpful to Mr. AH during this period. (Extend this question to focus on your specialty area, when possible).

Mr. AH developed severe headaches and diplopia and became increasingly lethargic, and his seizures increased in frequency despite anticonvulsant medication. He was given medication to reduce the frequency of vomiting.

h. Explain the specific rationale for each of his manifestations.

As the tumors increased in size, Mr. AH developed papilledema, and his vital signs indicated increased pulse pressure.

i. Explain the cause of each of these signs.

j. Describe the changes that are likely to occur as coma develops in Mr. AH.

CASE STUDY B
Multiple Sclerosis

WH, a woman of 36, has been diagnosed with multiple sclerosis. She has lost part of her left visual field and has weakness in her left leg. WH's mother had multiple sclerosis.

a. State the factors in the preceding description and the diagnostic tests that would indicate multiple sclerosis as a diagnosis in this case.

b. Describe the pathophysiology of multiple sclerosis.

c. State the possible locations of the lesions that have caused visual and motor deficits.

d. Describe the typical course of multiple sclerosis that WH can expect in future.

e. Suggest several measures that can be used to minimize exacerbations.

f. Explain why adequate nutrition and hydration are important in patients with chronic neurologic conditions. Include specific potential complications that can be so avoided.

g. Explain why a program of moderate activity is important for WH.

CASE STUDY C
Spinal Cord Injury

BL, age 17, has a compression fracture at C5 to C6, a result of diving from a bridge into a river and hitting a submerged rock. Fortunately, a companion who had training as a lifeguard rescued her and tried to minimize any secondary damage. In the emergency department, BL could not move her limbs nor sense touch, and lacked reflexes in her limbs.

a. Explain why caution is needed when handling a person with possible spinal cord injury.

b. Describe a compression fracture and how it can affect neurologic function.

c. Explain why reflexes are absent in BL at this early stage. What type of paralysis is present?

d. Explain why and how BL's respiratory function may be impaired at any time.

e. Explain why the full extent of permanent damage cannot be estimated in this initial period.

Surgery was performed to relieve pressure and stabilize the fracture site.

f. Describe several additional factors that may result in secondary damage to the spinal cord.

g. Explain the anticipated effect in the immediate period of this injury on BL's blood pressure and bladder function.

Several weeks later, routine examination indicated that some spinal cord reflexes were returning in the lower extremities.

h. Explain the significance of returning reflexes.

i. Explain why each of the following could develop in BL and state the early signs for each:

(1) pneumonia, (2) decubitus ulcer, (3) muscle atrophy, and (4) contracture.

j. Briefly describe how the risk of each of the above could be minimized.

Gradually more reflexes returned. Some muscle tone and movement associated with the shoulder and upper arm became apparent, but no other function returned.

k. Explain how the dermatomes can assist in detecting the functional areas.

l. Describe the change to be expected in bowel and bladder function as reflexes return. One day, BL suddenly developed a severe headache and blurred vision. Her blood pressure was 210/120 and pulse 62.

m. What has probably caused this effect, and what action needs to be taken?

n. Suggest the specific components for a rehabilitation program for BL. Expand your comments in areas of particular concern to you.

STUDY QUESTIONS

1. List the contents of the subdural space, subarachnoid space, and dura mater.

2. (a) Describe the specific location and list the functions of each of the following: auditory association area, prefrontal area, Broca's area, cerebellum, RAS. (b) Using Table 20–2 or 20–3 or Figure 20–1, describe the effects of damage to each area of the brain.

3. Draw a simple line diagram of the circle of Willis at the base of the brain by doing the following:
    a. Draw a line to show the division between the two hemispheres and label the top "frontal" and the bottom "occipital."
    b. In the lower half of the drawing, show the basilar artery dividing into two posterior cerebral arteries, and extend each down and to the side to the occipital lobes.
    c. Midway on the line and on either side of it, draw a circle showing each carotid artery.
    d. Draw two branches from each carotid: one extending upward toward the frontal lobe and one outward away from your line.
    e. Label the arteries you have drawn.
    f. Add the communicating arteries to complete the circle and label them.

4. (a) Explain why the circle of Willis is important in the cerebral circulation. (b) Predict the effects of obstruction of the left middle cerebral artery. (c) Explain why a constant supply of oxygen and glucose to the brain is necessary.

5. (a) Describe the characteristics of a spinal cord tract, using an example. (b) Differentiate an upper motor neuron from a lower motor neuron by location and function. (c) Describe a nerve plexus and how it affects nerve distribution. (d) Describe an acquired reflex and include an example.

6. Compare the location and three basic effects of the SNS and the PNS.

7. (a) Describe how the effects of deep coma differ from normal consciousness. (b) Describe the sites of damage that would cause left-sided hemiplegia, receptive aphasia, and loss of hearing.

8. (a) Describe the visual signs of increased ICP. (b) State the rationale for headache with ICP. (c) Describe what changes occur in vital signs (blood pressure, pulse, respiration) with rising ICP.

9. (a) State the common signs and symptoms of a frontal lobe tumor. (b) Predict the initial and progressive signs of a tumor growing in the left parietal lobe. (c) Compare the effects of similar-sized tumors in the occipital lobe and in the brainstem. (d) Explain why there are general signs of pressure with a brain tumor.

10. (a) Compare the pathophysiology and effects of transient ischemic attacks and CVAs. (b) Compare the origins and typical onset of the three categories of CVAs. (c) Describe several important factors in recovery from a CVA.

11. (a) List several causative organisms of meningitis and the age groups primarily affected by each. (b) Describe the significant signs of brain infection including signs of meningitis, brain abscess, and general signs of infection.

12. (a) Compare open and closed head injuries including a description of each, their effects, and their potential complications. (b) Describe the location, usual cause, and basic effect of an epidural hematoma.

13. (a) Compare the pathophysiology of communicating and noncommunicating hydrocephalus. (b) Explain why hydrocephalus occurs in adults.

14. Compare myelomeningocele with cerebral palsy with regard to etiology and effects on motor function and communication.

Box continued on following page

STUDY QUESTIONS *Continued*

15. (a) Describe the sequence of events in a generalized tonic-clonic seizure. (b) Define status epilepticus. (c) Explain why a focal seizure may occur in a person with a head injury.

16. Compare the pathophysiology and early signs of multiple sclerosis and Parkinson's disease.

17. Describe the changes occurring in the brain with Alzheimer's disease and its early effects on function.

18. (a) Describe two ways in which the spinal cord can be damaged in a fall. (b) Explain why it is difficult to predict the degree of permanent damage to the spinal cord during the first few days. (c) Describe the usual effects of transection of the spinal cord in the lumbar region immediately after injury and after recovery from spinal shock. Explain why there is a difference. (d) Describe the cause and effect of autonomic dysreflexia. How are the signs different from those of a stress response?

19. Compare depression and panic disorder in regard to
    a. classification
    b. two significant signs or symptoms
    c. recommended drug therapy

20. (a) Describe the function of each structure in the eye: sclera, cornea, lens, choroid, ciliary process. (b) Compare the signs of acute glaucoma, chronic glaucoma, cataract, and detached retina. (c) Describe the progress in sequence of a sound wave until it is identified in the brain. (d) State two ways in which otitis media can impair hearing permanently.

CHAPTER
21
Endocrine Disorders

KEY TERMS

adenoma
anabolic
antagonistic
atherosclerosis
autoimmune
catabolism
cataracts
cholesterol

ectopic
endemic
gangrene
gluconeogenesis
glucosuria
hyperglycemia
hypoglycemia
hypothalamus

iatrogenic
ketoacidosis
ketones
ketonuria
macroangiopathy
microangiopathy
negative feedback
neuropathy

nocturia
osteoporosis
polydipsia
polyphagia
polyuria
tetany
tropic

REVIEW OF THE ENDOCRINE SYSTEM

The major endocrine glands are scattered throughout the body and include the pituitary gland, the two adrenal glands, the thyroid gland, the four parathyroid glands, the endocrine portion of the pancreas, the gonads, the pineal gland, and the thymus (Fig. 21–1). There are also local hormones secreted in the digestive tract that regulate its secretions and motility. These hormones are discussed in Chapter 18. Endocrine glands secrete hormones directly into the blood. Hormones are chemical messengers that have either an amino acid (protein) structure or a steroid structure, synthesized from the lipid cholesterol. The hormones then circulate to target cells in other glands or tissues. After acting on the target cells, the hormones are metabolized or inactivated and excreted from the body to prevent excessive amounts from accumulating over a period of time. Table 21–1 provides a brief review of major hormones, their sources, and primary effects.

The release of hormones from glands is most fre-

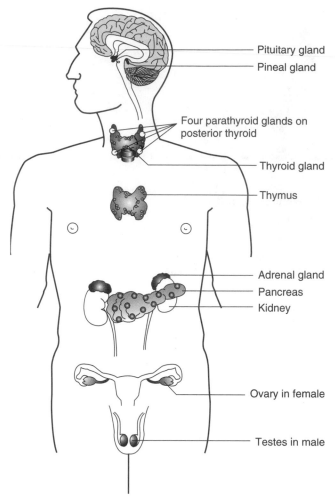

Pituitary gland

Pineal gland

Four parathyroid glands on posterior thyroid

Thyroid gland

Thymus

Adrenal gland

Pancreas

Kidney

Ovary in female

Testes in male

FIGURE 21-1. Location of the endocrine glands.

quently controlled by a **negative feedback** mechanism (Fig. 21–2). For example, as levels of glucose increase, the secretion of insulin increases. When glucose levels decrease, insulin secretion decreases. The endocrine and nervous system work together to regulate metabolic activities. Some hormones are controlled by the nervous system through the **hypothalamus** (e.g., epinephrine and norepinephrine). Together, the hypothalamus and pituitary gland comprise a more complex control system for some hormones (Fig. 21–3). The hypothalamus initially secretes releasing or inhibiting hormones such as thyrotropin-releasing factor (TRF), which acts on the pituitary gland to secrete thyroid-stimulating hormone (TSH). In some cases secretion is controlled by more than one mechanism (e.g., aldosterone). To assist in maintaining a well-controlled blood level of a substance such as calcium, a balance of hormones such as parathyroid hormone and calcitonin is required. These are **antagonistic** hormones and have opposing actions on serum calcium. Another variable affecting hormone levels in the body is the rate or timing of secretion. Some hormones, such as thyroid hormone,

are maintained at fairly constant levels, whereas others are released in large amounts intermittently as the demand occurs. Some hormones such as estrogen follow a cyclic pattern in women. ACTH and cortisol are secreted in a diurnal pattern, the highest levels occurring in the morning and the lowest levels at night. If an individual's sleep pattern changes, the hormonal secretion changes with it. However, any acute stress leads to the SNS overriding this pattern, resulting in a great outflow of ACTH and cortisol.

Thinkabout 21-1

a. A high-carbohydrate meal has what effect on insulin secretion and why?

b. Explain why it is beneficial for more than one hormone to control certain activities, e.g., blood pressure.

When determining the cause of a hormonal deficit or excess, it is necessary to check pituitary hormone levels as well as those of the target gland. For example, a deficit of thyroxine could result from a pituitary problem (decreased secretion of thyroid-stimulating hormone [TSH]) or from a problem in the thyroid gland. In the latter case, blood levels of TSH would be high while thyroxine levels would be low.

Thinkabout 21-2

a. Construct a feedback chart for the glucocorticoids (hydrocortisone).

b. Describe the effect on the natural secretion of hormone from the pituitary gland and the adrenal gland when large amounts of glucocorticoids are ingested.

ENDOCRINE DISORDERS

There are essentially two categories of endocrine problems—an excessive amount of hormone and a deficit of hormone. The manifestations of hormonal disorders reflect the actions of the hormone. The most common cause of endocrine disorders is the development of a benign tumor or **adenoma**. Adenomas may be secretory, causing excess hormone, or they may have a destructive effect on the gland, causing a hormonal deficit. Other causes of hormonal imbalances include congenital defects in the glands, hyperplasia or infection in the glands, abnormal immune reactions, and vascular problems. Frequently, endocrine disorders cause distinctive changes in the individual's physical appearance, which may be helpful in diagnosis.

Not all hormones are covered in this chapter. However, if the normal effects of a hormone are known, it is possible to predict the effects of an excess or deficit. Diagnostic tests and treatment follow similar patterns.

Diagnostic Tests

Levels of **tropic** hormones secreted by the pituitary gland as well as the levels of hormones secreted by the target gland must be evaluated to determine the source of an endocrine disorder (see Fig. 21–10). In some patients, an excessive amount of hormone may arise from an **ectopic** source such as a bronchogenic cancer rather than from a gland. In such cases, the levels of tropic hormones are low.

Blood tests are commonly used to check serum hormone levels, frequently making use of radioimmunoassay (RIA) methods or, more recently, immunochemical methods (enzyme-multiplied immunoassay technique [EMIT] or chemoluminescence). Twenty-four-hour *urine tests* are helpful for ascertaining daily levels of hormones or their metabolites rather than using a random level taken at a specific moment. *Stimulation* or *suppression* tests can be performed to confirm hyperfunction or hypofunction of a gland. *Scans, ultrasound,* and *magnetic resonance imaging (MRI)* are also helpful for checking the location and type of lesion that may be present. *Biopsy* is essential to eliminate the possibility of malignancy.

Treatment

Treatment depends on the cause of the problem. Hormone deficits may be treated with replacement

TABLE 21-1	Sources of Major Hormones and Primary Effects	
Hormone	**Source**	**Primary Effects**
Hypothalamic-releasing hormones	Hypothalamus	Stimuli to anterior pituitary to release specific hormone
Hypothalamic-inhibiting hormones	Hypothalamus	Decrease release of specific hormone by anterior pituitary
Growth hormone (GH, somatotropin)	Pituitary—anterior lobe (Adenohypophysis)	Stimulates protein synthesis
Adrenocorticotropic hormone (ACTH)	(Adenohypophysis)	Stimulates adrenal cortex to secrete primarily cortisol
Thyroid-stimulating hormone (TSH)	(Adenohypophysis)	Stimulates thyroid gland
Follicle-stimulating hormone (FSH)	(Adenohypophysis)	Females—stimulates growth of ovarian follicle and estrogen secretion Males—stimulates sperm production
Luteinizing hormone (LH)	(Adenohypophysis)	Females—stimulates maturation of ovum and ovulation Males—secretion of testosterone
Prolactin (PRL)	Pituitary posterior lobe (Neurohypophysis)	Stimulates breast milk production during lactation
Antidiuretic hormone (ADH, or vasopressin)	(Neurohypophysis)	Increases reabsorption of water in kidney
Oxytocin (OT)	(Neurohypophysis)	Stimulates contraction of uterus after delivery Stimulates ejection of breast milk during lactation
Insulin	Pancreas—beta cells of islets of Langerhans	Transport of glucose and other substances into cells Lowers blood glucose level
Glucagon	Pancreas—alpha cells	Glycogenolysis in liver Increases blood glucose level
Parathyroid hormone (PTH)	Parathyroid gland	Increases blood calcium level by stimulating bone demineralization and increasing absorption of Ca^{++} in the digestive tract and kidneys
Calcitonin	Thyroid gland	Decreases release of calcium from the bone to lower blood calcium level
Thyroxine (T_4) and triiodothyronine (T_3)	Thyroid gland	Increases metabolic rate in all cells
Aldosterone	Adrenal cortex	Increases sodium and water reabsorption in the kidney
Cortisol	Adrenal cortex	Anti-inflammatory and decreases immune response Catabolic effect on tissues Stress response
Norepinephrine	Adrenal medulla	General vasoconstriction
Epinephrine	Adrenal medulla	Stress response Visceral and cutaneous vasoconstriction Vasodilation in skeletal muscle Increases rate and force of heart contraction Bronchodilation

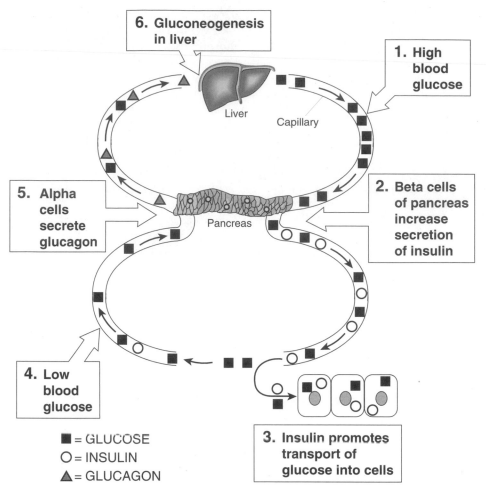

FIGURE 21-2. Negative feedback mechanism with glucose and insulin and glucagon.

therapy. Adenomas may be removed surgically or by radiation therapy. Removal may be essential when pressure from the mass causes additional problems. For example, pituitary tumors cause pressure inside the skull, compressing brain tissue.

PARATHYROID HORMONE AND CALCIUM

Hypoparathyroidism leads to *hypocalcemia,* or low serum calcium levels. Hypocalcemia affects nerve and muscle function in different ways. Low serum calcium levels result in weak cardiac muscle contractions but also increase the excitability of nerves, leading to spontaneous contraction of skeletal muscle. This causes muscle twitching and spasms, commonly known as **tetany**, which is usually observed first in the face and hands. Hypocalcemia does not weaken skeletal muscle contractions because sufficient calcium is stored in skeletal muscle cells. Cardiac muscle cells, on the other hand, do not have large stores of calcium but rely instead on calcium from the blood for contraction.

Hyperparathyroidism causes *hypercalcemia,* or high serum calcium levels. Hypercalcemia leads to forceful cardiac contractions. The most serious effects of hyperparathyroidism occur in the bone tissue. Increased parathyroid hormone (PTH) causes calcium to leave the bone, leading to **osteoporosis**, weakening the bone so that it fractures easily. Hypercalcemia also predisposes to kidney stones. Calcium metabolism is modified by other factors such as the presence of vitamin D and serum phosphate levels. Therefore, calcium imbalance may not be caused by hormone disorders. Serum levels of PTH and calcium may vary depending on the specific cause of the problem. For instance, in patients who are immobile or who have bone cancer, *hypercalcemia* may be present along with a *low* level of PTH (Fig. 21–4). In patients with severe renal disease, there is decreased activation of vitamin D in the kidneys (see Chapter 19). Vitamin D is essential for calcium absorption and metabolism. Renal failure also leads to retention of phosphate ion and hyperphosphatemia. Because calcium and phosphate have a reciprocal relationship, hypocalcemia results. In this case, hypocalcemia leads to *high* levels of PTH. Therefore, any changes in the bone, kidneys, or digestive tract are significant in determining the cause of calcium imbalance, as are serum levels of calcium, phosphate, and PTH.

Thinkabout 21–3

> a. Describe three ways in which increased secretion of PTH can increase blood levels of calcium.
>
> b. Describe the effect of increased calcitonin secretion on blood calcium levels.
>
> c. Explain how malabsorption of calcium from the intestine would affect serum calcium and serum PTH.
>
> d. Compare the effects of hypocalcemia on cardiac and skeletal muscle and explain the rationale for each.

INSULIN AND DIABETES MELLITUS

Diabetes mellitus is a very common chronic disorder. It is a major factor predisposing to strokes (CVA), heart attacks (MI), peripheral vascular disease, kidney failure, and blindness.

Diabetes mellitus is caused by a relative deficit of insulin secretion from the beta cells in the islets of Langerhans or by lack of response by cells to insulin (insulin resistance). In order to simplify the text, insulin deficit is used to cover both decreased secretion of the hormone and insulin resistance. Insulin is an **anabolic** hormone, and deficient insulin results in abnormal carbohydrate, protein, and fat metabolism because the transport of glucose and amino acids into cells is impaired as well as the synthesis of protein and glycogen. In turn, these metabolic abnormalities affect lipid metabolism. Many tissues in the body are adversely affected by diabetes. Some types of cells are not affected *directly* by the loss of insulin. Insulin is not required for transport of glucose into brain cells. This is fortunate, because neurons require glucose as

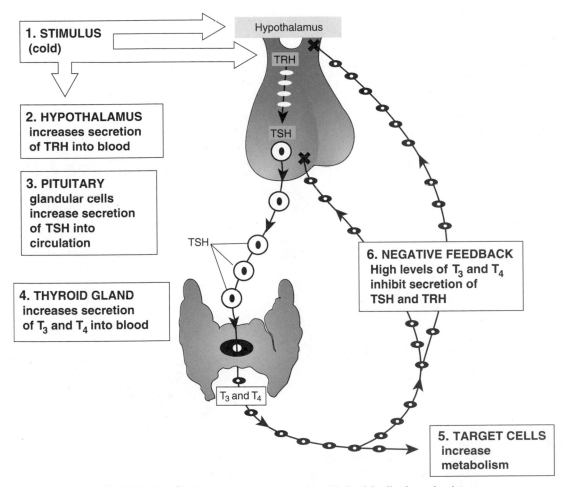

1. STIMULUS (cold)

Hypothalamus

TRH

TSH

2. HYPOTHALAMUS increases secretion of TRH into blood

3. PITUITARY glandular cells increase secretion of TSH into circulation

TSH

4. THYROID GLAND increases secretion of T_3 and T_4 into blood

T_3 and T_4

6. NEGATIVE FEEDBACK High levels of T_3 and T_4 inhibit secretion of TSH and TRH

5. TARGET CELLS increase metabolism

FIGURE 21–3. Hypothalamus-pituitary-thyroid gland feedback mechanism.

A. NORMAL CONTROL AND FEEDBACK OF CALCIUM

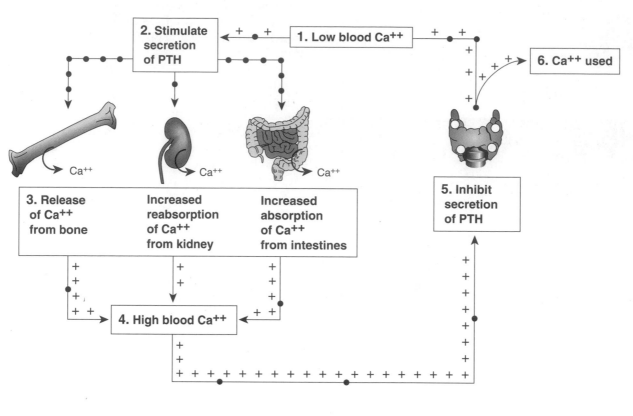

B. EFFECT OF IMMOBILITY ON SERUM Ca++ AND PTH

C. EFFECT OF RENAL DISEASE ON SERUM Ca++ AND PTH

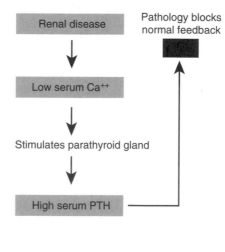

FIGURE 21–4. Calcium and PTH relationships. PTH, •; Ca++, +.

an energy source. In the digestive tract, insulin is not required for glucose absorption. Exercising skeletal muscle can utilize glucose without proportionate amounts of insulin. This can be significant because excessive exercise can deplete blood glucose and result in hypoglycemia. Conversely, exercise is helpful in controlling blood glucose levels in the presence of an insulin deficit.

Comparison of Type I (IDDM) and Type II (NIDDM)

There are two basic types of diabetes, types I and II (Table 21–2). Type I, or insulin-dependent diabetes mellitus (IDDM), sometimes called juvenile diabetes, is the severe form. It results from an absolute deficit of insulin in the body and requires replacement therapy. The amount of insulin required is equivalent to the metabolic needs of the body based on dietary intake and metabolic activity. Type II diabetes, or non–insulin-dependent diabetes mellitus (NIDDM), occurs with a relative or partial deficit of insulin. The supply of insulin is insufficient for the body's needs. This form of diabetes may be controlled by adjusting the need for insulin by reducing dietary intake or by stimulating the beta cells of the pancreas to produce more insulin. Type II is a milder form of diabetes. There are a number of other types of diabetes and glucose intolerance that vary in cause and severity. Gestational diabetes may develop during pregnancy and disappear following delivery of the child. In many cases, women who have gestational diabetes develop diabetes some years later. The following discussion focuses on types I and II.

Pathophysiology

An insulin deficit leads to a sequence of events:

INITIAL STAGE

1. Insulin deficit results in decreased transportation and use of glucose in many cells of the body.
2. Blood glucose levels rise (**hyperglycemia**).
3. Excess glucose spills into the urine (**glucosuria**) as the level of glucose in the filtrate exceeds the capacity of the renal tubular transport limits to reabsorb it.

TABLE 21–2 General Comparison of Type I (IDDM) and Type II (NIDDM) Diabetes

	Type I	Type II
Age at onset	Preadolescence (juvenile onset)	After age 30 (adult onset)
Onset	Acute	Insidious
Hereditary factors	Family history, possible autoimmune factor	Present in immediate family
Body weight	Thin	Obese
Plasma insulin level	Very low	Decreased
Treatment	Insulin replacement	Diet or oral hypoglycemic agents or insulin replacement
Occurrence of hypoglycemia or ketoacidosis	Frequent	Less common

4. Glucose in the urine exerts osmotic pressure in the filtrate, resulting in a large volume of urine to be excreted (**polyuria**) with loss of fluid and electrolytes (e.g., sodium) from the body tissues.
5. Fluid loss through the urine and high blood glucose levels draw water from the cells, resulting in dehydration (see Chapter 6).
6. Dehydration causes thirst (**polydipsia**).
7. Lack of nutrients entering the cells stimulates appetite (**polyphagia**).

Thinkabout 21–4

List the signs of developing diabetes.

If the insulin deficit is severe or prolonged, the process continues to develop, resulting in additional consequences. This occurs more frequently in persons with IDDM.

PROGRESSIVE EFFECTS

8. Lack of glucose in cells results in **catabolism** of fats and proteins, leading to excessive amounts of fatty acids and their metabolites known as ketones or ketoacids in the blood. **Ketones** consist of acetone and two organic acids—beta-hydroxybutyric acid and acetoacetic acid. Because the liver and other cells are limited in the amount of lipids, fatty acids, or ketones they can process completely within a given time, excessive amounts of ketones in the blood cause **ketoacidosis**. The ketoacids bind with bicarbonate buffer in the blood, leading to decreased serum bicarbonate and eventually to a decrease in the pH of body fluids. (Note that ketones can also accumulate in people on starvation diets.)

9. Some ketoacids are excreted in the urine (**ketonuria**), but as dehydration develops, the glomerular filtration rate in the kidney is decreased, and excretion of acids becomes more limited, resulting in decompensated metabolic acidosis, which has life-threatening potential (diabetic ketoacidosis [DKA] or diabetic coma).

Thinkabout 21–5

In people with diabetes mellitus, explain the reason for: (1) thirst, (2) acidosis, (3) polyuria.

Signs and Symptoms

In the early stage, fluid loss is significant. Polyuria is indicated by urinary frequency, which is often noticed by the patient at night (**nocturia**) with the excretion of large volumes of urine. Thirst and dry mouth occur in response to fluid loss. Weight loss may be noticeable. Appetite is increased. Typically, the three P's, polyuria, polydipsia, and polyphagia, herald the onset of diabetes. If the insulin deficit continues, the patient progresses to the stage of diabetic ketoacidosis.

Diagnostic Tests

Fasting blood glucose level, the glucose tolerance test, and the glycosylated hemoglobin test are used to screen people with clinical and subclinical diabetes. Patients with diabetes can monitor themselves carefully at home by taking a sample of capillary blood from a finger and checking it with a portable monitoring machine (glucometer). When performed regularly, this self-monitoring test helps to reduce the fluctuations in blood glucose levels and therefore the risk of complications. Urine tests for ketones are helpful for those who are predisposed to ketoacidosis. Arterial blood gas analysis is required if ketoacidosis develops. Serum electrolytes may be checked as well.

Treatment

Maintenance of normal blood glucose levels is important to minimize the complications of diabetes mellitus, both acute and chronic. Treatment measures depend on the severity of the insulin deficit and may change over time.

DIET

Therapy is based on maintaining optimum body weight (weight reduction may be necessary). This is particularly important for persons with NIDDM. Recommended diets include more complex carbohydrates (minimal amounts of simple sugars are advised) and adequate protein, and maintaining low cholesterol and low lipid levels. The total amount of food intake as well as the distribution of the constituents is important. Food intake must match available insulin and metabolic needs including activity level. Various methods of meal planning are available from the diabetic associations and local diabetic clinics to ensure that the patient ingests a good balance of the various nutrients and to provide information on exchange of food components without disruption of goals.

Thinkabout 21–6

How would omission of a meal affect blood glucose levels and insulin balance?

EXERCISE

A regular moderate exercise program is very beneficial to the diabetic. Exercise can increase the uptake of glucose by muscle substantially without an increase in insulin. It also assists in weight control, reduces stress, and improves cardiovascular fitness.

There is a risk that **hypoglycemia** may develop with exercise, particularly strenuous or prolonged exercise. The increased use of glucose by skeletal muscle plus the increased absorption of insulin from the injection site may lower blood glucose levels precipitously. Increasing carbohydrate intake by eating a snack to compensate for exercise can decrease this risk.

ORAL MEDICATIONS

Antidiabetic agents or oral hypoglycemic drugs such as glyburide are useful in the treatment of NIDDM when diet and exercise alone are not effective. These drugs stimulate the beta cells of the pancreas to increase insulin release. Frequently, a combination of diet, exercise, and oral hypoglycemic drugs can be used to treat mild forms of diabetes.

INSULIN INJECTIONS

Insulin can be used for replacement therapy. It must be injected subcutaneously because it is a protein that is destroyed in the digestive tract if taken orally. Insulin is standardized in units for subcutaneous administration and is produced in three forms: rapid-onset, short-acting (regular) insulin, intermediate-acting (Lente) insulin, and slow-onset, long-acting (protamine zinc [PZI]) insulin. The type of insulin used and its effective period can be important factors in predicting periods of potential hypoglycemia in individual patients, and food intake can be timed to coincide with peak insulin levels, thus avoiding hypoglycemia. Each patient has an individualized schedule of insulin administration. Injection sites must be rotated to minimize skin damage. Insulin types may be mixed for administration, and several injections may be required in one day. Continuous infusions using a small pump are favored by some diabetics. Some individuals develop allergies to insulin extracted from beef or pork pancreas. Human insulin synthesized by bacteria using recombinant DNA techniques is now available. Any transition from one type of insulin to another must be carefully monitored by a physician. Blood glucose levels should be checked at more frequent intervals during any changes. Insulin dosage may also require adjustment under special circumstances such as infection with high fever or vomiting, or at the time of surgery. Continuous control of blood glucose levels minimizes the risk of potential complications for the patient.

Complications

Many factors can lead to fluctuations in serum glucose levels and subsequent changes in cell metabolism throughout the body. These changes may result from variations in diet or physical activity, the presence of infections, or alcohol use. Complications may be acute (e.g., hypoglycemia) or chronic. Long-term complications such as vascular disease result from degenerative changes in the tissues.

ACUTE COMPLICATIONS

Hypoglycemia (Insulin Shock)

Hypoglycemia is precipitated by an excess of insulin, which causes a deficit of glucose in the blood (Fig. 21–5). It usually occurs in patients with IDDM, often quite suddenly, following strenuous exercise, an error in dosage, vomiting, or skipping a meal after taking insulin. The lack of glucose quickly affects the nervous system because neurons cannot use fats or protein as an energy source. The manifestations of hypoglycemia are

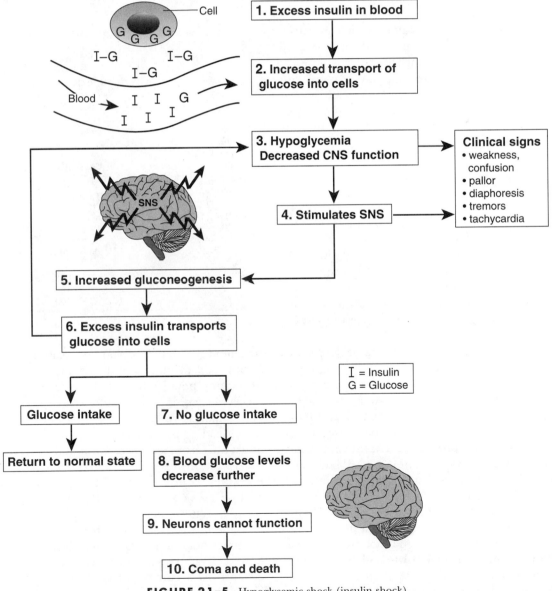

FIGURE 21–5. Hypoglycemic shock (insulin shock).

related directly to the low blood glucose levels, not to the high insulin levels. Many individuals are able to recognize their own response reactions. If hypoglycemia remains untreated, loss of consciousness, seizures, and death will follow.

One group of signs is related to impaired neurologic function resulting from lack of glucose. These signs include poor concentration, slurred speech, lack of coordination, and staggering gait. Persons with hypoglycemia are sometimes assumed to be intoxicated with alcohol. The second group of signs is related to stimulation of the sympathetic nervous system (SNS), resulting in increased pulse, pale, moist skin, anxiety and tremors.

Treatment consists of immediate administration of a concentrated carbohydrate, such as sweetened fruit juice or candy. If the person is unconscious, glucose or glucagon may be given parenterally (usually intravenously).

Hypoglycemia can be life threatening or can cause brain damage if it is not treated promptly. It is wise to verify that patients who have come for other treatments have eaten and taken the appropriate medications before the appointment to minimize the risk of a hypoglycemic episode during the appointment. Appointments should be scheduled so that meals are not unduly delayed or missed.

Diabetic Ketoacidosis

As indicated earlier, diabetic ketoacidosis (DKA) results from insufficient insulin, which leads to high blood glucose levels and mobilization of lipids. It is more common in patients with IDDM. Ketoacidosis usually develops over a few days and may be initiated by an infection or stress, which increases the demand for insulin in the body. It may also result from an error in dosage or overindulgence in food or alcohol.

The signs and symptoms of diabetic ketoacidosis are related to dehydration, ketoacidosis, and electrolyte imbalances (Table 21–3). Signs of dehydration include thirst, dry, rough oral mucosa, and a warm, dry skin. The pulse is rapid but weak and thready, and the blood pressure is low as the vascular volume decreases. Oliguria (decreased urine output) indicates that compensation mechanisms to conserve fluid in the body are taking place. Ketoacidosis leads to rapid, deep respirations (Kussmaul's respirations) and an acetone breath (a sweet, fruity smell). Lethargy and decreased responsiveness indicate depression of the central nervous system owing to acidosis and decreased blood flow. Nausea and vomiting result from electrolyte imbalances and increased ketone levels.

Metabolic acidosis develops as ketoacids bind with bicarbonate ions in the buffer, leading to decreased

TABLE 21–3 Progressive Effects of an Insulin Deficit (Diabetic Ketoacidosis)

Signs	Rationale
Early	
•Hyperglycemia	**Lack of insulin**
•Hunger (polyphagia)	Compensation for cell starvation
•Glucosuria	Glucose in filtrate exceeds tubule transport
•Polyuria	Osmotic diuresis due to glucosuria
•Thirst (polydipsia)	Response to water loss
•Weakness and weight loss	Loss of fluid and lack of glucose to cells
Progressive	
•Increasing hyperglycemia	Gluconeogenesis due to response by epinephrine, cortisol, and glucagon
•Dehydration	**Polyuria**
•Skin warm and dry; decreased turgor	Decreased interstitial fluid
•Oral mucosa rough and dry	Decreased interstitial fluid
•Eyeballs sunken and soft	Decreased interstitial fluid
•Decreased blood pressure	Decreased blood volume
•Pulse—rapid thready	Compensation—sympathetic nervous system
•Lethargy, weakness, confusion	Decreased oxygen and glucose to the brain resulting from hypovolemia. Also acidosis and electrolyte imbalance
•Ketoacidosis	**Catabolism of fats and protein**
•Serum bicarbonate and serum pH low	Compensation for acidosis
•Rapid, deep respirations (air hunger or Kussmaul respiration)	Compensation for acidosis
•Acetone breath—sweet, fruity odor	Acetone expired
•Ketonuria	Ketoacids excreted in urine
•Nausea, vomiting, weakness	Loss of Na^+, K^+, Cl^- in urine and ketonemia
Late	
•Coma	**Central nervous system depression due to acidosis and dehydration**

serum bicarbonate levels and decreased serum pH (see Chapter 6). Electrolyte imbalances include imbalances of sodium, potassium, and chloride. Signs include primarily abdominal cramps and nausea as well as lethargy and weakness. Actual serum values of electrolytes may be misleading because the proportion of water lost can affect the serum level even though the electrolytes were lost in the urine. Serum sodium is often low, but the potassium concentration may be elevated because of acidosis (see Chapter 6). If the condition remains untreated, central nervous system depression develops owing to the acidosis and dehydration, leading to *coma*. Treatment of diabetic ketoacidosis involves administration of insulin as well as replacement of fluid and electrolytes. Serum potassium levels may decrease when insulin is administered because insulin promotes transport of potassium into cells. Bicarbonate administration is essential to reverse the acidosis as well as specific treatment to resolve the causative factor of the diabetic ketoacidosis episode.

Thinkabout 21–7

a. Describe three signs that would help to differentiate someone with hypoglycemia from someone with diabetic ketoacidosis.

b. Describe and explain the loss of consciousness that occurs (1) with hypoglycemia and (2) with diabetic ketoacidosis.

Hyperosmolar Hyperglycemic Nonketotic Coma

Hyperosmolar hyperglycemic nonketotic coma (HHNC) develops more frequently in patients with NIDDM. Often the patient is an older person with an infection or one who has overindulged in carbohydrates, thereby using more insulin than anticipated. In these cases, hyperglycemia and dehydration develop because of the relative insulin deficit, but sufficient insulin is available to prevent ketoacidosis. Therefore, the condition may be difficult to diagnose initially. Severe cellular dehydration results in neurologic deficits, muscle weakness, difficulties with speech, and abnormal reflexes.

Thinkabout 21–8

Compare the characteristics of the urine and the effects on pulse and respiration of hypoglycemia, diabetic ketoacidosis, and hyperosmolar hyperglycemic nonketotic coma.

CHRONIC COMPLICATIONS

Degenerative changes occur in many tissues with both types of diabetes, particularly when blood glucose levels are poorly controlled. The insulin deficit and glucose excess cause a number of alterations in metabolic pathways involving carbohydrates, lipids, and proteins.

Vascular Problems

Changes occur in both the small and large arteries because of degeneration related to the metabolic abnormalities associated with diabetes (Table 21–4). **Microangiopathy,** in which the capillary basement membrane becomes thick and hard, causes obstruction or rupture of capillaries and small arteries and results in tissue necrosis and loss of function. Diabetic *nephropathy,* or vascular degeneration in the kidney glomeruli, eventually leads to chronic renal failure. *Retinopathy* is a leading cause of blindness (Fig. 21–6). Retinal changes can be observed through the pupil of the eye. **Macroangiopathy,** like **atherosclerosis,** affects the large arteries (see Chapter 16), thus leading to a high incidence of heart attacks, strokes, and peripheral vascular disease in diabetics. Obstruction of the arteries in the legs frequently results in ulcers on the feet and legs that are slow to heal and also in intermittent claudication (pain with walking), which greatly impairs mobility. Decreased blood flow also predisposes to frequent infection and gangrenous ulcers. In some cases, vascular problems necessitate amputation if **gangrene** develops.

Neuropathy

Peripheral neuropathy is a common problem for diabetics. It results from ischemia, decreased myoinositol content, and degenerative demyelination of peripheral nerves. This leads to impaired sensation, numbness, tingling, weakness, and muscle wasting. Autonomic nerve degeneration develops as well, leading to bladder incontinence, impotence, and diarrhea. The risks of tissue trauma and infection are greatly

TABLE 21–4 Vascular Problems with Diabetes	
Macroangiopathy	
•Myocardial infarction (heart attack)	Atherosclerosis in large arteries related to hyperlipidemia, hypertension, and degenerative changes in the intimal layer of the arterial wall.
•Cerebrovascular accident (stroke)	
•Peripheral vascular disease (ischemia, gangrene, and amputation affecting the legs)	
Microangiopathy	
•Kidneys Glomerulosclerosis Ischemia and chronic renal failure	Thickening of the capillary basement membrane, leading to occlusion or rupture
•Eyes Retinopathy Leads to blindness	Microaneurysms, neovascularization and fibrosis
•Nervous system Neuropathy in the central nervous system and peripheral nerves Decreased function of sensory, motor, and ANS fibers	*Note*—In addition to ischemia, there is also a metabolic abnormality that causes degeneration of myelin and deficit of *myo*-inositol, essential in the conduction of nerve impulses.

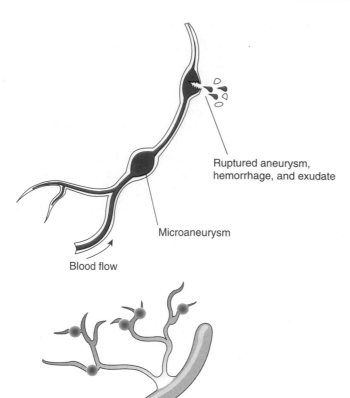

Ruptured aneurysm, hemorrhage, and exudate

Microaneurysm

Blood flow

Neovascularization with rupture and fibrosis

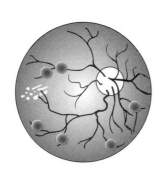

Retina with aneurysms and exudate

FIGURE 21–6. Diabetic retinopathy in the eye.

increased when vascular impairment and sensory impairment coexist.

Infections

Infections are more common and tend to be more severe in diabetics, probably because of the vascular impairment, which decreases tissue resistance, the delay in healing because of insulin deficit, and the increased glucose levels in body fluids, which support infection. The urinary tract is a common site of infection, particularly if bladder function is compromised, and predisposes the patient to cystitis and pyelonephritis. Vaginal and oral fungal infections occur frequently. Infections tend to persist and healing is slow, contributing to a high incidence of gangrene and amputation. Periodontal disease, infection in the tissues around the teeth, and dental caries (infection and decay in teeth) are more common in diabetics. Diabetics are also susceptible to tuberculosis, which is increasing in incidence.

Thinkabout 21–9

> a. Describe all the factors that may lead to a persistent infected ulcer on the foot in patients with diabetes.
> b. Suggest several precautions for foot care that should be taken by diabetics.

Cataracts

Clouding of the lens of the eye (**cataract**) is another degenerative process related to the abnormal metabolism of glucose, and it results in accumulated sorbitol and water in the lens, destroying the transparency. Cataracts may eventually lead to blindness and should be removed when they impair visual function.

Pregnancy

Complications for both the mother and the fetus may occur during pregnancy. Maternal diabetes may become more severe, control is more difficult with the continual hormonal and metabolic changes, and there is an increased incidence of spontaneous abortions and abnormalities in infants born to diabetic mothers. The newborn is usually greater than average in size. Good prenatal care decreases these risks.

PITUITARY HORMONES

Benign adenomas are the most common cause of pituitary disorders. They lead to two types of signs in the patient. One is the effect of the mass as it enlarges and causes pressure in the skull (increased intracranial pressure—see Chapter 20), and the second is the effect of the tumor on hormonal secretion. Signs of pressure on brain tissues include increasing headaches, visual defects, seizures, and drowsiness. The hormonal effects of the adenoma depend on which specific cells in the pituitary are affected. The tumor may secrete an excessive amount of a particular hormone (e.g., somatotropic cells secrete growth hormone [GH]). In some cases, the adenoma may destroy the pituitary cells, causing a deficit of a particular hormone (e.g., decreased ACTH and therefore decreased adrenal cortex activity). As mentioned before, it is important to determine the source of the hormonal imbalance, whether in the pituitary gland or the target gland. Untreated adenomas eventually destroy all types of cells, resulting in panhypopituitarism. Tumors are usually removed by surgery or radiation therapy.

Vascular thrombosis associated with obstetric delivery or other cardiovascular disorders may also damage the pituitary.

Growth Hormone

Dwarfism, or short stature, may be caused by a number of factors, one of which is a deficit of GH (somatotropin) or somatotropin-releasing hormone (Fig. 21–7). In some cases of pituitary adenomas, other types of pituitary cells are also affected, resulting in multiple deficits. Usually the pituitary dwarf has normal intelligence, normal body proportions, and some delay in skeletal maturation and puberty. Replacement therapy for GH deficiency is now available.

Gigantism, or tall stature, results from excess GH prior to puberty and fusion of the epiphyses (see Fig. 21–7).

Acromegaly refers to the effects of excess GH secretion in the adult, usually by an adenoma. The bones become broader and heavier, and the soft tissues grow, resulting in enlarged hands and feet, a thicker skull, and changes in the facial features (see Fig. 21–7). A protruding mandible or jaw (prognathia) and a large tongue (macroglossia) are common. Initially, the patient notices a need for a larger shoe or glove size. In addition, GH affects glucose metabolism and the effectiveness of insulin, resulting eventually in diabetes.

Thinkabout 21–10

Explain why longitudinal bone growth cannot occur in patients with acromegaly.

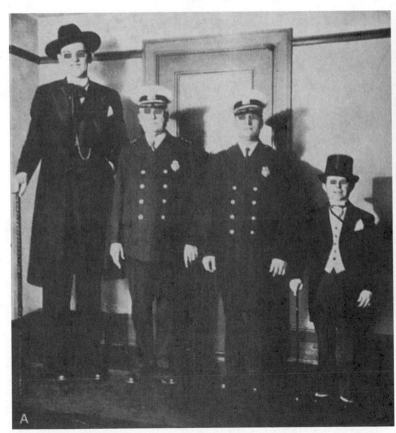

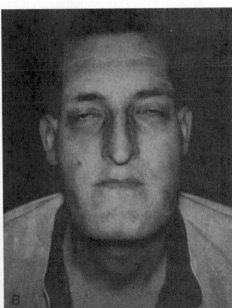

FIGURE 21–7. Effects of growth hormone. *A,* Comparison of *(from left to right)* gigantism, normal, and dwarfism. (From Thibodeau GA: Anatomy and Physiology. St. Louis, Times Mirror/Mosby College Publishing, 1987, pp. 392–393. Courtesy of Dr. Edmund Beard, Cleveland, Ohio.) *B,* Acromegaly. (Adapted from Rimon DL, et al: N Engl J Med 272:923, 1965. Copyright 1965, Massachusetts Medical Society. All rights reserved.)

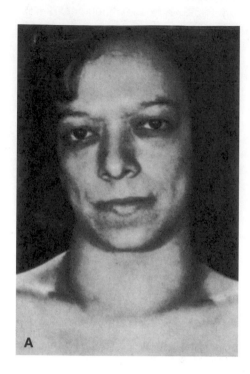

B. STRUCTURE OF THYROID HORMONES

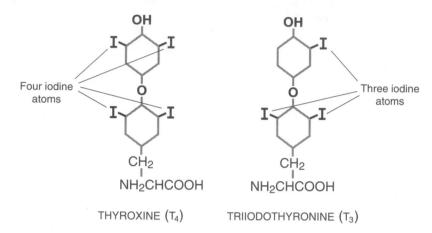

Four iodine atoms

Three iodine atoms

THYROXINE (T₄) TRIIODOTHYRONINE (T₃)

C. GOITER DEVELOPMENT

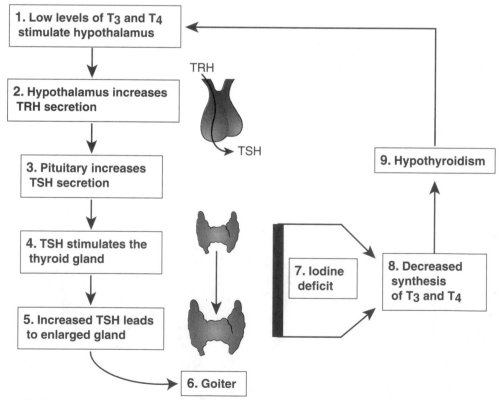

1. Low levels of T₃ and T₄ stimulate hypothalamus

2. Hypothalamus increases TRH secretion

TRH

TSH

3. Pituitary increases TSH secretion

4. TSH stimulates the thyroid gland

5. Increased TSH leads to enlarged gland

6. Goiter

7. Iodine deficit

8. Decreased synthesis of T₃ and T₄

9. Hypothyroidism

FIGURE 21-8. Endemic goiter and hypothyroidism. (*A* from Wilson JD, Foster DW: Williams Textbook of Endocrinology. 8th ed. Philadelphia, W.B. Saunders, 1992, p. 425.)

TABLE 21–5 General Comparison of Hypothyroidism and Hyperthyroidism

	Hypothyroidism	Hyperthyroidism
Serum levels of T_3 and T_4	Low	High
Metabolic rate	Low	High
Goiter	Present with endemic goiter	Present with Graves' disease
Skin	Pale, cool with edema	Flushed and warm
Temperature tolerance	Cold intolerance	Heat intolerance
Eyes		Exophthalmos
Cardiovascular	Bradycardia, enlarged heart	Tachycardia, increased blood pressure
Nervous system	Lethargic, slow intellectual functions	Restless, nervous, tremors
Body weight	Some weight increase with decreased appetite	Thin but increased appetite

ANTIDIURETIC HORMONE

Diabetes insipidus results from a deficit of ADH. Sometimes this condition results from renal tubules that do not respond to the hormone. The clinical manifestations include polyuria with large volumes of dilute urine and thirst, eventually causing severe dehydration. Replacement therapy for ADH is available.

Inappropriate ADH syndrome (SIADH) is due to excess ADH, which causes retention of fluid. In some cases, the additional ADH is secreted by an ectopic source (e.g., a bronchogenic carcinoma). The signs are related to the severe hyponatremia, which causes mental confusion and irritability. Diuretics and sodium supplements are used to correct the problem.

THYROID DISORDERS

Goiter

Goiter refers to an enlargement of the thyroid gland, which is often visible on the anterior neck. Goiters are caused by various hypothyroid and hyperthyroid conditions. A goiter can become very large, compressing the esophagus and interfering with swallowing, or it can cause pressure on the trachea. It can also be of cosmetic concern (Fig. 21–8A). *Endemic goiter* may affect large groups of people in a specific geographical area. It is a hypothyroid condition that occurs in regions where there are low iodine levels in the soil and food (e.g., mountainous areas or around the Great Lakes). Normally, iodine is "trapped" by the thyroid gland and used to synthesize triiodothyronine (T_3) and thyroxine (T_4) (see Fig. 21–8B). This dietary deficiency leads to low T_3

and T_4 (thyroid hormone) production and a compensatory increase in thyroid-stimulating hormone (TSH) from the pituitary, producing hyperplasia and hypertrophy in the thyroid gland (see Fig. 21–8C). The use of iodized salt has resolved this problem to a large extent. *Goitrogens* are foods that contain elements that block synthesis of T_3 and T_4, but increase TSH secretion. TSH causes hyperplasia of the gland and can promote goiter formation when such substances are ingested in large quantities. These foods include cabbage, turnips, and other related vegetables. Lithium and fluoride may also be goitrogenic.

Toxic goiter is a hyperthyroid condition resulting from hyperactivity of the thyroid gland, perhaps due to excessive stimulation by TSH, which produces a large nodular gland.

Hyperthyroidism (Graves' Disease)

Graves' disease occurs more frequently in women over 30 years of age and is related to an **autoimmune** factor. It is manifested by the signs of hypermetabolism, toxic goiter, and exophthalmos (Table 21–5). Exophthalmos results from increased tissue mass in the orbit pushing the eyeball forward. Exophthalmos is evident by the presence of protruding, staring eyes and decreased blink and eye movements (Fig. 21–9). If untreated, visual impairment may result from optic nerve damage or corneal ulceration. Graves' disease is treated by a course of radioactive iodine, surgical removal of the thyroid gland, or the use of antithyroid drugs. Following treatment, there is a risk that patients may develop hypothyroidism or hypoparathyroidism. Thyrotoxic crisis or thyroid storm is an acute situation in a patient with uncontrolled hyperthyroidism, usually precipitated by infection or surgery. It is life threatening because of the resulting hyperthermia, tachycardia, and heart failure and delirium.

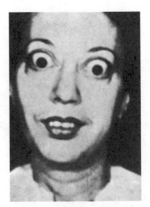

FIGURE 21–9. Hyperthyroidism showing exophthalmos. (From Wilson JD, Foster DW: Williams Textbook of Endocrinology. 8th ed. Philadelphia, W.B. Saunders, 1992, p. 426.)

A. PITUITARY TUMOR
(increased serum ACTH and cortisol)

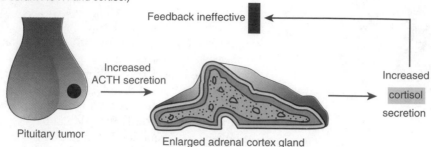

Feedback ineffective

Pituitary tumor

Increased
ACTH secretion

Enlarged adrenal cortex gland

Increased
cortisol
secretion

B. ADRENAL CORTEX TUMOR
(increased serum cortisol, decreased ACTH)

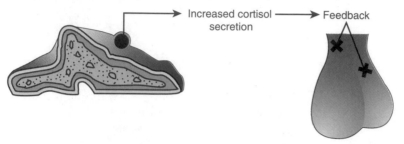

Increased cortisol
secretion

Feedback

Inhibit ACTH secretion

C. PARANEOPLASTIC SYNDROME
(increased serum ACTH and cortisol)

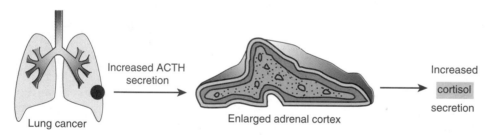

Lung cancer

Increased ACTH
secretion

Enlarged adrenal cortex

Increased
cortisol
secretion

D. IATROGENIC
(increased serum cortisol, decreased ACTH)

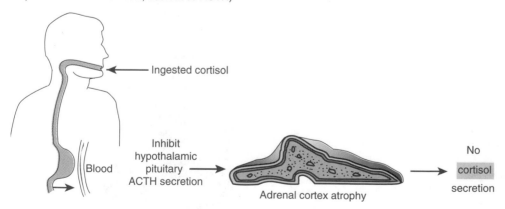

Ingested cortisol

Blood

Inhibit
hypothalamic
pituitary
ACTH secretion

Adrenal cortex atrophy

No
cortisol
secretion

FIGURE 21–10. Cushing's syndrome—causes and feedback effects.

Hypothyroidism

Mild hypothyroidism is very common and is easily treated by replacement doses of thyroid hormone. Signs of hypometabolism are listed in Table 21–5. Severe hypothyroidism occurs in several forms: *Hashimoto's thyroiditis*, a destructive autoimmune disorder; *myxedema*, severe hypothyroidism in adults; and *cretinism*, untreated congenital hypothyroidism, which may be related to iodine deficiency during pregnancy or may be a developmental defect. The thyroid gland may be nonfunctional or absent. Neonatal screening is standard in many areas of the country; it leads to early treatment and prevents the mental retardation that accompanies early hypothyroidism. Lack of treatment results in severe impairment of all aspects of growth and development because thyroid hormone affects the metabolism of all cells. For example, the child may have difficulty feeding, stunted skeletal growth, *extreme* lethargy, delayed tooth eruption, malocclusion, and a large protruding tongue. Myxedema refers to nonpitting edema manifested as facial puffiness and a thick tongue. Myxedema coma refers to acute hypothyroidism resulting in hypotension, hypoglycemia, hypothermia and loss of consciousness, a life-threatening complication occurring in undiagnosed or untreated elderly patients.

Diagnostic Tests

Current tests for thyroid disorders include checks of blood levels of T_4 and T_3 as well as serum TSH levels, the uptake of radioactive iodine (T_3 uptake test). Scans may be used to search for the presence of nodules. Antibody assays may also be required to confirm a specific diagnosis.

ADRENAL GLANDS

Adrenal Medulla

Pheochromocytoma is a benign tumor that secretes epinephrine, norepinephrine, and occasionally other substances. It is one of the "curable" causes of hypertension if it is diagnosed. The signs it produces—headache, heart palpitations, sweating, and anxiety, intermittent or constant—are related to elevated blood pressure.

Adrenal Cortex

Cushing's syndrome is caused by an excessive amount of glucocorticoids (e.g., hydrocortisone), usually related to a pituitary or adrenal tumor (Fig. 21–10A and B). About 15 percent of cases are due to an **ectopic** carcinoma that causes paraneoplastic syndrome (Fig. 21–10C) (see Chapter 5). A large number of cases result from **iatrogenic** conditions, such as administration of large amounts of glucocorticoids for many chronic inflammatory conditions (Fig. 21–10D) (see Chapter 2).

Cushing's syndrome causes a characteristic change in the person's appearance; obesity with a moon face and a heavy trunk with fat at the back of the neck (buffalo hump) and wasting of muscle in the limbs are typical features. The skin is fragile and may have red streaks as well as increased hair growth (Fig. 21–11). Other catabolic effects include osteoporosis and decreased protein synthesis, which delays healing. Metabolic changes include increased **gluconeogenesis** and insulin resistance, which may lead to glucose intolerance. High levels of glucocorticoids suppress the immune response and the inflammatory response and cause atrophy of the lymphoid tissue, predisposing the client to infection. Erythrocyte production is stimulated. Glucocorticoids can also cause emotional lability and euphoria.

The health care worker should be aware of the risk of infection in the patient with Cushing's syndrome and take precautions as necessary. Infection may be local or systemic (e.g., tuberculosis). There may be a decreased stress response in a patient with iatrogenic Cushing's syndrome because of atrophy of the adrenal cortex, and therefore the doses of medication may have to be increased before and during a stressful event. Similarly, dosage must be gradually reduced over a period of time to permit resumption of normal secretory function by the gland.

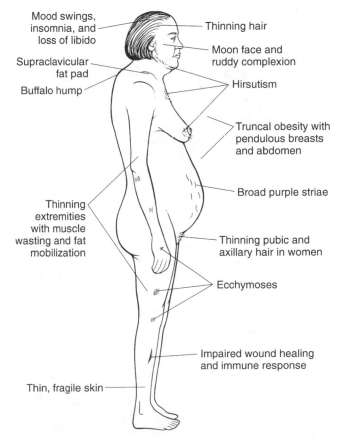

FIGURE 21–11. Cushing's syndrome—typical appearance. (From Monahan FD, Drake T, Neighbors M: Nursing Care of Adults. Philadelphia, W.B. Saunders, 1994, p. 1290.)

Thinkabout 21–11

Explain how diagnostic tests could distinguish a pituitary Cushing's syndrome from an adrenal Cushing's syndrome.

Addison's disease refers to a deficiency of adrenocortical secretions, the glucocorticoids, mineralocorticoids, and androgens. Viral infection is the common cause. Subsequently, an autoimmune disorder causes inflammation and destruction of the gland. The major effects of these hormonal deficits include decreased blood glucose levels, poor stress response, low serum sodium concentration, decreased blood volume and hypotension, decreased body hair due to lack of androgens, and hyperpigmentation in the extremities, skin creases, buccal mucosa, and tongue due to increased ACTH resulting from low cortisol secretion.

Replacement therapy with the necessary hormones controls the disease. Increased doses may be required in times of stress.

CASE STUDIES

CASE STUDY A
Diabetes Mellitus

Mr. F has had insulin-dependent diabetes for 15 years. He has just been admitted to the hospital with severe pyelonephritis, a kidney infection.

1. Explain why urinary tract infections are common in people with diabetes.
2. Mr. F has had the infection for a week and has developed a mild ketoacidosis because of the infection. Analysis of arterial blood gases indicates that his serum bicarbonate level is low and his serum pH is within the normal range.

Explain why infection may lead to ketoacidosis. Describe the characteristics of Mr. F's respirations that you would expect to observe during his experience with ketoacidosis. Include the rationale for your answer.

If Mr. F's serum pH decreases to a point below normal, how would that pH affect cell and organ function?

3. Mr. F is voiding large volumes of urine (polyuria). Explain the reason for this.

Describe three signs of excessive fluid loss.

4. During examination, it is noted that Mr. F has a large ulcerated area on his foot. It appears to have been there for some time. Mr. F said he had not noticed any discomfort in his foot.

Give one possible reason why Mr. F did not notice the ulcer.

Explain why the ulcer may not heal readily.

Explain why gangrene may develop in the foot at some time in the future.

Special shoes are to be ordered for Mr. F. State two other precautions Mr. F could take to prevent additional ulcers.

Mr. F will have to use crutches for a time. How could this affect his other foot and his arms?

5. Mr. F's vision has deteriorated in the last 3 years because of retinopathy.

Explain how retinopathy impairs vision.

Describe two problems related to diabetes that Mr. F might encounter because of his reduced vision.

CASE STUDY B
Cushing's Syndrome

Ms. C has a benign pituitary tumor that has caused Cushing's syndrome.

1. Describe the process by which a pituitary tumor causes Cushing's syndrome. Include the expected serum levels of any hormones.
2. Describe three major effects of Cushing's syndrome on the body. Include a sign of each effect.
3. Explain why Ms. C has neurologic signs such as headache and visual impairment.

STUDY QUESTIONS

1. Why may a spontaneous fracture occur in persons with hyperparathyroidism?

2. Compare the effects of hypocalcemia on skeletal muscle and on cardiac muscle.

3. Explain why a teenager with diabetes mellitus would be more likely than an older adult to have acute complications.

4. Compare the signs of diabetic ketoacidosis and hyperosmolar hyperglycemic nonketotic coma.

5. How would the characteristics of the urine differ in untreated diabetes mellitus and diabetes insipidus?

6. Compare three manifestations that differ in hyperthyroidism and hypothyroidism.

7. Explain why glucocorticoids are considered catabolic hormones and list two specific catabolic effects.

8. Explain why untreated Addison's disease could be life threatening.

9. Describe the effects of hyperaldosteronism.

10. State the hormone imbalance involved in each of the following and list two significant effects of each condition:
    a. gigantism
    b. cretinism
    c. pheochromocytoma
    d. myxedema
    e. acromegaly
    f. diabetes insipidus

CHAPTER
22
Musculoskeletal Disorders

KEY TERMS

acetylcholine	diaphysis	hypertrophy	osteocytes
anabolic steroids	electromyogram	hyperuricemia	osteoporosis
ankylosis	endosteum	ischemic	periosteum
arthroscopy	epiphysis	kyphosis	pseudohypertrophic
articulation	fascia	medullary cavity	scoliosis
atrophy	glycogen	metaphysis	synapse
cholinesterase	hematoma	myoneural junction	tetany
crepitus	hematopoiesis	osteoblasts	uveitis

REVIEW OF THE MUSCULOSKELETAL SYSTEM

Bone

The skeletal system provides rigid support for the body, particularly when it is in an upright position or is in motion. The skeletal framework determines the basic size and proportions of the body. Protection is provided for the viscera, such as the heart and lungs, and for fragile structures such as the spinal cord and brain. Bone also has important metabolic functions related to calcium metabolism and storage and to hematopoiesis in the bone marrow.

Bones may be classified by *shape*. Long bones, such as the humerus and femur, consist of a long hollow shaft with two bulbous ends. Short bones are generally squarish in shape and are found in the wrist and ankle. Flat bones occur in the skull and are relatively thin and often curved. Irregular bones, which have many projections and vary in shape, are represented by the vertebrae and the mandible. Individual bones have unique markings, which may be lines, ridges, processes or holes. Such landmarks provide for attachment of tendons or passage of nerves and blood vessels.

Bone is living connective tissue consisting of an intercellular matrix and bone cells. The matrix is organized in microscopic structural units called *haversian systems* or *osteons*, in which rings of matrix (lamellae) surround a haversian canal containing blood vessels (Fig. 22–1). The matrix is composed of collagen fibers and calcium phosphate salts (e.g., hydroxyapatite crystals), which provide a very strong and rigid structure. Mature bone cells, or **osteocytes,** lie between the rings of matrix in spaces called *lacunae.* Small passages termed canaliculi provide communication between the haversian canals and the lacunae. A dynamic equilibrium is maintained between new bone, which is constantly being produced by **osteoblasts,** and the resorption of old bone by *osteoclast* activity, in accordance with the various hormonal levels and the degree of stress imposed on the bone substance. The osteogenic or bone-producing cells, the osteoblasts, synthesize collagen and protein for the matrix and promote calcification. There are two types of bone tissue, which differ in density. *Compact* bone is formed when many haversian systems are tightly packed together, producing a very strong, rigid structure that forms the outer covering of bones. *Cancellous* or *spongy* bone is less dense and forms the interior structure of bones. Spongy bone lacks haversian systems but is made up of plates of bones bordering cavities that contain marrow.

A typical long bone consists of the **diaphysis,** a thin shaft, between two larger ends or epiphyses (see Fig. 22–1). The diaphysis is formed of compact bone surrounding a medullary cavity containing marrow. The **metaphysis** is the area where the shaft broadens into the **epiphysis.** The epiphysis is made up of spongy bone covered by compact bone. The epiphyseal cartilage or plate ("growth" plate) is the site of longitudinal bone growth in children and adolescents, such growth being promoted by growth hormone and sex hormones. Longitudinal bone growth ceases when the epiphyseal plate ossifies, becoming the epiphyseal line. However, bone may change in density or thickness at any time under the influence of hormones such as growth hormone, parathyroid hormone, or cortisol. The stress (weight-bearing or muscle tension) placed on the bone also affects the balance between osteoblastic and osteoclastic activity. With aging, bone loss is accentuated, resulting in decreased bone mass and density. **Osteoporosis** is common in older people, particularly women (see

Chapter 10). The end of each epiphysis is covered by hyaline cartilage (articular cartilage), which facilitates movement at points of **articulation** between bones. Except for the surface of the bone covered by articular cartilage, the bone is covered by **periosteum**, a fibrous connective tissue. The periosteum contains osteoblasts, blood vessels, nerves, and lymphatics, some of which penetrate into the canals in the bone. When the periosteum is stretched or torn, severe pain results. The **medullary cavity** is lined with **endosteum,** also containing osteoblasts. These osteoblasts are required for bone repair and remodeling as needed. At birth the medullary cavity in most bones contains red bone marrow in which **hematopoiesis** takes place. Gradually, yellow (fatty) bone marrow replaces red bone marrow in the long bones. In adults, red bone marrow is found in the cranium, bodies of the vertebrae, ribs, sternum, and ilia, the last two being the usual sites of bone marrow aspiration used in the diagnosis and monitoring of leukemias and blood dyscrasias.

Thinkabout 22–1

a. List three functions of bone.
b. Differentiate compact bone from cancellous bone.
c. Describe the characteristics of the
(1) periosteum
(2) epiphyseal plate
(3) metaphysis

Skeletal Muscle

Skeletal muscle has four basic functions—(1) to facilitate body movement by muscle contraction, (2) to maintain body position by continuing *muscle tone* (through constant partial muscle contractions), (3) to stabilize the joints and prevent excessive movement, and (4) to maintain body temperature by producing heat through muscle contraction. Skeletal muscle is considered to be under voluntary control, although some muscle activities occur without deliberate intent, such as respiratory movements, blinking, or certain facial expressions and postural adjustments.

Skeletal or *striated* muscle consists of bundles of muscle fibers covered by connective tissue. The striations or striped appearance results from the arrangement of the actin and myosin filaments within the muscle fibers. Muscle tissue is well supplied with nerves

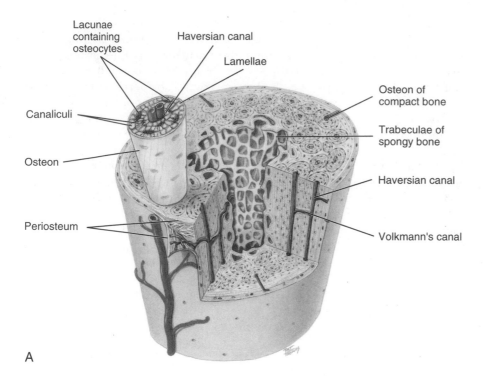

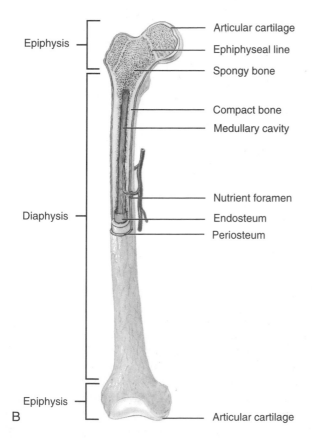

FIGURE 22–1. *A,* Structure of bone. *B,* Structure of a long bone. (From Applegate EJ: The Anatomy and Physiology Learning System. Philadelphia, WB Saunders, 1995.)

and blood vessels to fulfill its function. Each muscle fiber is an elongated muscle cell containing many mitochondria that supply energy for the contraction process. A muscle is stimulated to contract when an efferent impulse is conducted along a motor neuron to a muscle. The axon of the motor nerve branches as it penetrates a muscle so that each muscle fiber in the muscle receives a stimulus to contract at the same time.

At the **myoneural** (or neuromuscular) **junction**, where the **synapse** between the end of the motor nerve and the receptor site in the muscle fiber is located, the chemical transmitter **acetylcholine** is released (see Chapter 20). Following its release and the subsequent muscle contraction, acetylcholine is inactivated by the enzyme **cholinesterase**. Skeletal muscle relaxing drugs may act by blocking the muscle receptor sites, whereas muscle activity may be promoted by drugs that interfere with cholinesterase activity.

Each muscle cell contains myofibrils, which in turn are made up of smaller myofilaments consisting of the proteins actin and myosin. When the muscle fiber is stimulated, *calcium* ions are released from their storage site in the sarcoplasmic reticulum inside the muscle cell. Simultaneously, adenosine triphosphate (ATP) is broken down to adenosine diphosphate (ADP), providing energy, and the actin and myosin filaments slide over each other, resulting in shortening of the muscle cell (contraction). When the nerve stimulus ceases, calcium ions are actively transported (a step that also requires energy) back into the sarcoplasmic reticulum, and the muscle relaxes. During exercise, the blood vessels in the muscles are dilated to promote greater blood flow into the muscle, thus increasing the supply of oxygen and nutrients (glucose and fatty acids) to provide energy for the contraction and to remove metabolic wastes. Limited amounts of oxygen can be bound to *myoglobin* and stored in muscle fibers. Myoglobin is a red oxygen-binding protein, similar in structure to hemoglobin, that is present in muscle cells. **Glycogen**, a source of glucose, is also stored in muscle.

Aerobic respiration to produce ATP can be maintained in muscle fibers as long as adequate oxygen is made available from the myoglobin and the circulating blood. If the supply of oxygen does not meet the demand, the process of *anaerobic respiration* begins, using glucose as the primary energy source and incurring an oxygen debt (the amount of oxygen required to restore the muscle cell to its normal resting state, including converting lactic acid to pyruvic acid, glucose, or glycogen and replenishing stores of ATP). Anaerobic respiration produces lactic acid rather than carbon dioxide and smaller amounts of ATP. The accumulated lactic acid may cause local muscle pain and cramping during and immediately following exercise. A cramp is pain resulting from a strong muscle contraction or spasm, usually caused by local irritation from metabolic wastes. Muscle spasm reduces blood flow, thus leading to **ischemic** pain. Muscle soreness and pain that appears a day or so after strenuous exercise is often due to minor damage to muscle cells and subsequent inflammation. Also, during periods of strenuous physical activity and anaerobic metabolism, excessive lactic acid diffuses into the blood, lowering serum pH and causing metabolic acidosis. This state of acidosis leads to the increased respirations commonly observed during exercise, these respirations operating as a compensatory mechanism to reduce acidosis by decreasing carbon dioxide levels in the blood (see Chapter 6).

A muscle may be attached directly to the periosteum of a bone, but more often the connective tissue covering of the muscle (perimysium) extends to form a cordlike structure or *tendon,* which attaches each end of the muscle to the two bones that articulate at a joint. At a joint, one bone remains fixed, forming the *origin* of the muscle. The other bone attached to the same muscle is moved by the muscle contraction and is called the *insertion.* Ligaments form a direct attachment between two bones. Tendons and ligaments are composed of collagen fibers arranged in bundles, a structure that can withstand considerable stress. At the insertion point of tendons or ligaments there is a gradual transition from the connective tissue to the bone or cartilage. Tendons and ligaments have little blood supply, and therefore healing of these structures is difficult and slow. Muscles may work singly or in groups to perform a specific movement. Also, muscles at a site may be designated as *antagonists,* because one muscle opposes the action of another muscle, allowing movement in either direction. For example, at the elbow, the triceps brachii muscle functions as an extensor muscle, whereas the biceps brachii is a flexor muscle (Fig. 22–2A). Antagonistic muscles prevent excessive movement and provide more control of movements.

Skeletal muscle cells do not undergo mitosis and therefore cannot be replaced. However, muscle cells may undergo **hypertrophy** (increased size of the muscle cell) when the demands are increased, such as with regular exercise. *Aerobic* or *endurance* exercise, such as swimming or running, increases the muscle's capacity to work for a longer time without causing marked hypertrophy of the muscle. Such exercise increases the capillaries and blood flow in a muscle as well as the mitochondria and myoglobin content, thus improving efficiency and endurance. This type of exercise also promotes general respiratory and cardiovascular function. *Anaerobic* or resistance exercise such as weight lifting or bodybuilding regimens focuses on increasing muscle strength by increasing muscle mass (hypertrophy). It is helpful for those persons interested in developing strong muscles to incorporate some aerobic exercise into the training program to improve cardiopulmonary fitness as well as strength. **Anabolic steroids** are used by some athletes, bodybuilders, and others interested in changing the body image to increase muscle strength and mass. Anabolic steroids are synthetic hormones similar to testosterone, the male sex hormone. These synthetic hormones have been developed to increase the anabolic effects, or protein synthesis, and decrease the androgenic or male characteristics produced by these chemicals. Serious and sometimes life-threatening side effects are associated with the use of these substances, such as liver damage, cardiovascular disease, personality changes and emotional lability, and sterility. Unfortunately, this type of steroid is abused by many adolescents and young adults, including those involved in sports, those with eating disorders, and those with psychological problems related to body image and poor self-esteem. The use of anabolic steroids by participants in athletic competition has been banned by many organizations.

Skeletal muscle undergoes **atrophy,** in which muscle cell size is decreased, when the muscle is not used. Atrophy may occur when a fractured limb is placed in a cast or when the pain of arthritis limits movement. Atrophied muscle becomes weak and flaccid. Such *disuse atrophy* is also associated with immobilization and chronic illness (see Chapter 11). Atrophy may be secondary to nerve injury, with resultant flaccid paralysis.

As well, nutritional deficiencies, particularly protein, secondary to disorders such as anorexia or Crohn's disease, lead to atrophy. Skeletal muscle may also become weak owing to degenerative changes involving accumulations of fatty or fibrous tissue. With aging, muscle mass decreases owing to both a decrease in number of muscle cells and a decrease in size (diameter) of the fibers. Muscle strength generally diminishes as well (see Chapter 10), although this may vary with the individual's degree of activity and general health status.

Muscle twitch or **tetany** usually results from increased irritability of the motor nerves supplying the muscle. For example, hypocalcemia causes increased permeability of the nerve membrane and therefore increased or spontaneous stimulation of the skeletal muscle fibers, causing a contraction or spasm of the muscle. Note that sufficient calcium is stored and returned to storage in the skeletal muscle cell following contraction,

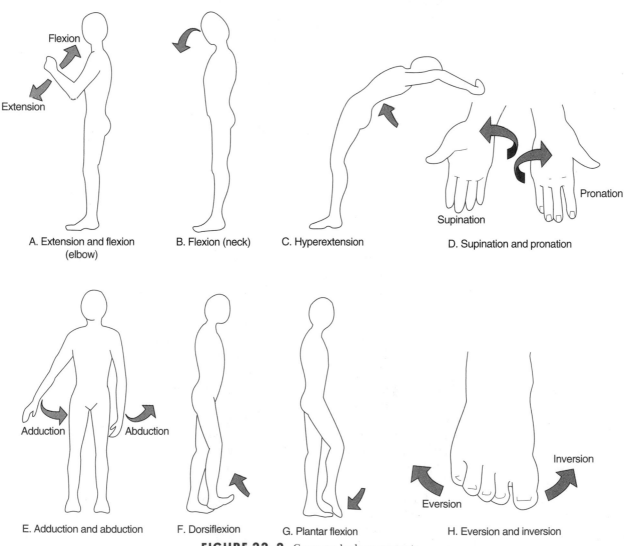

A. Extension and flexion (elbow)   B. Flexion (neck)   C. Hyperextension   D. Supination and pronation

E. Adduction and abduction   F. Dorsiflexion   G. Plantar flexion   H. Eversion and inversion

FIGURE 22-2. Common body movements.

and therefore hypocalcemia does not directly affect skeletal muscle function but rather its innervation.

Thinkabout 22–2

a. Explain why skeletal muscle cells contain many mitochondria.

b. Explain the purpose of shivering when one is cold.

c. What electrolyte is required for skeletal muscle contraction and what is its source?

d. Differentiate muscle hypertrophy from atrophy and give a cause of each.

e. Explain how an anticholinesterase drug affects skeletal muscle function.

f. When does anaerobic metabolism occur in skeletal muscle and what are the effects of this?

Joints

Joints or articulations between bones vary in the degree of movement allowed. The *synarthroses*, represented by the sutures in the skull, are immovable joints. Slightly movable joints, *amphiarthroses*, are joints in which the bones are connected by fibrocartilage or hyaline cartilage. Examples of this type of joint include the junction of the ribs and sternum, and the symphysis pubis. *Diarthroses* or *synovial* joints are freely movable joints and are the most common type of joint in the body. There are different types of diarthroses, allowing a variety of movements. For example, a hinge joint, providing flexion and extension, is found at the elbow, whereas a ball-and-socket joint at the shoulder provides a wide range of motion including rotation. Both hinge and gliding movements are found in the temporomandibular joint (TMJ), controlling the opening of the mouth. Common body movements are illustrated in Figure 22–2.

In a synovial joint, the ends of the bone are covered with *articular* (hyaline) *cartilage*, providing a smooth surface and a slight cushion during movement (see Fig. 22–8A). The joint cavity or space between the articulating ends of the bones is filled with a small amount of slippery *synovial fluid*, which facilitates movement. The synovial fluid prevents the articular cartilage on the two surfaces from damaging each other and also provides nutrients to the articular cartilage. The synovial fluid is produced by the *synovial membrane* (synovium), which

lines the joint capsule to the edge of the articular cartilages. The synovial membrane is well supplied with blood vessels. The *articular capsule* is composed of the synovial membrane and its outer covering, the *fibrous capsule*, a tough protective material that extends into the periosteum of each articulating bone (Sharpey's fibers). The capsule is reinforced by *ligaments*, straps across the joint that link the two bones, which support the joint and prevent excessive movement of the bones. There are some variations in structure in a few joints. The knee has additional moon-shaped fibrocartilage pads, termed lateral and medial *menisci*, which act to stabilize the joint. *Bursae* are fluid-filled sacs composed of synovial membrane and located between structures such as tendons and ligaments; they act as additional cushions in the joint. The TMJ, the only movable joint in the skull and face, has two synovial cavities and a central articular cartilage or meniscus. The *nerves* supplying a joint are those supplying the muscles controlling the joint. These motor fibers are accompanied by sensory fibers from *proprioceptor*s in the tendons and ligaments that respond to the changing tensions related to movement and posture. The joint capsule and ligaments are supplied with pain receptors. With aging, the cartilage in joints tends to degenerate and become thin, leading to difficulty with movement and potential changes in the alignment of bones.

Thinkabout 22–3

a. Name and describe the type of joint found in the skull.

b. Describe two structures in a joint that facilitate movement.

c. Describe the location and purpose of the synovial membrane.

Diagnostic Tests

In persons in whom trauma, tumors, or metabolic disease are suspected, bone abnormalities may be evaluated using x-ray films and bone scans. Serum calcium and phosphate levels may indicate metabolic changes perhaps secondary to renal disease or parathyroid hormone imbalance. Muscle disorders may be checked by determining levels of components such as serum creatine kinase, which is elevated in persons with many muscle diseases. Creatine kinase is an enzyme with an essential role in energy storage, which leaks out of damaged muscle cells into body fluids. **Electromyograms** (EMGs) measure the electrical charge associated with muscle contraction and are helpful in differentiating muscle disorders from neurologic disease. Also, there are devices that can determine the strength of individual muscle groups. Muscle biopsy is required to confirm the presence of some muscular disorders such as muscular dystrophy. Joints may be visualized by **arthroscopy** (insertion of a lens directly into the joint) or by magnetic resonance imaging (MRI), a noninvasive imaging procedure. Synovial fluid may be aspirated and analyzed to ascertain whether inflammation, bleeding, or infection is present.

TRAUMA

Fractures

A fracture is a break in the rigid structure and continuity of a bone (Fig. 22–3). Fractures can be classified in several ways. A *complete* fracture occurs when the bone is broken to form two or more separate pieces, whereas in an *incomplete* fracture the bone is only partially broken. An example of the latter is a *greenstick* fracture, common in the softer bones of children, in which the shaft of the bone is bent, tearing the cortical bone (outer layer of compact bone) on one side but not extending all the way through the bone. An *open* or compound fracture results when the skin is broken (Fig. 22–4). The bone

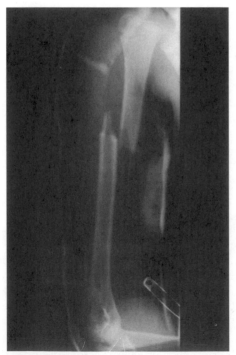

FIGURE 22–3. Fracture of the midshaft of the humerus. (Courtesy of Dr. Mercer Rang, The Hospital for Sick Children, Toronto, Ontario.)

fragments may be angled and may protrude through the skin. In open fractures there is more damage to soft tissue, including the blood vessels and nerves, and there is also a much higher risk of infection. In a *closed* fracture the skin is not broken at the fracture site. A *simple* fracture is a break in the bone in which the bone ends maintain their alignment and position. In a *comminuted* fracture there are multiple fracture lines and bone fragments. A *compression* fracture, common in the vertebrae, occurs when a bone is crushed or collapses into small pieces. An *impacted* fracture occurs when one end of the bone is forced into the adjacent bone. A *pathologic* fracture results from a weakness in the bone structure due to conditions such as a tumor or osteoporosis. The break occurs spontaneously or with very little stress on the bone. Fractures may also be classified by the direction of the fracture line. For example, a fracture across the bone is termed a *transverse* fracture; a break along the axis of the bone is a *linear* fracture; one at an angle to the diaphysis of the bone is an *oblique* fracture; and finally, a break that angles around the bone, usually due to a twisting injury, is called a *spiral* fracture (see Fig. 22–4).

PATHOPHYSIOLOGY

When a bone breaks, bleeding occurs from the blood vessels in the bone and periosteum. Bleeding and inflammation also develop around the bone because of soft tissue damage. This **hematoma** or clot forms in the medullary canal, under the periosteum, and between the ends of the bone fragments (Fig. 22–5). Necrosis occurs at the ends of the bone because the torn blood vessels are unable to continue delivery of nutrients. An inflammatory response develops as a reaction to the trauma and the presence of debris at the site. At fracture sites, the hematoma serves as the basis for a fibrin network into which granulation tissue grows. Many new capillaries extend into this tissue, and phagocytic cells (for removing debris) and fibroblasts (for laying down new collagen fibers) migrate to it. Also, chondroblasts begin to form cartilage. Thus, the two bone ends become splinted together by a *fibrocartilaginous callus* (collar) or *procallus*. This structure is not strong enough to bear weight but constitutes the preliminary bridge repair in the bone. Osteoblasts from the periosteum and endosteum begin to generate new bone to fill in the gap. Gradually the fibrocartilaginous callus is replaced by bone through extensive osteogenic activity, which forms a *bony callus*. Note that damaged bone is repaired by new bone formation, not by scar tissue. During subsequent months the repaired bone is *remodeled* by osteoblastic and osteoclastic activity in response to mechanical stresses on the bone. The excessive bone in the callus is removed, more compact bone is laid down, and eventually the bone assumes a normal appearance.

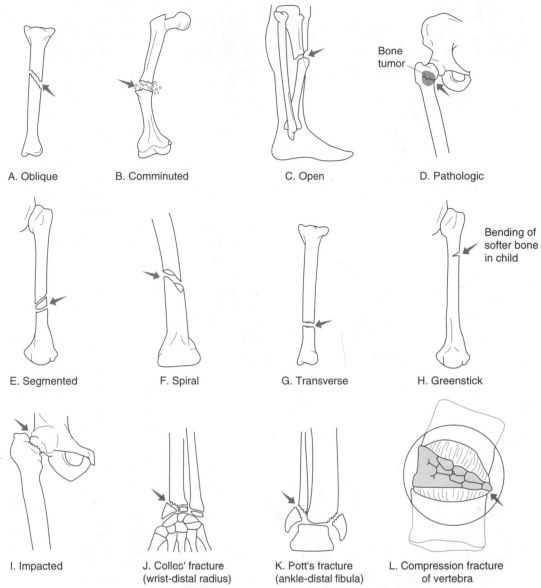

A. Oblique   B. Comminuted   C. Open   D. Pathologic

Bone tumor

E. Segmented   F. Spiral   G. Transverse   H. Greenstick

Bending of softer bone in child

I. Impacted   J. Colles' fracture (wrist-distal radius)   K. Pott's fracture (ankle-distal fibula)   L. Compression fracture of vertebra

FIGURE 22-4. Types of fractures.

Local complications may develop in patients who sustain severe injuries. In some cases, local pain and irritation cause strong muscle contractions or spasm at the fracture site. This muscle spasm pulls the bone fragments further out of position, causing angulation (deformity), rotation of a bone, or overriding of the bone pieces. Such abnormal movement of the bone causes more soft tissue damage, bleeding, and inflammation. *Infections* such as tetanus or osteomyelitis (see Chapter 8) are a threat in persons with compound fractures or when surgical intervention is required. In such cases, precautions include wound debridement, application of a windowed cast, and prophylactic antimicrobial therapy. Ischemia is a complication that develops in a limb following treatment as edema increases during the first 48 hours after the trauma and casting. If the peripheral area (e.g., the toes or fingers) becomes

pale or cold and numb or if the peripheral pulse has decreased or is absent, it is likely that the cast has become too tight and is compromising the circulation in the limb. The cast must be released quickly to prevent secondary tissue damage. During the later stages of healing it is also important that the cast not become too loose as edema decreases and muscle atrophies because the newly formed procallus may break down if there is any bone movement. Nerve damage, failure to heal (nonunion), healing with deformity (malunion), infection (osteomyelitis), and growth retardation in children due to epiphyseal plate damage are other possible complications. *Compartment syndrome* may develop shortly after the fracture occurs when there is more extensive inflammation, such as with crush injuries. Increased pressure of fluid within the **fascia**, the nonelastic covering of the muscle, compresses the nerves and blood ves-

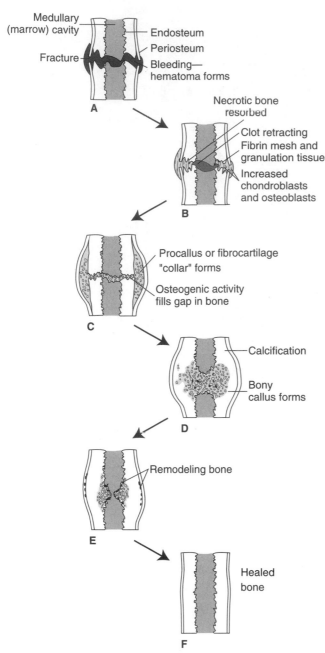

FIGURE 22-5. Healing of a fracture.

emboli, in combination with respiratory distress and severe hypoxia. Fractures in or near the joint may have long-term residual effects such as osteoarthritis or stunted growth if the epiphyseal plate is damaged in a child.

Many factors affect the *healing process* in bone. In children fractures usually heal in approximately 1 month; in adults the process requires 2 or more months. The amount of local damage done to the bone and to the soft tissue is a major determining factor. Extensive damage to the periosteum or blood vessels impairs healing. The more closely approximated the ends of the bone are, the smaller the gap to be filled and the faster the healing process. When necessary to prevent deformity, the bones must be realigned (reduced) in the proper position before healing can begin. It is most important to maintain immobilization of the bones to prevent disturbance or damage to the developing bridge of tissue. Any secondary problem such as infection at the site delays healing. Numerous systemic factors also affect the healing process in bone. For example, fracture repair is delayed in older persons and in individuals with circulatory problems, anemias, diabetes mellitus, or nutritional deficits as well as in those taking drugs such as glucocorticoids.

SIGNS AND SYMPTOMS

In some cases a fracture is clearly present, as in patients with compound fractures or an obvious deformity. Pain usually occurs immediately after the injury, although not always, if nerve function at the site is lost temporarily. Pain results from direct damage to the nerves by the trauma and from pressure and irritation due to the accumulated blood and inflammatory response. Severe pain may cause shock with pallor, diaphoresis, hypotension, and tachycardia. Nausea and vomiting sometimes occur. Swelling, tenderness at the site, or altered sensation are present but may occur with any type of injury. **Crepitus**, a grating sound, may be heard if the ends of the bone fragments move over each other (the limb should not be moved to test for this!).

DIAGNOSTIC TESTS

X-ray films are used to confirm the presence of a fracture.

TREATMENT

Immediate splinting and immobilization (first aid) of the fracture site is essential to minimize the risk of complications. If necessary, *reduction* of the fracture is performed to restore the bones to their normal position. *Closed* reduction is accomplished by exerting pressure and traction; *open* reduction requires surgery. Dur-

sels, causing severe pain and ischemia or necrosis of the muscle. The pressure effects may be aggravated by a cast. *Fat emboli* are a risk when fatty marrow escapes from the bone marrow into a vein within the first week after injury. Fat emboli are more common in patients with fractures of the pelvis or long bones such as the femur, particularly when the fracture site has not been well immobilized during transportation immediately after the injury. Fat emboli travel to the lungs (see Chapter 17), where they cause obstruction, extensive inflammation, and respiratory distress syndrome, and may disseminate into the systemic circulation as well. Frequently the first indications of a fat embolus are behavioral changes, confusion and disorientation associated with cerebral

ing surgery, devices such as pins or screws may be placed to fix the fragments in position; any necrotic or foreign material is removed, and the bone ends are aligned and closely approximated. Immobilization is attained by applying a cast or splints or by using traction. Traction involves the application of a force or weight pulling on a limb that is opposed by body weight. This force maintains the alignment of the bones, prevents muscle spasm, and immobilizes the limb. During the healing period, exercises are helpful to limit muscle atrophy in the immobilized area, maintain good circulation, and minimize joint stiffness or contractures.

Dislocations

A dislocation is the separation of two bones at a joint with loss of contact between the articulating bone surfaces (Fig. 22–6). Usually one bone is out of position while the other remains in its normal location. For example. the humerus is displaced from the shoulder joint. If the bone is only partially displaced, with partial loss of contact between the surfaces, the injury is termed *subluxation*. Trauma, such as a fall, is usually the cause of dislocations. In some cases, a fracture is associated with a dislocation, whereas in others, an underlying disorder such as a muscular disease or rheumatoid arthritis, or other damage such as torn ligaments, may predispose the individual to dislocation.

Dislocations cause considerable soft tissue damage including damage to the ligaments, nerves, and blood vessels as the bone is pulled away from the joint. Bleeding and inflammation result. Severe pain, swelling, and tenderness develop. Deformity and limited movement are usually evident. The diagnosis is confirmed by radiographs. Treatment consists of reduction to return the dislocated bone to its normal position, immobilization during healing, and therapy to maintain joint mobility. Healing is slow if the ligaments and soft tissue are extensively damaged.

Sprains and Strains

A tear in a *ligament* is called a *sprain*, and a tear in a *tendon* is referred to as a *strain*. Ligaments and tendons support the bones in a joint and can easily be torn when excessive force is exerted on a joint. In some cases, the ligaments or tendons can be completely separated from their bony attachments, a problem known as *avulsion*. Sprains and strains are quite painful and are accompanied by tenderness, marked swelling, and perhaps discoloration due to hematoma formation. Strength and range of movement in the joint are limited. Diagnosis requires radiographs and other tests to rule out the presence of a fracture and determine the extent of the damage.

When a tear occurs, inflammation and then granulation tissue develop at the site. Collagen fibers are formed that create links with the remaining tendon or ligament, and eventually the healing mass is bound together with fibrous tissue. A tendon or ligament requires approximately 6 weeks before it is strong again. Stress on a tendon in the early stage will reopen the tear and lead to the development of excessive fibrous tissue in the tendon and thus less strength, shortening and decreased flexibility at the joint. With severe damage to the tendons and ligaments, surgical repair may be necessary.

Thinkabout 22–4

a. Define each type of fracture:
(1) compound
(2) comminuted
(3) transverse
b. Describe the development of the fibrocartilaginous callus and its limitations.
c. Differentiate a dislocation from a sprain.

BONE DISORDERS

Osteoporosis

Osteoporosis is a common disorder characterized by a decrease in bone mass and density, combined with loss

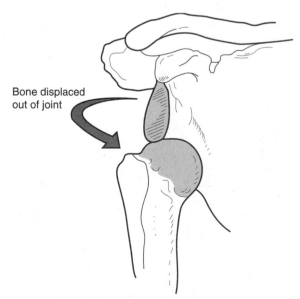

FIGURE 22–6. Dislocation.

Bone displaced out of joint

of bone matrix and mineralization (see Fig. 10–1). Bone resorption exceeds bone formation, leading to thin, fragile bones that are subject to spontaneous fracture, particularly in the vertebrae. Radiographs demonstrate the bone changes.

Osteoporosis occurs more frequently in older individuals, particularly in postmenopausal women with estrogen deficiency (see Chapter 10). Decreased mobility or a sedentary life style is another major factor in the development of osteoporosis. One limb or area of the body may be affected when it is immobilized because of conditions such as a fracture or an acute episode of rheumatoid arthritis. Or decreased osteoblastic activity and osteoporosis may be generalized throughout the skeletal system if a patient is on bed rest for a prolonged time with a chronic illness. Hormonal factors such as hyperparathyroidism, Cushing's syndrome, or continued intake of catabolic glucocorticoids such as prednisone may result in osteoporosis. Other contributing factors include deficits of calcium, vitamin D, or protein and smoking.

Back pain is a common sign of osteoporosis, associated with compression fractures of the vertebrae causing pressure on the nerves. **Kyphosis** and **scoliosis**, abnormal curvatures of the spine and loss of height, are characteristic of the vertebral changes seen with osteoporosis (see Figs. 8–1 and 8–2). Treatment for osteoporosis may include dietary supplements of calcium and vitamin D or protein, regular weight-bearing exercise, and estrogen supplements.

Rickets and Osteomalacia

These conditions result from a deficit of vitamin D or calcium during bone formation that prevents calcification of bone. The result is soft bone and rickets in children. Vitamin D is required for the absorption of calcium, and the lack of calcification of the cartilage forming at the epiphyseal plate leads to weak bones, often deformities, and the typical "bow legs." The child's height is usually below normal. Osteomalacia occurs in adults in whom poor absorption of vitamin D or sometimes calcium causes soft bones and resulting compression fractures. "Renal rickets" refers to osteomalacia associated with severe renal disease (see Chapter 19).

Paget's Disease (Osteitis Deformans)

Paget's disease is a progressive bone disease that occurs in adults older than 40 years. The cause has not yet been established, although a slow virus is suspected. Excessive bone destruction occurs with replacement of bone by fibrous tissue and abnormal bone. Structural abnormalities, evident on radiographs, and enlargement (or thickening) are apparent in the long bones, vertebrae, pelvis, and skull. In some cases, the disease is asymptomatic. Pathologic fractures are common. When the vertebrae are affected, compression fractures and kyphosis result. Skull involvement leads to signs of increased pressure such as headache and compression of cranial nerves. Paget's disease also causes cardiovascular disease and heart failure. Treatment goals are to reduce the risk of fractures and deformity.

Bone Tumors

The majority of primary bone tumors are malignant. Bone is also a common site of secondary tumors, particularly in the spine and pelvis. Metastatic tumors usually have spread from malignant tumors in the breast, lung, and prostate. *Osteosarcoma* (osteogenic sarcoma) is a primary malignant neoplasm that usually develops in the metaphysis of the femur, tibia, or fibula in children or young adults, particularly males. *Ewing's sarcoma* is another malignant neoplasm common in adolescents that occurs in the long bones. Both types of tumors grow quickly and metastasize to the lungs in the early stages of tumor development. Sometimes the tumor is revealed by pathologic fracture. Bone pain is the common symptom, a constant steady pain at rest as well as with activity that gradually increases in severity. An individual often feels the increased pain at night. Treatment may involve surgical amputation, excision with reconstruction surgery, chemotherapy, or radiation, or all of these. *Chondrosarcomas* arise from cartilage and are more common in adults older than 30 years. These tumors develop more gradually in the pelvic bone or shoulder girdle at the points of muscle attachment and eventually metastasize to the lung. Pain does not develop until late, and the tumors may remain silent until they are well advanced.

Thinkabout 22–5

a. Describe four contributing factors to osteoporosis in older women.

b. Explain how osteoporosis leads to loss of height.

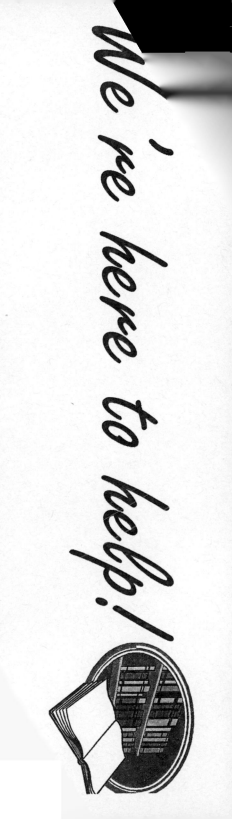

We're here to help!

Hours:

-Th..........	7am-Midnight
F	7am-5pm
Sat..................	10am-5pm
Sun............	1pm-Midnight

Check Out Periods:

Students ....3 weeks
(plus 3-week renewal)
Staff ....3 weeks
(plus 3-week renewal)
Community ....3 weeks
(plus 3-week renewal)
Faculty.............. 6 months
Adjuncts............ 3 months
(no renewals for faculty)

To Renew Books:

Go to "My Library Account"
via library website

Overdue Charges:

(New Policy - August 2006)
$1 per book, per day

PLNU Ryan Librar
(619)849-2312
circlib@pointlom
www.pointloma.ed

DISORDERS OF MUSCLE

Muscular Dystrophy

Muscular dystrophy (MD) is a group of inherited disorders characterized by degeneration of skeletal muscle. The disorders differ in type of inheritance, area affected, age at onset, and rate of progression. Common types are summarized in Table 22–1. Duchenne's or **pseudohypertrophic** muscular dystrophy is the most common type, affecting young male children. X-linked inheritance has been demonstrated in most cases of Duchenne's dystrophy. Serum creatine phosphokinase (CPK) is elevated in many but not all carriers of the abnormal gene and appears prior to the first signs.

The basic pathophysiology is the same in all types of muscular dystrophy. A metabolic defect in the muscle cell leads to degeneration and necrosis of the cell. Skeletal muscle fibers are replaced by fat and fibrous connective tissue (leading to the hypertrophic appearance of the muscle). Diagnosis is based on elevated CPK, which is raised before clinical signs appear, electromyography, and muscle biopsy. Muscle function is gradually lost.

With the Duchenne type of muscular dystrophy, early signs appear at around 3 years of age, when motor weakness and regression become apparent in the child. Initial weakness in the pelvic girdle causes a waddling gait and difficulty with climbing or attaining an upright position. The "Gower sign," in which the child pushes to an erect position by using the hands to climb up the legs, is a typical manifestation. The weakness spreads to other muscle groups and eventually to the shoulder girdle. Tendon reflexes are reduced. Vertebral deformities such as kyphoscoliosis and various contractures develop, and respiratory infections are common. The majority of patients with muscular dystrophy develop cardiac abnormalities, and many exhibit mild mental retardation. Death usually results by age 20 from respiratory or cardiac failure. If the patient chooses to use a ventilator in the event of respiratory failure, the life span can be prolonged substantially. Because no specific treatment is available, the goal is to maintain motor function as much as possible with moderate exercise and the use of supportive appliances.

Thinkabout 22–6

a. Describe the pathophysiologic changes in muscular dystrophy.
b. Explain how vertebral deformities develop in muscular dystrophy.

JOINT DISORDERS

There are many forms of arthritis that impair joint function, leading to various types of disability in all age groups.

Osteoarthritis

PATHOPHYSIOLOGY

Osteoarthritis may be called degenerative or noninflammatory joint disease. In this condition the articular cartilage of certain joints is damaged and lost through structural fissures and erosion resulting from excessive mechanical stress (Fig. 22–7). The surface of the cartilage becomes rough and worn, interfering with easy joint movement. Tissue damage appears to cause release of enzymes from the cells, which accelerates the disintegration of the cartilage. Eventually the subchondral bone may be exposed and damaged, and cysts and *osteophytes* or new bone spurs develop around the margin of the bone. Pieces of the osteophytes and cartilage break off into the synovial cavity, causing further irritation. The joint space becomes narrower, obvious on radiographs. There may be secondary inflammation of the synovium in response to altered movement and

TABLE 22–1	Types of Muscular Dystrophy			
Type	**Inheritance**	**Onset**	**Distribution**	**Progress**
Duchenne's	X-linked recessive (affects males)	2–3 years	Hips, legs, shoulder girdle (ascending)	Rapid
Fascioscapulohumeral (Laundouzy)	Autosomal dominant	Before age 20	Shoulder, neck, and face	Slow to moderate
Myotonic	Autosomal dominant (chromosome 19)	Birth to 50 years	Face, hands	Slow
Limb girdle	Autosomal recessive	All ages	Shoulders and pelvis	Varies

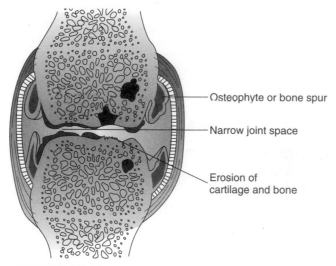

FIGURE 22–7. Pathophysiologic changes with osteoarthritis.

- Osteophyte or bone spur
- Narrow joint space
- Erosion of cartilage and bone

stress on the joint. No systemic effects are present with osteoarthritis.

ETIOLOGY

Osteoarthritis often develops in specific joints because of injury or excessive "wear and tear" on a joint. This is a common consequence of participation in sports and of certain occupations. Congenital anomalies of the musculoskeletal system may also predispose to osteoarthritis. Once the cartilage is damaged, joint alignment or the frictionless surface of the articular cartilage is lost. A vicious cycle ensues, because uneven mechanical stress is then applied to other parts of the joint. The large weight-bearing joints (e.g., the knees and hips) or specific joints that are subject to injury or occupational stress are frequently affected. In some cases of osteoarthritis there is a genetic component, and many cases are idiopathic.

SIGNS AND SYMPTOMS

The pain, which is often mild and insidious initially, is an aching pain that occurs with weight-bearing and movement. Pain becomes more severe as the degenerative process advances. Joint movement is limited. Frequently the joint appears enlarged and hard as the osteophytes develop. Walking becomes difficult if the joint is unstable, and the muscles atrophy, causing a predisposition to falls, particularly in older individuals. When the TMJ is involved, mastication becomes difficult, there is difficulty opening the mouth to speak or yawn, and preauricular pain may be quite severe. Crepitus may be heard. In some cases, other joints are affected as the individual exerts more stress on normal joints to protect the damaged joints.

Osteoarthritis is not a systemic disorder, and therefore there are no systemic signs or changes in serum levels. Diagnosis is based on exclusion of other disorders and radiographic evidence of joint changes consistent with the signs.

TREATMENT

Any undue stress on the joint should be minimized and adequate rest and additional support provided to facilitate movement. Ambulatory aids such as walkers are helpful. Other orthotic devices reduce the risk of deformity and help to maintain function. Analgesics may be required. Surgery is available to repair or replace joints such as the knee or hip.

Rheumatoid Arthritis

PATHOPHYSIOLOGY

Rheumatoid arthritis is considered a chronic systemic inflammatory disease based on an immunologic abnormality that is probably related to viral infection. Immune complexes activate an inflammatory response and subsequent tissue destruction. There are remissions and exacerbations leading to progressive damage to the joints. The disease often commences rather insidiously with symmetrical involvement of the small joints such as the fingers, followed by inflammation and destruction of additional joints (e.g., wrists, elbows, knees). Many individuals also have involvement of the upper cervical vertebrae and TMJ. The severity of the condition varies from mild to severe, reflecting the number of joints affected, the degree of inflammation, and the rapidity of progression.

In the affected joints, the first step is an immune reaction with deposit of immune complexes in the tissue, causing inflammation of the synovial membrane with vasodilation, increased permeability, and formation of exudate, causing the typical red, swollen, and painful joint (Fig. 22–8). This *synovitis* appears to result from the immune abnormality. *Rheumatoid factor (RF)*, an antibody against IgG, as well as other immunologic factors, is present in the blood in the majority of persons with rheumatoid arthritis. RF is also present in synovial fluid. After the first period of acute inflammation, the joint may appear to recover completely. During subsequent exacerbations, the process progresses. Inflammation recurs, synovial cells proliferate, and granulation tissue from the synovium spreads over the articular cartilage. This granulation tissue, called *pannus*, is destructive to the cartilage. The cartilage is *eroded* by enzymes from the pannus, and the pannus cuts off nutrients to the cartilage, normally supplied by the synovial fluid. Erosion of the cartilage creates an unstable joint. In time, the pannus between the bone ends becomes fibrotic, limiting movement and eventually causing *ankylosis* or joint fixation. During each exacerbation or acute period, inflammation and further damage occur in joints previously affected, and additional joints become affected by synovitis.

During this process, other changes frequently occur around the joint. The acute inflammation leads to disuse atrophy of the muscles and stretching of the tendons and ligaments, thus decreasing the supportive structures in the unstable joint. The alignment of the bones in the joint shifts, depending on how much cartilage has been eroded and the balance achieved between muscles. Eventually, deformity with subluxation develops. Various contractures and deformities such as ulnar deviation, swan neck deformity, or boutonnière deformity may present in the hands (Fig. 22–9), depending on the degree of flexion and hyperextension in the joints. On occasion, the inflammation and pain may cause muscle spasm, further drawing the bones out of normal alignment. Mobility is greatly impaired as the various joints become damaged and deformed. Walking becomes very difficult when the knees or ankles are affected.

The inflammatory process has other effects on the body. Rheumatoid or subcutaneous nodules may form on the extensor surfaces of the ulna. Nodules also may form on the pleura, heart valves, or eyes. These are small granulomas on blood vessels. Systemic effects are thought to arise from the circulating immune factors, causing marked fatigue, depression and malaise, anorexia, and low-grade fever. Iron deficiency anemia with low serum iron levels is common; it is resistant to iron therapy.

ETIOLOGY

The exact nature of the immunologic abnormality has not been determined, but it seems to be linked to several viral infections. RF is not present in all patients with rheumatoid arthritis and may be present in certain other disorders as well. Rheumatoid arthritis is more common in women than in men, and the incidence increases with aging.

SIGNS AND SYMPTOMS

Rheumatoid arthritis is insidious at onset, often becoming manifest as mild general aching and stiffness. Inflammation may be apparent in the fingers or wrists. It affects joints in a symmetrical (bilateral) fashion, and usually more than one pair is involved. The joints appear red and swollen and often are very sensitive to touch as well as painful. Joint stiffness occurs following rest, which then eases with mild activity as circulation through the joint improves. Joint movement is impaired by the swelling and pain. Frequently, daily activities become difficult, including dressing, food preparation, and oral hygiene. Malocclusion may develop from TMJ involvement as the condyle is damaged. With each exacerbation of disease, the function of the affected joints is further impaired as joint damage progresses. Eventually, the joint is no longer inflamed but is fixed and deformed (burnt out). The American Rheumatism Association has established criteria for diagnosis based

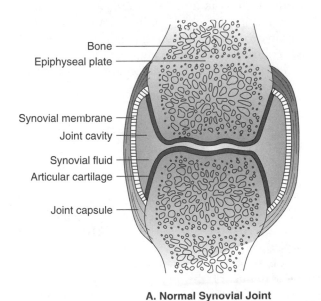

A. Normal Synovial Joint

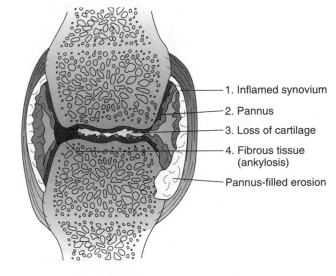

B. Pathologic Changes in Rheumatoid Arthritis

FIGURE 22-8. Pathophysiologic changes with rheumatoid arthritis.

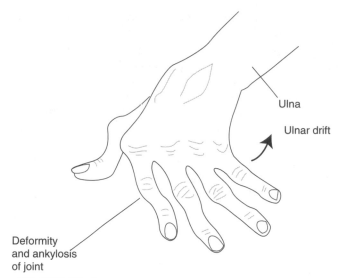

FIGURE 22–9. Deformity in a hand with rheumatoid arthritis.

on the manifestations and length of time they persist, for example, swelling of three joints for a minimum of 6 weeks.

Systemic signs are marked during exacerbations and include fatigue, anorexia, mild fever, and generalized aching.

TREATMENT

A balance between rest and moderate activity is suggested to maintain mobility and muscle strength while preventing additional damage to the joints. Physical therapy is an essential part of any treatment. During acute episodes, joints may require splinting to prevent excessive movement and maintain alignment. Appropriate body positioning and body mechanics when walking or moving also help to maintain function. Assistive devices such as wrist supports or padded handles with straps are available to help the patient cope with daily activities and to reduce contractures. The use of heat and cold modalities can be very effective when they are used correctly. For pain control, relatively high doses of the anti-inflammatory analgesic ASA (aspirin) or non-steroidal anti-inflammatory drugs (NSAIDs) may be required (see Chapter 2). In more severe cases, glucocorticoids may be used, orally or as intra-articular injections. Patients like the effects of glucocorticoids because the drug does promote a feeling of well-being and improves the appetite. However, there are a number of potential complications with long-term use of these drugs, so they should be used only during acute episodes or taken on alternate days at the lowest effective dose. Other drugs, such as gold compounds and immunosuppressants, are used in more resistant cases. Surgical intervention to remove pannus, reduce con-

tractures, or replace joints may be necessary to improve function.

Juvenile Rheumatoid Arthritis

Juvenile rheumatoid arthritis (JRA) is similar in some respects to the adult form of rheumatoid arthritis (see Chapter 8). There are several different types of JRA, and the onset of all of them is usually more acute than the adult form. Systemic effects are more marked, and the large joints are frequently affected. RF is not always present, but other abnormal antibodies such as antinuclear antibodies (ANA) may be present. The systemic form, sometimes referred to as Still's disease, develops with fever, rash, lymphadenopathy, and hepatomegaly as well as joint involvement. A second form of JRA causes polyarticular inflammation similar to that seen in the adult form. A third form of JRA involves four or fewer joints but causes **uveitis**, inflammation of the eye.

Septic (Infectious) Arthritis

Septic or infectious arthritis usually develops in a *single* joint. In some cases there is a history of minor trauma. Blood-borne bacteria are the source of the infection in most cases. *Staphylococcus aureus* and gonococcus are the two most common causative organisms, although anaerobic bacteria are becoming increasingly common. Septic arthritis may also develop from osteomyelitis (see Chapter 8), fractures, or joint-replacement surgery. The synovium is swollen, and a purulent exudate forms, leading to an edematous, red, and painful joint. Aspiration of synovial fluid followed by culture and sensitivity tests confirms the diagnosis. Immediate aggressive antimicrobial treatment is necessary to prevent extensive cartilage destruction and fibrosis of the joint.

Gout (Gouty Arthritis)

Gout results from deposits of *uric acid* crystals in the joint that then cause an acute inflammatory response. This form of joint disease is common in men older than 40. Uric acid is a waste product of purine metabolism, normally excreted through the kidneys. **Hyperuricemia** may develop if renal excretion is not adequate or if there is a metabolic abnormality, often a genetic factor such as a deficit of the enzyme uricase, leading to elevated levels of uric acid. A sudden increase in serum uric acid levels usually precipitates an attack of gout. When acute inflammation develops from uric acid deposits, the articular cartilage is damaged. The inflammation causes redness and swelling of the joint and severe pain. Attacks occur intermittently. Gout often affects a single joint such as the big toe. A *tophus* is a large hard nodule consisting of urate crystals that have been precipitated in soft tissue or bone, causing a local inflammatory reaction. Tophi usually occur a few years after the first attack of gout and may develop at joint bursae, on the extensor surfaces of the forearm, or on the pinnae of the ear. Treatment consists of reducing serum uric acid levels by drugs and dietary changes, depending on the underlying cause. Colchicine may be used during an acute episode, and allopurinol is used as preventive maintenance treatment. This normalization of serum uric acid levels is important because uric acid kidney stones are a threat in anyone with chronic hyperuricemia. Also, relief of the inflammation and pain associated with acute attacks by NSAIDs should be achieved as soon as possible.

Ankylosing Spondylitis

Ankylosing spondylitis is a chronic progressive inflammatory condition that affects the sacroiliac joints, intervertebral spaces, and costovertebral joints of the axial skeleton. Women tend to have peripheral joint involvement to a greater extent than men. It usually develops in persons 20 to 30 years of age and varies in severity. Remissions and exacerbations mark the course. The cause is unknown, but an immunologic basis is likely, given the presence of HLA-B27 antigen in the serum of most patients. In patients with ankylosing spondylitis the joints first become inflamed; then fibrosis and calcification or fusion of the joints follow. The result is ankylosis or fixation of the joints and loss of mobility. The inflammation begins in the lower back at the sacroiliac joints and progresses up the spine, eventually causing a typical "poker back." Kyphosis develops as a result of postural changes necessitated by the rigidity and loss of the normal spinal curvature. Osteoporosis is common and may contribute to kyphosis because of pathologic compression fractures of the vertebrae. Lung expansion may be limited at this stage as calcification of the costovertebral joints reduces rib movement.

Initially, low back pain and morning stiffness are evident. Pain is often more marked when lying down, and it may radiate to the legs similar to sciatic pain. The discomfort is relieved by walking or mild exercise. As calcification develops, the spine becomes more rigid, and flexion, extension, and rotation of the spine are impaired. Some individuals develop systemic signs such as fatigue, fever, and weight loss. Uveitis is a common additional problem.

Treatment is directed at relief of pain and maintenance of mobility. Sleeping in a supine position reduces the tendency to flexion, and an appropriate exercise program promotes muscle support. Anti-inflammatory drugs are useful during exacerbations of disease.

Thinkabout 22–7

a. Prepare a chart comparing osteoarthritis and rheumatoid arthritis with respect to pathophysiology, common joints affected, and characteristics of pain.

b. Describe two unique characteristics of septic arthritis.

c. Explain how the pathophysiologic changes in ankylosing spondylitis differ from those of rheumatoid arthritis.

CASE STUDIES

CASE STUDY A
Fracture

JR, age 17, has a compound fracture of the femur and is undergoing surgical repair.

1. Describe a compound fracture.
2. Give several reasons why it is important in this case to have immobilized the femur well before transporting JR to the hospital.
3. Explain why there is an increased risk of osteomyelitis in this case.
4. Explain why there is severe pain with this type of fracture.

The day after surgery JR's toes were numb and cold.

5. Explain the possible causes of the cold, numb toes.
6. Explain why appropriate exercise is important during healing of the fracture.
7. List four factors that would promote healing of this fracture.
8. Explain why the leg should be elevated during recovery.
9. Explain why, following the removal of the cast, JR can expect to feel some weakness and stiffness in the leg.

CASE STUDY B
Rheumatoid Arthritis

Ms WP is 42 and has had rheumatoid arthritis for 6 years. Her fingers are stiff and show slight ulnar deviation. She is now experiencing an exacerbation, and her wrists are red and swollen. She finds clothing or a touch on the skin over her wrists very painful. Her elbows and knees are also stiff and painful, especially after she has been resting. She is feeling extremely tired and depressed and has not been eating well.

1. Explain the reasons for the appearance and the pain occurring at her wrists.

2. Describe the factors contributing to the stiff, deformed fingers.

3. Explain why some activity relieves the pain and stiffness of rheumatoid arthritis.

4. Describe several factors contributing to the systemic symptoms noted in Ms WP.

5. Explain how each of the following drugs acts in the treatment of rheumatoid arthritis (see Chapter 2). a. NSAIDs b. Glucocorticoids

6. Predict the possible course of this disease in Ms WP.

STUDY QUESTIONS

1. Describe each of the following structures in a bone: (a) endosteum, (b) medullary cavity, (c) diaphysis of a long bone.

2. Define an irregular bone and give an example of one.

3. Where is red bone marrow found in adults? What is the purpose of red marrow?

4. (a) Describe the sources of energy for skeletal muscle contraction. (b) Explain the effect of a cholinergic blocking agent on skeletal muscle contraction (see Chapter 20). (c) Explain how anabolic steroid drugs affect skeletal muscle. (d) Describe the purpose and structure of a tendon. (e) Describe the outcome after part of a muscle has died.

5. (a) Describe the structures that stabilize and support a joint. (b) What type of joint is needed for the articulation between the ribs and sternum? What kind of mobility does it have? (c) Explain the meaning of the term *origin* as related to muscles at a joint.

6. (a) Describe each type of fracture: (i) compression fracture, (ii) pathologic fracture, (iii) spiral fracture. (b) Differentiate the procallus from the bony callus in the healing of a fracture.

7. Compare the changes and effects of a strain and a subluxation.

8. Compare the pathophysiology of osteoporosis, osteomalacia, and Paget's disease.

9. (a) Explain why the muscles of the legs of a child with Duchenne's muscular dystrophy appear large. (b) Explain why only boys are affected by Duchenne's muscular dystrophy. (c) Explain why a child with muscular dystrophy pulls himself up a flight of stairs.

10. Describe the characteristics of synovial fluid in (a) rheumatoid arthritis, (b) gout, (c) septic arthritis, and (d) osteoarthritis.

11. Explain why eating and coughing may be difficult in a person with severe ankylosing spondylitis.

CHAPTER

23

Skin Disorders

KEY TERMS

albinism	denuded	keratin	mitosis
alopecia	dermatome	larvae	paresthesia
atopic	erythematous	lichenification	pruritus
collagen	excoriation	melanin	sebum

REVIEW OF THE NORMAL SKIN

The skin or integument consists of two layers, the epidermis and the underlying dermis along with their associated appendages, such as hair follicles and glands (Fig. 23–1). The *epidermis* consists of five layers, which vary in thickness at different areas of the body. For example, facial skin is relatively thin, but the soles of the feet are protected by a thick layer of skin (primarily stratum corneum). There are no blood vessels or nerves in the epidermis. Nutrients and fluid diffuse into it from blood vessels in the dermis. The innermost layer of the epidermis is the stratum basale, located on the basement membrane. New squamous epithelial cells form by **mitosis** in the stratum basale, and one of each pair of cells then moves upward, forming, in turn, the stratum spinosum, the stratum granulosum, and the stratum lucidum (which is present primarily in thick skin), and eventually being shed from the outer layer, the stratum corneum. While they are in the stratum granulosum, **keratin,** a protein found in skin, hair, and nails, is deposited in these cells. Keratin prevents both loss of body fluid through the skin and entry of excessive water into the body as when swimming. The epithelial cells become flatter as they progress upward

413

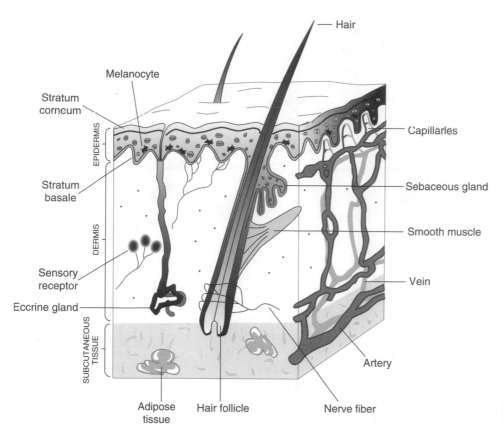

— Hair

Melanocyte

Stratum
corneum

EPIDERMIS

Capillaries

Stratum
basale

Sebaceous gland

DERMIS

Smooth muscle

Sensory
receptor

Vein

Eccrine gland

SUBCUTANEOUS
TISSUE

Adipose
tissue

Hair follicle

Nerve fiber

Artery

FIGURE 23-1. Diagram of the skin.

away from the dermis and eventually die from lack of nutrients. Thus, the stratum corneum, the top or outer layer of the epidermis, consists of many layers of dead, flat, keratinized cells that are constantly sloughed from the surface a few weeks after being formed in the basal layer.

The *dermis* is a thick layer of connective tissue that includes elastic and **collagen** fibers and varies in thickness over the body. These constituents provide both flexibility and strength in the skin and support for the nerves and blood vessels passing through the dermis. Many sensory receptors for pressure or texture, pain, heat, or cold are found in the dermis. The junction of the dermis with the epidermis is marked by papillae, irregular projections of dermis into the epidermal region. More capillaries are located in the papillae to facilitate diffusion of nutrients into the epidermis.

The epidermis also contains melanocytes, specialized pigment-producing cells. The amount of **melanin** or dark pigment produced by these cells determines skin color. Melanin production depends on genetic as well as environmental factors such as sun exposure (ultraviolet light). Melanin protects the skin from ultraviolet radiation. **Albinism** results from a recessive trait leading to a lack of melanin production; consequently, a person

with this trait has white skin and hair and lacks pigment in the iris of the eye. An additional pigment, carotene, gives a yellow color to the skin. Pink tones in the skin are increased with additional vascularity or blood flow in the dermis.

Embedded in the skin are the *appendages*, or accessory structures, the hair follicles, sweat and sebaceous glands, and the nails. The *hair follicles* are lined by epidermis that is continuous with the surface, the stratum basale producing the hair. Each hair follicle has smooth muscle attached to it, the arrector pili, which may be stimulated by emotion or exposure to cold, causing the hairs to stand upright ("on end") or creating small elevations on the skin ("goose bumps"). *Sebaceous* glands may be associated with hair follicles or may open directly onto the skin. These glands produce an oily secretion, **sebum,** which keeps the hair and skin soft and retards fluid loss from the skin. Secretions of sebum increase at puberty under the influence of the sex hormones. *Sweat glands* are of two types. Eccrine or merocrine glands are located all over the body and secrete sweat through pores onto the skin in response to increased heat or emotional stress. Apocrine sweat glands are located in the axillae, scalp, face, and external genitalia, and the ducts of these glands open into the hair follicles.

The secretion is odorless when formed, but bacterial action by normal flora on the constituents of sweat often causes odor to develop. A complex mix of resident flora is present on the skin, and the components differ in various body areas. Microbes are also present deep in the hair follicles and glands of the skin and may be a source of opportunistic infections (see section on burns in Chapter 2). Beneath the dermis is the *subcutaneous tissue or hypodermis*, which consists of connective tissue, fat cells, macrophages, fibroblasts, blood vessels, nerves, and the base of many of the appendages.

Skin has many functions. When unbroken, it provides the first line of defense against invasion by microorganisms and other foreign material. Sebum is acidic and inhibits bacterial growth. The resident flora of the skin is a deterrent to invading organisms. Skin also prevents excessive fluid loss and is important in controlling body temperature, using two mechanisms. Cutaneous vasodilation, which increases peripheral blood flow, and increased secretion and evaporation of sweat both have a cooling effect on the body (see Chapter 2). Sensory perception provided by the skin is important as a defense against environmental hazards, as a learning tool, and as a means of communicating emotions. Another important function of the skin is the synthesis and activation of vitamin D on exposure to small amounts of ultraviolet light.

Thinkabout 23–1

a. Describe three ways in which the dermis differs from the epidermis.

b. Describe how the basal layer of the epidermis is nourished.

c. Describe the role of sebaceous glands and eccrine glands.

d. Explain three ways the skin acts as a defense mechanism.

SKIN LESIONS

The characteristics of skin lesions are frequently helpful in making a diagnosis. Skin lesions may be caused by systemic disorders such as liver disease, systemic infections such as chickenpox (typical rash), or allergies to ingested food or drugs as well as by localized factors. Common types of lesions are illustrated in Figure 23–2 and defined in Table 23–1. The location, length of time the lesion has been present, and any changes occurring over time are significant. Physical appearance, including color, elevation, and texture, type of exudate, and the presence of pain or **pruritus** (itching) are also important considerations.

Some lesions such as tumors are usually neither painful nor pruritic and therefore may not be noticed. A few skin disorders such as herpes cause painful lesions. Pruritus is associated with allergic responses, chemical irritation due to insect bites, or infestations such as scabies. The mechanisms producing pruritus are not totally understood. It is known that release of histamine in a hypersensitivity response causes marked pruritus (see Chapter 3). Pruritus also may result from mild stimulation of pain receptors by irritants. Scratching a pruritic area usually increases the inflammation and may lead to secondary infection. Infection results from breaking the skin barrier, allowing microbes on the fingers (under the nails) or on the surrounding skin to invade the area. Infection may then produce scar tissue in the area.

Diagnostic Tests

Biopsy is an important procedure in the detection of malignant changes in tissue and provides a safeguard following removal of any skin lesion. Bacterial infections may require culture and staining of specimens; skin scrapings and other specific procedures (e.g., ultraviolet light) are necessary to detect fungal infections. Blood tests may be helpful in the diagnosis of allergic or abnormal immune reactions. Patch or scratch tests are also used to screen for allergens.

General Treatment Measures

Pruritus may be treated by antihistamines or glucocorticoids, administered topically or orally. Identification and avoidance of allergens reduce the risk of recurrence. With many skin disorders, extremes of heat or cold and contact with certain rough materials such as wool aggravate the skin lesions. Soaks or compresses using solutions such as Burow's solution (aluminum acetate) or colloidal oatmeal may cool the skin and reduce itching. Infections may require appropriate topical antimicrobial treatment. If the infection is severe, systemic medication may be preferred.

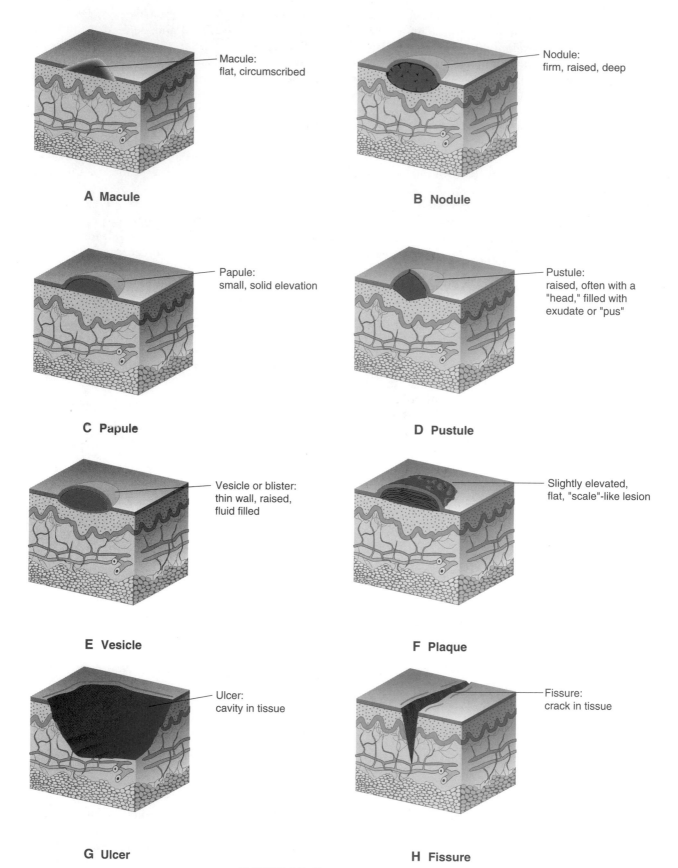

A Macule
Macule: flat, circumscribed

B Nodule
Nodule: firm, raised, deep

C Papule
Papule: small, solid elevation

D Pustule
Pustule: raised, often with a "head," filled with exudate or "pus"

E Vesicle
Vesicle or blister: thin wall, raised, fluid filled

F Plaque
Slightly elevated, flat, "scale"-like lesion

G Ulcer
Ulcer: cavity in tissue

H Fissure
Fissure: crack in tissue

FIGURE 23-2. Common skin lesions.

TABLE 23-1 Description of Some Skin Lesions

Macule	Small, flat, circumscribed lesion of a different color than the normal skin
Papule	Small, firm, elevated lesion
Nodule	Palpable elevated lesion; varies in size
Pustule	Elevated lesion, usually containing purulent exudate
Vesicle	Elevated thin-walled lesion containing clear fluid (blister)
Plaque	Large, slightly elevated lesion with flat surface, often topped by scale
Crust	Dry, rough surface or dried exudate or blood
Lichenification	Thick, dry, rough surface (leatherlike)
Keloid	Raised, irregular, and increasing mass of collagen resulting from excessive scar tissue formation
Fissure	Small, deep, linear crack or tear in skin
Ulcer	Cavity with loss of tissue from the epidermis and dermis, often weeping or bleeding
Erosion	Shallow, moist cavity in epidermis
Comedone	Mass of sebum and keratin and debris blocking the opening of a hair follicle

Thinkabout 23-2

a. Describe each of the following:
(1) macule
(2) vesicle
(3) pustule
b. Describe two causes of pruritus.
c. Explain why scratching a pruritic area may cause a scar.
d. Explain why cellular components of all resected skin lesions should be checked.

INFLAMMATORY DISORDERS

Contact Dermatitis

Contact dermatitis may be caused by exposure to an allergen or by direct chemical or mechanical irritation of the skin. *Allergic* dermatitis may result from exposure to any of a multitude of substances including metals, cosmetics, soaps, chemicals, and plants. Sensitization occurs on the first exposure (type IV cell-mediated hypersensitivity), and thereafter, on subsequent exposures, manifestations such as a pruritic rash develop at the site a few hours after exposure to that allergen. The location of the lesions is usually a clue to the identity of the allergen (Fig. 23–3). For example, poison ivy may cause lesions, often linear, on the ankles or hand, or a necklace may cause a rash around the neck. Typical allergic dermatitis is indicated by a pruritic, **erythema-** tous, and edematous area, which is often covered with small vesicles. Direct *chemical* irritation does not involve an immune response but is an inflammatory response caused by direct exposure to substances such as soaps and cleaning materials, acids, or insecticides. The skin is usually red and edematous and may be pruritic or painful. Removal of the irritant as soon as possible and reduction of the inflammation with topical glucocorticoids are usually effective.

Urticaria (Hives)

Urticaria results from a type I hypersensitivity reaction, commonly caused by ingested substances such as shellfish or certain fruits or drugs. The subsequent release of histamine causes the eruption of hard, raised erythematous lesions on the skin, often scattered all over the body. The lesions are highly pruritic. Occasionally hives also develop in the pharyngeal mucosa and may obstruct the airway, causing difficulty with breathing.

Atopic Dermatitis (Eczema)

Atopic eczema is a common problem in infancy and may persist into adulthood in some persons. Frequently the family history includes individuals with eczema, allergic rhinitis or hay fever, and asthma, indicating a genetic component. Chronic inflammation results from the response to allergens (Fig. 23–4). Eosinophilia and increased serum IgE levels indicate the allergenic basis for atopic dermatitis (type I hypersensitivity). In infants, the pruritic lesions are moist, red, vesicular, and covered with crusts. Involved areas are usually located symmetrically on the face, neck, extensor surfaces of the arms and legs, and buttocks. In adults, the affected skin appears dry and scaling with **lichenification** (thick and leathery patches), although it may be moist and red in the skin folds. Pruritus is common. Areas affected include the flexor surfaces of the arms and legs (e.g., antecubital areas) and the hands and feet. Identification of the causative agents and the use of topical glucocorticoids are helpful. Affected areas also become more sensitive to many irritants such as soaps and certain fabrics. Marked changes in temperature and humidity tend to aggravate the dermatitis, leading to more exacerbations in patients living in areas with dry winter months or hot, humid summers. Potential complications include secondary infections due to scratching and disseminated viral infections such as herpes. Antihistamines may reduce pruritus, and avoidance of skin irritants such as strong detergents or wool, a change to a hypoallergenic diet, and adequate moisturizing of the skin may reduce the inflammation. In severe

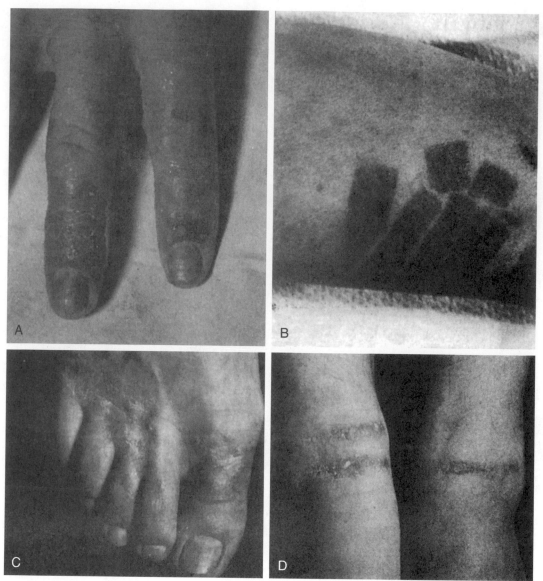

FIGURE 23–3. Various sources of contact dermatitis. *A,* Procaine dermatitis. *B,* Reaction to adhesive tape. *C,* Sensitivity to shoe leather. *D,* Sensitivity to leather shoe strap. (From Moschella SL, Hurley HJ: Dermatology, 2d ed. Vol. 1. Philadelphia, WB Saunders, 1985.)

cases, topical glucocorticoids may be used because severe pruritus may interfere with sleeping and eating, particularly in infants, which then further exacerbates irritability and stress.

Psoriasis

Psoriasis is a chronic inflammatory skin disorder of unknown origin, although it has a familial tendency. Onset usually occurs in the teen years, and the course is marked by remissions and exacerbations. Cases vary in severity. The rate of cellular proliferation is greatly increased, leading to thickening of the dermis and epidermis. Epidermal shedding may occur in 3 to 4 days rather than the normal several weeks. The lesion begins as a small red papule that enlarges. A silvery plaque forms while the base remains erythematous because of inflammation and vasodilation (Fig. 23–5). If the plaque is removed, small bleeding points are apparent. Lesions are commonly found on the face, scalp, elbows, and knees. Psoriatic arthritis is associated with psoriasis in some cases. Treatments that reduce cell proliferation include glucocorticoids, tar preparations, and, in severe cases, the antimetabolite methotrexate. Exposure to ultraviolet light is frequently part of the treatment regimen.

Lichen Planus

Lichen planus is an inflammatory condition of the skin and mucous membranes (Fig. 23–6). The cause is unknown, but the condition has been associated with certain drugs and chemicals. The lesions develop in adults and may last 1 to 2 years. Sometimes the disorder recurs. Basal cell degeneration is evident with reduced mitosis. The lesions are pruritic purplish papules of varying sizes and are found on the wrists, lower legs, and trunk. The papules are flat and white on top and have a slight depression. They become darker and may thicken as they persist. On the oral mucosa or on the vulva and vagina, lichen planus typically appears as an area of white lacy circles. Sometimes the oral lesions ulcerate, and chronic ulcerated lesions need to be monitored for malignancy. Treatment involves the use of topical gluco-corticoids.

Discoid (Cutaneous) Lupus Erythematosus

Discoid lupus erythematosus (DLE) is limited to the inflammatory skin disease. Systemic lupus erythemato-

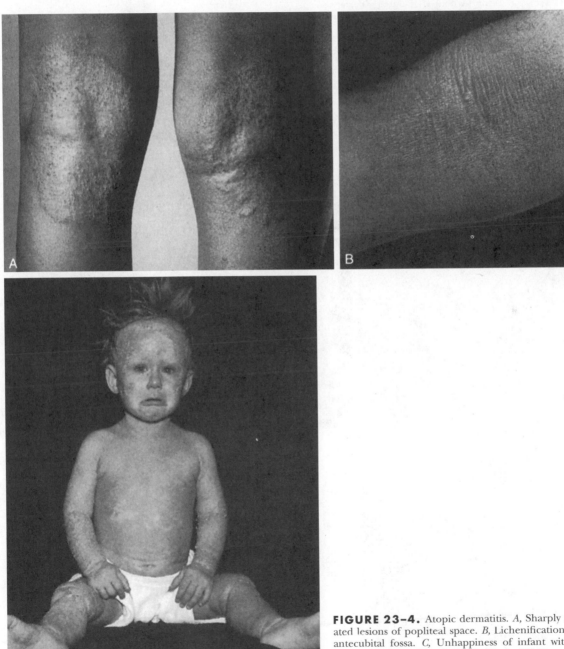

FIGURE 23–4. Atopic dermatitis. *A,* Sharply marginated excoriated lesions of popliteal space. *B,* Lichenification and thickening in antecubital fossa. *C,* Unhappiness of infant with extensive atopic dermatitis. (From Moschella SL, Hurley HJ: Dermatology, 2d ed. Vol. 1. Philadelphia, WB Saunders, 1985.)

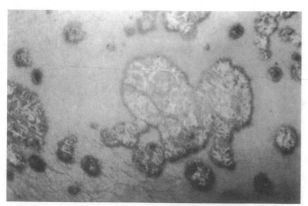

FIGURE 23–5. Psoriasis. (From Arnold HL, Odom RB, James WD: Andrews' Diseases of the Skin, 8th ed. Philadelphia, WB Saunders, 1990.)

plaque with a brown scale that involves the hair follicles. Eventually the lesion heals, often leaving scars and hypopigmentation. **Alopecia** (hair loss) is common in people with scalp lesions. Telangiectasia or dilated capillaries in the skin occurs on the palms of the hands and on the fingers. Raynaud's phenomenon, which involves intermittent vasospasm in the fingers (see Chapter 16), may be associated with DLE. Treatment of DLE includes topical glucocorticoids, use of antimalarial drugs such as chloroquine, and use of sunscreens to reduce the risk of exacerbations.

sus (SLE) is the multisystem disorder discussed in Chapter 3. DLE develops more commonly in women 30 to 40 years old, and an abnormal immune reaction appears to be the basis. There may be one or more lesions on areas of the face or body that are exposed to light. Most frequently, a butterfly pattern develops over the nose and cheeks (see Fig. 3–11). The lesion develops as a red

Pemphigus

Pemphigus is an *autoimmune* (see Chapter 3) disorder that comes in several forms—pemphigus vulgaris, pemphigus foliaceus, and pemphigus erythematosus. The severity of the disease varies among individuals. The autoantibodies disrupt the cohesion between the epidermal cells, causing blisters to form. In the most common form, pemphigus vulgaris, the epidermis separates above the basal layer. Blisters form initially in

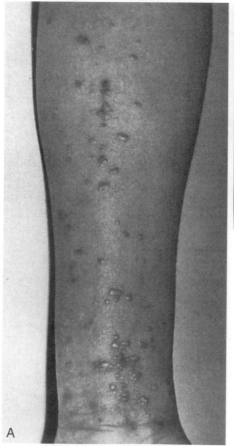

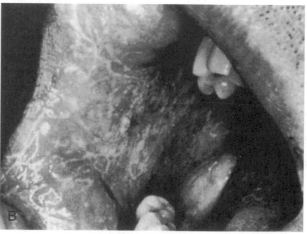

FIGURE 23–6. Lichen planus. *A*, Forearm; *B*, buccal mucosa.(From Arnold HL, Odom RB, James WD: Andrews' Diseases of the Skin, 8th ed. Philadelphia, WB Saunders, 1990.)

the oral mucosa or scalp and then spread over the face and trunk during the ensuing months. The vesicles become large and tend to rupture, leaving large **denuded** areas of skin covered with crusts. Systemic glucocorticoids such as prednisone and other immunosuppressants are used to treat pemphigus.

Scleroderma

Scleroderma may occur as a skin disorder, or it may be systemic, affecting the viscera. The cause is not known. Collagen deposits, inflammation, and fibrosis with decreased capillary networks develop in the skin, leading to hard, shiny, tight immovable areas of skin. The fingertips are narrowed and shortened, and Raynaud's phenomenon may be present, further predisposing the individual to ulceration and atrophy in the fingers. The facial expression is lost as the skin tightens, and movement of the mouth and eyes may be impaired (Fig. 23–7). The cutaneous form may spread to the viscera, eventually causing renal failure, intestinal obstruction, or respiratory failure.

Thinkabout 23–3

a. Describe the typical lesions of atopic dermatitis in the infant and adult in terms of their location and characteristics.

b. Describe the pathologic changes in the skin that occur with psoriasis.

c. Compare the characteristics of the oral and skin lesions of lichen planus.

d. Describe the development of the skin lesions of pemphigus vulgaris.

SKIN INFECTIONS

Bacterial Infections

CELLULITIS

Cellulitis is an infection of the dermis and subcutaneous tissue, usually arising secondary to an injury, a furuncle (boil), or an ulcer. The causative organism is usually *Staphylococcus aureus,* and the area becomes red, swollen, and painful. Antibiotics are usually necessary.

FURUNCLES (BOILS)

A furuncle is an infection, usually by *S. aureus,* which begins in a hair follicle (folliculitis) and spreads into the surrounding dermis. Common locations are the face, neck, and back. Initially, the lesion is a firm, red, painful nodule, which develops into a large, painful mass that frequently drains large amounts of pus. Squeezing boils can result in the spread of infection and cellulitis. For example, compression of furuncles in the nasal area may lead to thrombi or infection that spreads to the brain if the infected material reaches the cavernous sinus (a collecting point for venous blood from the face and brain) in the facial bones. *Carbuncles* are a collection of furuncles that form a large infected mass, which may drain through several sinuses or develop into an abscess.

IMPETIGO

Impetigo is a common infection in infants and young children. *S. aureus* may cause highly contagious infections in neonates, which is a threat in neonatal nurseries. In older children infection results primarily from *S. aureus* but, alternatively, may be caused by group A beta-hemolytic streptococci. The infection is easily spread by direct contact with the hands, eating utensils, or towels. Lesions commonly occur on the face and begin as small vesicles, which rapidly enlarge and rup-

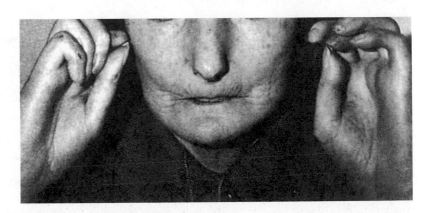

FIGURE 23–7. Scleroderma. (From Arnold HL, Odom RB, James WD: Andrews' Diseases of the Skin, 8th ed. Philadelphia, WB Saunders, 1990.)

ture to form yellowish-brown crusty masses. Underneath this characteristic crust, the lesion is red and moist and exudes a honey-colored liquid. Additional vesicles develop around the primary site. Pruritus is common, leading to scratching and further spread. Topical antibiotics may be used in the early stages, but systemic administration of these drugs is necessary if the lesions are extensive. Unfortunately, the number of antibiotic-resistant strains of *S. aureus* is increasing, resulting in local outbreaks of infection. Another concern with impetigo due to certain strains of streptococci is glomerulonephritis, which can develop if treatment is not instituted promptly (see Chapter 19).

Viral Infections

HERPES SIMPLEX (COLD SORES)

Herpes simplex virus type 1 (HSV-1) is the most common cause of cold sores or fever blisters, which occur on or near the lips. Herpes simplex type 2 is considered in Chapter 24, and herpatostomatitis is covered in Chapter 18. Both types of virus cause similar effects, and type 2 may cause oral as well as genital lesions. The primary infection may be asymptomatic, but the virus remains in a latent stage in the sensory nerve ganglion of the trigeminal nerve, from which it may be reactivated, causing the skin lesion (Fig. 23–8). Recurrence may be triggered by infection such as a common cold, sun exposure, or stress. Reactivation usually is indicated by a preliminary burning or tingling sensation along the nerve and at the site on the lips, followed by development of painful vesicles, which then rupture and form a crust. Spontaneous healing occurs in 2 to 3 weeks, but the acute stage and viral shedding may be reduced by the topical application of antiviral drugs such as acyclovir. The virus is spread by direct contact with fluid from the lesion. Viral particles may be present in the saliva for some weeks following healing of the lesion and therefore can spread the infection to the fingers, for example, if there is a break in the skin. A potential complication is spread of the virus to the eyes, causing keratitis (infection and ulceration of the cornea).

HERPES ZOSTER (SHINGLES)

Herpes zoster is caused by varicella-zoster virus (VSV) in adults. It occurs years after the primary infection of varicella or chickenpox, which usually occurs in childhood. Shingles usually affects one cranial nerve or one **dermatome**, a cutaneous area innervated by a spinal nerve (see Fig. 20–17) on one side of the body. Pain, **paresthesia**, and a vesicular rash develop in a line, unilaterally. This may occur on the face (e.g., following the trigeminal nerve) or along the path of a lumbar nerve from the spine extending around one side in the hip area (Fig. 23–9). The lesions persist for several weeks and then clear. In patients with immune deficiencies, the lesions tend to spread locally. Visual impairment has resulted from involvement of the ophthalmic division of the trigeminal nerve. In some cases, particularly in older individuals, neuralgia or pain continues after the lesions disappear. Antiviral medications such as acyclovir or vidarabine have provided some relief from symptoms.

Fungal Infections (Mycoses)

Fungal infections are diagnosed from scrapings of the skin processed with potassium hydroxide, which accentuates the spores and hyphae (filaments) of the fungal growth, which then becomes fluorescent in ultraviolet light. Most fungal infections are superficial because the fungi live off the dead keratinized cells of the epidermis. Specific antifungal agents are required to treat these infections. Candidal infections are discussed in Chapters 18 and 24.

TINEA

Tinea may cause several types of superficial skin infections (dermatophytoses or ringworm), depending on the area of the body affected. *Tinea capitis* is an infection of the scalp that is common in school-aged children. The infection may result from *Microsporum canis*, transmitted by cats and dogs, or by *Trichophyton tonsurans*, transmitted by humans. It manifests as a circular bald patch as hair is broken off above the scalp. Erythema or scaling may be apparent. Oral antifungal agents such as griseofulvin are recommended. *Tinea corporis* is a fungal infection of the body, particularly the nonhairy parts. The lesion is a round erythematous ring of vesicles or papules with a clear center (*ring*worm) scattered over the body. Pruritus or a burning sensation may be present. Topical antifungal medications such as tolnaftate or ketoconazole are effective. *Tinea pedis*, or athlete's foot, involves the feet, particularly the toes. *Trichophyton mentagrophytes* or *Trichophyton rubrum* are the usual causative organisms. This condition may be associated with swimming pools and gymnasia if appropriate precautions are not in place. The organisms may be normal flora that become opportunists, or spread easily from lesions under conditions of excessive warmth and moisture. The skin between the toes becomes inflamed and macerated with painful fissures (Fig. 23–10). The feet may have a foul odor. Secondary bacterial infection is common. Topical tolnaftate is usually effective. *Tinea unguium* or onychomycosis is an infection of the nails, particularly the toenails. Infection begins at the tip of

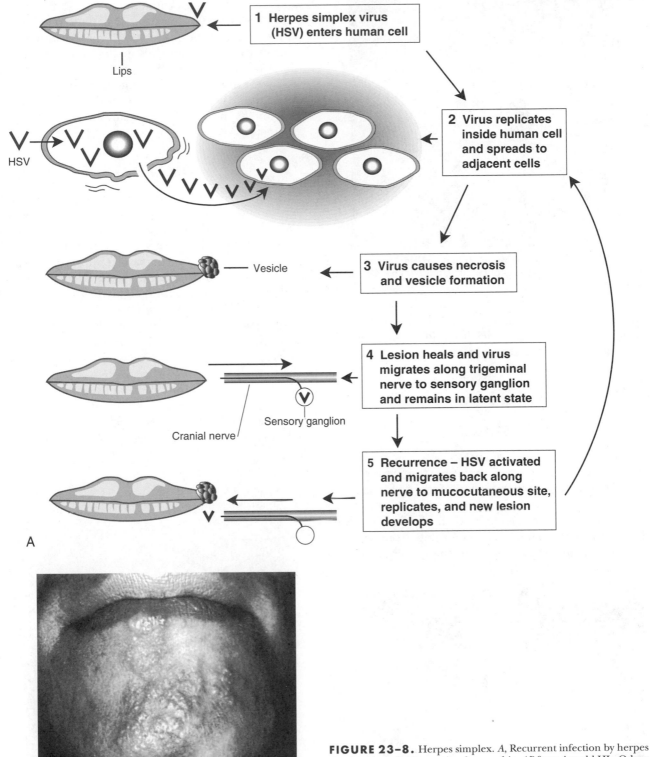

FIGURE 23–8. Herpes simplex. *A*, Recurrent infection by herpes simplex virus. *B*, Herpes simplex on chin. (*B* from Arnold HL, Odom RB, James WD: Andrews' Diseases of the Skin, 8th ed. Philadelphia, WB Saunders, 1990.)

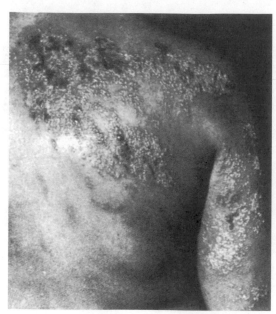

FIGURE 23-9. Herpes zoster. (From Arnold HL, Odom RB, James WD: Andrews' Diseases of the Skin, 8th ed. Philadelphia, WB Saunders, 1990.)

one or two nails, the nail turning first white and then brown. The nail then thickens and cracks, and the infection tends to spread to other nails.

Other Infections

SCABIES

Scabies is the outcome of an invasion by a mite, *Sarcoptes scabiei.* The female mite burrows into the epidermis, laying eggs over a period of several weeks as she moves along in the stratum corneum. The male dies after fertilizing the female, and the female dies after laying the eggs. The **larvae** emerging from the eggs migrate to the skin surface and then burrow into the

skin in search of nutrients. As the larvae mature into adults, the cycle is repeated. The burrows appear on the skin as tiny light brown lines, often with small vesicles and erythema. The inflammation and pruritus that result are caused by the damage done to the skin by the burrowing and the presence of mite fecal material in the burrow. Common sites include the areas between the fingers, the wrists, the inner surfaces of the elbow, and waist line. Topical treatment with lindane is effective. Mites can survive for only a short time away from the human host and are usually spread only by close contact.

PEDICULOSIS (LICE)

Pediculosis can take three forms in humans. *Pediculus humanus corporis* is the body louse, *Pediculus pubis* is the pubic louse, and *Pediculus humanus capitis* is the head louse (cooties). Lice are small brownish parasites that feed off human blood (humans are hosts only to human lice, not to animal lice) and cannot survive for long without the human host. Female lice lay eggs on hair shafts, cementing the egg firmly to the hair close to the scalp (Fig. 23–11). The egg or *nit* appears as a small whitish shell attached to a hair. After hatching, the louse bites the human host, sucking blood for its survival. The site of each bite is demonstrated by a macule or papule, which is highly pruritic owing to the mite saliva. The **excoriations** that result from scratching and visible nits provide evidence of infestation, the adult lice usually not being visible themselves. Topical lindane or per-

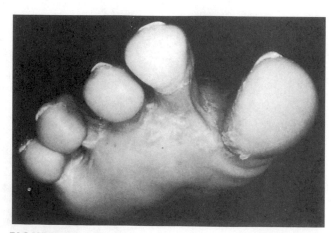

FIGURE 23-10. Tinea pedis. (From Arnold HL, Odom RB, James WD: Andrews' Diseases of the Skin, 8th ed. Philadelphia, WB Saunders, 1990.)

Head louse
(Pediculus humanus capitis)

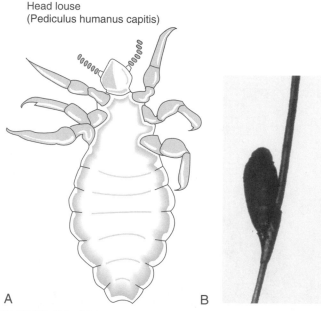

A   B

FIGURE 23-11. Pediculosis. *A,* Schematic representation of a louse. *B,* A nit attached to hair shaft. (*B* from Arnold HL, Odom RB, James WD: Andrews' Diseases of the Skin, 8th ed., Philadelphia, WB Saunders, 1990.)

methrin is used to treat lice. A fine-toothed comb can be used to remove empty nits from the hair. Clothing, linen, and the surrounding area need to be cleaned to prevent reinfection.

Thinkabout 23-4

a. Distinguish between tinea pedis and tinea capitis by location and lesion.
b. State one significant feature of the lesions of (1) impetigo, (2) herpes simplex.
c. State the causative organism of (1) shingles, (2) ringworm, (3) boils.
d. Explain why herpes simplex tends to recur.

SKIN TUMORS

Keratoses

Keratoses are benign lesions that are usually associated with aging. *Seborrheic keratoses* result from proliferation of basal cells, leading to an oval elevation that may be smooth or rough and is often dark in color. This type of keratoses is often found on the face or upper trunk. *Actinic keratoses* occur on skin exposed to ultraviolet radiation and commonly arise in fair-skinned persons.

The lesion appears as a pigmented scaly patch. Actinic keratoses may develop into squamous cell carcinoma.

Squamous Cell Carcinoma

Squamous cell carcinoma is similar to basal cell carcinoma in many respects (see Fig. 5–9). Skin cancer is easy to detect and treat and therefore should have a good prognosis. Squamous cell carcinoma is a painless malignant tumor of the epidermis; sun exposure is a major contributing factor. The lesions are found most frequently on exposed areas of the skin, such as the face and neck. Smokers also have a higher incidence of squamous cell carcinoma in the lower lip region and mouth. Scar tissue is also a source of carcinoma, particularly in the black population. Actinic keratoses predispose to in situ or intraepidermal squamous cell carcinoma, which usually remains limited to the epidermis for a long time. The invasive type of squamous cell carcinoma arises from premalignant conditions such as leukoplakia. Invasive carcinoma develops as a scaly, slightly elevated lesion with an irregular border and central ulceration (Fig. 23–12). The tumor grows relatively slowly in all directions at the site and then spreads to the regional lymph nodes.

Malignant Melanoma

This more serious form of skin cancer develops from the melanocytes and is increasing in incidence. The development of malignant melanoma depends

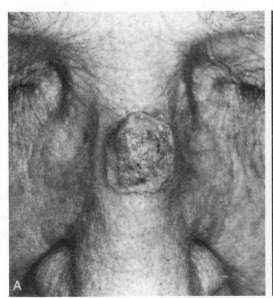
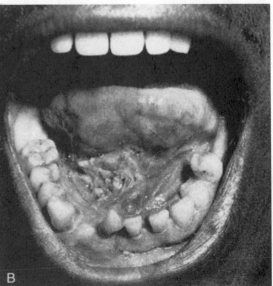

FIGURE 23-12. Squamous cell carcinoma. *A,* On the nose; *B,* on the floor of the mouth. (From Arnold HL, Odom RB, James WD: Andrews' Diseases of the Skin, 8th ed. Philadelphia, WB Saunders, 1990.)

on genetic factors, exposure to sunlight, and hormonal influences. Melanomas arise from melanocytes in the basal layer of the epidermis or from a nevus (mole), a collection of melanocytes. There are many types of nevi, most of which do not become malignant. Nevi that change shape, color, size, or texture or bleed are to be suspected. Malignant melanoma often appears as a multicolored lesion with an irregular border (Fig. 23–13). Melanomas grow quickly and metastasize first to the regional lymph nodes and then to other organs leading to a poor prognosis in many cases. When they are surgically removed, an extensive amount of tissue around and below the lesion is excised as well to ensure that all the malignant cells are removed.

Kaposi's Sarcoma

This type of skin cancer has come into prominence in recent years because of its association with human immunodeficiency virus (HIV) infection or acquired immunodeficiency syndrome (AIDS) (see Chapter 3). In immunosuppressed patients the cancer is quite common and may affect the viscera as well as the skin. Kaposi's sarcoma usually is a relatively rare cancer that occurs in older men originating from Eastern Europe or the Mediterranean area. The malignant cells arise from the endothelium in small blood vessels. The skin lesions commence as multiple purplish macules, often on the face, scalp, oral mucosa, or lower extremities. Initially, the lesions are nonpruritic and nonpainful. These lesions progress to form large irregularly shaped plaques or nodules, which may be darker in color, purplish or brownish (Fig. 23–14). In immunocompromised patients the lesions develop rapidly over the upper body and may become painful. Radiation and chemotherapy constitute the common treatment.

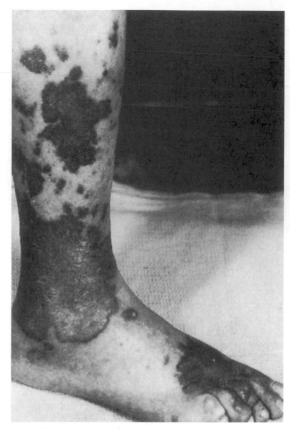

FIGURE 23–14. Kaposi's sarcoma. (From Arnold HL, Odom RB, James WD: Andrews' Diseases of the Skin, 8th ed. Philadelphia, WB Saunders, 1990.)

Thinkabout 23–5

a. Explain why squamous cell carcinoma has a better prognosis than malignant melanoma.
b. List skin disorders to which exposure to sunlight is a predisposing factor.
c. List the signs of possible malignant changes in a skin lesion.
d. Compare the characteristics of the typical lesion of squamous cell carcinoma, melanoma, and Kaposi's sarcoma.

CASE STUDIES

CASE STUDY A
Atopic Dermatitis

JW, age 5 months, has a moist erythematous rash on the cheeks, chest, and extensor surfaces of the arms

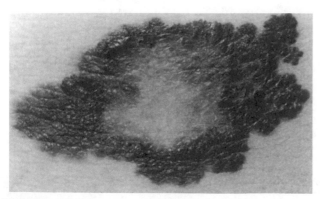

FIGURE 23–13. Malignant melanoma. (From Arnold HL, Odom RB, James WD: Andrews' Diseases of the Skin, 8th ed. Philadelphia, WB Saunders, 1990. Courtesy of Dr. Axel W. Hoke.)

caused by atopic dermatitis. She has a secondary bacterial infection on one cheek.

a. State the factors in the family history that would support a genetic predisposition to atopic dermatitis in this infant.

b. Explain why a secondary bacterial infection has probably developed.

c. List four factors that tend to aggravate atopic dermatitis.

d. Explain two ways in which administration of an antihistamine could help JW to sleep.

CASE STUDY B
Malignant Melanoma

Mr PX, age 45, had been swimming and was sitting on the beach when a friend commented on a dark reddish-black "pimple" with a rough surface on it on his upper back. Mr. PX said he had numerous moles on his body and it was not of concern. However, later he thought about the comment and saw his physician, who thought the lesion was suspicious and should be checked. The border and surface of the mass were irregular and it appeared to be quite thick. There was also a similar small lesion nearby. The lesion was diagnosed as a superficial spreading malignant melanoma, and further surgery was scheduled. Surgery revealed that the melanoma had penetrated through the dermis and had spread to the regional lymph nodes.

a. Explain the factors that make this lesion suspicious for cancer.

b. List the possible predisposing factors in this patient.

c. Predict the prognosis and the reasons for it in this case.

STUDY QUESTIONS

1. Describe the structure of a hair follicle, including any gland associated with it.

2. Describe the location of resident or normal flora related to the skin and its appendages.

3. State the location of nerves and blood vessels in the skin.

4. List the functions of the skin.

5. Define the terms papule, ulcer, and fissure.

6. Explain how glucocorticoids may reduce pruritus and give examples of conditions for which this drug may be helpful.

7. Compare the mechanisms and possible causes of allergic and irritant contact dermatitis.

8. Describe the skin lesion characteristic of DLE and the pathophysiologic basis for the disease.

9. Describe the manifestations of each of the following and state the causative agents for each: (a) shingles, (b) boils, (c) scabies, (d) scleroderma.

10. Prepare a list of contagious skin disorders.

11. Suggest a preventive measure that could reduce the risk of skin cancer.

12. Explain why allergic responses tend to recur.

13. Compare the characteristics of the exudate found in a furuncle and in herpes simplex.

14. Explain why Kaposi's sarcoma is more common in immunocompromised patients.

15. Explain the specific cause of pruritus with (a) scabies, (b) pediculosis, and (c) contact dermatitis.

KEY TERMS

anaplasia	ectopic	incontinence	micrometastases
dementia	exogenous	lactation	prostaglandin
differentiation	gonad	leukorrhea	semen
dyspareunia	gynecomastia	meatus	spermatogenesis
dysplasia	hirsutism	menarche	vesicle
dysuria			

DISORDERS OF THE MALE REPRODUCTIVE SYSTEM

Review of the Normal Male Reproductive System

STRUCTURE AND FUNCTION

The male **gonads**, the *testes*, are suspended by the spermatic cord in the s*crotum,* a sac outside the abdominal cavity (Fig. 24–1). The testes constantly produce sperm and the sex hormone testosterone. The scrotal sac consists of a layer of skin that is continuous with the skin of the perineal area plus an inner muscle layer and fascia. The scrotal covering is loose and falls into folds or rugae. A connective tissue septum separates the two testes within the scrotum. Each testis and attached epididymis is enclosed in the *tunica vaginalis,* a double-walled membrane with a small amount of fluid between the layers (see Fig. 24–3). The *spermatic cord* contains arteries, veins, and lymphatics for the testes (see Fig. 24–5). The testes are positioned outside the abdominal cavity to provide an optimum temperature for sperm production, 2 to 3°F (1 to 2°C) below normal body temperature. The scrotal muscle draws the testes closer to the body whenever the temperature drops. When the temperature climbs, the muscle relaxes, letting the testes drop away from the body. Higher temperatures for the testes in, for example, boys with undescended testes or men who constantly wear tight clothing, are considered a contributing factor to decreased sperm produc-

tion and infertility. The fetal testes descend from the abdominal cavity through the inguinal canal into the scrotum during the third trimester of pregnancy (see Fig. 24–2). At puberty, the testes mature and begin to produce sperm and testosterone under the influence of the gonadotropins secreted by the adenohypophysis. In addition to the testes, the male reproductive system includes an extensive duct system connected to accessory glands and structures, which form and transport the semen preparatory to ejaculation from the penis during sexual intercourse.

The testes consist of many lobules containing the *seminiferous tubules,* the "sperm factories" of the body. **Spermatogenesis** is a continuous process, which takes around 60 days. Efferent ducts conduct the multitudes of sperm into the *epididymis,* where the sperm mature. Peristaltic movements in the epididymis assist the sperm to move on into the *ductus deferens* (vas deferens) and then to the *ampulla,* where the now-motile sperm may be stored for several weeks until ejaculation occurs. Vasectomy, which is one method of birth control, involves obstructing the vas deferens to block the passage of sperm. When **semen** is formed at the time of emission, fluid containing many substances is gathered from the various accessory structures entering the ejaculatory duct and urethra. The *seminal vesicles,* located behind the bladder, provide a secretion that includes fructose to nourish the sperm. The *prostate gland,* which surrounds the urethra at the base of the bladder, adds an alkaline fluid to provide an optimum pH of around 6 for fertilization (the vaginal secretions and the initial

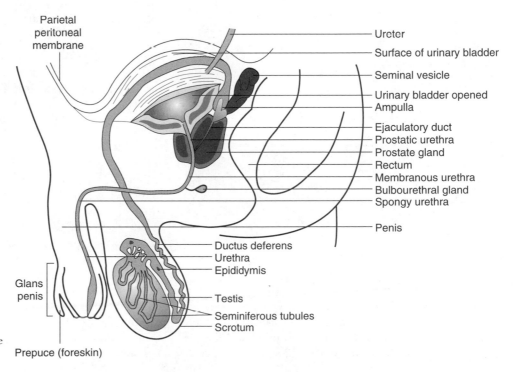

FIGURE 24-1. Anatomy of the male reproductive system.

sperm-containing fluid are acidic). Finally, the *bulbourethral glands* (Cowper's glands), situated near the base of the penis, secrete an alkaline mucus, which probably neutralizes any residual urine in the urethra. The total volume of semen ejaculated at one time is 2 to 5 mL; it consists primarily of fluid but contains several hundred million sperm.

HORMONES

Gonadotropic hormones released by the adenohypophysis or anterior pituitary gland include follicle-stimulating hormone (FSH), which initiates spermatogenesis, and luteinizing hormone (LH or interstitial cell-stimulating hormone [ICSH]), which stimulates testosterone production by the interstitial cells (Leydig's cells) in the testes. Testosterone is essential for the maturation of sperm. Serum levels of testosterone provide a negative feedback system for the continuous control of gonadotropin secretions, there being no cyclic hormones in males (see Chapter 21). Other functions of testosterone include the development and maintenance of secondary sex characteristics such as male hair distribution, deeper voice, and maturing of the male external genitalia. Also, testosterone is a steroid hormone that promotes protein metabolism and skeletal muscle development, influencing the physical changes seen in the adolescent male (see Chapter 8). These steroid hormones are being abused more frequently by both males and females who are athletes or are interested in body building or altered body image. Unfortunately, serious adverse effects are associated with such use, such as liver damage and damage to the reproductive structures.

Thinkabout 24–1

a. Describe the location and function of the (1) testis, (2) seminal vesicle, (3) epididymis.
b. Describe the source and feedback system of testosterone.

Infertility

Infertility or sterility affecting a couple's reproductive capacity may be caused solely by male conditions, solely by female conditions, or by combined male and female factors. Each of these categories occurs in approxi-

mately equal proportions. Male problems include changes in sperm or semen, hormonal abnormalities, or physical obstruction of sperm passage. Semen analysis assesses specific characteristics such as the number, normality, and motility of sperm. Penetration of the cervical mucus and the presence of sperm antibodies are also considered. Ductal obstructions may have resulted from congenital problems or scar tissue related to prior events such as infection. Hormonal imbalances may result from either pituitary disorders or testicular problems.

Congenital Abnormalities of the Penis

EPISPADIAS AND HYPOSPADIAS

Epispadias is a urethral opening on the dorsal (upper) surface of the penis, proximal to the glans. If the urethral defect extends proximally and affects the urinary sphincter, **incontinence** may result. Infections may result from stricture at the opening. In some cases, this condition is associated with *exstrophy of the bladder*, which is a failure of the abdominal wall to form across the midline.

Hypospadias is a urethral opening on the ventral (under) surface of the penis. If the opening occurs in the proximal section of the penis, it is considered more severe and may be accompanied by *chordee*, ventral curvature of the penis. Other abnormalities such as cryptorchidism are often associated with hypospadias. Surgical reconstruction, which may be performed in stages, is recommended for both these abnormalities to provide normal urinary flow and normal sexual function.

Disorders of the Testes and Scrotum

CRYPTORCHIDISM

Maldescent of the testis or cryptorchidism occurs when one of the testes fails to descend into the normal position in the scrotum during the latter part of pregnancy (Fig. 24–2). The testis may remain in the abdominal cavity or discontinue the descent at some point in the inguinal canal or above the scrotum. In some cases, the testis assumes an abnormal position outside the scrotum; this is called an ectopic testis. In many cases, spontaneous descent occurs during the first year after birth. The reason for maldescent is not fully understood. Possible factors include hormonal abnormalities, a short spermatic cord, or a small inguinal ring. If the testis remains undescended, the seminiferous tubules degenerate, and spermatogenesis

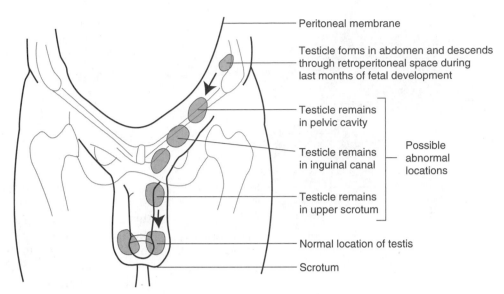

Peritoneal membrane

Testicle forms in abdomen and descends through retroperitoneal space during last months of fetal development

Testicle remains in pelvic cavity

Testicle remains in inguinal canal

Possible abnormal locations

Testicle remains in upper scrotum

Normal location of testis

Scrotum

FIGURE 24-2. Cryptorchidism and possible positions of the undescended testis.

is impaired. Of concern is the increased risk of testicular cancer in cryptorchid testes. Therefore, surgical positioning of the testes in the scrotum at an early age is advisable.

HYDROCELE, SPERMATOCELE, AND VARICOCELE

Hydrocele occurs when excessive fluid collects in the potential space between the layers of the tunica vaginalis (Fig. 24–3). This may occur around one or both testes. Hydrocele may occur as a congenital defect in a newborn when peritoneal fluid accumulates in the scrotum. This fluid may be reabsorbed in time. The fluid may continue to escape from the peritoneal cavity if the proximal portion of the processus vaginalis does not close off as expected following descent of the testes. Usually the scrotum fills with more fluid during the day, becoming larger and firmer, and then the fluid subsides during the night. The other common finding in an infant in whom the processus vaginalis remains open is an inguinal hernia, which is a loop of intestine that passes through the abnormal opening (see Fig. 18–18 in Chapter 18). Such a hernia may lead to intestinal obstruction. Surgical repair is recommended if the opening remains patent or herniation persists because there is a risk that the herniated intestinal loop may become strangulated.

Acquired hydrocele may result from scrotal injury, an infection or a tumor, or unknown causes. These hydroceles are more common after middle age. Large amounts of fluid may compromise the blood supply to the testis, requiring aspiration.

Spermatocele is a cyst that develops between the testis and the epididymis outside the tunica vaginalis, which contains fluid and sperm. It may be related to an

abnormality of the tubules. If the cyst is large, it may be surgically removed.

A *varicocele* is a dilated vein in the spermatic cord, usually on the left side. It frequently develops after puberty and results from lack of valves in the veins, permitting backflow of blood and increased pressure in the veins. Varicocele may be mild, and scrotal support minimizes the heavy feeling. If it is extensive, the varicocele is painful or tender and leads to infertility because of the impaired blood flow to the testes and decreased spermatogenesis. In this case, surgical treatment of the abnormal veins is necessary

Torsion of the testis occurs when the testis rotates on the spermatic cord, compressing the arteries and veins. Ischemia develops, and the scrotum swells. Immediate treatment is required manually and surgically to restore blood flow to the testis. Testicular torsion frequently occurs during puberty, both spontaneously and following trauma.

Inflammation and Infections

PROSTATITIS

Prostatitis may be present as an acute or chronic condition, and as a bacterial infection or nonbacterial inflammation. Bacterial prostatitis is usually associated with urinary tract infection (UTI) due to invasion by coliform bacteria from the intestines (see Chapter 19). The cause of the common nonbacterial form of prostatitis and prostatodynia (painful prostate) has not been established. The prostate is somewhat protected from ascending infection by the flushing action of urination and ejaculation and by an intact mucous membrane. Also, the prostatic secretions contain antimicrobial factors. However, the close association of the male repro-

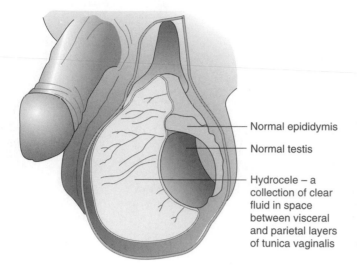

Normal epididymis

Normal testis

Hydrocele – a collection of clear fluid in space between visceral and parietal layers of tunica vaginalis

A. Hydrocele

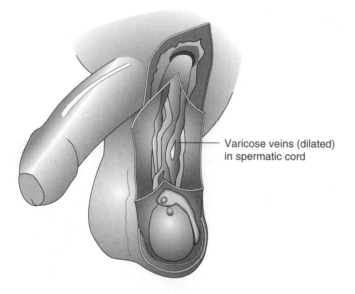

Varicose veins (dilated) in spermatic cord

B. Varicocele

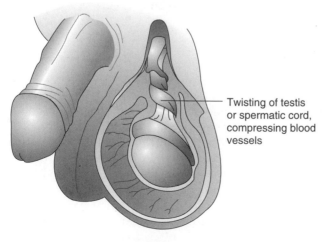

Twisting of testis or spermatic cord, compressing blood vessels

C. Torsion of testis

FIGURE 24–3. Abnormalities of the scrotum.

ductive tract with the urinary tract, including the continuous mucosa, promotes the spread of infection through the structures, and prostatitis is closely associated with UTI.

Pathophysiology

Acute bacterial prostatitis causes a tender, swollen gland, typically soft and boggy. The urine contains large quantities of microorganisms and leukocytes. Expressed prostatic secretions also contain many organisms, confirming the source of the infection. However, this process may be painful and may actually spread the infection in severe cases. Nonbacterial prostatitis is indicated by large numbers of leukocytes in the urine and secretions, although the prostate gland is not markedly enlarged. In patients with chronic prostatitis the prostate is only slightly enlarged, irregular, and firm because fibrosis is more extensive. In most cases of prostatitis the urinary tract is infected, and other parts of the reproductive tract may be involved as well (e.g., epididymitis).

Etiology

Acute bacterial prostatitis is usually an *ascending* infection (it progresses up the urethra) and is caused primarily by *Escherichia coli* but sometimes by *Pseudomonas*, *Proteus*, or *Streptococcus faecalis*. It is common in young men in association with UTI but also occurs frequently in older men with benign prostatic hypertrophy. Chronic prostatitis is usually related to chronic or recurrent UTI caused by *E. coli*. Infection may also result from instrumentation such as catheterization or sometimes from hematogenous spread (through the blood).

Signs and Symptoms

Both acute and chronic infections are manifested by dysuria, urinary frequency, and urgency. Low back pain or lower abdominal discomfort may be present. Severe inflammation in the prostate may cause obstruction of the urinary flow through the urethra, resulting in a decreased urinary stream, hesitancy in initiating urination, incomplete bladder emptying, and nocturia or frequency. Systemic signs include fever, malaise, anorexia, and muscle aching. With nonbacterial prostatitis, the urinary signs are present, often intermittently, but the systemic signs are less marked.

Treatment

Antibacterial drugs are recommended for bacterial infections. For chronic infections, drugs such as the sulfonamides, which can better penetrate prostatic tissue, are recommended; they are taken for a prolonged period, perhaps a month, to ensure total eradication of the causative organisms. Nonbacterial prostatitis can be treated by anti-inflammatory drugs as well as prophylactic antibacterials.

Thinkabout 24–2

> a. Define (1) epispadias, (2) hydrocele.
> b. Compare the typical signs of acute bacterial prostatitis, chronic bacterial prostatitis, and acute nonbacterial prostatitis.

Tumors

BENIGN PROSTATIC HYPERTROPHY

Pathophysiology

Benign prostatic hypertrophy (BPH) is a very common disorder in older men, varying from mild to severe forms. Although called hypertrophy, the change is actually hyperplasia of the prostatic tissue with formation of nodules surrounding the urethra; these changes lead to compression of the urethra and variable degrees of urinary obstruction (Fig. 24–4). This hyperplasia appears to be related to an imbalance between estrogen and testosterone that results from the hormonal changes associated with aging. No connection between BPH and prostatic carcinoma has been identified. Rectal examination reveals an enlarged gland. Incomplete emptying of the bladder because of the obstruction leads to frequent infections. If significant obstruction and urinary retention develop in the patient, surgical intervention, using one of several techniques, is required.

Signs and Symptoms

The initial signs indicate obstruction of urinary flow. Hesitancy, dribbling, and decreased force of the urinary stream are direct results of the narrowed urethra. Incomplete bladder emptying leads to frequency, nocturia, and recurrent urinary tract infection.

CANCER OF THE PROSTATE

Prostate cancer is very common in men older than 50 years and ranks high as a cause of cancer death. Statistically, it is second to lung cancer as a cause of these deaths in men.

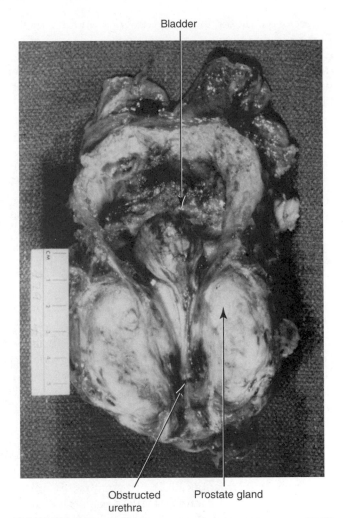

FIGURE 24–4. Benign prostatic hypertrophy. (Courtesy of R.W. Shaw, M.D., North York General Hospital, Toronto, Ontario.)

Pathophysiology

Most tumors are adenocarcinomas arising from the tissue near the surface of the gland (rather than in the central area, as in BPH). There may be more than one focus of neoplastic cells. Tumors vary in degree of cellular differentiation; the more undifferentiated or anaplastic tumors are much more aggressive, growing and spreading at a faster rate. Many tumors are androgen dependent. Metastasis to bone occurs relatively early and involves the spine, pelvis, ribs, and femur. In most cases, the cancer has spread before diagnosis. The tumor may spread to the pelvic lymph nodes, liver, adrenal glands, and lungs. Staging is based on four categories: stage A is a small, nonpalpable, encapsulated tumor; stage B is a palpable tumor confined to the prostate; stage C is a tumor that has extended beyond the prostate; and stage D implies the presence of distant metastases.

Etiology

The cause has not been determined, although an environmental factor appears to be involved. Prostatic cancer is common in North America and northern Europe but not in countries farther east. The incidence is higher in the black population than in whites, indicating a possible genetic factor. Also, a hormonal factor has a role in the development of prostatic cancer. It has been noted that BPH does not precede carcinoma.

Signs and Symptoms

A hard nodule in the periphery of the gland, often in the posterior lobe, may be detected on rectal examination. The tumor tends not to cause early urethral obstruction because of its location. As the tumor develops, some obstruction does occur, producing signs of hesitancy, a decreased stream, urinary frequency, or bladder infection (cystitis).

Diagnostic Tests

Ultrasonography and biopsy confirm the diagnosis. Two serum markers are helpful—prostate-specific antigen (PSA), which provides a useful screening tool for early detection as well as supportive data for the diagnosis, and prostatic acid phosphatase, which is elevated when metastatic cancer is present. Bone scans are useful for detecting early metastases.

Treatment

Surgery and radiation are the treatments of choice. When the tumor is androgen sensitive, orchiectomy (removal of the testes) or hormonal therapy may be suggested to reduce testosterone levels.

CANCER OF THE TESTES

The majority of tumors that occur in the testes are malignant, arising from germ cells. Although it is not common, concern has been expressed because testicular cancer occurs primarily in the 15- to 35-year-old age group, and the incidence is increasing. Certain types of testicular cancer may occur in other groups, such as younger children or older males. Testicular cancer is the most common solid tumor in young men. For this reason, regular monthly testicular self-examination (TSE) is recommended to check for an unusual hard mass.

Pathophysiology

Testicular cancer may originate from one type of cell, for example, a seminoma, or it may be mixed, consisting of cells from a variety of sources and with varying degrees of differentiation (Fig. 24–5). A common mixed tumor is a teratoma, derived from one or more of the germ cell layers, combined with an embryonal

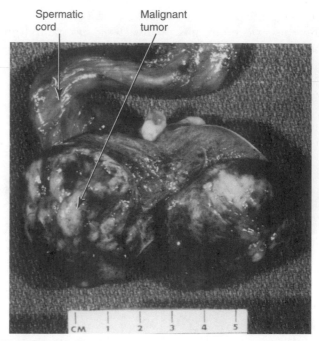

FIGURE 24–5. Cancer of the testes—spermatic cord and left testis with mixed embryonal teratoma and choriocarcinoma. (Courtesy of R.W. Shaw, M.D., North York General Hospital, Toronto, Ontario.)

carcinoma, which has poorly differentiated cells. Some malignant tumors secrete human chorionic gonadotropin (hCG) or alpha-fetoprotein (AFP), which serves as a useful serum marker for both diagnosis and follow-up monitoring. Some testicular neoplasms spread at an early stage, for example, choriocarcinoma, whereas others such as seminomas remain localized for a more prolonged period. Testicular tumors follow a typical pattern when spreading, first appearing in the common iliac and para-aortic lymph nodes and then in the mediastinal and supraclavicular lymph nodes. Metastases spreading through the blood to the lungs, liver, bone, and brain occur at a later time. Several staging systems are used, based on the extent of the primary tumor, the degree of lymph node involvement (retroperitoneal or otherwise), and the presence of distant metastases.

Etiology

This tumor has a familial incidence, and there is a possible relationship with infection or trauma. However, the primary established predisposing factor is *cryptorchidism*, or maldescent of the testes.

Signs and Symptoms

Testicular tumors present as a hard painless mass, usually unilateral. The testis may be enlarged or may feel heavy. Eventually, there may be a dull aching pain in the lower abdomen. In some cases, hydrocele or epididymitis may develop because of inflammation, or gynecomastia may become evident if hormones are secreted by the tumor.

Diagnostic Tests

Because biopsy encourages the spread and recurrence of the tumor, diagnosis is based on other tests, such as computed tomography scans and lymphangiography, and the presence of tumor markers (e.g., AFP and hCG).

Treatment

Treatment of testicular cancer using a combination of surgery (orchiectomy), radiation therapy, and chemotherapy has greatly improved the prognosis. Orchiectomy does not usually interfere with sexual function. However, fertility may be reduced by radiation and chemotherapy.

Thinkabout 24-3

a. Compare BPH and prostatic cancer in terms of the characteristic location of the tumor and the early signs.

b. List the factors predisposing to testicular cancer.

c. Describe the early signs of cancer of the testes.

d. Explain why bone scans are important in determining the prognosis of prostatic cancer.

DISORDERS OF THE FEMALE REPRODUCTIVE SYSTEM

Review of the Normal Female Reproductive System

STRUCTURE AND FUNCTION

The female external genitalia or *vulva* include the mons pubis, the labia, the clitoris, and the vaginal orifice. The *mons pubis* consists of the adipose tissue and hair covering the symphysis pubis. The *labia majora*, the outer fold, and the *labia minora* inside it are long, thin folds of skin extending back and down from the mons pubis, protecting the orifices. Sebaceous glands and sweat glands are located in the folds. The *clitoris* is a small projection of erectile tissue located anterior to the urethra. It is analogous to the male penis and is very sensitive to touch. In the *vagina*, the entryway to the reproductive tract, the orifice or introitus is situated between the urethral **meatus** (anterior) and the anus (posterior) (Fig. 24–6). The vagina is a muscular, distensible canal extending upward from the vulva to the cervix. It is lined with a mucosal membrane and falls in rugae or folds, allowing expansion during coitus or childbirth. The mucosa consists of stratified squamous epithelial cells, which are hormone sensitive. Following menopause and the decline in estrogen secretions, the mucosa becomes thin and fragile. *Bartholin's glands* (the greater vestibular glands) are located on either side of the vaginal orifice and secrete mucus in response to sexual stimulation to facilitate penile penetration into the vagina during intercourse. *Skene's glands*, located by the external urethral meatus, also secrete mucus to keep the tissues moist. Both of these sets of mucus-secreting glands are easily obstructed and infected. **Leukorrhea**, the normal vaginal discharge, is produced by these glands; the secretions are relatively clear or whitish and contain mucus and sloughed cells. The amount fluctuates during the menstrual cycle. Before puberty and after menopause vaginal pH is around 7, but during the reproductive years it is more acidic, between 4 and 5, due to an increased population of *Lactobacillus*. The acidic pH and the thickness of the epithelium provide protection against infection.

The upper vagina surrounds the *cervix*, which is the lower part or neck of the uterus. The *endocervical canal* is the passageway between the internal *os* of the cervix at the uterine end and the external os at the vaginal end. The external os is a small opening filled with thick mucus that acts as a barrier to vaginal flora attempting to ascend into the uterus. The lining of the endocervical canal is continuous with that of the uterus and the vagina but differs in composition. The endocervical canal is lined with columnar epithelial cells, which change to squamous epithelium in the vagina. The point of change is known as the *transformation zone* or *squamous-columnar junction*, and this is the common site of cervical dysplasia and cancer. The *uterus* is a muscular sac within which a fertilized ovum may be implanted and develop. The pear-shaped body of the uterus is called the corpus. It is loosely suspended by ligaments in the pelvic cavity to allow for expansion during pregnancy. Normally it is anteverted or tipped forward, resting on the urinary bladder. The uterine wall is made up of three layers: the outer perimetrium or parietal peritoneum, the thick, middle layer of smooth muscle or myometrium, and the inner endometrium. The endometrium consists of a functional layer that is responsive to hormones during the menstrual cycle and an underlying basal layer that is responsible for the regeneration of the endometrium following menses.

The two *fallopian tubes* (oviducts) originate near the top of the uterus, just under the fundus, the top part of

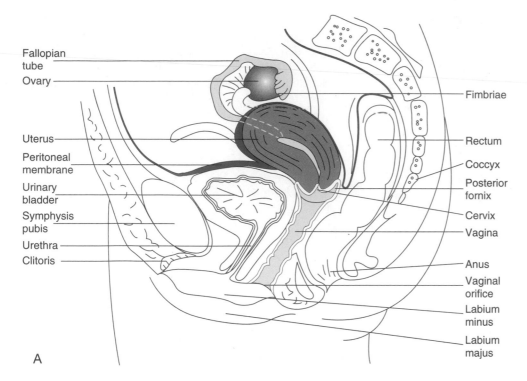

Fallopian tube
Ovary
Uterus
Peritoneal membrane
Urinary bladder
Symphysis pubis
Urethra
Clitoris

Fimbriae
Rectum
Coccyx
Posterior fornix
Cervix
Vagina
Anus
Vaginal orifice
Labium minus
Labium majus

A

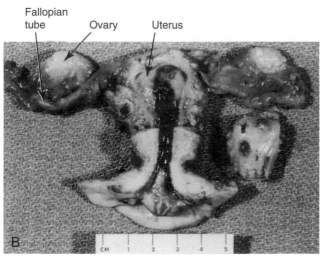

Fallopian tube   Ovary   Uterus

B

FIGURE 24-6. *A*, Anatomy of the female reproductive system. *B*, Ovaries, fallopian tubes, uterus, and vagina of a postmenopausal woman. (*B*, Courtesy of R.W. Shaw, M.D., North York General Hospital, Toronto, Ontario.)

the corpus. Each tube curves up and out, ending in a flared opening over the ovary. This end portion has a fringe of *fimbriae*, moving fingerlike projections that draw the released ovum into the tube. Cilia and peristaltic movements in the fallopian tube continue to move the ovum toward the uterus. Usually the ovum is fertilized by a sperm in the distal fallopian tube, and then it continues on to the uterus, where it is implanted at a suitable site in the endometrium.

The female gonads are the *ovaries,* which produce the *ova,* one each month during the reproductive years between **menarche** and menopause. The two ovaries are suspended by ligaments, one on either side of the uterus. These ovaries supply the female gamete, the *ovum,* and the sex hormones for the female, primarily

estrogen and progesterone, on a cyclic basis (Fig. 24–7).

The female breast plays a significant role in the reproductive system. It responds to cyclic hormonal changes and is responsible for **lactation**, the provision of breast milk to the newborn. Mammary tissue develops under the influence of increased estrogen secretion, commencing at puberty. The breast consists of 15 to 20 lobes supported by ligaments. Muscle and fatty tissue are interspersed among the lobes and their subunits, the lobules and the acini. The *acini* are the basic functional units of the breast tissue, consisting of epithelial cells that secrete milk and contracting cells that move the milk into ducts. The breast tissue also has a system of collecting and ejecting ducts for milk that culminate in openings in the nipple. The breast is well supplied with blood vessels, lymphatics, and nerves. Sebaceous glands are found in the areola, the pigmented tissue surrounding the nipple. During the menstrual cycle, the higher estrogen and progesterone levels increase both the vascularity of the breast and the proliferation and dilation of the ducts, leading to increased fullness and tenderness of the breasts premenstrually. It is recommended that breast self-examination be performed shortly after the conclusion of menses, when hormone levels are low and the breasts are small and less nodular. This examination should be performed at the same time each month to allow comparison of the normal characteristics of the breast. Post-

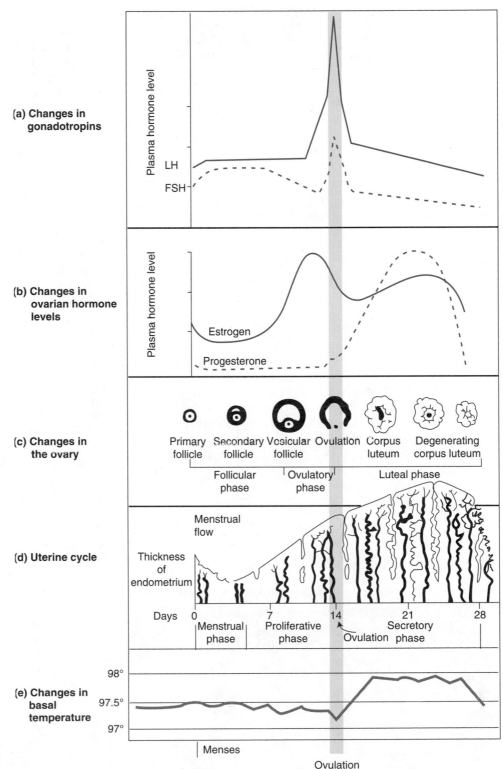

FIGURE 24-7. Graphs illustrating changes occurring during the menstrual cycle.

menopausally, examination should be done at regular intervals.

HORMONES AND THE MENSTRUAL CYCLE

Hormonal secretions, release of ova, and associated endometrial changes occur in a cyclic pattern in women during the reproductive years (see Fig. 24–7). The average cycle is 28 days, but a range of 21 to 45 days is found. Some women experience irregular cycles. The cycle begins with menstruation or menses, the sloughing of the endometrial tissue that occurs when implantation of the ovum has not occurred. This stage is followed by the endometrial proliferation stage, when increasing FSH is secreted by the anterior pituitary gland, resulting in maturation of an ovarian follicle. This maturing follicle secretes estrogen, causing proliferation or thickening of the functional layer of the endometrium. At midpoint, as LH levels greatly increase, ovulation takes place with release of the mature ovum. The ovarian follicle is now converted by LH into the corpus luteum, which increases production of progesterone. Progesterone enhances the development of endometrial blood vessels and glycogen-secreting glands in preparation for the implantation of a fertilized ovum. If fertilization does not occur, estrogen and progesterone levels drop, and the corpus luteum and endometrium degenerate, resulting in menstruation.

Hormonal levels fluctuate considerably in the female during the cycle, a result of complex interactions involving the hypothalamus, the anterior pituitary, and the ovary (see Chapter 21). The feedback mechanism involves estrogen and progesterones acting on the anterior pituitary gland to control the release of LH and FSH. The changes in hormone levels and in basal body temperature (early morning) that occur during the cycle may be useful in determining the anticipated time of ovulation or fertile periods in women.

Thinkabout 24–4

a. Describe the location and structure of (1) the ovary, (2) the cervix, and (3) the labia.

b. Describe the lining of the reproductive tract in sequence from the vagina through the fallopian tubes.

c. At what time in the menstrual cycle is the level of the following hormones high, and what is the effect of this elevation?

(1) LH

(2) progesterone

Infertility

As indicated previously, infertility may be caused by abnormalities in the female partner, by a combination of factors in both male and female partners, or by abnormalities in the male. A couple is considered infertile after a year of unprotected intercourse fails to produce a pregnancy. There are many possible causes of decreased fertility. In the female, infertility may be associated with hormonal imbalances resulting from altered function of the hypothalamus, anterior pituitary gland, or ovaries. This may occur following the use of oral contraceptives. For example, the feedback system may not be functioning or may be suppressed by stress, or the ovaries may be abnormal (e.g., in the Stein-Leventhal syndrome). Structural abnormalities may prevent pregnancy, for example, a small or bicornuate (divided) uterus. The fallopian tubes may be obstructed by scar tissue resulting from infection or endometriosis. Access of viable sperm may be reduced by a change in vaginal pH due to infection or the use of douches, by excessively thick cervical mucus, or by the development of antibodies in the female to particular sperm. A broad range of tests is available to assess each group of factors in a progressively more detailed manner. The woman's general health status is investigated to rule out any systemic causes. The patient may record basal body temperature, times of intercourse, and menstrual cycles to determine the optimal time for fertilization. Physical abnormalities may be assessed by means of a pelvic examination and by tests such as ultrasound, computed tomography scans, or laparoscopy. Hysteroscopy is another method of detecting uterine abnormalities. Tubal insufflation (using gas and a pressure measurement) or a hysterosalpingogram (radiograph with contrast material) can ascertain the patency of the tubes and uterus. Evaluation of hormone levels throughout the cycle requires extensive testing. Other possible factors such as cervical mucus and the presence of sperm antibodies require specific tests. Frequently, a combination of factors contributes to infertility, and therefore it is best to conduct a range of tests.

Structural Abnormalities

The normal position of the uterus is slightly *anteverted* (tipped forward) and *anteflexed* (bent forward over the bladder), with the cervix downward and back. The position of the uterus may vary because of a minor congenital anatomic alteration, childbirth, or a pathologic condition such as scar tissue or a tumor. In most cases, there are no deleterious effects. In some cases, infertility may result if the cervix is not positioned appropriately to facilitate the passage of sperm. Often malposition does not cause any symptoms. Marked retroversion may cause back pain, dysmenorrhea, and **dyspareunia**. Examples of uterine displacement are shown in Figure 24–8*A*. A *retroverted* uterus is tipped backward. The uterus may be excessively curved or bent, either retroflexed (bent backward) or anteflexed (bent forward).

With aging or excessive stretching or trauma, the supporting ligaments, fascia, and muscles for the uterus, bladder, and rectum may become weakened (*pelvic relaxation*), and these organs shift out of their normal position in the pelvis. Factors predisposing to this condition include difficult childbirth including prolonged labor, multiple births, birth of a large baby, and repeated pregnancies separated by short intervals. A genetic component also appears to be a factor. The effects often become apparent some years after the original injury has occurred, usually around menopause, when the decreasing hormonal levels contribute further to tissue atrophy. More than one structure may be affected in any one individual.

Uterine displacement or *prolapse* is the descent of the cer-vix or uterus into the vagina (see Fig. 24–8*B*). Prolapse is classified as first degree if the cervix drops into the vagina, second degree if the cervix lies at the introitus and the corpus is in the vagina, and third degree (procidentia) if the uterus and cervix protrude through the vaginal orifice. Although the early stage may be asymptomatic, the more advanced stages cause discomfort and a feeling of heaviness in the vagina. Protrusion of the cervix causes irritation and infection in the cervix. Prolapse may be treated by surgery or by using a pessary to maintain the uterus in position.

A cystocele is a protrusion of the bladder into the anterior wall of the vagina (see Fig. 24–8*C*). The bladder cannot be emptied completely, and recurrent cystitis is common. *A rectocele* is a protrusion of the rectum into the posterior wall of the vagina (see Fig. 24–8*D*). The mass may be small or large enough to drop into the vaginal introitus. Interference with defecation and a feeling of pressure in the pelvis are the common indicators. Rectocele and cystocele, if severe, require surgical repair.

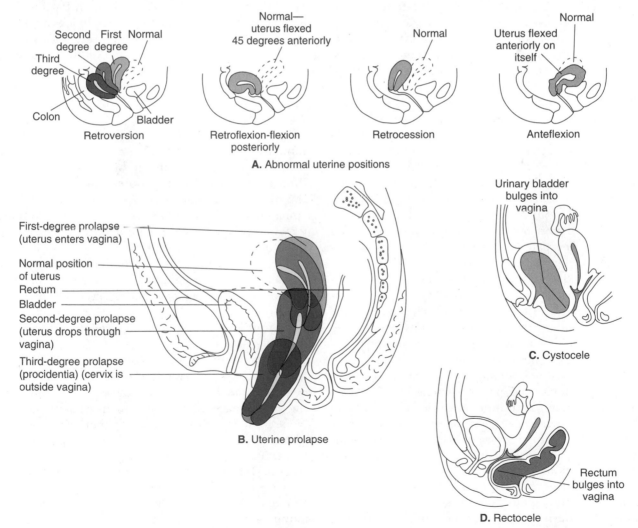

A. Abnormal uterine positions

B. Uterine prolapse

C. Cystocele

D. Rectocele

FIGURE 24–8. Structural abnormalities of the uterus.

Menstrual Disorders

MENSTRUAL ABNORMALITIES

Amenorrhea, or absence of menstruation, may be primary or secondary. In the primary condition, menarche has never occurred. This may result from a genetic disorder such as Turner's syndrome (a chromosome abnormality, XO, in which the ovaries do not function). Congenital defects affecting the hypothalamus, central nervous system, or pituitary, or congenital absence of the uterus and congenital uterine hypoplasia (infantile uterus) may also interfere with the normal process. Secondary amenorrhea is the cessation of menstruation in an individual who previously experienced cycles. It frequently results from an impediment in the hypothalamic-pituitary axis. The hypothalamus may be suppressed by conditions such as tumors, stress, sudden weight loss, eating disorders, or participation in competitive sports, leading to reduced body fat. Systemic factors such as anemia or chemotherapy may also cause secondary amenorrhea.

Dysmenorrhea refers to painful menstruation and may be primary or secondary. Primary dysmenorrhea has no organic foundation and develops when ovulation commences. The majority of women experience some discomfort, but for many the pain is sufficient to interrupt normal activities. In many cases, dysmenorrhea is relieved following childbirth. The severe cramping pain is related to the excessive release of **prostaglandin** ($PGF_{2\alpha}$) during endometrial shedding. This prostaglandin causes strong uterine muscle contractions and ischemia. Pain develops 24 to 48 hours before or at the onset of menses and lasts for 24 to 48 hours. In addition, nausea and vomiting, headache, and dizziness may accompany the cramps as the prostaglandins enter the systemic circulation. Some relief may be afforded by the use of a heating pad, exercise, or medications such as ibuprofen or naproxen (nonsteroidal anti-inflammatory drugs [NSAIDs]), which inhibit prostaglandin synthesis. An alternative treatment is the use of oral contraceptives, which lead to anovulatory cycles that are not painful. Secondary dysmenorrhea results from pelvic disorders such as endometriosis, uterine polyps or tumors, or pelvic inflammatory disease.

Abnormal menstrual bleeding is a common concern. Examples of abnormal patterns include *menorrhagia* (increased amount and duration of flow), *metrorrhagia* (bleeding between cycles), *polymenorrhea* (short cycles of less than 3 weeks), or *oligomenorrhea* (long cycles of more than 6 weeks). The usual cause of an altered pattern is lack of ovulation; however, this condition may also result from hormonal disorders such as thyroid abnormalities or pathologic conditions such as tumors. Any change in pattern is significant and should be investigated.

Premenstrual syndrome (PMS) is a condition that begins a week or so before the onset of menses and ends with the onset of menses. The cause is not understood, although research in this area continues. Common manifestations include breast tenderness, weight gain, abdominal distention or bloating, irritability, emotional lability, sleep disturbances, depression, headache, and fatigue. Some women have increased mental concentration and activity, whereas others are lethargic. Treatment measures are tailored to the individual and may include hormonal therapy and the use of diuretics or antidepressants as necessary.

ENDOMETRIOSIS

Endometriosis is the presence of endometrial tissue outside the uterus on structures such as the ovaries, ligaments, or colon (Fig. 24–9). On occasion, it may affect distant sites such as the lungs. This **ectopic** endometrium responds to cyclic hormone variations, growing during the proliferation and secretory stages of the menstrual cycle and then degenerating, shedding, and bleeding. Because there is no exit point for this blood, and blood is irritating to tissues when it does not belong there, local inflammation and pain result. This inflammation recurs with each cycle and eventually causes the development of fibrous tissue, which may cause adhesions and obstruction of the involved structures, such as the urinary bladder or colon. When the uterus is pulled out of its normal position (e.g., into retroversion) by adhesions, infertility frequently results. The fallopian tube may be blocked or the ovary covered by fibrous tissue, preventing movement of the ovum into and through the tube. When endometrial tissue occurs on the ovary, a "chocolate cyst" develops, a fibrous sac containing old brown blood (see Fig. 24–9B). Although it may be possible to palpate nodular tissue, the diagnosis is confirmed by laparoscopy.

The most common manifestation of endometriosis is dysmenorrhea. The pain may persist throughout menses and typically becomes more severe each month. Dyspareunia, or painful intercourse, may occur if the vagina and supporting ligaments are affected by adhesions.

The cause of endometriosis has not been established. Proposed mechanisms include migration of endometrial tissue up through the fallopian tubes into the peritoneal cavity during menstruation, development from embryonic tissue at other sites, spread of endometrium through the blood or lymph, or transplantation of tissue during surgery such as a cesarean section. Treatment measures include hormonal suppression of the endometrial tissue, with relief of the pain associated with the monthly cycle, or surgical removal of the ectopic endometrial tissue. Pregnancy and lactation also result in amenorrhea and atrophy of

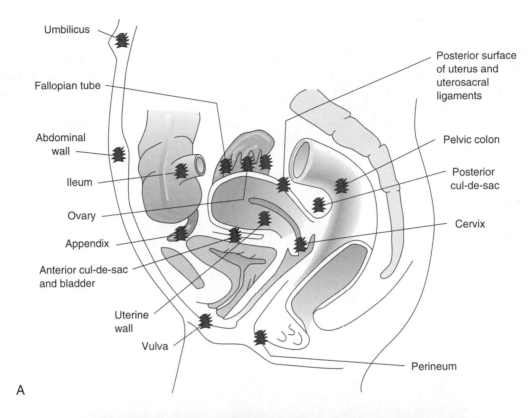

Umbilicus

Fallopian tube

Abdominal wall

Ileum

Ovary

Appendix

Anterior cul-de-sac and bladder

Uterine wall

Vulva

Posterior surface of uterus and uterosacral ligaments

Pelvic colon

Posterior cul-de-sac

Cervix

Perineum

A

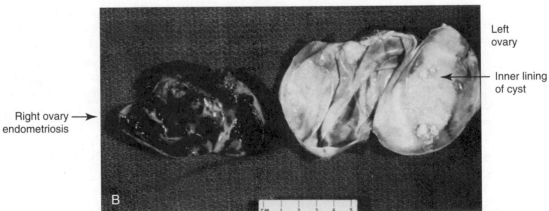

Right ovary endometriosis

Left ovary

Inner lining of cyst

B

FIGURE 24–9. Endometriosis. *A*, Possible ectopic sites. *B*, Endometriosis involving the right ovary (chocolate cyst) and left ovary showing the inner lining of a large cyst with excrescences. (*B*, Courtesy of R.W. Shaw, M.D., North York General Hospital, Toronto, Ontario.)

the ectopic tissue. These measures do not cure endometriosis, but they do delay further damage and alleviate the symptoms.

Thinkabout 24–5

a. Describe each of the following: (1) second-degree uterine prolapse, (2) cystocele, (3) retroversion of the uterus.
b. Differentiate the following terms from one another: dysmenorrhea, premenstrual syndrome, and menorrhagia.
c. Explain the process by which endometriosis can cause infertility.

Infections

Many infections of the vagina and cervix are considered sexually transmitted diseases and are included in the section on these diseases later in this chapter.

CANDIDIASIS

Candidiasis is one form of vaginitis. It is a yeast infection caused by *Candida albicans* (*Monilia*) and usually occurs as an opportunistic infection. Infection may follow antibiotic therapy for an unrelated bacterial infection elsewhere in the body (which creates a more alkaline pH) or may develop because of decreased resistance (e.g., in immune-deficiency states) or increased glycogen or glucose levels in the secretions (e.g., with pregnancy, use of oral contraceptives, or diabetes). Candidiasis causes red and swollen pruritic mucous membranes and a thick, white, curd-like discharge. White patches may adhere to the vaginal wall. **Dysuria** (painful urination) and dyspareunia (painful intercourse) may be present. An antifungal agent such as nystatin is effective treatment. To prevent recurrence, the predisposing factors need to be addressed.

PELVIC INFLAMMATORY DISEASE

Pelvic inflammatory disease (PID) is an infection of the reproductive tract, particularly the fallopian tubes and ovaries. The condition includes cervicitis (cervix), endometritis (uterus), salpingitis (fallopian tubes), and oophoritis (ovaries). The infection may be acute or chronic. PID is a common problem and is a matter of concern because of the potential acute complications such as peritonitis and pelvic abscess as well as the long-term problems of infertility and the high risk of ectopic pregnancy.

Pathophysiology

The infection usually originates as a vaginitis or cervicitis and often involves several causative bacteria. The microbes ascend through the uterus into the fallopian tubes (Fig. 24–10). The tubal walls become edematous, and the lumen is filled with purulent exudate, effectively obstructing the tube and restricting drainage into the uterus. The exudate drips out of the fimbriae onto the ovary and surrounding tissue. The peritoneal membranes attempt to localize the infection initially, but peritonitis may develop (see Chapter 18). Abscesses may form as the inflammatory response struggles to contain or wall off the infection. Pelvic abscesses may be life threatening if not quickly drained surgically. The most common cause of death in women with PID is septic shock. Adhesions and strictures are common sequelae; they affect the tubes and ovaries, leading to infertility or ectopic pregnancy (implantation of the fertilized ovum in the fallopian tube). Adhesions or scar tissue may also affect the surrounding structures such as the colon.

Etiology

The majority of infections arise from sexually transmitted diseases such as gonorrhea (*Neisseria gonorrhoeae*) and chlamydiosis (*Chlamydia trachomatis*). Multiple organisms are present in many cases. Potential agents include *Bacteroides*, *Gardnerella vaginalis*, streptococci, *E. coli*, *Pseudomonas*, and *Haemophilus influenzae*. A prior episode of vaginitis or cervicitis, often with few signs, frequently precedes the development of PID. Infection is likely to become acute during or immediately following menses, when the endometrium is more vulnerable. PID may also result from insertion of an intrauterine device (IUD, a contraceptive device) or other instrument contaminated by organisms from the lower reproductive tract or other source. Any instrument is likely to traumatize the tissue, providing a portal of entry for bacteria. Occasionally, infection in the reproductive tract may result from blood-borne organisms or from an infection in the peritoneal cavity related to conditions such as appendicitis. Infection may also be associated with abortion or childbirth. Historically, this was the feared complication of illegal abortions or deliveries under primitive conditions. The uterus may be perforated by objects such as IUDs or trauma, creating inflammation and infec-

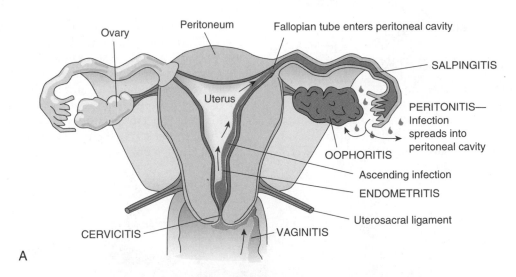

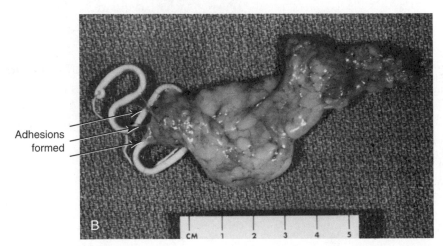

FIGURE 24-10. Pelvic inflammatory disease. *A,* Spread of infection. *B,* Uterus perforated by intrauterine device (IUD) leads to localized inflammation in peritoneal cavity and omentum, forming adhesions around IUD. (*B,* Courtesy of R.W. Shaw, M.D., North York General Hospital, Toronto, Ontario.)

tion in the peritoneal cavity and subsequent adhesions (see Fig. 24–10*B*).

Signs and Symptoms

Lower abdominal pain is usually the first indication of PID. Pain may be sudden and severe or gradually increasing in intensity. Characteristically, it is a steady pain that increases with walking. Tenderness is common during pelvic examination. Purulent discharge is evident at the cervical os. Dysuria may be noted. Fever and leukocytosis depend on which causative organisms are involved. Peritonitis is indicated by increasing abdominal distention and rigidity.

Treatment

Aggressive treatment with appropriate antibiotics such as cefoxitin and doxycycline is required. Recurrent infections are common, and therefore it is recommended that sexual partners be treated with antibiotics and that follow-up examinations be scheduled to ensure complete eradication of the infection.

Thinkabout 24-6

a. Describe three factors predisposing to vaginal candidiasis.

b. Explain how infection in the vagina can cause PID.

c. List the signs of PID and the reasons for them.

d. Give three reasons why PID is considered a serious condition.

Benign Tumors

LEIOMYOMA (FIBROIDS)

A leiomyoma is a benign tumor of the myometrium, the cause of which is unknown. These uterine tumors are very common in women during the reproductive years and tend to shrink following menopause. As benign tumors, they are not considered precancerous.

They are classified by location, developing in the uterine wall (intramural), beneath the endometrium (submucosal), or under the serosa (subserosal). The two latter forms may develop as polyps, the submucosal type projecting inward into the uterine cavity and the subserosal type growing outward into the pelvic cavity. Fibroids usually occur as multiple well-defined but unencapsulated masses, which vary widely in size (Fig. 24–11). Large leiomyomas degenerate in the central re-

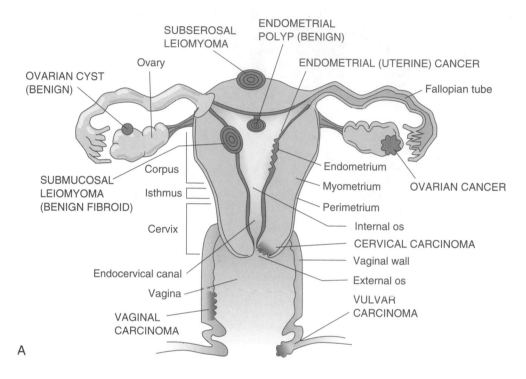

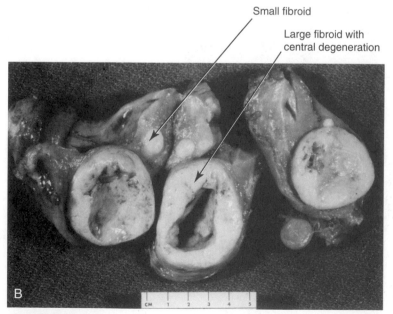

FIGURE 24–11. Leiomyomas. *A,* Types of benign uterine fibroids. *B,* Multiple leiomyomas of different sizes. The cut section of the large tumor shows central degeneration. (*B,* Courtesy of R.W. Shaw, M.D., North York General Hospital, Toronto, Ontario.)

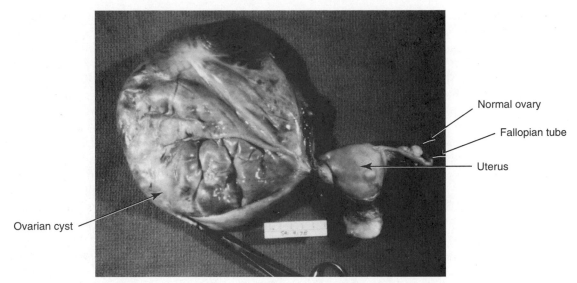

FIGURE 24-12. A large ovarian cyst. (Courtesy of R.W. Shaw, M.D., North York General Hospital, Toronto, Ontario.)

gion, undergoing necrosis and forming cysts. These benign tumors are hormone dependent, growing rapidly during pregnancy and decreasing in size with increasing fibrosis after menopause. Fibroids are often asymptomatic until they grow large enough to be palpated. Abnormal bleeding such as menorrhagia may be an indicator of fibroid development. Large tumors may cause pressure on adjacent structures, leading to urinary frequency or constipation and a heavy sensation in the lower abdomen. Large fibroids may interfere with implantation of the fertilized ovum or the course of pregnancy

OVARIAN CYSTS

A variety of types of cysts occur frequently on the ovaries. Follicular and corpus luteal cysts are common and develop unilaterally in both ruptured and unruptured follicles. They are usually multiple, small, fluid-filled sacs located under the serosa covering the ovary. On occasion, a cyst may become large enough to cause discomfort or menstrual irregularities (Fig. 24–12). Bleeding resulting from rupture can cause more serious inflammation in the peritoneal cavity and requires surgical intervention.

In *polycystic ovarian syndrome,* or Stein-Leventhal syndrome, large ovaries covered with cysts develop. Associated hormonal abnormalities include elevated androgen, estrogen, and LH levels and decreased FSH levels. The usual fluctuations or peaks in FSH and LH are missing. Ovulation does not occur. The basic problem is a dysfunction in the hypothalamic-pituitary control system. The cause is unknown, although in some women an inherited factor has been demonstrated. Young women manifest **hirsutism**,

amenorrhea, and infertility. Medications such as clomiphene, an antiestrogen agent, may stimulate ovulation, or surgical wedge resections of the ovaries may help to control the hormone levels. Oral contraceptives are used to reduce androgen secretions and masculinization effects.

FIBROCYSTIC BREAST DISEASE

Also called benign breast disease, fibrocystic breast disease or physiologic nodularity includes a broad range of breast lesions. There is some confusion between the normal physiologic changes in the breast that occur during the menstrual cycle and abnormal or pathologic changes. Fibrocystic disease refers to the presence of nodules or masses in the breast tissue that change during the menstrual cycle in response to fluctuating hormone levels, particularly estrogen. Three categories of lesions have been designated, based on the risk of development of breast cancer. One category is nonproliferative lesions, which include microcysts and fibroadenomas. These are not considered precancerous. The second category includes proliferative lesions (with epithelial hyperplasia in the ducts) in which there are no atypical cells. The risk in this group increases if there is also a family history of breast cancer. The third category, a small one, is the one that requires monitoring, particularly if a family history of breast cancer is present. These lesions show proliferative changes with atypical cells. Fibroadenomas are specific benign tumors that usually appear as a singular, movable mass. These are usually excised. Breast biopsy can detect atypical cells and can differentiate benign from malignant cells.

The changes occurring in fibrocystic disease include

formation of multiple cysts, fibrosis, increased acini, and hyperplasia in both breasts in response to cyclic hormonal changes such as estrogen. The cysts or nodules feel firm and movable and vary in size during the cycle. The effects are more marked before menstruation, the breasts becoming heavy, painful, and tender. Treatment is largely symptomatic but may include dietary changes such as reduction of caffeine and fat intake and drugs such as the androgen danazol. Drainage of large cysts may be necessary.

Malignant Tumors

Neoplasms of the breast, cervix, and uterus are covered in this section. Ovarian cancer is discussed in Chapter 5.

CARCINOMA OF THE BREAST

Pathophysiology

Malignant tumors develop in the upper outer quadrant of the breast in approximately half the cases; the central portion of the breast is the next most common location. Most tumors are unilateral, although bilateral primary tumors may develop in some cases. There are different types of breast carcinomas, but the majority arise from cells of the ductal epithelium. This cancer infiltrates the surrounding tissue and frequently adheres to the skin, causing dimpling. The tumor becomes *fixed* when it adheres to the muscle or fascia of the chest wall. The malignant cells spread at an early stage, first to the nearby lymph nodes. Tumors in the upper outer quadrant and central breast area spread to the axillary lymph nodes. In most cases, several nodes are affected at the time of diagnosis. Widespread dissemination follows quickly, including metastases to the lungs, brain, bone, and liver. Tumor cells are graded on the basis of the degree of **differentiation** or **anaplasia** (see Chapter 5). The tumor is then staged based on the size of the primary tumor, the involvement of lymph nodes, and the presence of metastases. The presence of estrogen or progesterone receptors on the tumor cells is a major factor in determining how to treat the individual cancer. Such a tumor is hormone dependent because its growth is enhanced by the particular hormone.

Etiology

Carcinoma of the breast is a common malignancy in women and a major cause of death. Rarely, breast cancer occurs in males. The incidence of breast carcinoma continues to increase after age 20, and more women are developing the malignancy at a younger age. A strong genetic predisposition has been supported by the identification of specific genes related to breast cancer. Familial occurrence that is proportional to the numbers of affected relatives and the closeness of the relationships has been well documented. The other major factor in the etiology is hormones—specifically, exposure to high estrogen levels. Circumstances such as a long period of regular menstrual cycles (for example, from an early menarche to late menopause), nulliparity (no children), and delay of the first pregnancy appear to promote cancer development. The role of **exogenous** estrogen in oral contraceptives or postmenopausal supplements remains controversial. Current formulations for oral contraceptives have considerably reduced the risks. Other factors predisposing to breast carcinoma include fibrocystic disease with *atypical* hyperplasia, prior carcinoma in the uterus or in the other breast, and exposure of the chest to radiation (particularly in young women).

Signs and Symptoms

The usual initial sign is a single, small, hard, painless nodule. The mass is freely movable in the early stage but later becomes fixed. Other signs as the tumor becomes more advanced include dimpling of the skin, retraction of or discharge from the nipple, and a change in breast contour. Biopsy confirms the diagnosis of malignancy.

Treatment

Surgery, combined with radiation and chemotherapy, provides effective treatment for many cases. Surgical removal of the tumor, involving minimal tissue loss as in a lumpectomy, is the preferred method, although a more radical approach involving a mastectomy may be necessary in some cases. In addition, the appropriate lymph nodes are removed according to the existing lymphatic pathway from the tumor. Subsequent surgical reconstruction may be desired by some patients. Chemotherapy and radiation are useful for eradicating any undetected **micrometastases** remaining in such a high-risk cancer and are used as palliative measures as well. If the tumor proves to be responsive to a hormone, postoperative therapy includes removal of the hormonal stimulation. In a premenopausal woman, the ovaries are removed. A hormone-blocking agent reduces the risk of cancer recurrence in postmenopausal women. The prognosis is relatively good for tumors without nodal involvement, but as the number of lymph nodes affected by the cancer increases, the prognosis becomes more negative. Breast cancer may recur many years later, but generally the longer the time elapsed without recurrence, the lower the risk.

Breast self-examination (BSE) is recommended for all women older than 20 years as a preventive measure. Indeed, most tumors are discovered by women during BSE. Mammography is used as a routine screening tool because it can detect lesions before they become palpable or masses deep in the breast tissue.

Thinkabout 24-7

a. Compare the signs of fibrocystic disease and breast cancer.

b. Explain why chemotherapy and radiation may be recommended following surgery for breast cancer even when no lymph nodes appear to be involved.

c. Explain the recommended treatment for estrogen-dependent breast cancer in premenopausal and postmenopausal women.

CARCINOMA OF THE CERVIX

The number of deaths from cervical cancer has declined markedly with the increased use of the Papanicolaou (Pap) smear for screening and early diagnosis while the cancer is still in situ. However, the number of cases of *carcinoma in situ* has increased in the United States. The average age at onset for carcinoma in situ is 35, whereas invasive carcinoma manifests at approximately age 45. These age ranges seem to be dropping because more cases seem to be occurring in younger women.

Pathophysiology

The early changes in the cervical epithelial tissue consist of **dysplasia**, which is initially mild but becomes progressively more severe. This dysplasia usually occurs at the junction of the columnar cells with the squamous epithelial cells of the external os of the cervix (the transformation zone). The majority of cervical carcinomas arise from squamous cells. Cervical intraepithelial neoplasia (CIN) is graded from I to III based on the amount of dysplasia and the degree of cell differentiation. Grade III CIN consists of carcinoma in situ in which many disorganized, undifferentiated, abnormal cells are present (severe dysplasia).

Because the time span from mild dysplasia to carcinoma in situ may be 10 years, there are many opportunities for detection in this early stage. The Pap smear allows an examination of scrapings of the cervical cells and those that slough from the site and are present in the local secretions. These cells indicate the presence of dysplasia long before any signs of cancer appear. Carcinoma in situ is noninvasive but is followed by the *invasive* stage. Invasive carcinoma has varying charactersistics, sometimes appearing as a protruding nodular mass or perhaps an ulceration and sometimes infiltrating the wall. Eventually, all characteristics are present in the lesion. As the carcinoma spreads in all directions into the adjacent tissues, including the uterus and the vagina, it may also invade the uterine wall and extend into the ligaments, bladder, or rectum. Metastases to lymph nodes or distant sites occur rarely and at a very late stage. Staging of the carcinoma begins with stage 0, representing carcinoma in situ; stage 1 represents cancer restricted to the cervix; and stages 2 to 4 indicate further spread to the surrounding tissues.

Etiology

Cervical cancer is strongly linked to oncogenic sexually transmitted diseases such as herpes simplex virus type 2 (HSV-2) and human papillomavirus (HPV). The virus may exert direct effects on the host cell or may cause an antibody reaction; increased viral antibodies have been associated with the increasing dysplasia. High-risk factors for cervical carcinoma include multiple sexual partners, promiscuous partners, participation in sexual intercourse during the early teen years, and a patient history of sexually transmitted disease. Other environmental factors, such as smoking, are being studied.

Signs and Symptoms

Cervical cancer is asymptomatic in the early stage but can be detected by the Pap test. The invasive stage is indicated by slight bleeding or spotting or a slight watery discharge. Anemia or weight loss may accompany the local signs.

Treatment

Biopsy is used to confirm the diagnosis. Surgery combined with radiation (either an implant of radioactive material or external radiation—see Chapter 5) is the recommended treatment. The 5-year survival rate is 100% when the carcinoma is still in situ. The prognosis for the patient with invasive carcinoma depends on the extent of spread of the cancer.

Thinkabout 24–8

a. Explain the following terms and give an example of each:
(1) dysplasia
(2) carcinoma in situ
(3) carcinogenic
(4) invasive
b. Explain how viruses can be carcinogenic.
c. Explain why vaginal bleeding or abnormal discharge indicates a more advanced stage of cervical cancer.

CARCINOMA OF THE UTERUS (ENDOMETRIAL CARCINOMA)

Carcinoma of the uterus remains a common cancer in women older than 40 years, the majority of cases occurring in the 55- to 65-year age range. A simple screening test is not available for this cancer. However, the early indicator is bleeding, which in a postmenopausal woman would be a significant sign demanding investigation.

Pathophysiology

The majority of endometrial carcinomas are adenocarcinomas arising from the glandular epithelium. The malignant changes develop from endometrial hyperplasia, with the cells gradually becoming more atypical. Excessive estrogen stimulation appears to be the major factor in the development of hyperplasia. This cancer is a relatively slow-growing tumor and may infiltrate the uterine wall, leading to a thickened area, or it may mushroom out into the endometrial cavity. Eventually, the tumor mass fills the interior of the uterus and extends through the wall into the surrounding structures. Endometrial cancers are graded from 1, indicating well-differentiated cells, to grade 3, indicating poorly differentiated cells. Staging of the cancer is based on the degree of localization; in stage 1, tumors are confined to the body of the uterus; in stage 2, cancer is limited to the uterus and the cervix; in stage 3, the cancer has spread outside the uterus but remains within the true pelvis; and in stage 4, the tumor has spread to the lymph nodes and distant organs.

Etiology

Individuals with a history of increased estrogen levels have an increased incidence of uterine cancer. Exogenous estrogen taken by postmenopausal women is associated with an increased risk of endometrial cancer, and currently the recommended dosage of estrogen has been reduced to minimize this danger. Other causes of hyperestrinism include infertility or the earlier ingestion of sequential oral contraceptives. The current practice of combining estrogen with progestin reduces the risk of hyperplasia. There is also an increased incidence of cancer in obese persons, those with diabetes, and those with other endocrine abnormalities.

Signs and Symptoms

Painless vaginal bleeding or spotting is the key sign of endometrial cancer because it erodes the surface tissues. The Pap smear is not a dependable assessment tool for detecting abnormal endometrial cells. Direct aspiration of uterine cells provides a more accurate cell sample. Late signs of malignancy include a palpable mass, discomfort or pressure in the lower abdomen, and bleeding following intercourse.

Treatment

Surgery and radiation constitute the usual treatment measures. The prognosis is relatively good if the cancer is well localized at the time of diagnosis.

Thinkabout 24–9

a. Differentiate a uterine fibroid from uterine cancer.
b. Explain why the cure rate for cervical cancer is much better than that for ovarian cancer (refer to Chapter 5).
c. List the tumors whose development is influenced by hormones.

SEXUALLY TRANSMITTED DISEASES

Sexually transmitted diseases (STDs), formerly called venereal diseases, encompass a broad range of infectious diseases that are spread by sexual contact. The incidence of STDs is rising, and the actual figures are probably much higher than those stated because many cases of STD are not reported. The increased numbers have been attributed to societal changes in many countries. These changes include factors such as increased participation in premarital sex, particularly among young adults; an increased divorce rate; and an increased number of sexual partners of some individuals. Many people do not take protective measures against STD, especially when they take oral contraceptives. In addition to the standard STDs such as gonorrhea, syphilis, and chlamydial infection, there is evidence that infections such as hepatitis B may be spread by sexual contact.

There are many concerns about STDs. Immunity against recurrent infection is not achieved during the first infection with many STDs, and therefore recurrent infections are common. Because more than one STD may be present in any one individual at a given time, careful testing and diagnosis to uncover the presence of second infections are necessary. Frequently, STDs are asymptomatic, particularly in women, thus promoting the spread of infection by persons who are unaware that they are carrying the microbes. No cure is available for viral STDs such as herpes or human immunodeficiency virus (HIV; see discussion of HIV-AIDS in Chapter 4), although drugs are available that may help to limit the infection. More drug-resistant microorganisms are becoming apparent, thus increasing the inherent risks associated with STDs. Infections may be transmitted by an infected mother to the fetus or newborn, which frequently results in congenital defects or death for the child. In this section, several of the more common STDs are discussed.

Bacterial Infections

CHLAMYDIAL INFECTION

Chlamydial infection is considered one of the most common STDs. The pathogen is the bacterium *Chlamydia trachomatis*, a gram-negative obligate intracellular parasite, which requires a host cell to reproduce. As in gonorrhea, chlamydiae invade the epithelial tissue of the urogenital tract, causing inflammation. In males this becomes evident as urethritis (nongonococcal urethritis) and epididymitis. Manifestations of urethritis include dysuria and a whitish discharge, although some cases are asymptomatic. Epididymitis manifests as a painful swollen scrotum, usually unilateral, accompanied by fever. Proctitis (rectal inflammation with bleeding and discharge) may occur in anyone practicing anal intercourse. Females experience urethritis, bartholinitis, cervicitis, and salpingitis. Signs of urethritis include dysuria and urinary frequency. Infection in Bartholin's glands causes a purulent discharge and cyst formation. Cervicitis may be asymptomatic, or a purulent discharge with inflamed tissues may be evident at the cervical os. Spread to the fallopian tubes leads to the development of PID, a common complication. Newborns may be infected during passage through the cervix and vagina, resulting in infection in the eyes (conjunctivitis) or in the lungs due to aspiration of infected secretions (pneumonia). The usual treatment for chlamydial infection is tetracycline or doxycycline for the infected person and any sexual partners.

GONORRHEA

Gonorrhea is caused by *N. gonorrhoeae*, a gram-negative aerobic diplococcus (gonococcus). Many strains of *N. gonorrhoeae* have become resistant to penicillin and tetracycline. The bacteria use pili to attach to the epithelial cells and then damage the mucosa, causing an inflammatory reaction and formation of a purulent exudate. The most common site of inflammation in males is the urethra, which results in dysuria and a purulent urethral discharge. Epididymitis may follow. In females, the infection usually involves the endocervical canal and frequently is asymptomatic. It may also affect Skene's and Bartholin's glands, causing more visible manifestations. PID, a serious complication, frequently follows as the infection ascends along the mucosa. Females may experience infection in the anus and rectum when infected exudate spreads from the vagina. Orogenital contact leads to pharyngeal infection manifested as pharyngitis, tonsillitis, or lymphadenopathy. The newborn may become infected during the birth process, resulting in the eye infection called ophthalmia neonatorum. Considering the resistant strains of the organism, the suggested drugs are ceftriaxone and doxycycline. Culture and sensitivity tests may be required to determine effective drugs.

SYPHILIS

The causative organism of syphilis is *Treponema pallidum*, an anaerobic spirochete (so called because of its corkscrew shape). Dark-field microscopy is required for identification. Serum antibodies also provide a diagnostic test. Syphilis is a systemic infection that consists of four stages, and the organism can be isolated from lesions in the first two stages. The primary stage is identifiable by the presence of a *chancre*, a painless, firm, ulcerated nodule that develops at the point of contact on the skin or mucosa about 3 weeks after exposure. The organisms reproduce in the chancre and initiate an immune response. This lesion heals spontaneously (without treatment) in several weeks. Such lesions are frequently missed because they may not be visible (e.g., in the cervix in the female) and are asymptomatic. Regional lymphadenopathy may also be present in this stage. By this time the organisms have entered the general circulation, and if untreated, the second stage of the infection begins with a widespread symmetrical rash, usually maculopapular and reddish, on the skin and mucous membranes, particularly the palate. This typical rash may be found on the palms of the hands and the soles of the feet. Mucous patches (a loose, white, necrotic material) may appear on the tongue. General signs of infection—malaise, low-grade fever, sore throat, stomatitis, and anorexia—are common. Again, these lesions are self-limiting and disappear spontaneously in a few weeks.

The patient then enters the latent stage, which may persist for years. Sometimes the skin lesions recur, but usually the person is asymptomatic, although serologic evidence of disease remains. Some untreated patients never develop tertiary syphilis, and treatment has reduced the incidence of this stage. The typical lesion of this stage is the *gumma*, an area of necrosis and fibrosis. Bone gummas lead to destruction (e.g., in the hard palate) and pathologic fractures, whereas gummas in the liver manifest as nodules similar to those of cirrhosis. The cardiovascular system is most frequently affected by gummas, showing damage to the arterial wall and development of aortic aneuryms. Neurosyphilis damages the central nervous system, resulting in **dementia**, blindness, and motor disabilities (tabes dorsalis).

The other concern with syphilis is the development of congenital syphilis if the fetus is infected after the fourth month of gestation. The child may die in utero or survive with active infection or multiple abnormalities, particularly in the bones (e.g., saddlenose). Malformations of the teeth (e.g., Hutchinson's incisors and mulberry molars) are typical. Inflammation and fibrosis damage the liver and lungs.

Syphilis is transmitted by contact with exudate from the skin and mucosal lesions or by body fluids, including semen, blood, and vaginal secretions during sexual contact. It is likely that syphilis can be transmitted during the first few years of the latent stage as well as during the first two stages. Long-acting penicillin is effective in treating the infection.

Thinkabout 24–10

a. Name the causative organisms for chlamydial infection, gonorrhea, and syphilis.

b. Explain how salpingitis may develop in persons with chlamydial infection.

c. Compare syphilis and gonorrhea in terms of the early signs, distribution of organisms, and potential long-term effects if untreated.

d. Give two reasons why STDs are difficult to control (i.e., why it is difficult to reduce the incidence).

Viral Infections

HIV-AIDS has been described under Infections in Chapter 4. Antiviral agents reduce the severity of the acute stage of infection by inhibiting viral reproduction and shedding of viruses, but they do not eradicate the infection.

GENITAL HERPES

Herpes genitalis is usually caused by HSV-2, although some cases result from HSV-1. HSV-1 is the agent that also causes herpes labialis, or cold sores, and may cause genital lesions if oral sex is practiced or if it is autoinoculated by the hands. Usually a tingling and burning sensation at the site precedes the appearance of the actual lesion. The lesion characteristic of herpes is a **vesicle** (blister) surrounded by an erythematous area. The vesicle ruptures after several days, leaving a painful ulcerated area and watery exudate. Eventually a crust forms over the ulcer, and it heals spontaneously in 3 to 4 weeks. In women, the lesion is usually found on the cervix and urethra. Men have lesions on the penis, scrotum, or urethra. Vesicles may also appear on the buttocks or thighs. Systemic signs may be present during the acute stage, including fever, headache, and lymphadenopathy.

Following this acute stage, the herpes virus usually migrates along the dermatome to the dorsal sacral root ganglion and there enters a latent stage. Body secretions may contain viruses for a time after the visible lesion heals. When reactivated, the virus migrates back to the mucosa or skin and enters the host cells for replication, forming a new vesicle. Reactivation may be triggered by many factors such as respiratory infections or stress. Recurrent herpes is more common with HSV-2 than with HSV-1. Prodromal signs of recurrence, such as tingling or burning, signal recurrence before the lesion appears. The fluid in the vesicles contains many viruses and may spread the infection to the eyes or skin elsewhere if caution and careful handwashing are not practiced. Active lesions in the vagina or cervix may transmit herpes virus to an infant during a vaginal delivery, frequently causing death or severe CNS damage. Acyclovir, an antiviral agent, may be applied topically or taken orally to reduce the active stage of infection.

CONDYLOMATA ACUMINATA (GENITAL WARTS)

HPV causes genital warts, an STD that is increasing in frequency. HPV is a circular, double-stranded DNA virus. There are many types of HPV, of which several affect the genital tract. The incubation period for this infection may be as long as 6 months, and the disease may be asymptomatic, depending on the location of the lesions. The condylomata, or warts, vary in appearance from soft, fleshy projections or cauliflowerlike masses to flat lesions to small pointed masses. Flat condylomata require preliminary treatment with acetic acid before they can be visualized. Biopsy is useful in differentiating condylomata from other causes of dysplasia or hyperkeratoses. In women the lesions may be present in the cervix or vagina, and in men they frequently are found on the penis. Certain strains of HPV are considered carcinogenic and predispose to carcinoma of the cervix, vulva, and penis. Genital warts may be removed by a number of different methods but tend to recur.

Protozoan Infection

TRICHOMONIASIS

Trichomoniasis is caused by *Trichomonas vaginalis*, an anaerobic flagellated protozoa, an extracellular parasite. The infection is usually asymptomatic in men, the organisms residing primarily in the urethra. In women the infection may be subclinical and then flare up when the microbial balance of the vagina shifts. Trichomoniasis vaginalis is a localized infection, the organism attaching to the squamous epithelium of the vaginal and urethral mucosa and to Bartholin's glands. Active infection causes a copious yellowish, foul-smelling discharge as well as inflammation and itching of the mucosa. Systemic treatment of both partners is necessary with drugs such as metronidazole.

Thinkabout 24–11

a. Name the causative organism and its classification for
  (1) trichomoniasis
  (2) genital herpes
b. Compare the early manifestations of chlamydial infection, syphilis, and genital herpes.
c. Explain why genital herpes tends to recur.

CASE STUDIES

CASE STUDY A
Benign Prostatic Hypertrophy

Mr H, age 71, presented to his physician with dysuria, urinary frequency, and urgency. Following urinalysis, cystitis was diagnosed. Benign prostatic hypertrophy was noted.

a. What is the purpose of the prostate gland?
b. Describe the changes that occur in the prostate with BPH and the reason for these changes.
c. Explain how BPH predisposes to cystitis (refer to Chapter 19).

The infection was treated with antibacterial drugs, and Mr H was asked to return for follow-up.

d. List the manifestations of BPH, along with the reasons for them, that Mr H is likely to experience as the disease continues to develop.

As the disease progresses, Mr H is reluctant to consider surgical treatment.

e. Is there a high risk of developing a prostatic malignancy if treatment is delayed?

CASE STUDY B
Breast Cancer

Mrs AT, age 52, felt a small, hard, painless lump in the upper outer quadrant of her left breast during a regular breast self-examination. Her mother and a cousin had had breast cancer. Mrs AT has no children and still has menstrual cycles. After seeing her physician and having a mammogram, a biopsy was scheduled, which confirmed that the nodule was malignant.

a. List the factors in the patient's history that increase the risk of developing breast cancer.
b. Describe other possible signs of breast cancer
c. Explain why this lump is not typical of a benign condition.
d. A lumpectomy was performed, and a number of axillary lymph nodes were removed. Explain why the axillary lymph nodes were removed.
e. The tumor cells tested positive for estrogen receptors. Explain the significance of this information and the implications for Mrs AT.
f. Mrs AT's lung and bone scans were negative. Explain the purpose of these scans.
g. Only two of the axillary lymph nodes were positive for tumor cells. The prognosis appeared good, but the oncologist recommended a course of radiation and chemotherapy (refer to Chapter 5). Explain why additional treatment is recommended in this case.
h. Explain why Mrs AT will have an increased risk of infection after she starts the radiation and chemotherapy treatments.
i. Explain why Mrs AT will have to undergo frequent mammograms and checkups for the next few years.

CASE STUDY C
Gonorrhea and PID

PJ, age 23 years, tested positive for gonorrhea 6 months ago. She had no signs of infection, but her partner had been diagnosed and was being treated for gonorrhea. In this case, the penicillinase-producing organisms proved to be resistant to penicillin, and treatment continued with ceftriaxone.

a. Describe the usual signs of gonorrhea in a male.

b. Explain the meaning of the term drug-resistant as it relates to microbes and how it might be determined (see Chapter 4).

Six months later, PJ was admitted to the emergency department with severe abdominal pain and vomiting. A purulent cervical discharge was obvious, and initial examination of the exudate indicated infection by *N. gonorrhoeae* as well as several other microorganisms. A tentative diagnosis of PID was given.

c. Describe how gonorrhea leads to PID.

d. Explain why peritonitis is a potential complication of PID.

e. Give several reasons why infertility may be a sequela to PID.

STUDY QUESTIONS

1. Describe the structure and function of the (a) scrotum, (b) spermatic cord, (c) prostate gland.

2. List the functions of testosterone.

3. Describe the altered function resulting from (a) hypospadias, (b) cryptorchidism.

4. Explain why BPH occurs in older males.

5. List the signs of BPH.

6. Compare the typical sites of metastasis for prostatic and testicular cancer.

7. State and explain one significant effect of cystocele.

8. Explain the cause of pain resulting from (a) endometriosis, (b) primary dysmenorrhea.

9. Explain the potential problem resulting from the break in continuity between the fallopian tubes and the ovaries.

10. Describe the structure and purpose of each layer in the uterine wall.

11. Describe the defenses against infection in the female reproductive tract.

12. Describe the effects of increased estrogen secretion during the menstrual cycle.

13. Describe the causative organism and the manifestations of vaginal candidiasis.

14. Explain how an abscess may develop with PID.

15. Explain why most forms of fibrocystic breast disease are not considered precancerous, but some lesions require monitoring.

16. List the disorders characterized by pain related to the menstrual cycle.

17. Define the terms invasive and metastatic and give an example of each from the reproductive disorders.

18. Compare the early signs and the reasons for them of (a) cervical cancer, (b) uterine cancer, (c) ovarian cancer (refer to Chapter 5).

19. List three hormone-dependent reproductive disorders and describe the role of the hormone in each case.

20. Name and describe the characteristics of the organism causing chlamydial infection.

21. Explain, using specific examples, two reasons why STDs may go undetected.

22. Describe the manifestations of the secondary stage of syphilis.

23. Explain how antiviral agents may reduce the transmission of herpes simplex virus.

24. List the STD and the organism that causes a (a) chancre, (b) vesicle, (c) gumma, (d) purulent exudate, (e) pharyngitis, (f) wart.

READY REFERENCE 1

Anatomic Terms

The following diagrams and terms are useful in describing body position and movement as well as the location of structures in the body (see the first figure illustrating body planes).

PREFIX OR ROOT (COMBINING FORM) USED IN ANATOMIC TERMS

ab away from
ad toward
ante before, forward

bi two

caud lower part or tail
cephal top or head
cervic, cervico neck
circum around
contra opposite
crani head

en, endo in
ex, exo out

mono one

post after, behind

retro behind

sub below or under

version to turn

DIRECTIONAL TERMS

afferent moving toward
anterior front or abdominal surface

contralateral opposite side

distal far from the center or point of attachment
dorsal back surface

efferent moving away
external outside

inferior lower part, beneath
internal inside
ipsilateral same side

lateral toward the side

medial toward the midline

posterior toward the back
prone lying on the abdominal surface
proximal near the center or point of attachment

superior above, upper part
supine lying flat on the back

ventral front or belly surface

BODY PLANES

coronal a line extends from side to side, dividing the front and back halves of the body

midsagittal a line from superior to inferior along the midline, dividing the right and left halves of the body

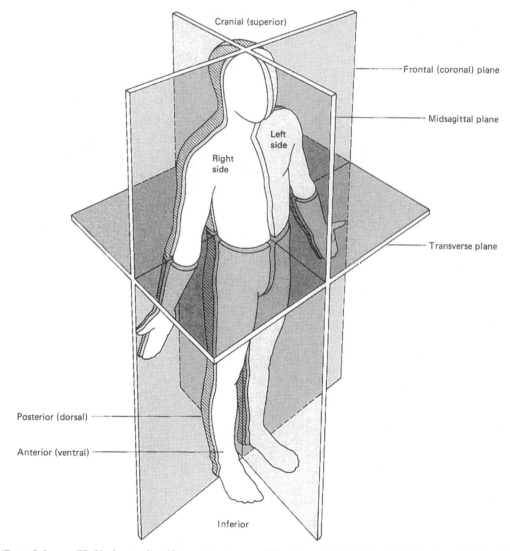

(From Solomon EP: Understanding Human Anatomy and Physiology. Philadelphia, W.B. Saunders, 1987, p. 12.)

sagittal a vertical line from superior to inferior at any point that divides the body into right and left parts

transverse a line dividing the upper and lower halves of the body

BODY CAVITIES

abdominal cavity below the diaphragm; contains the stomach, intestines, pancreas, and liver

dorsal cavity cranial cavity and vertebral cavity

pelvic cavity most inferior cavity, containing the urinary bladder, rectum, and uterus

thoracic cavity above the diaphragm; contains the heart, lungs, esophagus, trachea, aorta, and venae cavae

ventral cavity thoracic cavity

BODY REGIONS

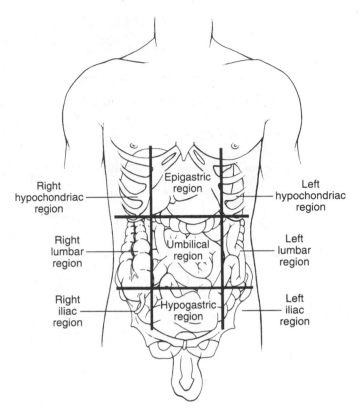

From Dowd SB, Wilson BG: Encyclopedia of Radiographic Positioning. Philadelphia, W.B. Saunders, 1995, pp. 5, 6.)

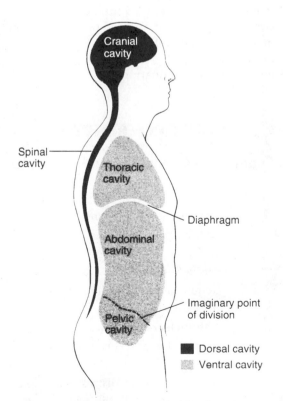

From Leonard PC: Building a Medical Vocabulary. 3rd ed. Philadelphia, W.B. Saunders, 1993, p. 52.)

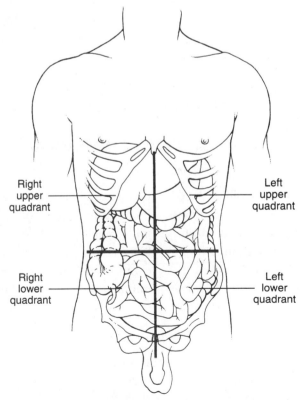

From Dowd SB, Wilson BG: Encyclopedia of Radiographic Positioning. Philadelphia, W.B. Saunders, 1995, pp. 5, 6.)

READY REFERENCE 2

Conversion Tables

TEMPERATURE

To convert Fahrenheit to Centigrade:

Subtract 32 from the number of °F and multiply by $\frac{5}{9}$:

$$(X°F - 32) \times \tfrac{5}{9} = Y°C$$

To convert Centigrade to Fahrenheit:

Multiply the number of °C by $\frac{9}{5}$ and add 32:

$$(Y°C \times \tfrac{9}{5}) + 32 = X°F$$

Equivalents	°F	°C
	95.0	35.0
	96.0	35.5
	97.0	36.1
	98.0	36.7
Normal body temperature	98.6	37.0
	99.0	37.2
	100.0	37.8
	101.0	38.3
	102.0	38.9
	103.0	39.4
	104.0	40.0

$$1°C = 1.8°F$$
$$0°C = 32°F \text{ (freezing point of water)}$$
$$20°C = 68°F \text{ (room temperature)}$$
$$100°C = 212°F \text{ (boiling point of water)}$$

UNITS OF MEASUREMENT (APPROXIMATE)

Common Units

nano	one billionth	nanogram	ng	10^{-9} g
micro (µ)	one millionth	microgram	µg	10^{-6} g
milli	one thousandth	milligram	mg	10^{-3} g
kilo	one thousand	kilogram	kg	10^{3} g
centi	one hundredth	centimeter	cm	10^{-2} m
		millimeter	mm	10^{-3} m

Conversion Factors

To Convert	Multiply by
centimeters to inches	0.39
inches to centimeters	2.54
meters to feet	3.28
feet to meters	0.305
fluid ounces to milliliters	30
milliliters to fluid ounces	0.03
liters to quarts	1.06
quarts to liters	0.95
gallons (U.S.) to liters	4.4
grams to ounces	0.035
ounces to grams	28
pounds to grams	453.6
kilograms to pounds	2.2
grains to grams	0.065
calories to joules	0.23

Some Equivalents

1 grain (apothecary) = 65 mg (metric) = 0.035 ounce
15 grains = 1 g
437.5 grains = 28.3 g = 1 ounce
453.6 g = 1 pound or 16 oz
1 kg = 32 ounces or 2.2 pounds
1 dram (apothecary) = 4 ml
30 ml = 1 fluid ounce
1 liter = 2.1 pints or 1 quart

Equivalents for Household Measures

1 teaspoon = 4 ml
1 tablespoon = 15 ml or 0.5 fluid ounce
1 cup = 240 ml = 8 fluid ounces = 0.5 pint
1 quart = 960 ml = 4 cups = 2 pints
1 fluid ounce = 30 ml
1 liter = 1.06 quart
1 inch = 2.5 cm

READY REFERENCE 3

Common Abbreviations and Acronyms

ABGs	arterial blood gases
ACTH	adrenocorticotropic hormone
ADH	antidiuretic hormone
ADLs	activities of daily living
AFP	alpha-fetoprotein
AIDS	acquired immune deficiency syndrome
AKA	also known as
ANA	antinuclear antibodies
aPTT or APTT	activated partial thromboplastin time
ARDS	adult respiratory distress syndrome
ASA	aspirin, acetylsalicylic acid
ATP	adenosine triphosphate

b.i.d.	twice daily
BM	bowel movement
BMR	basal metabolic rate
BP	blood pressure
BPH	benign prostatic hypertrophy
BSA	body surface
CA	cancer
Ca^{2+}	calcium ion
CAD	coronary artery disease
CAT or CT scan	computerized axial tomography or computed tomography
CBC	complete blood count
CCU	coronary care unit
CDC	Centers for Disease Control and Prevention
CF	cystic fibrosis
CHF	congestive heart failure
Cl^-	chloride ion
CNS	central nervous system
COPD	chronic obstructive pulmonary disease
CPR	cardiopulmonary resuscitation
C&S	culture and sensitivity test
CSF	cerebrospinal fluid
CVA	cerebrovascular accident (stroke)
CVP	central venous pressure
D5W	intravenous solution of 5% glucose in water
D&C	dilation and curettage of the uterus
DNA	deoxyribonucleic acid
DNR	do not resuscitate
DPT	diphtheria, pertussis, and tetanus vaccine
Dx	diagnosis
EBV	Epstein-Barr virus
ECF	extracellular fluid
ECG	electrocardiogram
ECT	electroconvulsive therapy
EEG	electroencephalogram
EPS	extrapyramidal signs
FUO	fever of undetermined origin
Hb or Hgb	hemoglobin
HBV	hepatitis B virus
HDL	high-density lipoprotein

HIV	human immunodeficiency virus
HLA	human leukocyte antigen
HPV	human papillomavirus
h.s.	at bedtime
HSV	herpes simplex virus
I&O	intake and output of fluids
ICU	intensive care unit
IDDM	insulin-dependent diabetes mellitus
IgG	immunoglobulin G (gamma globulin)
IM	intramuscular injection
IRDS	infant respiratory distress syndrome
IV	intravenous injection
K^+	potassium ion
LDL	low-density lipoprotein
LLQ	left lower quadrant
LMP	last menstrual period
LOC	loss of consciousness
MAOI	monoamine oxidase inhibitor (antidepressant drug)
MD	muscular dystrophy
MI	myocardial infarction (heart attack)
MMR	measles, mumps and rubella vaccine
MRI	magnetic resonance imaging (test)
MS	multiple sclerosis
Na^+	sodium ion
NIDDM	noninsulin-dependent diabetes mellitus
NMR	nuclear magnetic resonance test
NPO	no food or fluid (nothing) by mouth
NSAID	nonsteroidal anti-inflammatory drug
OD	overdose or right eye
OTC	over-the-counter (availability of drugs, e.g., ASA [aspirin])
Pao_2	partial pressure of oxygen in arterial blood
p.c.	after meals
Pco_2	partial pressure of carbon dioxide
pH	hydrogen ion concentration (acidity)
PID	pelvic inflammatory disease
PKU	phenylketonuria
PMN	polymorphonuclear leukocyte (polys, neutrophil)

PMS	premenstrual syndrome
p.o.	by mouth
p.r.n.	as needed
PT	physical therapy or prothrombin time pro time
PTT	partial thromboplastin time
PVC	premature ventricular contraction
q.d.	each day
q.i.d.	four times a day
RBC	red blood cell (erythrocyte)
RLQ	right lower quadrant
ROM	range of motion
SC	subcutaneous injection
SIDS	sudden infant death syndrome
SL	sublingual
SOB	shortness of breath
stat	at once, immediate
STD	sexually transmitted disease
T&A	tonsillectomy and adenoidectomy
TB	tuberculosis
TIA	transient ischemic attack
t.i.d.	three times a day
TPN	total parenteral nutrition
TPR	temperature, pulse, respiration

URI	upper respiratory infection
UTI	urinary tract infection
VS	vital signs
WBC	white blood cell (leukocyte)

READY REFERENCE 4

Common Diagnostic Tests

The following list of diagnostic tests is not intended to be comprehensive but rather to indicate the range of basic tests available for the diagnosis and monitoring of disease processes and effectiveness of treatment. A brief description is included for some of the procedures. Additional highly specialized tests may be offered in certain institutions. New techniques and more accurate equipment are constantly being developed. Test results are now available more rapidly with the use of multiple analyzers and computers. However, older procedures and equipment may be used by some centers.

IMAGING TECHNOLOGY OR RADIOLOGY

RADIOGRAPH OR X-RAY FILM. Ionizing radiation provides an image on film of bones and soft tissues that varies in density with the absorption of the x-rays striking the tissues (see Fig. 22–3 and *A* and *B*, below).

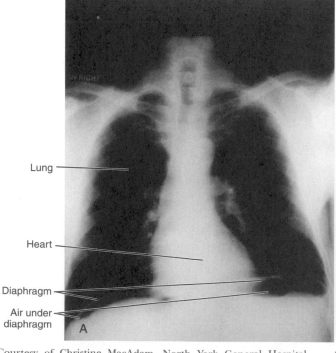

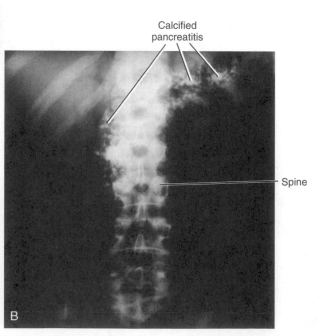

(Courtesy of Christine MacAdam, North York General Hospital, Toronto, Ontario.)

(Courtesy of Christine MacAdam, North York General Hospital, Toronto, Ontario.)

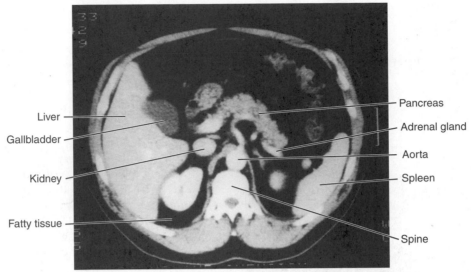

Liver
Gallbladder
Kidney
Fatty tissue
Pancreas
Adrenal gland
Aorta
Spleen
Spine

(Courtesy of Christine MacAdam, North York General Hospital, Toronto, Ontario.)

- *Plain x-ray films* are used as a preliminary screen for problems such as fractures or pneumonia.
- *Contrast medium* may be used (e.g., barium swallow or barium enema) to illustrate digestive tract abnormalities in more detail. In angiography various contrast media are used to examine the blood vessels.
- *In mammography* low-dose x-ray films are used to detect lesions in breast tissue.

COMPUTED TOMOGRAPHY (CT SCAN, formerly computerized axial tomography or CAT scan). A cross-section of tissues is provided by a scanning machine taking x-ray films in a series of shots from all directions (360 degrees); these measure differences in tissue density. A computer processes and compiles the readings to produce an image (above).

ULTRASONOGRAPHY (ULTRASOUND). High-frequency sound waves that bounce off body structures are used. The echoes reflect differences in the structures, which are analyzed and then visualized (below). This test is useful because it does not involve radiation, is noninvasive, is considered safe during pregnancy, and is inexpensive. It is limited by its low penetration.

- Doppler ultrasound assesses the blood flow in arteries and veins by measuring sound waves reflected from moving red blood cells.
- Echocardiography measures the efficiency of heart valves and heart function.

Magnetic Resonance Imaging (MRI)

MRI makes use of a magnetic field surrounding the body and the hydrogen (water) content of the body. Radio waves provide the energy source. Relative tissue densities are calculated by computer to produce an image (see p. 460). MRI is noninvasive and safe because it does not use ionizing radiation or injected contrast media. It provides more detailed visualization and can project past bone; therefore, it is particularly useful for visualization of neurologic and cardiovascular abnormalities.

NUCLEAR SCANNING

Nuclear medicine tests involve tracking the distribution of a radioactive tracer substance (radionuclide or radioisotope) in the body. A substance that is normally used in the body such as iodine or phosphate is labeled with a very small amount of radioactive material and administered to the patient. A scanning procedure then follows the material through the body to the appropriate tissue—for example, iodine to the thyroid gland or

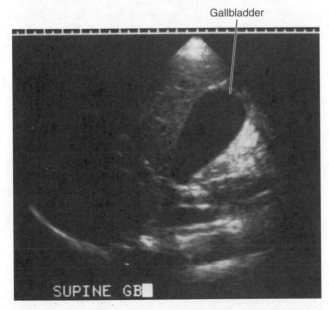

Gallbladder

SUPINE GB

(Courtesy of Christine MacAdam, North York General Hospital, Toronto, Ontario.)

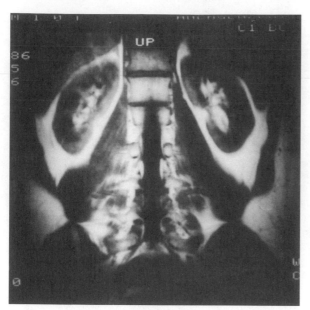

(Courtesy of Christine MacAdam, North York General Hospital, Toronto, Ontario.)

phosphate to bone. Abnormalities of distribution function of the tissue can be detected by this process. For example, a "hot spot" indicates increased uptake of the radioactive material.

- *Positron emission tomography (PET)* involves radioisotopes used with a scanner and computer to provide a cross-sectional image of a tissue such as the brain. This method is used to determine biochemical changes in the tissue.

DETERMINATIONS OF ELECTRICAL ACTIVITY

ELECTROCARDIOGRAM (ECG, EKG). By attaching electrodes to the chest and limbs of a patient, the conduction system of the heart can be assessed. The rate, rhythm, and characteristics of the contractions can be recorded by the machine. Typical abnormal patterns assist in the diagnosis of myocardial infarctions, cardiac dysrhythmias, electrolyte imbalances, and digoxin toxicity.

- Holter monitoring uses a portable ECG device to monitor cardiac activity in ambulatory patients while they continue their daily activities. The patient wears a small recording device attached to electrodes on the chest for a 24-hour period.

Stress Test (Exercise Electrocardiography)

Electrocardiographic measurements and blood pressure are monitored during a period of controlled exercise on a treadmill or stationary bicycle to determine the cardiac response to increased workload. The test is useful in detecting early coronary artery disease, in checking post-MI cardiac function, and in assessing the effectiveness of medication. It may also be used prior to establishing an individual's fitness or exercise program.

Electroencephalogram (EEG)

The electrical activity of the neurons in the brain is determined by electrodes attached to the scalp, which are then recorded as waves by the machine. Abnormal patterns may result from seizure disorders, tumors, or injuries. Absence of electrical activity in all parts of the brain may be used to confirm brain death.

PULMONARY FUNCTION TESTS

Both pulmonary volumes and capacities (e.g., tidal volume, total lung capacity) can be measured using a spirometer, a machine into which the patient breathes through a mouthpiece. These tests assist in diagnosing specific respiratory disorders, response to treatment, or progression of chronic disorders.

BLOOD TESTS
Hematologic Testing

Blood is checked for its components and for its blood clotting capability (hemostasis). Depending on the particular test, blood may be procured from a vein or a small puncture on the fingertip.

- *Complete blood count (CBC)* is used to check the count and characteristics of all formed elements or cells (erythrocytes, leukocytes, and thrombocytes). This examination is useful in the diagnosis of anemias or leukemias.
- *White blood cell differential count,* often referred to as a "differential count," determines whether there has been a change in the proportions of leukocytes and may provide a clue to the cause of a problem. For example, an increase in eosinophils usually indicates an allergic response.
- *Bone marrow aspiration* may be used to confirm abnormalities related to the production of blood cells such as megaloblastic anemia or leukemia.
- *Blood culture and sensitivity* may be performed if bacteremia or unknown infection is present.
- *Blood clotting tests* evaluate various clotting times (e.g., prothrombin time) and serum levels of the clotting factors (e.g., fibrinogen). These tests may be used to determine deficits of individual factors or to monitor anticoagulant treatment.
- *Hemoglobin electrophoresis* is used to detect the presence of abnormal hemoglobin (e.g., HbS).
- *Serum-ferritin* level indicates the level of iron storage.
- *Glycosylated hemoglobin* test is used to monitor control of diabetes mellitus.

Blood Chemistry Testing

Automated electronic systems are now in widespread use. They make use of computerized multiple analyzers that can process a number of determinations rapidly and in some cases indicate the cause of a problem or suggest additional tests.

Blood chemistry tests evaluate arterial blood gases (ABGs) for acid-base balance or oxygen levels and measure serum hormone levels (e.g., ACTH), serum cholesterol and lipoproteins such as high-density lipoprotein (HDL), serum electrolytes (e.g., Ca^{2+}, K^+, Na^+, Cl^-), serum glucose, serum enzymes and isoenzymes (to determine the site of infarction or inflammation or to monitor the spread of a malignant tumor), and serum levels of bilirubin, urea, or ammonia. Special methods such as chromatography may be used for amino acid determinations.

Immunodiagnostic Tests

Major changes are occurring in this area as improved methods are being developed to assess serum antigen and antibody levels. Current methods make use of precipitation or agglutination reactions, immunofluorescence tests or enzyme-linked immunosorbent assay (ELISA). Immunologic testing is used for many purposes such as the diagnosis and monitoring of the course of hepatitis, diagnosis of HIV infection, screening for infection during pregnancy (the TORCH test), ABO blood typing, and assistance in the diagnosis of diseases resulting from immunologic abnormalities (e.g., antinuclear antibodies in systemic lupus erythematosus or rheumatoid factor in rheumatoid arthritis).

- *Skin tests,* scratch or patch tests, are simple local tests based on immune responses. They are used to check for specific allergies or for exposure to microbes (e.g., Mantoux test for tuberculosis).

CHROMOSOME ANALYSIS. Chromosome analysis, including techniques used in cytogenetics and molecular biology, is used to examine the chromosomes and DNA to determine chromosome abnormalities in affected individuals or carriers, to determine paternity, or in forensic science. Gene mapping and subsequent development of tests for various genetic defects is a current major project. Blood cells are commonly used for this type of testing, but other sources of cells, such as fetal cells in amniotic fluid, may also be used.

Therapeutic Drug Monitoring

Serum drug levels are checked in patients in whom there is a narrow therapeutic range of a drug or who have severe renal or liver disease or potential drug interactions.

URINE TESTS

ROUTINE URINALYSIS. Urinalysis is used to check the physical and chemical characteristics of a freshly collected urine specimen. Physical examination of the specimen includes its appearance and specific gravity. Color of urine may be altered by drugs or diet. Chemical analysis includes pH and presence of abnormal constituents such as protein or ketones, as well as electrolyte levels and wastes such as urea. Microscopic examination determines the presence of cells or urine casts. Tests such as creatinine clearance are used to determine the glomerular filtration rate. Pregnancy tests make use of urine levels of human chorionic gonadotropin. Patients who have diabetes mellitus or are on certain diets may monitor their own urine for ketones.

CEREBROSPINAL FLUID TESTS

Cerebrospinal fluid is collected by means of a lumbar puncture. The pressure is measured, and the fluid is examined for appearance, protein and glucose levels, and the presence of cells or microorganisms.

FECAL TESTS

A fecal specimen is checked for its physical characteristics such as color and consistency. Stool cultures are used to check for parasites as well as other microbial content. Chemical tests include tests for lipids, enzymes such as trypsin, mucus, and occult blood. Microscopic examination assesses factors such as the presence of leukocytes (abnormal).

MICROBIOLOGIC TESTS

Any body fluids or exudates from lesions may be examined for the presence of microorganisms, which then may be identified. Body fluids may include sputum, blood, urine, stool, semen, gastric aspirate, or cervical scrapings. Microscopy may involve the use of different types of microscopes (dark-field, phase contrast, electron), depending on the site of examination and the type of microbe being checked. Stains such as Gram's stain may be used to assist with identification. Cultures, using a medium suitable for the specific organism, and sensitivity tests to determine the most effective drugs, are common procedures. Organisms such as viruses require living tissue for culture, a more complex and time-consuming procedure.

ENDOSCOPIC EXAMINATION

Endoscopy is used to visualize lesions or structures directly by inserting a tube into the body through an opening (e.g., trachea) or through the body wall. This procedure may facilitate a diagnosis or be used to obtain a specimen (tissue or fluid) for further examination and diagnosis (e.g., a biopsy) or to perform simple surgery (e.g., remove cartilage debris from a knee joint). Examples of endoscopic examinations include bronchoscopy, cystoscopy, proctosigmoidoscopy, arthroscopy, and laparoscopy.

Index

Note: Page numbers in *italics* indicate figures; those followed by t indicate tables.

pH Scale

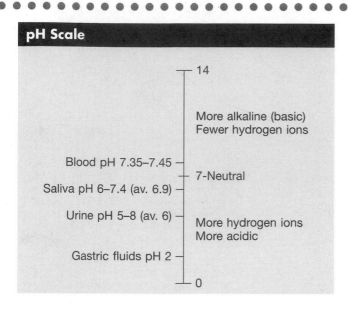

14

More alkaline (basic)
Fewer hydrogen ions

Blood pH 7.35–7.45

7-Neutral

Saliva pH 6–7.4 (av. 6.9)

Urine pH 5–8 (av. 6)

More hydrogen ions
More acidic

Gastric fluids pH 2

0

BLOOD COAGULATION FACTORS

FACTOR	NAME	INFORMATION
I	Fibrinogen	Plasma protein synthesized in liver: forms fibrin
II	Prothrombin	Plasma protein synthesized in liver (vitamin K required): forms thrombin
III	Tissue thromboplastin	Released from damaged tissue (extrinsic pathway) and platelets (intrinsic pathway); phospholipid involved in activation of clotting process
IV	Calcium ions	Required for many stages of coagulation process
V and VI	Proaccelerin; labile factor or accelerator globulin	Synthesized in liver: used in prothrombin activation
VII	Proconvertin; serum prothrombin conversion accelerator (SPCA)	Synthesized in liver (vitamin K required); used in extrinsic pathway
VIII	Antihemophilic factor (AHF)	Deficit causes hemophilia A
IX	Plasma thromboplastin component (PTC), Christmas factor, antihemophilic factor B	Synthesized in liver (vitamin K required)
X	Stuart factor	Synthesized in liver (vitamin K required); required for both extrinsic and intrinsic pathways
XI	Plasma thromboplastin antecedent (PTA), antihemophilic factor C	Synthesized in liver; used for activation of intrinsic pathway
XII	Hageman factor	Required in activation of intrinsic pathway
XIII	Fibrin stabilizing factor (FSF)	From platelets—cross-links fibrin to stabilize clot